AF326831

Maximizing Healthcare Delivery and Management through Technology Integration

Tiko Iyamu
Cape Peninsula University of Technology, South Africa

Arthur Tatnall
Victoria University, Australia

A volume in the Advances in Healthcare
Information Systems and Administration (AHISA)
Book Series

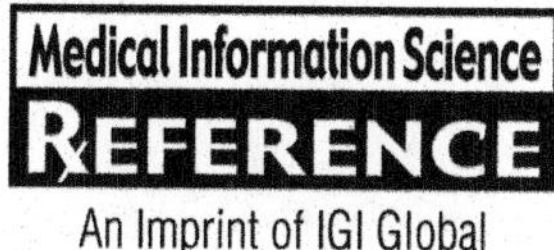

Medical Information Science
REFERENCE
An Imprint of IGI Global

Managing Director: Lindsay Johnston
Managing Editor: Keith Greenberg
Director of Intellectual Property & Contracts: Jan Travers
Acquisitions Editor: Kayla Wolfe
Production Editor: Christina Henning
Development Editor: Courtney Tychinski
Cover Design: Samantha Barnhart

Published in the United States of America by
    Medical Information Science Reference (an imprint of IGI Global)
    701 E. Chocolate Avenue
    Hershey PA, USA 17033
    Tel: 717-533-8845
    Fax: 717-533-8661
    E-mail: cust@igi-global.com
    Web site: http://www.igi-global.com

Library of Congress Cataloging-in-Publication Data

Maximizing healthcare delivery and management through technology integration / Tiko Iyamu and Arthur Tatnall, Editors.
     pages cm
  Includes bibliographical references and index.
  Summary: "This book presents scholarly research on the integration of ICT within the health services sector, featuring comprehensive coverage on a range of topics from technical and non-technical perspectives"-- Provided by publisher.
  ISBN 978-1-4666-9446-0 (hardcover) -- ISBN 978-1-46666-9447-7 (ebook) 1. Medical care--Technological innovations. 2. Medical technology--Management. I. Iyamu, Tiko. II. Tatnall, Arthur.
  R855.3.M39 2016
  610.285--dc23
                                        2015028219

This book is published in the IGI Global book series Advances in Healthcare Information Systems and Administration (AHISA) (ISSN: 2328-1243; eISSN: 2328-126X)

British Cataloguing in Publication Data
A Cataloguing in Publication record for this book is available from the British Library.

For electronic access to this publication, please contact: eresources@igi-global.com.

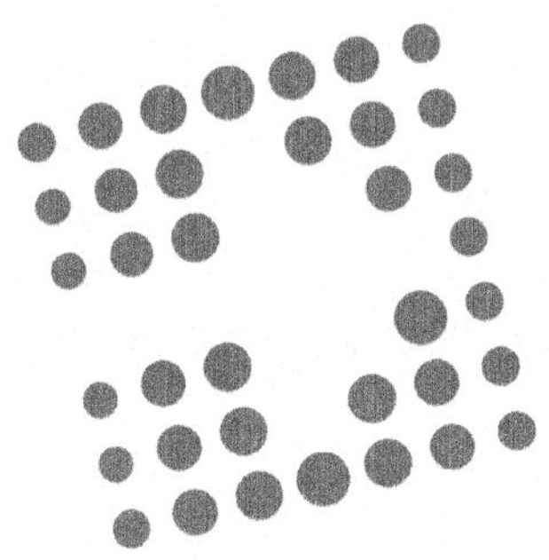

Advances in Healthcare Information Systems and Administration (AHISA) Book Series

Anastasius Moumtzoglou
Hellenic Society for Quality & Safety in Healthcare and P. & A. Kyriakou Children's Hospital, Greece

ISSN: 2328-1243
EISSN: 2328-126X

MISSION

The **Advances in Healthcare Information Systems and Administration (AHISA) Book Series** aims to provide a channel for international researchers to progress the field of study on technology and its implications on healthcare and health information systems. With the growing focus on healthcare and the importance of enhancing this industry to tend to the expanding population, the book series seeks to accelerate the awareness of technological advancements of health information systems and expand awareness and implementation.

Driven by advancing technologies and their clinical applications, the emerging field of health information systems and informatics is still searching for coherent directing frameworks to advance health care and clinical practices and research. Conducting research in these areas is both promising and challenging due to a host of factors, including rapidly evolving technologies and their application complexity. At the same time, organizational issues, including technology adoption, diffusion and acceptance as well as cost benefits and cost effectiveness of advancing health information systems and informatics applications as innovative forms of investment in healthcare are gaining attention as well. **AHISA** addresses these concepts and critical issues.

COVERAGE

- IT Applications in Health Organizations and Practices
- Telemedicine
- Management of Emerging Health Care Technologies
- IT Security and Privacy Issues
- Pharmaceutical and Home Healthcare Informatics
- Measurements and Impact of HISA on Public and Social Policy
- Rehabilitative Technologies
- IS in Healthcare
- Clinical Decision Support Design, Development and Implementation
- Role of Informatics Specialists

IGI Global is currently accepting manuscripts for publication within this series. To submit a proposal for a volume in this series, please contact our Acquisition Editors at Acquisitions@igi-global.com or visit: http://www.igi-global.com/publish/.

Titles in this Series

For a list of additional titles in this series, please visit: www.igi-global.com

Flipping Health Care through Retail Clinics and Convenient Care Models
Amer Kaissi (Trinity University, USA)
Medical Information Science Reference • copyright 2015 • 306pp • H/C (ISBN: 9781466663558) • US $245.00
(our price)

Healthcare Informatics and Analytics Emerging Issues and Trends
Madjid Tavana (La Salle University, USA) Amir Hossein Ghapanchi (Griffith University, Australia) and Amir Talaei-Khoei (University of Technology, Sydney, Australia)
Medical Information Science Reference • copyright 2015 • 325pp • H/C (ISBN: 9781466663169) • US $235.00
(our price)

Laboratory Management Information Systems Current Requirements and Future Perspectives
Anastasius Moumtzoglou (Hellenic Society for Quality and Safety in Healthcare, Greece & P. & A. Kyriakou Children's Hospital, Greece) Anastasia Kastania (Athens University of Economics and Business, Greece) and Stavros Archondakis (Military Hospital of Athens, Greece)
Medical Information Science Reference • copyright 2015 • 354pp • H/C (ISBN: 9781466663206) • US $245.00
(our price)

Cloud Computing Applications for Quality Health Care Delivery
Anastasius Moumtzoglou (Hellenic Society for Quality and Safety in Healthcare, Greece & P. & A. Kyriakou Children's Hospital, Greece) and Anastasia N. Kastania (Athens University of Economics and Business, Greece)
Medical Information Science Reference • copyright 2014 • 342pp • H/C (ISBN: 9781466661189) • US $245.00
(our price)

Achieving Effective Integrated E-Care Beyond the Silos
Ingo Meyer (empirica, Germany) Sonja Müller (empirica, Germany) and Lutz Kubitschke (empirica, Germany)
Medical Information Science Reference • copyright 2014 • 366pp • H/C (ISBN: 9781466661387) • US $245.00
(our price)

Social Media and Mobile Technologies for Healthcare
Mowafa Househ (College of Public Health and Health Informatics, King Saud Bin Abdulaziz University for Health Sciences, Saudi Arabia) Elizabeth Borycki (University of Victoria, Canada) and Andre Kushniruk (University of Victoria, Canada)
Medical Information Science Reference • copyright 2014 • 372pp • H/C (ISBN: 9781466661509) • US $245.00
(our price)

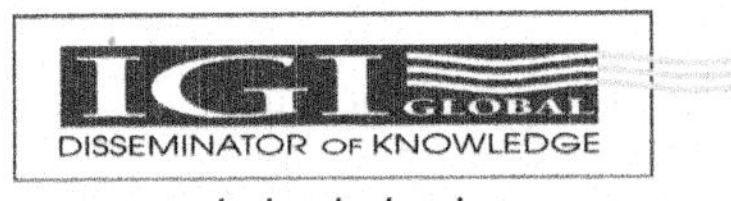

www.igi-global.com

701 E. Chocolate Ave., Hershey, PA 17033
Order online at www.igi-global.com or call 717-533-8845 x100
To place a standing order for titles released in this series, contact: cust@igi-global.com
Mon-Fri 8:00 am - 5:00 pm (est) or fax 24 hours a day 717-533-8661

Editorial Advisory Board

Table of Contents

Detailed Table of Contents

    Hoda Moghimi, RMIT University, Australia
    Nilmini Wickramasinghe, Deakin University & Epworth HealthCare, Melbourne, Australia
    Jonathan L. Schaffer, Cleveland Clinic, USA

Rapid increase of service demands in healthcare contexts today requires a robust framework enabled by IT (information technology) solutions as well as real-time service handling in order to ensure superior decision making and successful healthcare outcomes. Contemporaneous with the challenges facing healthcare, we are witnessing the development of very sophisticated intelligent tools and technologies such as Business Analytics techniques. Therefore, it would appear to be prudent to investigate the possibility of applying such tools and technologies into various healthcare contexts to facilitate better risk detection and support superior decision making. The following serves to do this in the context of Total Hip and Knee Arthroplasty and Congenital Heart Disease.

    Tiko Iyamu, Cape Peninsula University of Technology, South Africa
    Sharol Sibongile Mkhomazi, Tshwane University of Technology, South Africa

In every living being, health is essentially important, and as such, requires attention. Health related matters are at one point or the other embedded into humans' strategic, tactical and operational activities. However, due to human complexity, manifesting from factors such as food consumption and weather effect, healthcare services have increasingly become essential to individuals, groups and organisations in their daily life activities. As healthcare services increase in significance, the knowledge acquired and used in carrying out its services also becomes vital. The management of knowledge has increased in its relevance over the years. This could be attributed to the complexity in human activities. Thus, the management of knowledge has many challenges, which are never straight forward, and does not always produce positive result. Based on the challenges, it is critical to understand the enabling and constraint scenery of knowledge management. This article applied Structuration Theory to examine the different types of knowledge within the healthcare environment, using one of South African healthcare service providers as a case. This was done in order to gain better understanding on how certain knowledge are managed to give the result that they do. A better understanding of how knowledge is acquired and used within the healthcare environment would assist practitioners and managers, including Government and academic researchers in their roles and responsibilities.

Chapter 3

H. G. Sandeep Patil, Manipal University, India
Ajit N. Babu, Saint Louis University, USA &Center for Advancement of Global Health, India
P. S. Ramkumar, Applied Cognition Systems Pvt Ltd, India

Non-invasive medical measurements have expanded into several types of diagnostic and monitoring activities in health care delivery. They are being used in handling a number of non-infectious diseases such as diabetes, asthma, hypertension, congestive heart failure, cardiac arrhythmia, etc., as well as infectious diseases such as cholera, malaria, etc.. Non-Invasive Medical Devices (NIMDs) are naturally preferred over invasive methods considering patient convenience, reduced patient risk, increased speed, and operational simplicity. However non-invasive methods are often perceived to be less accurate than their invasive counterparts. Over the last decade, technological advances and mathematical techniques have improved significantly, challenging this perception across the board. The chapter will discuss this important transformation in health care diagnostics and monitoring. The chapter will also provide further insight into some of the currently available non-invasive measurement products and explore how futuristic techniques and technology trends which have great potential to transform healthcare into a significantly different paradigm than the one we experience today.

Chapter 4

Suama Hamunyela, Namibia University of Science and Technology, Namibia
Tiko Iyamu, Cape Peninsula University of Technology, South Africa

Many patients are often associated with various types of health related records, needing care and attentions. Healthcare system is intended for all that live in the country. Normally, there is spread of people across the geographical locations, of both the rural and urban communities. Even though the healthcare service is intended to spread across the country, the services are not always available as individuals require it. Hence, there is need for Mobility of healthcare services at both primary and secondary healthcare levels, particularly in the developing countries such as Namibia. In Namibia, the population is scantly spread far apart in the average of about 175 kilometres between major towns, necessitating movements of individuals and groups, particularly the old, poor, and nomadic people. The challenge is, healthcare records in the country are not centralised or virtualised, making accessibility into patients' records difficult or impossible. As a result, healthcare service delivering is challenged. This chapter explored the possibility healthcare services through virtualisation or centralisation as empowered by different translation of activities. The objectives of the study were to identify and discuss actors in the mobility of healthcare services. Mobility in this paper refers to the availability of services to the nomadic patients. The study employed the qualitative approach, within which data was gathered from primary healthcare services providers using open-ended questionnaires. The moments of Translation from the perspective of ANT was used a lens to analyse the data to examine and understand the power and factors which could influences mobility of healthcare service in Namibia.

Chapter 5
An Investigation of the Role of Using IS/IT in the Delivery of Treatments for ADHD in

Bader Binhadyan, RMIT University, Australia & Ministry of Education, Saudi Arabia
Nilmini Wickramasinghe, Deakin University & Epworth HealthCare, Melbourne, Australia

Over the last decade, the popularity of incorporating advances in information systems and information technology (IS/IT) has been steadily growing. IS/IT can improve the delivery for better intervention and treatment with many different mental illnesses; however, there appears to be great potential for IS/IT in the context of young adults with mental disorders such as Attention Deficit Hyperactivity Disorder (ADHD). ADHD affects approximately 11% of the university population; negatively impacting students' academic performance, study skills, and social life. The study design outlined in this paper suggests a possibility for the role of IS/IT in the delivery of treatments and management of ADHD in university students to be examined with the view to introduce IS/IT into the traditional treatment context. This research involves collecting data from psychologists in the form of semi-structured interviews and a grounded theory methodology using multiple cases is adopted.

Chapter 6
Radio Frequency Identification Technology in an Australian Regional Hospital: An Innovation

Chandana Unnithan, Victoria University, Australia
Arthur Tatnall, Victoria University, Australia

Australian hospitals had begun exploring Radio Frequency Identification, a wireless automatic identification and data capture technology for improving the quality of their services towards the end of 2000s. After many an unsuccessful pilots, a breakthrough for large hospitals came in 2010, with a key learning rendered by a large regional hospital that not only experimented with the technology, but also have made it all pervasive in their operations. In this chapter, we present the case study, through an innovation translation perspective, focusing on the socio-technical factors captured through elements of Actor-Network Theory.

Chapter 7

Phathutshedzo Nemutanzhela, Namibia University of Technology, Namibia
Tiko Iyamu, Cape Peninsula University of Technology, South Africa

On one hand, healthcare has taken the centre stage of attention in recent years, due to many more activities of both natural and manmade. On another hand, the use of mobile technologies is increasingly growing across the world, particularly in developing countries. Mobile devices, including phones and computers are becoming significant ICT tools for many activities and process of healthcare service delivery in both urban and rural areas, by organisations and individuals, literates and educated. Also, both businesses (organisations) and individuals are involved in the delivering and accessibility (recipient) of healthcare services at different levels and locations. The nature of the diverse tribes and languages within some developing countries make it difficult to deliver or receive the services which are provided by some Healthcare organisations. This is so because particular language, such as English, as in the case of South Africa, is often used for communication. Even though majority of the citizens make use of Mobile devices (such as cellular phones), the media of communication exchange is English language. Due to the sensitivity, confidentiality, and private nature of healthcare information and services, a one-on-one and the use of language which the patient is comfortable with is critical. Otherwise, the services and objectives of the healthcare organisations continue to be challenged. As such, there is need to address the semantics of language through the use of electronic devices for healthcare services.

Chapter 8

Catherine Han-Lin, Deakin University, Melbourne, Australia
Angela Wei Hong Yang, RMIT University, Melbourne, Australia
Siddhi Pittayachawan, RMIT University, Melbourne, Australia
Nilmini Wickramasinghe, Deakin University & Epworth HealthCare, Melbourne, Australia

Chinese Medicine (CM) has become increasingly demanding globally. Recent World Health Organisation traditional and complementary medicine strategy of integrating CM to Western Medicine (WM) indicates that it is crucial that CM developments have strong literature, scientific, and evidence-based medical approval and support. To achieve this, there is a need to form a synthesis foundation or platform for future studies. This chapter serves to discover this synthesis that is suitable for CM by discussing the basics of inquiring and Knowledge Management (KM) systems. It suggests that CM should follow a combination of Hegelian and Kantian inquiring systems with the support of Singerian and Leibnizian inquiring systems and KM features. This proposed synthesis is one of the first, if not the first study to apply Churchman's inquiring systems into the context of CM and differentiate them from WM.

Chapter 9

V. Horner, University of South Africa, South Africa
A. Coleman, University of South Africa, South Africa

Implementation of guidelines in the health system is a complex and considerable undertaking. After the health administration has developed guidelines, a dissemination strategy needs to be put in place. Dissemination involves distribution of printed guidelines booklets, training of health care providers, provision of the equipment needed for implementing the guidelines, improvements to facilities, and supervision and monitoring by managers. This chapter reports on the Basic Antenatal Care Information System (Bacis) study in South Africa which pertains to an e-health decision support systems that is intended as an aid for nurses and managers at primary health care. The Bacis program study is important because there are few published studies from developing countries on implementation of e-health decision support systems at primary health care and their effectiveness in improving care.

Chapter 10

Quazi Omar Faruq, Victoria University, Australia

The influence of ICT in General Practice varied from a solo practice to a GP specialist of a primary healthcare team. Different factors influence the GP to use ICT. After 2nd World War the national legislative requirement influenced more to adopt ICT, of which most important is the Medicare or Medicaid payment and also the richness of the environment (measured by network readiness index). Shift to group practice or corporate level practice requires ICT support to handle automated actions (i.e. completing repetitive jobs, answering frequently asked questions by webpage). Role of telecommunication and IT service providers, and that of entrepreneurs for information management are also discussed. While discussing the challenges in implementing ICT in future model of GP service it focuses on the slow usage of computer and other IT products by doctors, as noted in the past decades.

Chapter 11

Ronald Karon, Namibia University of Science and Technology, Namibia

The use of Health Information Systems (HIS) is considered to be a major contributing factor to healthcare service delivery. However, the utilisation of HIS which includes use and management is critically challenging in the public health sector in many developing countries. The manifestation of the challenges results in poor service delivery, which includes patient deaths. This is the main motivation for this study, to investigate how HIS can be used to improve service delivering in the hospitals from developing countries perspective. The study was carried out in Namibia, using two hospitals in the public healthcare. The study adopted the qualitative case study. The study revealed that the use of parallel systems, lack of systems integration, lack of portable devices and users' incompetency are some of the factors which impact the use and management of HIS in hospitals.

Chapter 12

Amir Manzoor, Bahria University, Pakistan

Implementation of RFID technology-based healthcare services is on the rise. The purpose of this chapter is a thorough, systematic review of the existing literature to provide a discussion of current trends and future directions in this domain. Findings indicate that tracking is the key RFID enabling function. Automatic data collection and transfer is an RFID function also frequently used in relation to assets, staff, and patients. Finally, RFID is employed for sensing, most often in relation to patients, but also to assets. The chapter concludes by highlighting future research directions where the deployment of RFID technology is likely to transform the healthcare sector.

Chapter 13

Putu Wuri Handayani, Universitas Indonesia, Indonesia
Puspa Indahati Sandhyaduhita, Universitas Indonesia, Indonesia
Achmad Nizar Hidayanto, Universitas Indonesia, Indonesia
Ave Adriana Pinem, Universitas Indonesia, Indonesia
Haya Rizqi Fajrina, Universitas Indonesia, Indonesia
Kasiyah M. Junus, Universitas Indonesia, Indonesia
Indra Budi, Universitas Indonesia, Indonesia
Dumilah Ayuningtyas, Universitas Indonesia, Indonesia

Implementing Hospital Information System is an ultimately important practice that should be performed by hospitals in order to deliver accurate, timely, complete, and easily accessible data/information in an integrated manner. Given the specific characteristics of Indonesia, the objective of this research is to design an Information System Architecture as part of the Enterprise Architecture based on The Open Group Architecture Framework in order to support the Hospital Information System implementation in Indonesia. This research focuses on the hospitals basic processes, viz. the emergency processes, the inpatient processes and the outpatient processes. The integration aspect of the architecture should connect the hospitals with other related stakeholders. This research is a qualitative study by conducting interviews and observations in three government public hospitals, several directorate generals of the Indonesian Ministry of Health and a representative from the WHO. The result of this research is an integrated Information System Architecture model.

Chapter 14

Paraskevas Vezyridis, University of Nottingham, UK
Stephen Timmons, University of Nottingham, UK
Heather Wharrad, University of Nottingham, UK

Clinical information systems are increasingly used in emergency departments across the English National Health Service. The implementation outcome is unpredictable and success is not guaranteed. This study identifies facilitating social and technical factors for implementing an Emergency Department Information System. This is a qualitative study, using interviews with 28 emergency department clinicians, administrators and managers. Project management documents, user guides, design blueprints and internal reports were also analysed. Lessons learned include the importance of acquiring an established, customised and user-friendly system, attracting funding, establishing communication channels between stakeholders, developing detailed implementation plans and tailored training programmes, investing in peer-support, and analysing the workflow impact of the system. Socio-technical factors, both in and out of the hospital, influenced the success of the implementation. By being systematic in addressing these socio-technical factors certain implementation barriers can be overcome.

Chapter 15

Irja N. Shaanika, Namibia University of Science and Technology, Namibia

In developing countries, Health Information Systems (HISs) are increasingly used to enable and support both clinical and administrative processes for healthcare services. The use of the HISs in developing countries' healthcare centres is influenced and impacted by humans' interactions which manifests from culture and traditions. Due to the diverse nature of culture and traditions, it is near impossible to have single formula in addressing the patients' needs. As a result, the aim to improve quality of healthcare through HISs is challenged, and many stakeholders do not seem to understand the problem. The challenge continues to significantly contribute to poor service delivery, as the need for healthcare services increases. This study focused on the interaction between the healthcare professionals and the HISs, to understand how and why the challenges of using the ICT systems exist. This includes examining the implication, and how the challenges impact the recipients of healthcare services.

The adoption of health information systems and the integration of healthcare data and systems into efficient cross-institutional collaboration workflows of stakeholders (e.g., medical providers such as physicians, hospitals, clinics, labs, etc.) is a challenging problem for the healthcare domain. This chapter studies the way that well-established software engineering concepts and architectural styles can be employed to satisfy requirements of the healthcare domain and ease health information exchange (HIE) between stakeholders. Towards this goal, this chapter proposes a hybrid HIE architecture (HHIEA) that leverages the studied styles that include service-oriented architecture, grid computing, publish/subscribe paradigm, and data warehousing to allow the health information systems of stakeholders to be integrated to facilitate collaboration among medical providers. To demonstrate the feasibility and utility of the HHIEA, a realistic regional healthcare scenario is introduced that illustrates the interactions of stakeholders across an integrated collection of health information systems.

Rabies is a neurodegerative viral zoonotic disease that affects all warm blooded animals. It is estimated that about 99% of human rabies cases are caused by dog bites. High prevalence of rabies has been reported in different parts of Tanzania. The disease has continued to cause public health threat to the communities due to weak passive and active surveillance systems. The data piloted in this study was based on the information gathered from Kilosa district. The geo information collected was used to develop a geospatial based system that can easily show the hotspots of rabies. The use of WEB GIS is likely to strengthen disease surveillance in Kilosa and other Districts of Tanzania. This approach offers a model for sharing both human and animal diseases surveillance information. Adoption of this approach is likely to increase awareness and timely response to rabies incidences.

Foreword

Many people consider health informatics as innovation concept in the future and not a concept of continuous improvisation of health processes and systems. The attitude has led to extensive knowledge sitting in academic research output on how health information technology has been used to improve health care across the globe. Therefore reading this book will enable the readers to understand and interpret the process of improvisation of health care delivery processes in relation to adverse health incidences in various regions and settings of this world.

The chapters in this book bring to bear the opportunities in the health care delivery industry and the need for multidisciplinary and interdisciplinary empirical research where findings make health care accessible and affordable. The researchers who have immensely contributed chapters have not only brought readers and other researchers closer to creative, innovative thinking and ways to improve health care delivery in the different countries, but have also brought it closer to effective technology-in-practice in underdeveloped countries.

It is imperative that with today's knowledge economy where technology is mushrooming, contributions such as the chapters in this book compel technology architects and systems developers to take a cue from where health care delivery will need the power of informatics.

Also, it is interesting to note how social theories have been used to help the readers to understand how socially constructed health phenomena have been interpreted. Furthermore, where system theory has been used, the underpinning principles of process and systems integration have been made critical for low cost and accessible health care. This is of course, represents an admirable approach as it serves to teach, stabilize, and give meaning and future direction to immerging and existing researchers in the health informatics discipline.

This book is recommended for both practitioners and researchers in the health care delivery industry. It can further be used as the basis for further research in an attempt to improve access to affordable health care in developing countries. The book should assist in the conscious development of future health care practitioners and researchers in health informatics.

Michael Twum-Darko
Cape Peninsula University of Technology, South Africa
May 2015

Preface

INFORMATION AND COMMUNICATION TECHNOLOGIES AND HEALTHCARE

Many Information and Communications Technology (ICT) practitioners, including healthcare professionals and managers, find themselves struggling and challenged with problems of integration, consolidation, configuration, development, technology planning, software management, management of hardware and processes. These widely shared problems have remained within the healthcare environment across the globe over the last decade.

The need for improved healthcare services continues to increase in both developing and developed countries around the world and in consequence, governments along with various non-governmental and private organisations continue to strive to improve upon the healthcare services that they provide to their citizens and clients. In this book factors influencing the delivery of healthcare services have therefore been explored from both technical and non-technical perspectives, making use of case studies from a number of different countries.

Healthcare information systems and related technologies are now widely used to support and improve both clinical and administrative process in the provision of healthcare services. As revealed in this book, information systems and technologies aim to promote the quality of healthcare through improving access to information and its use as well as to its transmission and storage. Through improved information systems and technologies, accuracy of information will be improved and data-related errors will be reduced as well as improving decision making by practitioners and managers of healthcare services.

This book presents details of how various information systems and technologies are used to examine, understand and provide solutions to some of the challenges that are currently experienced by both healthcare service providers and receivers. The need for reliable and accurate information which continues to prevail in the healthcare sector makes the roles and actions of the agents (both technical and non-technical) even more critical. The impacts of various technologies for healthcare services are covered in the book.

Empirically, the book reveals that the activities and processes within the healthcare sector are not as straightforward as some agents had originally expected. This complexity is attributed to the fact that healthcare data comes from many different sources, is used for various purposes, and has numerous different users. Another factor that makes the data even more complicated is its heterogeneous nature in its form, accessibility and storage. The book pays great attention to heterogeneity and roles of agents in the use and management of information systems and technologies for the delivery of healthcare services. The inevitably diverse nature of agents and the structure of the healthcare sector in many countries all work to increase this complexity as a societal phenomenon. The healthcare sector in some countries, particularly in developing countries, adopts and uses only minimal technologies. This can often be attributed to lack of know-how and accessibility.

The book presents a combination of the factors, rigour and relevance related to healthcare and technology from the perspectives of in-depth theory and practice, looking at how information technology can add value to the development of healthcare in a bid to continually improve services. The quality and the credibility that are instilled in the delivery of healthcare services through rigour and relevance increase the level of stakeholder confidence. This book will therefore benefit both academics and professionals in the healthcare sector in the continued process of improving the services to healthcare through information systems and technologies. This includes the development of human skills in the area of healthcare informatics.

The book is truly international with authors from Australia, USA, South Africa, India, Namibia, Tanzania, Pakistan, Indonesia, UK and Cyprus, and chapters covers a diverse set of issues ranging from healthcare risk management and non-invasive data acquisition to rabies surveillance.

The first chapter: 'Intelligent Risk Detection in Healthcare Contexts of Hip and Knee Athroplasty and Paediatric Congenital Heart Disease' was contributed by Hoda Moghimi and Nilmini Wickramasinghe from Epworth Healthcare and RMIT University, Melbourne, Australia and Jonathan L. Schaffer from Cleveland Clinic, USA. The chapter notes that a rapid increase of service demands in healthcare contexts today requires a robust framework enabled by information and communication technology (ICT) solutions as well as real-time service handling in order to ensure superior decision making and successful healthcare outcomes. With the challenges facing healthcare, at the same time in other areas we are witnessing development of sophisticated intelligent tools and technologies such as Business Analytics techniques and so it would be prudent to investigate the possibility of applying such tools and technologies into various healthcare contexts to facilitate better risk detection and support superior decision making. The chapter discusses this in the context of Total Hip and Knee Arthroplasty and Congenital Heart Disease.

Next, Sharol Sibongile Mkhomazi from Tshwane University of Technology, South Africa and Tiko Iyamu from University of the Western Cape, South Africa discuss: 'Managing Knowledge towards Enabling Healthcare Service Delivery'. The chapter describes how, at one point or another, health-related matters are embedded into strategic, tactical and operational activities of In every living being including humans. Healthcare services have increasingly essential to individuals, groups and organisations in their daily life activities due to factors such as food consumption and weather effect. This chapter applies Structuration Theory to examine the different types of knowledge within the healthcare environment, using one of South African healthcare service providers as a case study example so as to gain better understanding on how knowledge is managed.

'Non-invasive Data Acquisition and Measurement in Bio-Medical Technology' by Sandeep Patil HG from Manipal University, India, Ajit N. Babu from Saint Louis University, USA and Ramkumar PS, Applied Cognition Systems Pvt Ltd, Bangalore, India looks at how non-invasive medical measurements have expanded into several types of diagnostic and monitoring activities in health care delivery, including handling a number of non-infectious diseases such as diabetes, asthma, hypertension, congestive heart failure and cardiac arrhythmia, as well as infectious diseases such as cholera and malaria. Non-Invasive medical devices are preferred over invasive methods for considerations of patient convenience, reduced patient risk, increased speed and operational simplicity. Non-invasive methods are often perceived to be less accurate than their invasive counterparts, but over the last decade, technological advances and mathematical techniques have improved significantly, challenging this perception across the board.

Suama Hamunyela from Namibia University of Science and Technology then discusses: 'Healthcare Services for Nomadics through a Mobile Framework'. In many counties both the rural and urban communities are spread across geographical locations and there is significant mobility of individuals and groups within the country. Even though healthcare services are intended to spread across the whole country these services are not always as mobile as individuals are, creating a need for mobility of healthcare services at both primary and secondary healthcare levels, particularly in the developing countries such as Namibia.

The following chapter: 'An Investigation of the Role of Using IS/IT in the Delivery of Treatments for ADHD in University Students', is by Bader Binhadyan from RMIT University, Melbourne, Australia and Nilmini Wickramasinghe from RMIT University and Epworth HealthCare, Australia. Their chapter points out how, over the last decade, the popularity of incorporating advances in information systems and information technology into healthcare has been steadily growing. ICT can improve the delivery of better intervention and treatment in relation to many different mental illnesses, but there appears to be great potential for its use in the context of young adults with mental disorders such as Attention Deficit Hyperactivity Disorder (ADHD) which affects approximately 11% of the university population. It negatively impacts students' academic performance, study skills, and social life. This chapter outlines a study that suggests a possible role for ICT in the delivery of treatments and management of ADHD in university students. Their research involved collecting data from psychologists in the form of semi-structured interviews and a grounded theory methodology using multiple cases.

Chandana Unnithan and Arthur Tatnall from Victoria University, Melbourne, Australia next present a chapter titled: 'Radio Frequency Identification Technology in an Australian Regional Hospital'. In the chapter they present a case study of a large an Australian regional hospital, focusing on socio-technical factors, through an innovation translation perspective informed by Actor-Network Theory. Radio Frequency Identification (RFID) a wireless automatic identification and data capture technology and in the last few years Australian hospitals have been exploring use of RFID for improving the quality of their services. After many unsuccessful pilots a breakthrough for large hospitals came in 2010 when a large regional hospital began not only experimented with the technology, but also making it all pervasive in their operations. The chapter presents a case study of the use of RFID in this hospital.

Again returning to mobile technology, Phathutshedzo Nemutanzhela and Tiko Iyamu from University of the Western cape, Cape Town, South Africa present: 'Introducing Mobile Device for Health Services: the Semantics of Language Translation'. They point out how healthcare has taken centre stage of attention in recent years, due to many activities, both natural and man-made. The use of mobile technologies including phones and computers is increasingly growing across the world, and particularly in developing countries. ICT and mobile devices have become significant tools for many activities and process of healthcare service delivery in both urban and rural areas, and are used by organisations and individuals. The nature of the diverse tribes and languages within some developing countries makes it difficult to deliver or receive the services which are provided by some Healthcare organisations and this is particularly so because languages such as English in the case of South Africa are often used for communication and the media of communication exchange is English language. Due to the sensitivity, confidentiality and private nature of healthcare information and services, a one-on-one use of a language with which the patient is comfortable is critical as otherwise services and objectives of the healthcare organisations continue to be challenged. The chapter then stresses that there is need to address the semantics of language through the use of electronic devices for healthcare services.

Chinese Medicine has come into increasing demanding globally in recent times and is a fascinating topic. Catherine Han-Lin, Angela Wei Hong Yang and Siddhi Pittayachawan from RMIT University along with Nilmini Wickramasinghe from RMIT University and Epworth HealthCare, Melbourne, Australia offer a chapter titled: 'Utilisation of Health Information Technology to Support Clinical Operation of Chinese Medicine'. They note that a recent World Health Organisation traditional and complementary medicine strategy of integrating Chinese Medicine to Western Medicine indicates that it is crucial that Chinese Medicine developments have strong literature, scientific, and evidence-based medical approval and support and to achieve this there is the need to form a synthesis foundation or platform for future studies. This chapter serves to discover a synthesis that is suitable for Chinese Medicine by discussing the basics of inquiring and Knowledge Management systems. The authors suggest that Chinese Medicine should follow a combination of Hegelian and Kantian inquiring systems with the support of Singerian and Leibnizian inquiring systems and kn owledge management features. They claim that this proposed synthesis is one of the first, if not the first study to apply Churchman's inquiring systems into the context of Chinese Medicine and differentiate them from Western Medicine.

'Strengthening Implementation of Guidelines at Primary Health Care: Decision support in primary health care', by Vincent Horner and Alfred Coleman from the University of South Africa, discusses how decision support systems can support healthcare. The authors begin by noting that the implementation of guidelines in the health system is a complex and considerable undertaking, as after health administration has developed guidelines, a dissemination strategy needs to be put in place. This dissemination involves distribution of printed guidelines booklets, training of nurses, provision of the equipment needed for implementing the guidelines, improvements to facilities and supervision and monitoring by managers. The chapter reports on the Basic Antenatal Care Information System (Bacis) study in South Africa which relates to an e-health decision support systems that is intended as an aid for nurses and managers at primary health care. This Bacis program study is important because there are few published studies from developing countries on implementation of e-health decision support systems at primary health care and their effectiveness in improving care.

Perhaps the most obvious aspect of healthcare to many people is their General Practitioner (Family Doctor). Different factors influence the General Practitioner (GP) to use ICT. The next chapter, by Quazi Omar Faruq from Victoria University, Melbourne, Australia: 'General Practitioners' Adoption and Use of ICT' discusses the issue of how the influence of ICT in General Practice varies from a solo practice to a GP specialist of a primary healthcare team. In Australia, national legislative requirements influenced more GPs to adopt ICT, of which most important was Medicare or the Medicaid payment. The shift to group practice or corporate level practices requires ICT support to handle automated actions like completing repetitive jobs and answering frequently asked questions. The role of telecommunication and IT service providers, and that of entrepreneurs for information management are discussed in the chapter. While discussing the challenges in implementing ICT in GP service it focuses on the slow uptake of computers and other IT products by doctors over the past decade.

Ronald Karon from Namibia University of Science and Technology next offers a chapter on: 'Utilisation of Health Information Systems for Service Delivery in the Namibian Environment'. The author begins with the statement that the use of Health Information Systems is considered to be a major contributing factor to healthcare service delivery but that this, which includes use and management, is critically challenging in the public health sector in many developing countries, resulting in poor service delivery including patient deaths. The main motivation for the reported study was to investigate how Health Information Systems can be used to improve service delivering in the hospitals from a developing country perspective. The study was carried out in Namibia, using two hospitals in the public healthcare sector and involved a qualitative case study which revealed that the use of parallel systems, lack of systems integration, lack of portable devices and users' incompetency are some of the factors which impact the use and management of Health Information Systems in hospitals.

The term 'Rabies' is one that strikes fear into many people's minds and a chapter by Anna Geofrey from Sokoine University of Agriculture, Tanzania discusses 'A Web Based System for Rabies Surveillance in Kilosa District'. She points out that Rabies is a viral zoonotic disease that affects all warm blooded animals and that the rabies virus belongs to the Lyssavirus genus of the family Rhabdoviridae, and order Mononegavirales. Ninety nine percent of human rabies cases are caused by dog bites but weak surveillance systems, attributed to lack of proper records and co-ordinated mass vaccination programs of domestic dogs, poor reporting systems, detection of rabid animals, mapping of endemic areas and prompt response to treatment of rabies victims in Kilosa compound the problem. The chapter describes a project whose objective is to improve the communication of rabies surveillance information by enhancing awareness and supporting a more rapid and timely response to rabies incidences through a web based system. The data for this project is based on the information gathered from various print and electronic resources and also on data collected from the Kilosa district through questionnaires and interview. Result showed that the false perception that rabies impacts on society are low is due to under-reporting and limited awareness of the disease burden.

'RFID Applications in Healthcare-State-of-the-Art and Future Trends' by Amir Manzoor from Bahria University in Pakistan a thorough, systematic review of the existing literature discussing current trends and future directions in this domain. Implementation of RFID technology-based healthcare services is on the rise and findings indicate that tracking is the key RFID enabling function. Automatic data collection and transfer is an RFID function also frequently used in relation to assets, staff, and patients and is also employed for sensing, most often in relation to patients, but also to assets. The chapter concludes by highlighting future research directions where the deployment of RFID technology is likely to transform the healthcare sector.

The next chapter 'Integrated Hospital Information System Architecture Design in Indonesia' was contributed by from Universitas Indonesia: Putu Wuri Handayani, Puspa Indahati Sandhyaduhita, Achmad Nizar Hidayanto, Ave Adriana Pinem, Haya Rizqi Fajrina, Kasiyah M. Junus, Indra Budi and Dumilah Ayuningtyas. Implementing Hospital Information Systems is an important practice that should be performed by hospitals in order to deliver accurate, timely, complete, and easily accessible information in an integrated manner. Given the specific characteristics of Indonesia, the objective of the research described in this chapter was to design an Information System Architecture as part of the Enterprise Architecture based on The Open Group Architecture Framework in order to support Hospital Information System implementation in Indonesia. This research focused on hospital basic processes such as emergency processes, in-patient processes and out-patient processes and found that the integration aspect of the architecture should connect the hospitals with other related stakeholders. The reported research was a qualitative study which involved conducting interviews and observations in three government public hospitals, several directorate generals of the Indonesian Ministry of Health and a representative from the WHO. The result of this research is an integrated Information System Architecture model.

The chapter: 'Lessons Learned from the Implementation of an Emergency Department Information System' is by Paraskevas Vezyridis from Frederick University in Cyprus and Stephen Timmons and Heather Wharrad from the University of Nottingham, UK. The chapter describes how Clinical Information Systems are increasingly being used in emergency departments across the English National Health Service, but that the implementation outcome of this is unpredictable and its success is not guaranteed. The chapter reports a qualitative study, using interviews with 30 emergency department clinicians, administrators and managers. Project management documents, user guides, design blueprints and internal reports were also analysed. The reported study identifies facilitating social and technical factors for implementing an Emergency Department Information System. Lessons learned from the study include the importance of acquiring an established, customised and user-friendly system, attracting funding, establishing communication channels between stakeholders, developing detailed implementation plans and tailored training programmes, investing in peer-support and analysing the workflow impact of the system. The study also found that socio-technical factors, both in and out of the hospital, influenced the success of the implementation but by being systematic in addressing these socio-technical factors certain implementation barriers can be overcome.

A chapter by Irja N Shaanika from Namibia University of Science and Technology is concerned with human interactions in the use of ICT in healthcare. Titled: 'Human Interaction in the Use of Health Information Systems: A Case of a Developing Country' the chapter begins by stating that in developing countries, Health Information Systems are increasingly used to enable and support both clinical and administrative processes for healthcare services, but that the use of these systems in developing countries' healthcare centres is influenced and impacted by humans' interactions which manifests from culture and traditions. Due to the diverse nature of culture and traditions, it is near impossible to have single formula in addressing the patients' needs and as a result the aim to improve quality of healthcare through Health Information Systems is challenged with many stakeholders not able to understand the problem. As the need for healthcare services increases this challenge continues to significantly contribute to poor service delivery. This study focused on the interaction between the healthcare professionals and the Health Information Systems in order to understand how and why the challenges of using the ICT systems exist. This includes examining the implications and how the challenges impact the recipients of healthcare services.

'Toward Integrating Healthcare Data and Systems: A Study of Architectural Alternatives' is a chapter by Timoteus B. Ziminski, Steven A. Demurjian and Eugene Sanzi from the University of Connecticut, USA and Thomas Agresta from University of Connecticut Health Center, USA. In the chapter they point out that the adoption of health information systems and the integration of healthcare data and systems into efficient cross-institutional collaboration workflows of stakeholders, including physicians, hospitals, clinics and labs a challenging problem for the healthcare domain. Their chapter studies the way that well-established software engineering concepts and architectural styles can be employed to satisfy requirements of the healthcare domain and ease health information exchange between stakeholders. The chapter proposes a hybrid health information exchange architecture that leverages the studied styles that include service-oriented architecture, grid computing, a publish/subscribe paradigm and data warehousing to allow the health information systems of stakeholders to be integrated to facilitate collaboration among medical providers. To demonstrate the feasibility and utility of this, a realistic regional healthcare scenario in introduced that illustrates the interactions of stakeholders across an integrated collection of health information system

The final chapter: 'On Piloting a Web-Based Rabies Surveillance System for Humans and Animals' also deals with Rabies. Maulilio J. Kipanyula, Anna Geoffrey, Kadeghe Fue and Camilius Sanga from Sokoine University of Agriculture, Tanzania. They describe how there is a high prevalence of reported rabies in different parts of Tanzania and how the disease has continued to cause a public health threat to communities due to weak passive and active surveillance systems. The data reported in this study was based on the information gathered from various sources and those collected from the Kilosa district council through interviews. The geo information collected was used to develop a geospatial based system that can easily show the hotspots of rabies and the use of web-based interactive maps is likely to strengthen disease surveillance in the area and offers an opportunity for application of such technologies throughout Tanzania. This approach offers a model for sharing both human and animal diseases surveillance information and adoption of this approach is likely to increase awareness and a timely response to rabies incidences. The results from the analysis showed that the false perception that rabies impacts on society are low is due to under-reporting and limited awareness of the disease burden.

It is important to provide empirical insights on the utilisation of ICT in healthcare services. The goal of this book is to consider various aspects of the use of ICT in healthcare, ranging from uptake of ICT to the use of RFID in equipment tracking. This includes the development, implementation and diffusion of technologies for healthcare purposes and also the roles and account of agents in systems and healthcare technologies deployments.

The recent contributions of ICT to healthcare have been enormous and ICT continues to offer huge opportunities for improved service. ICT is now used in a large range of areas in healthcare from diagnostics and delivery to administration. We hope that this book will encourage even greater use of this technology in order to further improve healthcare services.

Tiko Iyamu
Cape Peninsula University of Technology, South Africa

Arthur Tatnall
Victoria University, Australia

Chapter 1
Intelligent Risk Detection in Healthcare Contexts of Hip and Knee Athroplasty and Paediatric Congenital Heart Disease

Hoda Moghimi
RMIT University, Australia

Nilmini Wickramasinghe
Deakin University & Epworth HealthCare, Melbourne, Australia

Jonathan L. Schaffer
Cleveland Clinic, USA

ABSTRACT

Rapid increase of service demands in healthcare contexts today requires a robust framework enabled by IT (information technology) solutions as well as real-time service handling in order to ensure superior decision making and successful healthcare outcomes. Contemporaneous with the challenges facing healthcare, we are witnessing the development of very sophisticated intelligent tools and technologies such as Business Analytics techniques. Therefore, it would appear to be prudent to investigate the possibility of applying such tools and technologies into various healthcare contexts to facilitate better risk detection and support superior decision making. The following serves to do this in the context of Total Hip and Knee Arthroplasty and Congenital Heart Disease.

INTRODUCTION

For some diseases, surgery is not always a final cure and it result in a considerably high rate of disabilities, as well as the possibility of co-morbidities (Goossens, Apers, Gewillig, Budts, & Moons, 2013; Tabbutt et al., 2012); for example, types of cancer and even the development of bowel diseases. Naturally, this also has a direct adverse impact on patients and their families (Landolt, Buechel, & Latal, 2011). Hence,

DOI: 10.4018/978-1-4666-9446-0.ch001

decision-making regarding major surgery is multi-faceted and complex (Noyes, Masakowski, & Cook, 2012; Sox, Higgins, & Owens, 2013).

To facilitate the surgical decision making process, we suggest the application of real time intelligent risk detection decision support would be beneficial. We proffer a suitable solution which combines the application of data mining tools followed by Knowledge Discovery (KD) techniques to score key surgery risk levels, assess surgery risks and thereby help medical professionals to make appropriate decisions.

The aim of this chapter is to outline how it might be possible to improve the outcomes and benefits of surgical interventions and support a healthcare value proposition of excellence for patients, their families, providers, healthcare organizations and society by developing an intelligent risk detection framework to improve surgery decision making processes. While such strategies have been used in other industries (i.e. banking and finance) (Bhambri, 2011; Pulakkazhy & Balan, 2013), it appears that this is one of the first studies focused on healthcare contexts. We focus on the contexts of Total Hip and Knee Arthroplasty and Congenital Heart Disease (CHD) in children to illustrate the potential of this approach.

BACKGROUND

Clinical Decision Support Systems (CDSS) are computer driven technology solutions, developed to provide support to physicians, nurses and patients using medical knowledge and patient-specific information (De Backere, De Turck, Colpaert, & Decruyenaere, 2012). Decision Support systems can be found in widely divergent functional areas. However, in e-health contexts, key features such as intelligent timing, multidimensional views of data and calculation-intensive capabilities become important features given the need for real time outcomes and the multi-spectral nature of care teams (Wickramasinghe, Chalasani, & Koritala, 2012). Hence, systems for healthcare must give advice and support rather than decision making replacing that of clinical staff.

Studies have already proved that CDSS enhance quality, safety and effectiveness of medical decisions through providing higher performance of the medical staff and patient care as well as more effective clinical services. A variety of CDSS programs designed to assist clinical staff with drug dosing, health maintenance, diagnosis, and other clinically relevant healthcare decisions have been developed for the medical workplace (Haug, Gardner, Evans, Rocha, & Rocha, 2007). On the other hand, patients' demand for participation in medical decisions has been increasing (Kuhn, Wurst, Bott, & Giuse, 2006). Therefore, to be respectful of patients and parents/guardians participation and decisions, shared decision-making (SDM) between health care professionals, patients, parents and guardians is widely recommended today (Lai, 2012). SDM is defined as the active participation of both clinicians and families in treatment decisions, the exchange of information, discussion of preferences, and a joint determination of the treatment plan (Barry & Edgman-Levitan, 2012; Charles, Gafni, & Whelan, 1997; Légaré et al., 2011; Makoul & Clayman, 2006).

Although SDM is supported in many disease management domains, some concerns and issues still remain regarding the adoption of SDM solutions such as a perception among some practitioners that the ultimate responsibility for treatment should remain under their authority (Edwards & Elwyn, 2009; Schauer, Everett, del Vecchio, & Anderson, 2007). Moreover, client capacity to participate in decisions (O'Brien, Crickard, Rapp, Holmes, & McDonald, 2011), identifying the SDM components (Sheridan, Harris, & Woolf, 2004; T. van der Weijden et al., 2011) as well as SDM user acceptance (Scholl et al., 2011)are main issues to promote this type of CDCS in the healthcare contexts. However, SDM also has some limitations; for example, SDM is appropriate for situations in which two or more medically reasonable choices exist (O'connor et al., 2009), regardless of whether the degree of risk is high or low (Whitney, McGuire, & McCullough, 2003). Therefore, SDM is not appropriate in these cases while still patients or their families would like to have participation in the care process. Hence, more studies are needed to deepen the understanding of interactions between patient decision aid use and the patterns of patient-practitioner communication as well as format issues such as web-based delivery of patient decision aids. (Cousin, Schmid Mast, Roter, & Hall, 2012; Flight, Wilson, Zajac, Hart, & McGillivray, 2012; O'connor et al., 2009; Parsons et al., 2012).

Research on shared decision making is under way (Barry & Edgman-Levitan, 2012; Deegan & Drake, 2006), but much more is needed in this area. Moreover, it is critical to address the importance of asking right questions in shared decision making process before looking for a right answer, as asking the wrong questions in clinical cases can generate seemingly right answers, but these answers may not be enough to reflect or predict real-life scenarios (Horwitz, Abell, Christian, & Wivel, 2014).

Medical decisions always have to be made in a trade-off between benefit and risk. Unfortunately, many decisions are based upon an incorrect knowledge of risk (Trudy van der Weijden et al., 2011). In addition, different viewpoints concerning risks can result in different optimal choices because of different perspectives (Hsu, Tseng, Chiang, & Chen, 2012). Therefore, the following suggest that an Intelligent Risk Detection (IRD) model which attempts to facilitate and provide decision support for clinicians and patients regarding the treatment risk factors might be beneficial.

To understand the current state and potential for intelligent risk detection, as a first step, more than 500 relevant publications in the period 2003 to 2013 were reviewed. These focused on surgical decision efficiency and/or detecting surgical risk factors. Almost 350 of these publications focused on Information Systems and Health Informatics. From this literature review, the following issues and challenges were identified:

- Lack of communication facilitators to share decisions between clinicians, and between clinicians and patients or their families, in order to support clinical decisions by understanding the treatment risk factors and anticipated outcomes (Bates et al., 2003).
- Lack of some specific Socio-technical components of people, process, technology and environment in healthcare to make a successful implementation of a new technology to address data importance and accuracy issues (Gosain & Kumar, 2009; Kuhn et al., 2006)
- Lack of a dynamic risk assessment system, in the healthcare context (Fortinsky et al., 2004; Gambrill & Shlonsky, 2000; Greenland, 2012; Pancorbo-Hidalgo, Garcia-Fernandez, Lopez-Medina, & Alvarez-Nieto, 2006; Ryan et al., 2012; Twetman, Fontana, & Featherstone, 2013)
- Lack of a multidimensional risk detection model/algorithm (Anderson, Brodie, Vincent, & Hanna, 2012; Aylin, Bottle, & Majeed, 2007; Gran, Fredriksen, & Thunem, 2004; Staal, Hermanns, Schrijvers, & van Stel, 2013; Trucco & Cavallin, 2006).

This in turn makes a real time intelligent risk detection framework the preferred choice. Thus, our study proposes an intelligent application for high-level surgery risk detection and outcome prediction to support surgical decisions. The model is designed based on two steps of the decision making process (surgical and personal) and, includes a decision support system which is suitable for high concentration prediction. Continual model updates inherent in the proposed system results in adaptive and more accurate risk detection and outcome prediction capabilities as compared to a fixed model.

THE CURRENT STUDY

Through this study, it is noted that while data mining is being utilized in various healthcare contexts including applications of text mining and secondary uses for data (Safran et al., 2007), infection control (Iakovidis, Tsevas, Savelonas, & Papamichalis, 2012), physician order entry and electronic health records (Harshberger et al., 2011) and even in the identification of high risk patients (Marschollek et al., 2012) the application of data mining and BI for risk detection is at a nascent state. However, the lack of interaction between healthcare industry practitioners and academic researchers makes it hard to discover surgical risks, and limits opportunities for the application of Business Intelligence and Business Analytics (BI/BA) techniques, and hence weakens the value that knowledge discovery and data mining methods may bring to healthcare risk detection.

In the context of surgical risk detection many dimensions and perspectives (Haga, Ikejiri, Takeuchi, Ikenaga, & Wada, 2012) are of importance and these mainly focus on pathological process, physiological variables, some general health perceptions, social paradigm and also quality of life (Rizzo & Kintner, 2013). Naturally, detecting the risk factors in all of these dimensions is not easy or trivial but based on two approaches to assess the risks, with contribution of clinical experts; this research aims to cover these main dimensions.

Research Design and Methodology

Throughout this research a mixed method approach is conducted incorporating well established qualitative and quantitative data collection techniques. Qualitative and quantitative data are collected by two distinct method; namely, individual semi-structured interviews and questionnaires.

SOLUTIONS AND RECOMMENDATIONS

To capture the inherent complexities of surgery interventions, the conceptual model has been developed. Integral to this model are the two steps of decision making defined over the three key phases of the decision making process for the surgery (Figure 1). The first type of decision making is called "surgical decision making" and is primarily associated with the surgeons while the second type is called "personal decision making" as it is primarily associated with the patients or their family.

Figure 1. The Conceptual Model.
Source: adapted from (Moghimi, Seif Zadeh, Cheung, & Wickramasinghe, 2011)

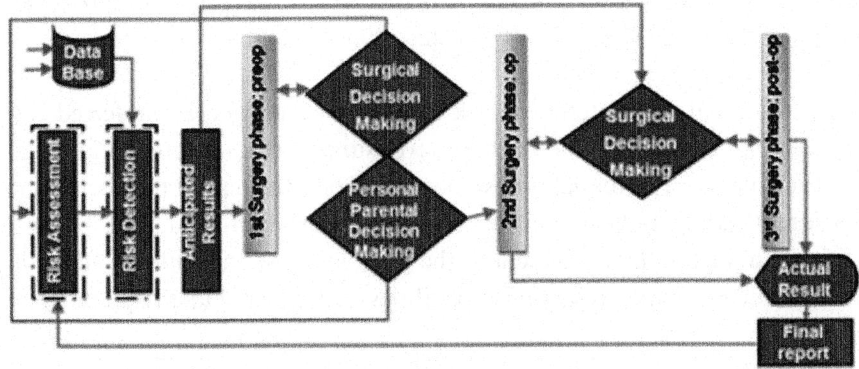

Risk Assessment and Detection

Detecting risk factors based on a risk assessment process using BI tools is a useful way to assess improvements in surgery (Larrazabal et al., 2007). Therefore, after first identifying important risk factors in the literature, we will seek expert input at two distinct stages to address this subject. The specific stages involved in the risk assessment process include the following: In the first stage, the specialists in an expert group of clinicians and surgeons are presented with risk factors identified from the literature. The experts will then nominate (or introduce) some main risk categories or dimensions as well as risk factors to be used in the surgical decision making process. In the next stage, the expert group is asked to assess the risk factors and also evaluate the effects of these factors in surgery outcomes. It is also important to document the surgeons' and specialists' recommendations and advice in order to improve the Model.

To incorporate an intelligent technology into the proposed risk assessment process, data mining tasks followed by knowledge discovery will be trained. In the research case, the data types have a significant impact on the data mining tasks. Hence, after completing the data collection phase, techniques such as neural networks and association rules will be used. After the risk assessment process, applying the necessary data mining techniques, and the development and implementation of the model, a database of the patients' data will be used in order to detect risk factors.

Applying Anticipated and Actual Results

To evaluate a risk detection process in the proposed conceptual model, the actual results will be compared with the anticipated results. This provides feedback to assess the accuracy of the process and also provide appropriate modification as new factors are identified. Lastly, the BI reporting tools will be used to create a final report to show important items, and finally apply them to the risk assessment process, for subsequent iterations of evaluations.

CASE STUDIES

To illustrate the benefits of our proposed IRD Model, we look at two specific healthcare contexts: case one, Orthopaedic interventions and case two, Congenital Heart Disease. The following serves to examine the technical and conceptual layers of the IRD Model and also defines some of the associated knowledge driven healthcare services which are supported by the IRD model in order to facilitate superior healthcare delivery.

Case 1: Incorporating IRD Model to Total Hip and Knee Arthroplasty (THA/TKA)

In general, Total Hip and Knee Arthroplasty are successful solutions for people experiencing pain associated with degenerative joints (Malviya et al., 2011). In fracture care for broken hips however, there are other risk factors involved which impact on both the choice of treatment and on patient outcomes (Malviya et al., 2011). This makes the decision process connected with this surgery of significant importance. In addition hip and knee replacements continue to undergo innovation with improvement in technology and it needs to be monitored (Moghimi, Zadeh, Schaffer, & Wickramasinghe, 2012). Taken together, this serves to underscore that performance management in this context is clearly complex, de-

Table 1. The role of IRD components to improve performance management in hip and knee arthroplasty

IRD Components	Improvements Subjects	Description (How)
Balanced scorecard	• To improve financial issues • To improve clinical issues	By developing relevant measurements and KPIs
Service line analysis and reporting	• To improve financial issues • To improve clinical issues • To improve physiological issues • To improve prosthetic issues	By making analytical and multidimensional reports
Health and wellness service line management	• To improve biomedical issues • To improve physiological issues	By real-time monitoring and controlling patients' clinical conditions
On-Line Analytical Processing (OLAP)	To improve biomedical issues	By making ad-hoc and real-time analytical reports

pendent on multi spectral data and information and has far reaching consequences. Therefore, our IRD Model should be an effective and efficient solution in such a context.

Thus, to illustrate the role for our IRD Model, we have categorized the hip and knee arthroplasty, particularly for hip and knee replacement, into four key components as follows in an attempt to systematically capture four key risk factors (Moghimi & Wickramasinghe, 2012):

- **Prosthetic Issues:** Specific to implant that may impact on the outcome of surgery.
- **Financial Issues:** Regarding the costs of these devices in relationship to outcome and type of surgery
- **Physiological and Co-Morbidities:** Patient specific issues that may impact on the outcome of surgery
- **Clinical Issues:** To medical/provider intervention that may impact on the outcome of the surgery.

Table 1 then, serves to illustrate how the key BA techniques can then be transformed and translated into a specific context; in this instance the context of the hip and knee arthroplasty specifically focussing on hip and knee arthroplasty. Implicit in this conceptualisation is that the proposed IRD Model is sufficiently flexible to cover all process from pre-operative, operative and post-operative. In so doing it will then provide most benefit to all key stakeholders.

Case 2: Incorporating IRD Model to the Congenital Heart Disease (CHD)

Congenital Heart Disease (CHD), as a common health problem affecting many children around the world (Marino et al., 2012), is involved a multi-faceted set of considerations including the immediate medical result, the ongoing increased risk of sudden death, exercise intolerance, neuro developmental and psychological problems as well as long-term impacts on the family unit (Long, Galea, Eldridge, & Harris, 2012). This multi-faceted consideration is important because of the far reaching consequences that can result post-surgery or even mortality or morbidity.

The decision making process in the context of CHD surgery can be divided into three broad phases. In the first phase, or pre-operative phase, the surgeon, having received information about the patient and his/her medical condition, needs to make a decision relating to whether surgery is the best medical option. Once this decision is made but before surgery, the parents must then decide whether to accept or reject the surgeon's decision in consideration of the predicted outcomes. Typically, parents have met many medical staff before they meet the cardiac surgeon. Thus, already at stage one, two key decisions must be made. Once parents and surgeons have agreed to proceed, in phase two, critical decisions pertaining to the unique situations that may arise during the surgery must be addressed. For example, in CHD cases sometimes due to the clinical conditions, surgeons have to change the shunt size during the surgery and regarding this ad-hoc decision, they have to choose the best suitable shunt size with fewer risks, in a very short time. Finally, in the post-operative phase, or phase three, decision making is primarily done at two levels; a) strategies to ensure a sustained successful result for the patient during aftercare and beyond, and b) a record of lessons learnt for use by clinicians in future similar cases.

To clarify the function of the decision making framework across CHD surgery for this study, we summarize current surgery steps and the associated decision making process in one of the common CHD classifications; Hypoplastic Left Heart Syndrome (HLHS) in Figure 2. HLHS patients, usually have three types of surgery during their childhood treatment period, called Norwood, BCPC and Fontan (Hoffman & Kaplan, 2002). These are most recent surgeries suggested to patients in different age and conditions. However, the Norwood surgery is still much more complex and risky with a high rate of mortality and morbidity (Hoffman & Kaplan, 2002). Many factors are likely to be responsible for the improvement in operative survival following the Norwood procedure. These factors include improved surgical techniques, improved peri-operative management, and improved anaesthetic techniques. Despite the improving outcome, early survival for these children is still significantly lower than for other forms of heart disease, which require neonatal surgical intervention (Tabbutt et al., 2012).

In the case of HLHS, it would be diagnosed, either in pre or neonatal and the newborn should be operated, as soon as possible. Hence, as demonstrated at Figure 2, in pre-operative step, the first surgery should be organized by cardiologists and surgeons through making a complex decision regarding the best time and techniques to carry out the surgery. Also, during the surgery surgeons have to make some semi-structured as well as ad hoc decisions such as choosing the best shunt size. In post-operative step, considering the patient conditions, surgeons should make a decision for another surgery or any other clinical treatment. In addition, they should plan a periodic assessment to assess the patient conditions.

Figure 2. Flow Diagram of Key Steps With CHD Surgery (Highlighted boxes in the current procedure represent proposed situations to use the IRD Model)
(Adapted from (Moghimi, Schaffer, & Wickramasinghe, 2014))

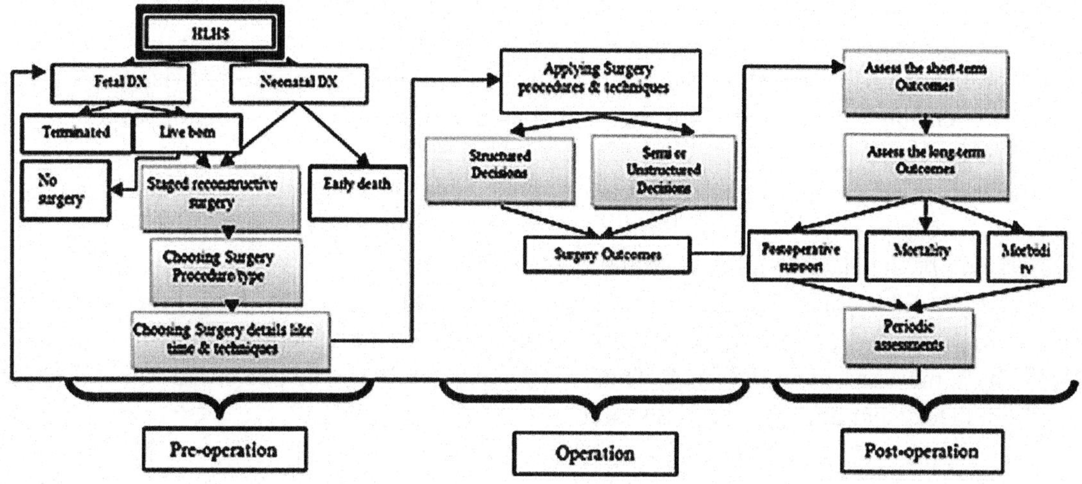

Thus, our proposed IRD Model will be a valuable Model to apply in the highlighted steps in all three surgery phases and surgery types to predict the operation results by detecting risk factors to assist parents as well as surgeons to make superior decisions.

FUTURE RESEARCH DIRECTIONS

This research cannot attempt to determine all actual risk versus actual benefit. This is because long term risks and rare occurrences are not currently possible to identify using randomized controlled trials, these risks and occurrences can only be identified by using methods that were specifically developed for large, observational and longitudinal data sets. This study therefore can only explore the main components of a surgical intelligent risk detection framework to improve clinical decision efficiency.

Although this study supports the benefits of such an intelligent application for healthcare contexts, many issues regarding its implementation into specific healthcare contexts such as Congenital Heart Disease (CHD) and Hip and Knee Arthroplasty remain to be examined. Therefore, the next phase for this research is prototyping and simulation of the solution to trial the model in a selected clinical environment.

DISCUSSION AND CONCLUSION

This study has outlined an exploratory research study aimed at trying to examine the potential benefits of combining a real time intelligent risk detection solution with decision support in a healthcare context. The outcomes from this exploratory research include, early identification of risk factors, providing superior decision support, developing key performance indicators to detect the surgery risk factors, predicting surgical results to identify patients at risk during surgery, standardizing clinical risk assessment and management processes to facilitate superior health outcomes, developing a risk profile for patients, improving risk information sharing, developing a true picture of risk categories and factors, creating a "Risk Aware" alarm to control the risk factors and monitoring the risk factors by using dashboards.

Emphasizing the importance of knowledge sharing between clinicians as well as between clinicians and patients; clinicians' involvement during systems development; acceptability and capability of the system and high demand of outcome predictions to improve decision efficiency are the major contribution to practice.

Providing analytical report to clinicians and patients in three phases of preoperative, operative and post-operative, through different and secure access level, is the other advantages of the IRD model.

In addition, using KPIs as a set of metrics not only is a novel idea to control the risk factors, finding the level and defining their relationships, but it also enables effective monitoring of several key items during surgery.

Another advantage of the proposed IRD model that should be noted is its continuous nature. Most importantly, by comparing anticipated results and actual outcomes and also performing risk auditing, risk factors will be amended to improve future predictions.

A further and final important feature of the proposed IRD model is the integration of the three IT solutions to solve a clinical issue in the definition and assessment of "outcomes" in patients with CHD, combined by some assessment measures. Thus, we believe it will also be one of the valuable contributions to both theory and practice of this research.

REFERENCES

Anderson, O., Brodie, A., Vincent, C. A., & Hanna, G. B. (2012). A systematic proactive risk assessment of hazards in surgical wards: A quantitative study. *Annals of Surgery, 255*(6), 1086–1092. doi:10.1097/SLA.0b013e31824f5f36 PMID:22504280

Aylin, P., Bottle, A., & Majeed, A. (2007). Use of administrative data or clinical databases as predictors of risk of death in hospital: Comparison of models. *BMJ: British Medical Journal, 334*(7602), 1044. doi:10.1136/bmj.39168.496366.55 PMID:17452389

Barry, M. J., & Edgman-Levitan, S. (2012). Shared Decision Making—The Pinnacle of Patient-Centered Care. *The New England Journal of Medicine, 366*(9), 780–781. doi:10.1056/NEJMp1109283 PMID:22375967

Bates, D. W., Kuperman, G. J., Wang, S., Gandhi, T., Kittler, A., Volk, L., & Middleton, B. et al. (2003). Ten commandments for effective clinical decision support: Making the practice of evidence-based medicine a reality. *Journal of the American Medical Informatics Association, 10*(6), 523–530. doi:10.1197/jamia.M1370 PMID:12925543

Bhambri, V. (2011). Application of data mining in banking sector. *International Journal of Clothing Science and Technology, 2*(2).

Charles, C., Gafni, A., & Whelan, T. (1997). Shared decision-making in the medical encounter: What does it mean?(or it takes at least two to tango). *Social Science & Medicine. Social Science & Medicine, 44*(5), 681–692. doi:10.1016/S0277-9536(96)00221-3

Cousin, G., Schmid Mast, M., Roter, D. L., & Hall, J. A. (2012). Concordance between physician communication style and patient attitudes predicts patient satisfaction. *Patient Education and Counseling, 87*(2), 193–197. doi:10.1016/j.pec.2011.08.004 PMID:21907529

De Backere, F., De Turck, F., Colpaert, K., & Decruyenaere, J. (2012). *Advanced pervasive clinical decision support for the intensive care unit*. Academic Press.

Deegan, P., & Drake, R. (2006). Shared decision making and medication management in the recovery process. *Psychiatric Services (Washington, D.C.), 57*(11), 1636–1639. doi:10.1176/ps.2006.57.11.1636 PMID:17085613

Edwards, A., & Elwyn, G. (2009). *Shared decision-making in health care: Achieving evidence-based patient choice*. Oxford University Press.

Flight, I. H., Wilson, C. J., Zajac, I. T., Hart, E., & McGillivray, J. A. (2012). Decision support and the effectiveness of web-based delivery and information tailoring for bowel cancer screening: an exploratory study. *JMIR Research Protocols, 1*(2), e12.

Fortinsky, R. H., Iannuzzi-Sucich, M., Baker, D. I., Gottschalk, M., King, M. B., Brown, C. J., & Tinetti, M. E. (2004). Fall-Risk Assessment and Management in Clinical Practice: Views from Healthcare Providers. *Journal of the American Geriatrics Society, 52*(9), 1522–1526. doi:10.1111/j.1532-5415.2004.52416.x PMID:15341555

Gambrill, E., & Shlonsky, A. (2000). Risk assessment in context. *Children and Youth Services Review*, *22*(11), 813–837. doi:10.1016/S0190-7409(00)00123-7

Goossens, E., Apers, S., Gewillig, M., Budts, W., & Moons, P. (2013). *Evaluating quality of life after correction of a cardiac defect*. Academic Press.

Gosain, A., & Kumar, A. (2009). *Analysis of health care data using different data mining techniques*. Paper presented at the Intelligent Agent & Multi-Agent Systems, 2009. IAMA 2009. International Conference on. doi:10.1109/IAMA.2009.5228051

Gran, B. A., Fredriksen, R., & Thunem, A. P.-J. (2004). *An approach for model-based risk assessment. In Computer Safety, Reliability, and Security* (pp. 311–324). Springer. doi:10.1007/978-3-540-30138-7_26

Greenland, P. (2012). Should the resting electrocardiogram be ordered as a routine risk assessment test in healthy asymptomatic adults? *Journal of the American Medical Association*, *307*(14), 1530–1531. doi:10.1001/jama.2012.441 PMID:22496268

Haga, Y., Ikejiri, K., Takeuchi, H., Ikenaga, M., & Wada, Y. (2012). Value of general surgical risk models for predicting postoperative liver failure and mortality following liver surgery. *Journal of Surgical Oncology*, *106*(7), 898–904. doi:10.1002/jso.23160 PMID:22605669

Harshberger, C. A., Harper, A. J., Carro, G. W., Spath, W. E., Hui, W. C., Lawton, J. M., & Brockstein, B. E. (2011). Outcomes of computerized physician order entry in an electronic health record after implementation in an outpatient oncology setting. *Journal of Oncology Practice*, *7*(4), 233–237. doi:10.1200/JOP.2011.000261 PMID:22043187

Haug, P. J., Gardner, R. M., Evans, R. S., Rocha, B. H., & Rocha, R. A. (2007). Clinical decision support at Intermountain Healthcare. *Clinical Decision Support Systems*, 159-189.

Hoffman, J. I., & Kaplan, S. (2002). The incidence of congenital heart disease. *Journal of the American College of Cardiology*, *39*(12), 1890–1900. doi:10.1016/S0735-1097(02)01886-7 PMID:12084585

Horwitz, R. I., Abell, J. E., Christian, J. B., & Wivel, A. E. (2014). Right answers, wrong questions in clinical research. *Science Translational Medicine, 6*(221), 221fs225-221fs225.

Hsu, W.-K., Tseng, C.-P., Chiang, W.-L., & Chen, C.-W. (2012). Risk and uncertainty analysis in the planning stages of a risk decision-making process. *Natural Hazards*, *61*(3), 1355–1365. doi:10.1007/s11069-011-0032-1

Iakovidis, D. K., Tsevas, S., Savelonas, M. A., & Papamichalis, G. (2012). Image analysis framework for infection monitoring. *Biomedical Engineering. IEEE Transactions on*, *59*(4), 1135–1144.

Kuhn, K., Wurst, S., Bott, O., & Giuse, D. (2006). Expanding the scope of health information systems. *IMIA Yearbook of Medical Informatics*, 43-52.

Lai, P. (2012). Shared decision making. *Surgical Practice*, *16*(4), 127–127. doi:10.1111/j.1744-1633.2012.00623.x

Landolt, M. A., Buechel, E. V., & Latal, B. (2011). Predictors of parental quality of life after child open heart surgery: A 6-month prospective study. *The Journal of Pediatrics, 158*(1), 37–43. doi:10.1016/j.jpeds.2010.06.037 PMID:20688338

Larrazabal, L. A., Jenkins, K. J., Gauvreau, K., Vida, V. L., Benavidez, O. J., Gaitán, G. A., . . . Castañeda, A. R. (2007). Improvement in Congenital Heart Surgery in a Developing Country: The Guatemalan Experience. *Circulation is published by the American Heart Association, 116*, 1872-1877.

Légaré, F., Stacey, D., Pouliot, S., Gauvin, F. P., Desroches, S., Kryworuchko, J., & Gagnon, M. P. et al. (2011). Interprofessionalism and shared decision-making in primary care: A stepwise approach towards a new model. *Journal of Interprofessional Care, 25*(1), 18–25. doi:10.3109/13561820.2010.490502 PMID:20795835

Long, S. H., Galea, M. P., Eldridge, B. J., & Harris, S. R. (2012). Performance of 2-year-old children after early surgery for congenital heart disease on the Bayley Scales of Infant and Toddler Development. *Early Human Development, 88*(8), 603–607. doi:10.1016/j.earlhumdev.2012.01.007 PMID:22336496

Makoul, G., & Clayman, M. L. (2006). An integrative model of shared decision making in medical encounters. *Patient Education and Counseling, 60*(3), 301–312. doi:10.1016/j.pec.2005.06.010 PMID:16051459

Malviya, A., Martin, K., Harper, I., Muller, S. D., Emmerson, K. P., Partington, P. F., & Reed, M. R. (2011). Enhanced recovery program for hip and knee replacement reduces death rate: A study of 4,500 consecutive primary hip and knee replacements. *Acta Orthopaedica, 82*(5), 577–581. doi:10.3109/17453674.2011.618911 PMID:21895500

Marino, B. S., Lipkin, P. H., Newburger, J. W., Peacock, G., Gerdes, M., Gaynor, J. W., & Johnson, W. H. et al. (2012). Neurodevelopmental Outcomes in Children With Congenital Heart Disease: Evaluation and Management A Scientific Statement From the American Heart Association. *Circulation, 126*(9), 1143–1172. doi:10.1161/CIR.0b013e318265ee8a PMID:22851541

Marschollek, M., Gövercin, M., Rust, S., Gietzelt, M., Schulze, M., Wolf, K.-H., & Steinhagen-Thiessen, E. (2012). Mining geriatric assessment data for in-patient fall prediction models and high-risk subgroups. *BMC Medical Informatics and Decision Making, 12*(1), 19. doi:10.1186/1472-6947-12-19 PMID:22417403

Moghimi, H., Schaffer, J., & Wickramasinghe, N. (2014). *Exploring The Possibilities For Intelligent Risk Detection In Healthcare Contexts* Paper presented at the ECIS Workshop, Tel Aviv.

Moghimi, H., Seif Zadeh, H., Cheung, M., & Wickramasinghe, N. (2011). *An intelligent risk detection framework using business intelligence tools to improve decision efficiency in healthcare contexts.* Paper presented at the Seventeenth Americas Conference on Information Systems (AMCIS).

Moghimi, H., & Wickramasinghe, N. (2012). *Improving e-performance management in healthcare using intelligent IT solutions. In Critical Issues for the Development of Sustainable E-health Solutions* (pp. 3–15). Springer. doi:10.1007/978-1-4614-1536-7_1

Moghimi, H., Zadeh, H., Schaffer, J., & Wickramasinghe, N. (2012). Incorporating intelligent risk detection to enable superior decision support: The example of orthopaedic surgeries. *Health Technology, 2*(1), 33–41. doi:10.1007/s12553-011-0014-z

Noyes, J., Masakowski, Y., & Cook, M. (2012). *Decision making in complex environments.* Ashgate Publishing, Ltd.

O'Brien, M. S., Crickard, E. L., Rapp, C., Holmes, C., & McDonald, T. (2011). Critical issues for psychiatric medication shared decision making with youth and families. *Families in Society, 93*(3), 310–316. doi:10.1606/1044-3894.4135

O'connor, A., Bennett, C., Stacey, D., Barry, M., Col, N., Eden, K., . . . Khangura, S. (2009). Decision aids for people facing health treatment or screening decisions (Review). *The Cochrane Collaboration published in the Cochrane Library, 3.*

Pancorbo-Hidalgo, P. L., Garcia-Fernandez, F. P., Lopez-Medina, I. M., & Alvarez-Nieto, C. (2006). Risk assessment scales for pressure ulcer prevention: A systematic review. *Journal of Advanced Nursing, 54*(1), 94–110. doi:10.1111/j.1365-2648.2006.03794.x PMID:16553695

Parsons, S., Harding, G., Breen, A., Foster, N., Pincus, T., Vogel, S., & Underwood, M. (2012). Will shared decision making between patients with chronic musculoskeletal pain and physiotherapists, osteopaths and chiropractors improve patient care? *Family Practice, 29*(2), 203–212. doi:10.1093/fampra/cmr083 PMID:21982810

Pulakkazhy, S., & Balan, R. (2013). Data mining in banking and its applications-a review. *Journal of Computer Science, 9*(10), 1252–1259. doi:10.3844/jcssp.2013.1252.1259

Rizzo, V. M., & Kintner, E. (2013). The utility of the behavioral risk factor surveillance system (BRFSS) in testing quality of life theory: An evaluation using structural equation modeling. *Quality of Life Research: An International Journal of Quality of Life Aspects of Treatment, Care and Rehabilitation, 22*(5), 987–995. doi:10.1007/s11136-012-0228-1 PMID:22797867

Ryan, P. B., Madigan, D., Stang, P. E., Marc Overhage, J., Racoosin, J. A., & Hartzema, A. G. (2012). Empirical assessment of methods for risk identification in healthcare data: Results from the experiments of the Observational Medical Outcomes Partnership. *Statistics in Medicine, 31*(30), 4401–4415. PMID:23015364

Safran, C., Bloomrosen, M., Hammond, W. E., Labkoff, S., Markel-Fox, S., Tang, P. C., & Detmer, D. E. (2007). Toward a national framework for the secondary use of health data: An American Medical Informatics Association White Paper. *Journal of the American Medical Informatics Association, 14*(1), 1–9. doi:10.1197/jamia.M2273 PMID:17077452

Schauer, C., Everett, A., del Vecchio, P., & Anderson, L. (2007). Promoting the value and practice of shared decision-making in mental health care. *Psychiatric Rehabilitation Journal, 31*(1), 54–61. doi:10.2975/31.1.2007.54.61 PMID:17694716

Scholl, I., Loon, M. K., Sepucha, K., Elwyn, G., Légaré, F., Härter, M., & Dirmaier, J. (2011). Measurement of shared decision making–a review of instruments. *Zeitschrift für Evidenz. Fortbildung und Qualität im Gesundheitswesen, 105*(4), 313–324. doi:10.1016/j.zefq.2011.04.012

Sheridan, S. L., Harris, R. P., & Woolf, S. H. (2004). Shared decision making about screening and chemoprevention. *American Journal of Preventive Medicine, 26*(1), 56–66. doi:10.1016/j.amepre.2003.09.011 PMID:14700714

Sox, H. C., Higgins, M. C., & Owens, D. K. (2013). *Medical decision making.* John Wiley & Sons. doi:10.1002/9781118341544

Staal, I. I., Hermanns, J., Schrijvers, A. J., & van Stel, H. F. (2013). Risk assessment of parents' concerns at 18 months in preventive child health care predicted child abuse and neglect. *Child Abuse & Neglect, 37*(7), 475–484. doi:10.1016/j.chiabu.2012.12.002 PMID:23352082

Tabbutt, S., Ghanayem, N., Ravishankar, C., Sleeper, L. A., Cooper, D. S., Frank, D. U., & Goldberg, C. S. et al. (2012). Risk factors for hospital morbidity and mortality after the Norwood procedure: A report from the Pediatric Heart Network Single Ventricle Reconstruction trial. *The Journal of Thoracic and Cardiovascular Surgery, 144*(4), 882–895. doi:10.1016/j.jtcvs.2012.05.019 PMID:22704284

Trucco, P., & Cavallin, M. (2006). A quantitative approach to clinical risk assessment: The CREA method. *Safety Science, 44*(6), 491–513. doi:10.1016/j.ssci.2006.01.003

Twetman, S., Fontana, M., & Featherstone, J. D. (2013). Risk assessment–can we achieve consensus? *Community Dentistry and Oral Epidemiology, 41*(1), e64–e70. doi:10.1111/cdoe.12026 PMID:24916679

van der Weijden, T., van Veenendaal, H., Drenthen, T., Versluijs, M., Stalmeier, P., Loon, M. K., & Timmermans, D. (2011). Shared decision making in the Netherlands, is the time ripe for nationwide, structural implementation? *Zeitschrift für Evidenz. Fortbildung und Qualität im Gesundheitswesen, 105*(4), 283–288. doi:10.1016/j.zefq.2011.04.005

van der Weijden, T., van Veenendaal, H., Drenthen, T., Versluijs, M., Stalmeier, P., Loon, M. K.-, & Timmermans, D. et al. (2011). Shared decision making in the Netherlands, is the time ripe for nationwide, structural implementation? *Zeitschrift für Evidenz. Fortbildung und Qualität im Gesundheitswesen, 105*(4), 283–288. doi:10.1016/j.zefq.2011.04.005

Whitney, S. N., McGuire, A. L., & McCullough, L. B. (2003). A typology of shared decision making, informed consent, and simple consent. *Annals of Internal Medicine, 140*(1), 54–59. doi:10.7326/0003-4819-140-1-200401060-00012 PMID:14706973

Wickramasinghe, N., Chalasani, S., & Koritala, S. (2012). *The role of healthcare system of systems and collaborative technologies in providing superior healthcare delivery to native american patients.* Paper presented at the System Science (HICSS), 2012 45th Hawaii International Conference. doi:10.1109/HICSS.2012.582

KEY TERMS AND DEFINITIONS

Business Analytics: Developing new insights and understanding of business performance based on data and statistical methods.

Clinical Decision Support Systems: Clinical decision support system (CDSS) is an expert system software to assist health professionals in decision making process to improve decision efficiency.

Congenital Heart Disease (CHD): Is a defect in the structure of the heart and great vessels that is present at birth.

Hip and Knee Arthoplasty: A primary hip and knee arthoplasty occurs when the native joint surface(s) are replaced with artificial implants.

Predictive Analytic: Predictive analytics is defined as a variety of statistical techniques to analyse current and historical facts to make predictions about future.

Risk Detection: The ability to capture clinical risks at the earliest time.

Chapter 2
Managing Knowledge towards Enabling Healthcare Service Delivery

Tiko Iyamu
Cape Peninsula University of Technology, South Africa

Sharol Sibongile Mkhomazi
Tshwane University of Technology, South Africa

ABSTRACT

In every living being, health is essentially important, and as such, requires attention. Health related matters are at one point or the other embedded into humans' strategic, tactical and operational activities. However, due to human complexity, manifesting from factors such as food consumption and weather effect, healthcare services have increasingly become essential to individuals, groups and organisations in their daily life activities. As healthcare services increase in significance, the knowledge acquired and used in carrying out its services also becomes vital. The management of knowledge has increased in its relevance over the years. This could be attributed to the complexity in human activities. Thus, the management of knowledge has many challenges, which are never straight forward, and does not always produce positive result. Based on the challenges, it is critical to understand the enabling and constraint scenery of knowledge management. This article applied Structuration Theory to examine the different types of knowledge within the healthcare environment, using one of South African healthcare service providers as a case. This was done in order to gain better understanding on how certain knowledge are managed to give the result that they do. A better understanding of how knowledge is acquired and used within the healthcare environment would assist practitioners and managers, including Government and academic researchers in their roles and responsibilities.

1. INTRODUCTION

Many organisations take cognizance and seriously the value of knowledge in enhancing their capacity to compete and adapt to change (Bevern, 2003). As a result, some organisations are attentive to manage-

DOI: 10.4018/978-1-4666-9446-0.ch002

ment knowledge to make a difference.

According to Lee and Lee (2007), knowledge management (KM) is aimed to strengthen public service effectiveness, so as to serve the society better. The need for KM is based on a paradigm shift in the business environment, where knowledge is considered central to organisational performance.

In the last two decades, KM has received increasing attention in the field of healthcare. This could be attributed to the sensitive nature, and the increasing needs of healthcare services. Similar to other disciplines, healthcare operations depend, and are influenced by available data. Data within the healthcare environmental is often voluminous. This could be attributed to the high volume of information such as electronic medical records, clinical trial data, and hospital records that flows in the healthcare environment (Omary et al., (2009). The voluminous data require different types of knowledge for effective and efficient management.

Many research studies have been conducted on KM's benefits, implications, and effects on healthcare service delivery. The study by Khorasani et al (2012) emphasised that KM in healthcare is critical, particularly, in developing the necessary capacity amongst professionals, in order for them to be able to manage the required and available knowledge. In managing knowledge within the healthcare environment, there is need to understand the factors which impact, influences, as well as the drivers within the environment, which contribute to clinical, strategic and tactical decision-making.

The objective was to gain better understanding of how knowledge impact (enables and constrain) on healthcare service delivery within the healthcare environment, particularly in developing countries. The research question was what are the factors which influence the management of knowledge within the healthcare environment? The examination of enablement and constraint was possible through Structuration Theory (ST), mainly through its focus on production and reproduction of events and activities.

The ST also focus on double hermeneutic process, where people, upon reflection of day-to-day activities, are able to influence the structure within which they operate (Giddens, 1984). Giddens (1984) further argued that this is done by either reproducing current practices or by changing them. In structuration, structure are rules and resources (Iyamu & Roode, 2010). Based on knowledge, or through management of knowledge, rules and resources that stem within healthcare organisations are produced and reproduced overtime.

2. KNOWLEDGE MANAGEMENT

There is no accepted single definition of knowledge management (KM). However most of the definitions adopted by different scholars represent knowledge management as a social and learning process which facilitate organisational growth and competitiveness. KM is a process which could be used by individuals, organisations or communities facilitate improvement of events and activities in their environment (Weber, 2007). This includes leveraging data and information that are gathered, organised, managed, and shared. Hasanali (2002) describe knowledge management as a set of strategies and approaches which denotes a definite structure or a way of doing things that enables the flow of information to the right person at the right time.

There are two types of knowledge, tacit and explicit knowledge. Tacit knowledge is derived from experience and trusted sources while explicit knowledge comes from documented sources (Chunharas, 2006). This means that the use of both explicit and tacit knowledge, knowledge management is intended to help an organisation to deliver the right information to the right place and person at the right time.

In Bali and Dwivedi (2007), it is argued that KM places value on the tacit knowledge that individuals hold within an organisation.

The fundamental distinction in KM is between the activities that involve the application of existing knowledge and those that generate new knowledge (Bate & Robert, 2002). KM activities results in what Lee et al (2005) refer to, as knowledge circulation process. The types of knowledge include the following:

- **Knowledge Creation:** It deals with a variety of knowledge, whether tacit or explicit and is accelerated by encouraging synergistic interrelations of individuals from diverse background. Knowledge accumulation. All individuals in the form must have access to the base to obtain the relevant knowledge to aid in their work and decision making.
- **Knowledge Sharing:** Which promotes diffusion of knowledge and also contributes to making the work process astute and knowledge-intensive.
- **Knowledge Utilization:** Can occur at all levels of management activities in firms: one of the popular forms of knowledge utilization is to adopt the best practice from other leading organizations, uncover relevant knowledge, and apply it (O' Dell & Grayson, 1998).
- **Knowledge Internalisation:** Which may occur when individual workers discover relevant knowledge, obtains it and then applies it.

Irrespective of the type, knowledge is a result of agent action, which is produced and reproduced overtime. The action is enabling and constraining in nature.

3. STRUCTURATION THEORY

Structuration theory (ST) is concerned with the influence of human interaction on social life, which impact rules, communication and power relationship, as they are produced and reproduced within structure (Giddens, 1984). The theory outlines some of the social processes which are involved in the evolution of societal aspects. In Giddens (1984) view, the theory was developed to gain an understanding of how social practices are ordered across time and space. If the actions of actors in social practice become reasonably stable over time and space, then routines or practices in which actors habitually engage are developed (Rose, 1998).

Cultural context is important in ST as it is generated and re-generated through the interplay of action and structure also referred to as the duality of structure (Giddens, 1986). The basis of the duality lie in the relationship which the agency has with the structure, thus action and structure cannot be conceived of apart from one another. Therefore they are not independent of each other. In understanding how knowledge is managed within the Healthcare environment, we followed the agents and structures that drive and influence the processes and activities.

3.1. Agents and Knowledge

Agents are guided by the organisational policies and procedures as well as unarticulated expertise and experience that reside within individual workers (Wickramasinghe, Gupta & Sharma, 2005). Humans are knowledgeable agents operating in specific context, and that "every member of a society must know a great deal about the workings of that society by virtue of his or her participation in it" (Giddens, 1984).

In the context, Khorasani et al. (2012) argued that it is therefore cooperation amongst agents within the healthcare organisation is vital in order to deliver quality of care, crucially.

3.2. Structure

In ST, structure are both rules and resources, as defined by Giddens (1984). Through action, rules and resources are used to produce and reproduce social system. These rules and resources mediate in that they are what tie social relations together and they are what actors use to create, sustain, or transform relations across time and in space. In order to draw on rules and resources, awareness of the agents is required. According to Giddens (1984), structure are both the medium and outcomes of a process.

The most important application of ST lies in the recognition of structure and agency as duality that cannot be conceived apart from one another, a relationship that draws on interdependence. Thus human action is enabled and constrained by structure, but structure is also the result of human action.

4. METHODOLOGY

In an exploratory nature, the case study approach as described by Yin (2009) was employed to investigate how knowledge is acquired, used and managed within healthcare environment..

The information that is used in this study was gathered within a period of six months, between February and August, 2012. This was done through our active observation and participation of processes and activities in the organisation. Also, 19 professional and administrative managers in the organisation participated in the study, though semi-structured interviews.

The observation technique was adopted in order to understand the manner in which practitioners verbally expressed themselves, and how they respond to activities. Also, the observation was considered useful for the study so as to witness surgical operations which is sometime different in theoretical expression.

The organisation that was used in the study is a healthcare service provider in South Africa. The organisation prefers to be anonymous due to the sensitive nature of their services to the general public. In respect to the code of ethic within which the study was carried out, we decided to be silent about the name of the organisation. This has also limited us from providing much information about the individual organisation, so as not to give away the identity.

Based on the quality and depth of data, the empirical inquiring as gathered in the study, it was enough to draw the conclusions that we did.

5. STRUCTURATION VIEW: KNOWLEDGE MANAGEMENT IN HEALTHCARE

Based on the analysis and interpretation of our data, and review of literature such as Khorasani et al. (2012), four types of knowledge are considered to be very critical in the healthcare services. They include Practitioner knowledge, Resources knowledge, Process knowledge, and Organisational knowledge. Activities of Orthopaedists' which happened during the study, in the organisation used as the case study are used as example.

Knowledge is required in the different areas of specialisation of healthcare services, and they complement each other. The need for these types of knowledge is influenced, driven, and determined by how they are used, stored and managed. The management of knowledge within the healthcare environment is therefore influenced by the intensive and sensitive nature of the services. As a result, management of knowledge for healthcare services requires distinct and specialisation in processes and activities.

5.1 Practitioner Knowledge

This is the knowledge of areas of specialisation which were specifically required by the practitioners such as Orthopaedists to executive their activities, and deliver service in the organisation. The area of specialisation defined the network of operationalisation of duties by the personnel in the organisation. Within the network, actors established relationship, through which interest groups were formed. This relationship was used to foster knowledge acquisition, use and sharing.

Orthopaedists have deeper knowledge of musculoskeletal disorders, which include fractures, and chronic systemic disorders such as loss of bone density or lupus erythematosus. For example, during the study, when it came to treatment of Orthopaedic patent, medical information about the patient was not freely available to other practitioners (non Orthopaedists) including the General Practitioner who initially examined the patient. This could be an act of unconsciousness. Also, this could also be attributed to the knowledge of resources that are used by Orthopaedists whose accesses are limited to other practitioners.

5.2 Resource Knowledge

This type of knowledge is of operational facilities. The availability of this type of knowledge made it possible for decisions making, which was required by the practitioners in order for them to execute their activities and service delivery. Through the relationship that was established by the actors, their interaction within the network, understanding of operational facilities became critical in enabling the effectiveness of healthcare delivery.

During the study, an Orthopaedist carried out treatment on bone replacement on patient. The same treatment was carried out on another female patient at another day, using the same medical resources. A senior practitioner expressed his view as: that is based on the Orthopaedist knowledge of the available resources. The Orthopaedist operation took into account multiple inputs which were dependent on his knowledge, and it is not possible to automate to them. Also, the same processes were repeated for both patients.

5.3 Process Knowledge

This is the knowledge of actions which was undertaken by actors to produce change in their operations. This type of knowledge was also used to bring development that was required by actors to execute their tasks and activities. However, the change or development process were often manipulated by, or carried out by actors within networks (of social system). During the development or change process, cultures was born, which profoundly influenced the actors' conducts and performances within the social system. The culture shaped the social practices (thoughts, feelings and behaviours) of the actors within the organisation.

5.4 Organisational Knowledge

This is the type of knowledge which helped actors with an understanding of their organisation and the industry in general. It came from different sub-units within the networks that had value in operationalising their events and activities. This involved information flows which were pragmatically used to enhance the performance of the organisation. It also involved the know-how of individuals and groups within the social system in which the find themselves in the organisation.

Unfortunately, the organisation was not able to produce a stock of knowledge in the form of repository that contains how much knowledge (based on experiments and their outcome) each Orthopaedist have on their profession. This could have formed part of the organisational knowledge.

The focus of the use of Structuration theory was to understand why certain knowledge is required; how the knowledge is applied in the manner that they do; and the impact and implication of the knowledge in its application. *According to Giddens (1984), every member of a society must know a great deal about the workings of that society by virtue of his or her participation in it.* Knowledge is acquired, and made use of, based on the relationship, which is the ability to understand and expressive of the object or subject.

Through the lens of Structuration Theory, it is revealing that for the above mentioned knowledge to exist and function, it would have to be within social system (network). This is based on the fact that where there are agents, knowledge do not exist, vice versa. Knowledge that is not put to use in order to make a difference cannot be considered as one.

The four knowledge types (Practitioner knowledge; Resources knowledge; Process knowledge; and Organisational knowledge) which were discussed and presented above are now interpreted and drawn into one single entity as Networks of Relationship within the context of healthcare service delivery.

6. NETWORKS RELATIONSHIP

There existed different types of networks within the healthcare organisation that was used in the study. The relationships that were form amongst the actors in the organisation were heterogeneous in nature. The networks influenced and shaped the outcome of healthcare service delivery, through conscious and unconscious actions of the actors. In the delivering of healthcare services, networks such as communicative platform, cultural, and resource are formed.

6.1 Communication Network of Relationship

Communication was carried out by actors within a network, in the course of operationalising events in their duties t provider service. Communication and sharing of information in the delivery of services was critical mainly due to societal need for healthcare. What was even more important was what (content) was communicated; how they were communicated; and understood them.

Actors who belonged to the same network seemed to communicate and understand each other better than others who were external or not recognised to be part of the network. The communication was influenced by the interest of the communicators, and the receivers. The content of the communication was always interpreted before usage. Also, the interpretation was informed by understanding, as well as the interest of the receivers. The understanding and interest of both the communicator and receiver determines the enabling or constraining use of the information and knowledge acquired and shared.

6.2 Cultural Network of Relationship

Culture was considered very important in the management of knowledge within the organisation. This was attributed to traditional heritage in South Africa, which has similarity with other African countries. It is a factor which has been practiced overtime, and within network of people, which are often people of the same tribal origin, or ethnicity. Personnel with the organisation were interconnected based on their cultural beliefs, which shaped their relationship.

According to Giddens (1984), agents (such as people) have the capacity to make a difference through their interaction within structure, which they belong. Within such frame, we observed and analysed similar actions, whereby agents constantly produced and reproduced actions which were both constraining and enabling in the delivering of healthcare service to the community. For example, some specialist responded to certain nurses that they did with others.

The health sector involves a range of key agents such as patients, suppliers, practitioners and administrators, who often form a particular cultural belief. The interaction among these agents shaped and determined what was considered as relevant knowledge. Therefore the practices and activities that they undertook could not exist independently of cultural belief, directly or indirectly, within the social context in which they found themselves

6.3 Resources Network of Relationship

Resources were critical in making knowledge management a success or failure in the organisation. Resources were the means through which intentions of the personnel were realised, and some goals of the organisation were accomplished in delivering healthcare services by the organisation. Also, power was expressed and exercised by knowledgeable agents in the course of interaction within the network.

Power depends upon the mobilisation of resources (such as people, technology and knowledge) which reflected in the way that the interests of different actors were represented within the networks of the organisation in providing healthcare services to the communities. This included the way in which different actors accessed and granted access to resources in the organisation.

Thus, the accessibility d and utilisation of resources depended upon the relationship amongst the personnel (agents) within the organisational networks. The approach was not all negative as some of the senior managers explored the avenue for organisational benefit. For example, some teams were created based on relationship amongst employees, and through this, there was improvement on information flow, use and management, which was said to increased in efficiency and effectiveness of healthcare service delivery.

The different types, including the networks within which personnel formed relationship as discussed above, were influenced by certain factors. The factors were actions which were produced and reproduced overtime and space in the course of providing service to the communities.

7. FACTORS INFLUENCING HEALTHCARE KNOWLEDGE MANAGEMENT

In order to gain better understanding of how knowledge could effectively be managed to improve healthcare service delivery, the influencing factors must be established and understood. The management approach was intended to accelerate knowledge culture in the organisation. The organisation expected the culture to cover how information flows, as well as their practices of events in their activities and services to the communities.

People, process and technology are considered to be the focal actors in the management of events and activities. The three (people, process and technology) components interconnect, and they depend on each other. The components were critical in providing services to the communities in the South African environment. None of the resources can be responsible for supporting Knowledge management in isolation within the organisation. According to Iyamu and Adelakun (2008), there are underlying relations between these three resources and they cannot be treated in isolation. Even though their argument was in the context of information technology, the same applies, and in the same vein, they can contribute to success or failure of KM in healthcare organisation.

Medical Doctors and Nurses and other personnel were knowledge facilitators in the organisation. They used technologies to deliver and facilitate knowledge within the organisation. For example, groups email was created to share information and manage available knowledge in delivering service. Furthermore, email was enabled and supported through devices such as Mobile phones.

This implies that personnel acquired assessed certain knowledge with the assistance of technology, through processes that were defined by the organisation. Based on the knowledge on the acquired knowledge, an understanding amongst the personnel is formed. The understanding helped the personnel to provide carried out their tasks and provide services to the communities in the country.

Organisational processes tend to improve as knowledge is shared and leveraged among organisational members. An efficient KM approach is a valuable way for helping individuals within organisation to exploit all the available knowledge sources.

8. HEALTHCARE SERVICES: MANAGING KNOWLEDGE

The management of knowledge was an easy task to undertake, according some personnel in the organisation. Both Medical Doctors and Nurses attributed difficulty in managing knowledge to human factor which was unpredictable. This is primary because no person or organisation has absolute power over another person or their employees. As a result, the management of knowledge enables, and at the same time constrains depending on the interest of the actors with the network.

The management of knowledge enabled, and at the same time constrained the services which were provided by the healthcare organisation. This happened direct and through unintended actions of humans, in groups or individually in the organisation. Humans' actions were often driven by interest as enacted by power, which was based on the relationship that the different agents upheld in their networks.

Based on our analysis, using the lens of Structuration Theory, the enablement and constraint of management of knowledge in providing healthcare services was drawn from network of relationship and power relationship within the organisation. As depicted in Figure 1 below, the management of Practitioner knowledge, Resources knowledge, Process knowledge, and Organisational knowledge was enabled and constrained by network relationships which were informed, influenced, and manifested by recursive actions during communication; in the practice of culture; and use of resources by the personnel of the organisation.

Figure 1 is a Framework which exhumes how different factors were connected in enabling and constraining the management of knowledge in providing healthcare services in South Africa. It consists of two connective schemes, network relationship and power relationship. The network relationship as it

Figure 1. Factors to Managing knowledge

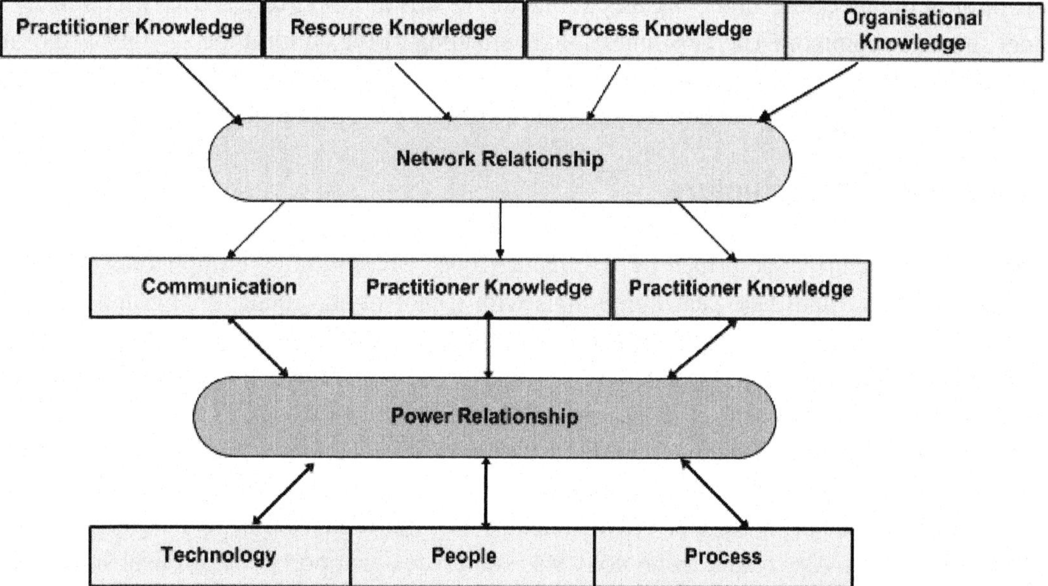

impacted the management of knowledge within the context of healthcare service delivery was discussed above. The discussion that follows focuses on power relationship, how it impact, through enablement and constraints, the management of knowledge in the organisation's delivering of healthcare services.

8.1. The Roles of Human and Culture

Knowledge, as enacted by individuals and groups had significant roles in the organisation's healthcare service delivery. The significant effect was recursively produced overtime before this study. As a result, it needed to be shared and well managed, according to some of the employees of the organisation. Otherwise, as perceived by some of the personnel (both Medical Doctors and Nurses), it would become only a constraining vehicle as opposed to enabler. Personnel in the organisation were one of the key vehicles, which were used for knowledge sharing. Unfortunately, the personnel's actions and reactions were often unpredictable. However, it is easier to assess people's permanent interest. They used the power bestowed upon them to achieve their individual or group interest. Power was often embedded into organisational process or technology as enacted by reliance and relevance to service delivery.

Managing knowledge in the organisation was conducted through processes, which were formulated by personnel. KM built upon professional teamwork by actively engaging personnel at different levels and units in the organisation. Through knowledge sharing and stimulation of learning some of the managers in the organisation anticipated that service quality would improve.

Some of the personnel were aware of the fact that their actions have significant influence and impact on the services, which the organisation delivers to the communities. This was so because knowledge management was a process which depended upon people in order to make it useful in the organisation. Thus, knowledge-sharing culture was built by people's participation, interest and willingness to share information for others' consumption in the organisation.

The interaction which took place amongst individuals and groups described the type of culture that was built in organisation. In the organisation, culture was an important factor, which many of the personnel shared in common. The personnel's understanding of the cultural factor consisted of norms, values, attitudes and beliefs. According to DeLong and Fahey (2000), norms and values drive subsequent behaviours by providing the social context through which people communicate and act.

8.2. Technology Infrastructure

Technology infrastructure is described by Nyrhinen (2006) as technology components (such as communication technology and data) that individuals with technical and managerial competence use, in order to produce actions such as standards, policies and procedures. Importantly, IT was intended to enable effectuating the knowledge-based view in the delivering of service in the organisation. This was to further and foster improvement of healthcare service delivery. However, IT sometimes constrained their activities of the organisational process. For example, critical healthcare related decision depended on data which required authorisation before it could be retrieved from the information system.

Technology was crucial in their effort to transforming the organisation to building a knowledge sharing cultural system. As a result, technology was employed to supports both clinical and administrative decision-making process in delivering healthcare services to the communities. Without technology infrastructure, the organisation had finds it difficult, or couldn't have been able to enable its employees to share information on a large scale. At the same time, technology could be used to prevent employees from accessing information.

8.3. Process and Organisational Policies

Managing knowledge was mainly a process of automation of existing activities, events and tools. Due to the sensitive nature of the organisation's business, process was strictly defined by legal norms such as organisational policies and procedures.

Actors were guided by the organisation's policies and procedures as well as unarticulated expertise and experience that resided within individual workers' domain. The organisation's policies and procedures were important catalysts in information sharing and management, as well as ensuring efficient and effective use of information within an organisation.

The effectiveness of healthcare service delivery through knowledge sharing necessitated collaboration among stakeholders who were involved in the delivery of healthcare services. This is subject to explicit involvement of stakeholders in enforcing implementation of knowledge management in healthcare service delivery.

9. CONCLUSION

In the article, management of knowledge and healthcare service are linked together, and viewed through the lens of Structuration Theory. The article help us gain better understanding of the knowledge factors which have enabling and constraining influence and impact on healthcare delivery. Some of the factors were known, but some of the healthcare practitioners and information systems personnel take them for granted. This is mainly because they didn't understand the implications, potentially. As such, the article benefits knowledge managers, healthcare practitioners and information systems personnel. Also, it would benefits IS researchers who would be interested in carrying out extended studies which is based on the article, in the areas of knowledge management, health informatics, and information systems.

The article invigorated the criticality of managing knowledge, through its examination of the social context. The understanding drawn from the article would help the managers and other practitioners to take cognisance, thereby perform their duties better, taking into cognisance of actors' influencing factors. Otherwise, recursive of actions of the current state would be observed, continuously manifest to challenges.

REFERENCES

Bali, R. K., & Dwivedi, A. N. (2007). *Healthcare Knowledge Management.* Springer. doi:10.1007/978-0-387-49009-0

Bate, S. P., & Robert, G. (2002). Knowledge Management and communities of practice in the private sector: Lessons for modernizing the National Health Service in England and Wales. *Public Administration Journal, 80*(4), 643–663. doi:10.1111/1467-9299.00322

Chunharas, S. (2006). An interactive integrative approach to translating knowledge and building a "learning organisation" in health services management. *Bulletin of the World Health Organization, 84*(8), 652–657. doi:10.2471/BLT.05.026922 PMID:16917653

DeLong, D. W., & Fahey, L. (2000). Diagnosing cultural barriers to knowledge management. *The Academy of Management Executive, 14*(4), 113–127.

Giddens, A. (1984). *The Constitution of society: Outline of the theory of Structuration.* Berkeley, CA: University of California Press.

Giddens, A. (1986). *Situation of society: Outline of the theory of structuration.* Uninversity of Carlifornia Press.

Hasanali, F. (2002*). Critical success factors of Knowledge Management.* Available online: http://polaris.umuc.edu/mts/TMAN/TMAN_636/articles/csfs.pdf

Iyamu, T., & Adelakun, O. 2008. The impact of non-technical factors on Information Technology Strategy and E-business. In *Proceedings of the 12th Pacific Asia Conference on Information Systems (PACIS).* Academic Press.

Iyamu, T., & Roode, D. (2010). The use of Structuration and Actor Network Theory for analysis: A case study of a financial institution in South Africa. *International Journal of Actor-Network Theory and Technological Innovation, 2*(1), 1–26. doi:10.4018/jantti.2010071601

Khorasani, E., Darab, M. G., Yarmohammadian, M., & Afshari, S. (2012). Knowledge based health system in the age of Knowledge Management. *Proceedings of the 3rd International Conference on Information Management and Evaluation.* Ankara, Turkey: Academic Press.

Lee, K. C., Lee, S., & Kang, I. W. (2005). KMPI: Measuring knowledge management performance. *Information & Management Journal, 42*(3), 469–482. doi:10.1016/j.im.2004.02.003

Lee, Y. C., & Lee, S. K. (2007). Capabilities, processes and performance of knowledge management: A structural approach. Research Articles. *Human Factors Ergonomics and Manufacturing Journal, 17*(1), 21–41. doi:10.1002/hfm.20065

Nyrhinen, M. (2006). *IT Infrastructure: Structure, properties and processes*. Helsinki School of Economics, Finland. Working paper, W-403. HSE Print.

O'Dell, C., & Grayson, C. J. (1998). If only we knew what we know: Identification and transfer of internal best practices. *California Management Review, 40*(3), 154–174. doi:10.2307/41165948

Omary, Z., Lupiana, D., Mtenzi, F. & Wu, B. (2009). *Challenges to E-Healthcare Adoption in Developing Countries: A Case Study of Tanzania*. Academic Press.

Rose, J. (1998). Evaluating the contribution of Structuration Theory to the Information Systems discipline, In *Proceedings of the 6th European Conference on Information Systems (ECIS)*, Aix-en-Provence, France.

Van Beveren, J. 2003. Does health care for knowledge management? *Journal of Knowledge Management, 7* (1), 90-95.

Weber, R. O. (2007). Knowledge Management in Call Centres. *Electronic Journal of Knowledge Management, 5*(3), 333–346.

Wickramasinghe, N., Gupta, J. N. D., & Sharma, S. K. (2005). *Creating Knowledge-Based Healthcare Organizations*. Idea Group Inc. doi:10.4018/978-1-59140-459-0

Yin, R. K. (2009). *Case Study Research, Design and Methods* (3rd ed.). Newbury Park, CA: Sage Publications.

Chapter 3
Non-Invasive Data Acquisition and Measurement in Bio-Medical Technology:
An Overview

H. G. Sandeep Patil
Manipal University, India

Ajit N. Babu
Saint Louis University, USA &Center for Advancement of Global Health, India

P. S. Ramkumar
Applied Cognition Systems Pvt Ltd, India

ABSTRACT

Non-invasive medical measurements have expanded into several types of diagnostic and monitoring activities in health care delivery. They are being used in handling a number of non-infectious diseases such as diabetes, asthma, hypertension, congestive heart failure, cardiac arrhythmia, etc., as well as infectious diseases such as cholera, malaria, etc.. Non-Invasive Medical Devices (NIMDs) are naturally preferred over invasive methods considering patient convenience, reduced patient risk, increased speed, and operational simplicity. However non-invasive methods are often perceived to be less accurate than their invasive counterparts. Over the last decade, technological advances and mathematical techniques have improved significantly, challenging this perception across the board. The chapter will discuss this important transformation in health care diagnostics and monitoring. The chapter will also provide further insight into some of the currently available non-invasive measurement products and explore how futuristic techniques and technology trends which have great potential to transform healthcare into a significantly different paradigm than the one we experience today.

DOI: 10.4018/978-1-4666-9446-0.ch003

INTRODUCTION

Non-invasive medical measurements have expanded into several types of diagnostic and monitoring activities in health care delivery. They are being used in handling a number of non-infectious diseases such as diabetes, asthma, hypertension, congestive heart failure, cardiac arrhythmia, etc., as well as infectious diseases such as cholera, malaria, etc.. Non-Invasive Medical Devices (NIMDs) are naturally preferred over invasive methods considering patient convenience, reduced patient risk, increased speed, and operational simplicity. Over the last decade, technological advances and mathematical techniques have improved greatly, challenging this perception across the board, from complex measurements such as a magnetic-resonance-imaging (MRI) or a simple arm-cuff based blood pressure recording. Adopting advances in electronic communication and computing, these important developments have been able to decouple the acquisition, processing, analysis, reporting and archival aspects of medical measurements, which were earlier all packed into a single box. This has enabled significant reduction of cost and enlarged the reach of medical care for early detection and prevention of diseases. This is particularly important since delay in detection and intervention can increase health care costs and worsen clinical outcomes.

Underlying the sensing, processing and presentation technologies is a notable adoption of advanced computing and communication methods which were simply not available on a large scale a decade ago. Owing to these developments, it has become possible to shift a large portion of processing that used analog hardware into equivalent software implementation of the same functionalities. This not only enables the system more environmentally stable, repeatable and flexible but also makes patient-end equipment affordable by containing only the technology to acquire sensory data and relay patient data to a remote processing center, which host software that can handle the processing, storage and distribution of data. At the remote processing center, data from thousands of patients can be processed together on common computing platforms, thereby reducing cost of the robust backend infrastructure, through aggregation of demand. Earlier, the medical equipment in use directly displayed results mandating physical proximity of the patient, doctor/nurse and the equipment to each other in order to measure and check the results. This is no longer required with the advent of the processing center, since the results can be transmitted to wherever the doctor/nurse/patient is available and presented to them on low cost computers and mobile phones. This is a major leap in enabling continuum of care from the hospital to the home of the patient, coupled with convenience and cost saving. This has allowed many patients to self-manage their own routine measurements and report automatically to the care taker. Over all the change seems to be in three major aspects – the shift from hardware implementations to their software equivalents, the shift from all-in-one boxed solutions to function-specific modularity, and shift from individual processing systems to aggregated computing. This chapter will discuss several innovative methods of bio-medical sensing, processing and presentation that may be used in transitioning from hospital to home based tele-diagnostics and monitoring. The chapter will also provide further insight into some of the currently available non-invasive measurement products and explore how futuristic techniques and technology trends which have great potential to transform healthcare into a significantly different paradigm than the one we experience today. But first, it is important to categorize various biomedical equipment based on the type of bio-medical parameters they are used to measure, some which are identified in Table 1.

Although an exhaustive coverage of all types of biomedical parameters and equipment is out the scope of this chapter, some of the highly used measures and equipment are discussed in detail in the further sections.

Table 1. Vital parameters, their sensory element and equipment used to measure them

Biomedical Parameter	Sensory Element	Typical Equipment
Blood Glucose	Infra spectrum	Glucometer
Blood Oxygen	Infra-Red spectrum	SPO2
Blood Pressure	pressure	NIBP
Respiration Rate	Bio-potentials	ECG
Heart Rate	bio-potentials / Pressure	ECG / NIBP
Arrhythmia	bio-potentials	ECG
Internal organ characteristics	XRAY	XRAY / MRI
Internal organ characteristics	Magneto-resonance	MRI
Internal organ characteristics	Ultrasonic spectrometry	US scanner/ US Doppler
Retina/Cornea/other eye parts	Photo image	Fundus camera
Skin resistance	Bio potentials	
Ear	Audio spectrum	Otoscope
Lung function	pressure	Spirometer
Heart function	Sound	Stethoscope
Hemoglobin	spectrum	
Bone density	XRAY	XRAY
Brain function	Bio-potentials	EEG
Brain Function	Magneto resonance	MRI
Internal Organ characteristics	Imaging	Virtual Endoscope

BACKGROUND

Non-invasive medical measurements have expanded into several types of diagnostic and monitoring activities in health care delivery. They are being used in handling a number of non-infectious diseases such as diabetes, asthma, hypertension, congestive heart failure, cardiac arrhythmia, etc., as well as infectious diseases such as cholera, malaria, etc. Non-Invasive Medical Devices (NIMDs) are naturally preferred over invasive methods considering patient convenience, reduced patient risk, increased speed, and operational simplicity. However non-invasive methods are often perceived to be less accurate than their invasive counterparts. Over the last decade, technological advances and mathematical techniques have improved significantly, challenging this perception across the board, from complex measurements such as a magnetic-resonance-imaging (MRI) or a simple arm-cuff based blood pressure recording. Adopting advances in electronic communication and computing, these significant developments have been able to decouple the acquisition, processing, analysis, reporting and archival aspects of medical measurements, which were earlier all packed into a single box. This has enabled significant reduction of cost and enlarged the reach of medical care for early detection and prevention of diseases. This is particularly important since delay in detection and intervention can increase health care costs and worsen clinical outcomes. It is also important to note that while people spend a relatively insignificant amount of their life-time in a hospital, hospitalization lands majority of the population in financial struggle throughout their life time. Disease incidence rate far outstrips the available supply in terms of hospitals, skilled doctors and nurses in most parts of the world, especially in the developing countries. Thanks to the innovations in the area of non-invasive detection, it is possible for adoption in much larger scale at much lesser cost and skill levels and induce a paradigm shift to move from hospital-based, curative care to home-based preventive care

NON INVASIVE MEASUREMENTS

Noninvasive Blood Glucose Measurement

Diabetes is one of the greatest worldwide health challenges of the twenty-first century, given that it is irreversible, it can affect all parts of the human body. There are over 340 million diabetic people and the age of incidence has also come down from 60+ to 40+ and the diabetic population is trending to double in the next couple of decades. Management of the disease mandates closely monitoring blood-glucose levels and maintaining blood glycaemic control through medicine, exercise and diet throughout a person's post-diabetic life span. Consistent monitoring remains a challenge in practice for many diabetic patients owing to its invasive methods of measurement, cost and external dependence to take measurements periodically. Conventional invasive methods of extracting a drop of blood by pricking their finger yields the highest accuracy, but invokes patient reluctance due to the associated physical pain and some patients fear infections due to repeated ruptures. In the recent years handheld, battery operated glucometers costing about $100 have been developed to be operated by patients themselves, although they are less accurate than their laboratory counterparts, as it may suffice to detect if there is a significant deviation needing detail investigation and doctor consultation. However, these devices also involve pricking and employ a use-and-throw glucose measuring strip (typically 1$ per strip) that may add significant cost over person's diabetic life span. At a global level, this translates to a cost of about $1Billion annually on the glucose strip alone, even if patients are to be checked 3 times per year. Hence the dire need for an alternate affordable non-invasive measurement technology.

Non-invasive techniques for diabetes have been of great interest and have been the most sorted topic for research because of the emergence of diabetes as a major epidemic. NI determination of glucose will promote more frequent testing, allows tighter control of diabetes, and delays the onset of diabetes complications and their associated health care costs.

Among non-invasive detection techniques, optical methods have received considerable attention given the fact that glucose displays significant absorption in Mid-infrared radio spectrum. Several methods have been explored to measure blood glucose reliably and accurately amid of noise and artefacts due to other elements in and around blood. These methods have faced limitations in achievable wavelength and safe intensity of laser, poor penetration of light, smudging of information due to scattering in the subject media, and some devices even lead to causing skin irritations.

Non-invasive blood glucose (BG) monitoring has been important factor in the healthcare paradigm, given the enormous demand in both numbers and the positive impact it would bring to diabetics.

Table 2 gives an insight to various commercially available devices for measuring blood glucose.

Figure 1. The various methods of NI glucose measurement

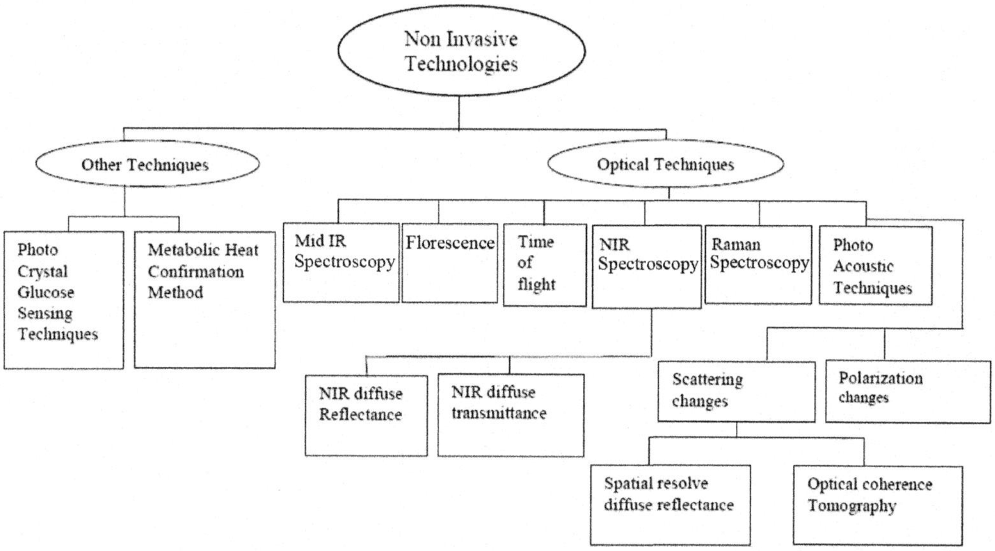

Non Invasive Technologies
Other Techniques
Optical Techniques
Photo Crystal Glucose Sensing Techniques
Metabolic Heat Confirmation Method
Mid IR Spectroscopy
Florescence
Time of flight
NIR Spectroscopy
Raman Spectroscopy
Photo Acoustic Techniques
NIR diffuse Reflectance
NIR diffuse transmittance
Scattering changes
Polarization changes
Spatial resolve diffuse reflectance
Optical coherence Tomography

Table 2. List of commercially available glucose monitoring devices

Device	Approvals	Technology
GlucoWatch by Cygnus Inc.	FDA -2001-2002	Iontophoresis
Diasensor1 by BICO Inc.	CE Mark in 2000	Near infrared spectroscopy
Pendra by Pendragon Medical Ltd.	CE Mark in 2003	Impedance spectroscopy
Aprise by Glucon Medical Ltd.	In Progress	Ultrasound technology/ photoacoustic spectroscopy
Glucoband by Calisto Medical Inc.	In Progress	Impedance spectroscopy
GlucoTrack by Integrity Applications Ltd.	FDA	Ultrasound technology
OrSense Ltd.	NONE	Near infrared spectroscopy
SpectRx Inc.	Not approved yet	Fluid harvesting
SugarTrac by LifeTrac Systems Inc.	Not Yet	Near infrared spectroscopy
Symphony by Sontra Medical Corp.	No information	Fluid harvesting
Dream Beam by Futrex Medical Instrumentation Inc	Not approved	Near infrared spectroscopy
GluCall by KMH Co. Ltd.	No information	Iontophoresis
GluControl GC3001 by ArithMed GmbH	No recent information found	Near infrared spectroscopy
Hitachi Ltd.	In progress	Thermal spectroscopy
Sysmex Corporation	No information	probably iontophoresis
TouchTrak Pro 200 by Samsung Fine Chemicals Co. Ltd.	No information	NIR spectroscopy

Table 3. Non invasive devices

Device	Company	Technology	Approval
Pronto-7	Masimo	Pulse Oximeter	FDA
Glasswing	Orsense	Occlusion Spectroscopy	FDA
ToucHb	Biosense	Pulse Oximeter	NA

Courtesy: www.masimo.com, www.orsense.com, www.biosense.in

Non Invasive Determination of Anemia

Anemia is a condition in which number of red blood cells or their oxygen carrying capacity is insufficient to meet the physiological needs which vary by age, sex, altitude, smoking and pregnancy. Deficiency in iron thought to be the main cause of anemia around the world. Anemia continues to be one of the most serious problem in the world. It is estimated that nearly 1.6 billion people suffer from Iron Deficiency worldwide. The main victims of anemia are pregnant women and children especially in the developing countries. Effective screening of IDA both in children and pregnant women has not been successful especially in the developing countries due to various methods used for the screening. Generally, medical and nutritional practitioners assume that both hemoglobin and hematocrit are equally useful in detecting anemia and that they can be used interchangeably for anemia screening. Currently, most commonly used method for hemoglobin concentration measurement is by collecting venous blood from a finger prick and transferring it to a disposable cuvette which is then placed in a suitable analyzer and the hemoglobin is measured spectrophotometrically. Attempts to develop more accurate, easier-to-use, and sustainable hemoglobin detection technologies have been under way for many years. Noninvasive technologies have been of special interest, and with recent advances in technology and expertise and continued concern about the risks of blood-borne diseases, there have been renewed efforts among researchers and manufacturers to develop such technologies (Table 3).

Blood Oxygen (Oxygen Saturation)

The concentration of oxygen in the blood is measured in as SpO2 (Peripheral capillary oxygen saturation). It is the measurement of percentage of hemoglobin binding sites in the bloodstream occupied by oxygen. Normal blood oxygen levels in humans is 95 – 100 percent. Less than 90 percent is considered to be hypoxemia and below 80 percent would result in organ failure.

The most common way measuring oxygen saturation is pulse oximetry which is a non-invasive technique. The percentage of blood that is loaded with oxygen is displayed on the monitor of the pulse oximeter. This is based on red (600-750 nm) and infrared light (850-1000 nm) absorption characteristics of oxygenated and deoxygenated hemoglobin. Absorption of infrared light is more in oxygenated hemoglobin and it allows red light to pass through. Conversely deoxygenated hemoglobin absorbs red light and infrared light to pass through.

Pulse oximeters have wide range of applications as individual oxygen saturation readings where hypoxia may be a factor especially in elderly person. It is used as replacement for blood gas analysis in many clinical situations. Pulse oximeters are now used routinely in critical care, anesthesiology, and A&E departments, and are often found in ambulances. A brief survey on the available pulse oximeters is shown in Table 4.

Blood Pressure

Blood pressure or the arterial blood pressure has been one of the principal vital signs, which is the pressure exerted by circulating blood upon the walls of blood vessels. It is measured as systolic pressure or the diastolic (mm Hg). Table 5 gives the classification of blood pressure for adults.

Sphygmomanometer is the device used to measure arterial pressureColumn of mercury is used to measure the circulating pressure. The noninvasive and oscillometric measurements are simpler and quicker than invasive measurements, require less expertise in fitting, have virtually no complications, and are less unpleasant and painful for the patient. However low accuracy has been a matter of concern.

The oscillometric technique is a blood pressure monitoring method where pulse waves (caused by arterial pulsation) and not sounds are detected. Oscillometric methods are used for long term measurement. It uses an electronic pressure sensor (transducer) fitted in to detect blood flow. In practice, the pressure sensor is a calibrated electronic device with a numerical readout of blood pressure. NIBP or non-invasive blood pressure monitoring is normally used to describe oscillometric method.

Arrhythmia

A problem in rate or rhythm of the heartbeat is called arrhythmia. An anomaly in the heart rate can be considered in two scenarios, either the heart beating too fast known as tachycardia or heart beating too slow known as bradycardia. During arrhythmia heart may not be able to supply or pump enough blood to organs which in turn may lead to serious complication.

Relating human heart to an electrical system, each heart beat is an electrical signal which traverses across the heart. The contraction and pumping of blood is due to this movement of electrical signal in the heart. The origin of the signal is in sinoatrial node (SA), located in the upper right chamber which is also called as right atrium. The movement of the signal to atria lead in contraction and pumping of the blood to lower chambers (ventricles). The signal from atria ventricular node travels to bundle of His

Table 4. Commercially available pulse oximeters

Oximeter	Manufacturer	Operating Temp	Display Screen
Drive PulseOx	SPO Medical	39° to 107° F	Liquid Crystal
DigiO2 Finger Pulse Oximeter	Graham-Field	41° to 104° F	Color LED
Digit Finger Pulse Oximeter	Smiths-Medical	32° to 131° F	Red LED
Digit-Ox II Pulse Oximeter	Probasics	N/A	Color LED
9500 Onyx Pulse Oximeter	Nonin	32° to 104° F	Red LED
CMS-50D Fingertip Pulse Oximeter	Contec Medical	50° to 104° F	Color LED
Go-2 Achieve Fingertip Pulse Oximeter	Nonin	41° to 104° F	Liquid Crystal

Courtesy: http://justoximeters.com/

Table 5. Disorders due to varied blood pressure as seen in systolic and diastolic modes

Category	Systolic, mm Hg	Diastolic, mm Hg
Hypotension	Less than 90	< 60
Desired	90–119	60–79
Prehypertension	120–139	80–89
Stage 1 hypertension	140–159	90–99
Stage 2 hypertension	160–179	100–109
Hypertensive emergency	Above 180	≥ 110

Figure 2. Digital BP meter
Courtesy: http://ae.hartmann.info/883.php

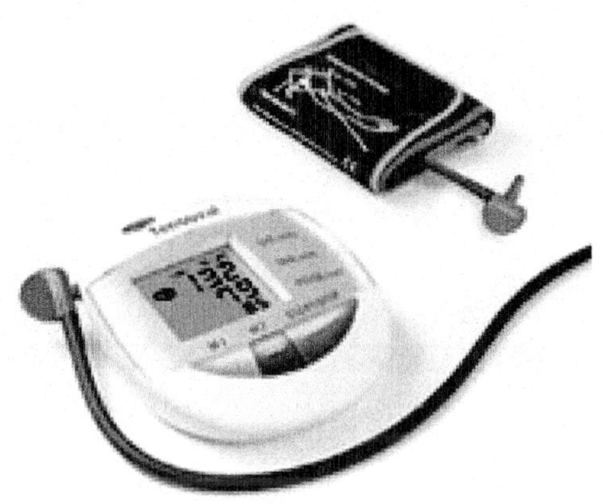

Table 6. Commercially available BP meters

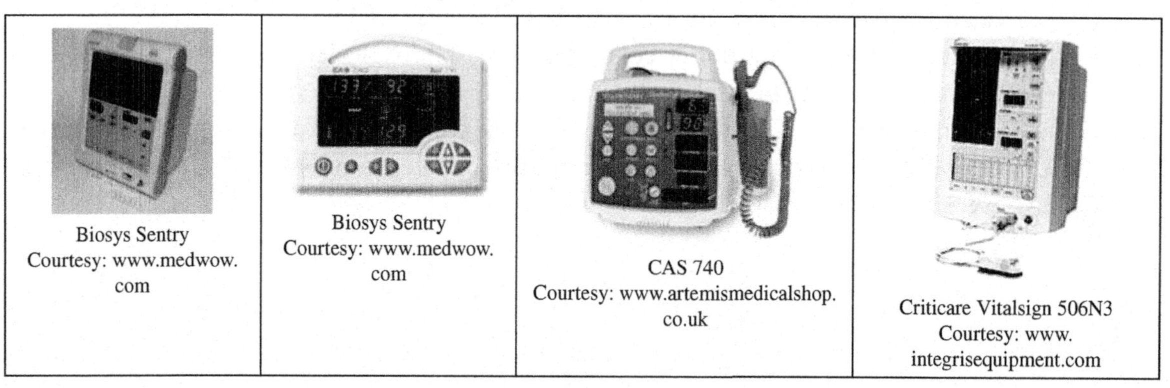

Biosys Sentry Courtesy: www.medwow.com	Biosys Sentry Courtesy: www.medwow.com	CAS 740 Courtesy: www.artemismedicalshop.co.uk	Criticare Vitalsign 506N3 Courtesy: www.integrisequipment.com

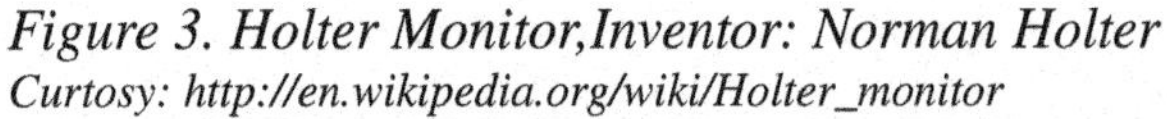

Figure 3. Holter Monitor,Inventor: Norman Holter
Curtosy: http://en.wikipedia.org/wiki/Holter_monitor

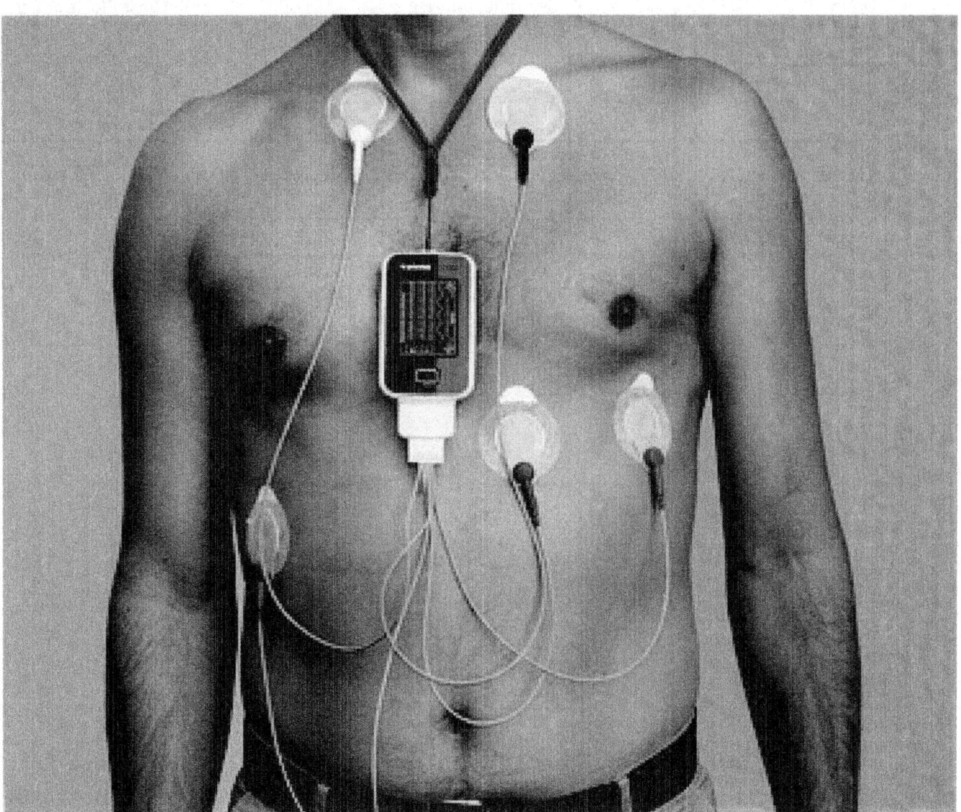

which divides into left and right bundles. The signal then moves to ventricles through these branches leading to contraction and pumping the blood to lungs and other parts of the body. Any anomaly in the entire process would lead to arrhythmia.

Various methods and devices have been adopted to diagnose and report arrhythmia in real time.

- **Electrocardiogram (EKG/ECG):** This device uses electrodes connected to chest and the recording is done to produce graphical representation of heart rhythms. Normally 10 electrodes are used.
- **Echocardiogram:** A graphical representation of electrical impulses of the heart which are in the form of videotaped images. They are also called as cardiac ultrasounds.
- **Holter Monitoring:** A portable device connected to chest through electrodes. Five adhesive electrodes are connected and heart rhythms are recorded (Figure 3).
- **Event Recorder:** It's a portable device used for people who do not experience arrhythmia often. The device also called as loop recorder as it loops two minutes record to memory which are continually overwritten (Figure 4).

Figure 4. Cardiac Event recorder
Courtesy: ALBA medical

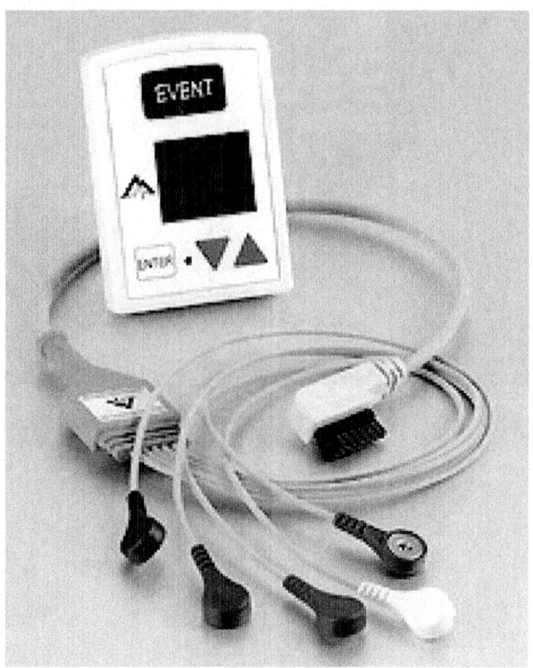

Internal Organ Characteristics

Ultrasound Scan

Sound wave with frequency above the hearing range i.e. above 20kHz is called ultrasound. One of the prime application of ultrasound is in medical imaging. Ultrasound images are constructed by sending ultrasound pulses to tissues and organs by a transducer. The reflection or echoes of the sound are recorded and displayed as images.

Ultrasonography or medical sonography is a medical imaging technique used to visualize internal organs. Radiologists and sonographers have been using this as a diagnostic tool to image the human body. Ultrasound technique is relatively inexpensive and portable when compared magnetic resonance imaging (MRI) and computed tomography.

Figure 5. Frequency bands indicating types of spectrum

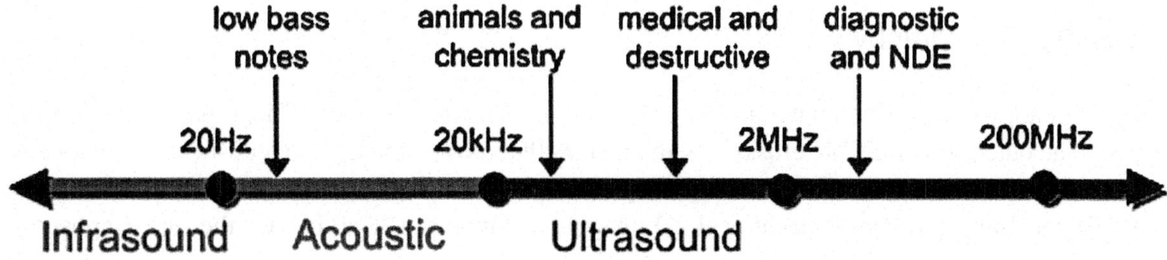

Figure 6. Typical Ultrasound images

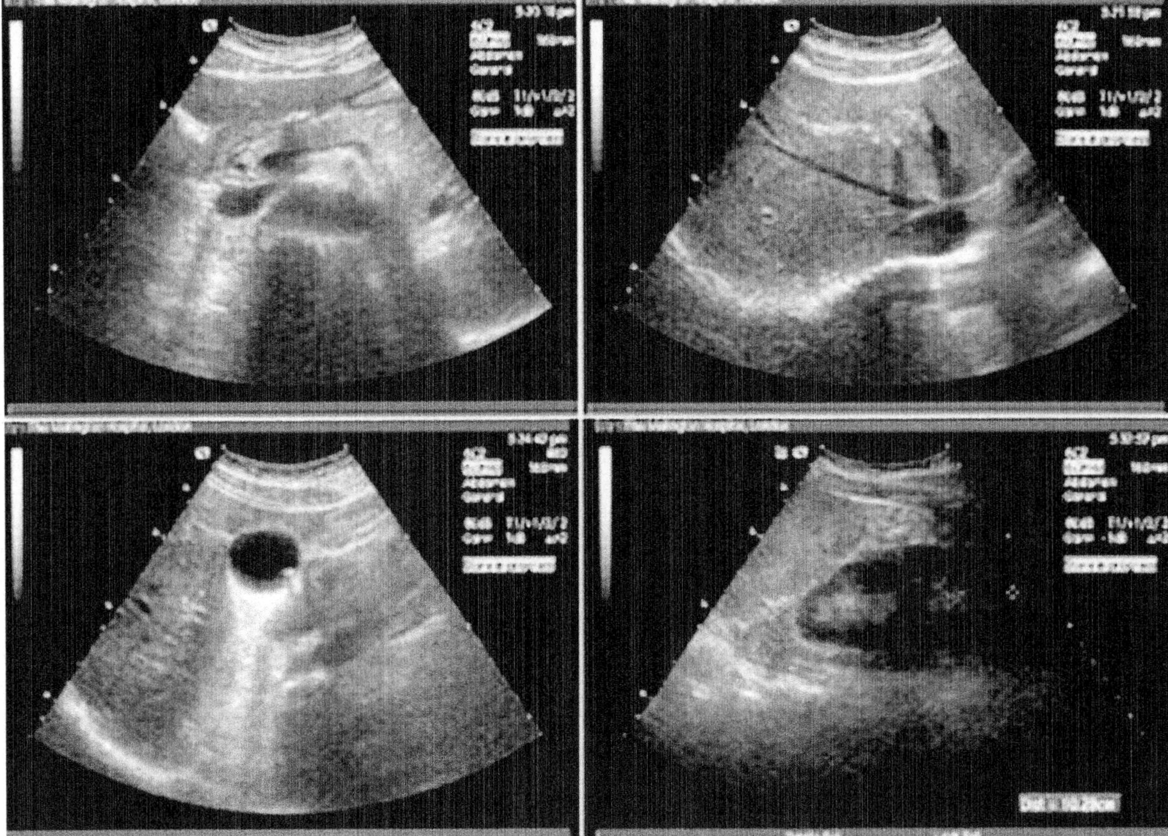

AN ULTRASOUND OF AN ABDOMEN

One of the key advantages of the ultrasound scanners is that its paradigm shift in moving from typical wired clinical settings to hand held devices to wireless ultrasounds. This shift will enable access to public at large especially in the developing world. The biggest advancement in ultrasound world is real time imaging of the internal anatomy of the human body, volume rendering and real time 3D view of the images. There has been lot of efforts in fusion technologies also, for example, synchronization of ultrasound images with magnetic resonance imaging (MRI) and computed tomography (CT) images to detect lesions which are hard to find otherwise. These advancement in ultrasound technology has made it more attractive to clinical application, thanks to noninvasiveness, affordability and lack of radiation. Figures 7 and 8 show a typical portable clinical ultrasound and a hand held mobile ultrasound respectively.

Computed Tomography

It's a technology that uses computer processed Xrays as source and produce tomographic images of the organs. The outcomes of CT are cross sectional images that are used in both diagnostic and therapeutic issues in medicine. Volume of data rendered by CT is based on the organs ability to block the x-ray beam. When compared with conventional 2D imaging techniques, CT eliminates the superimposition

Figure 7. Ultrasound
Courtesy: www.medwow.com

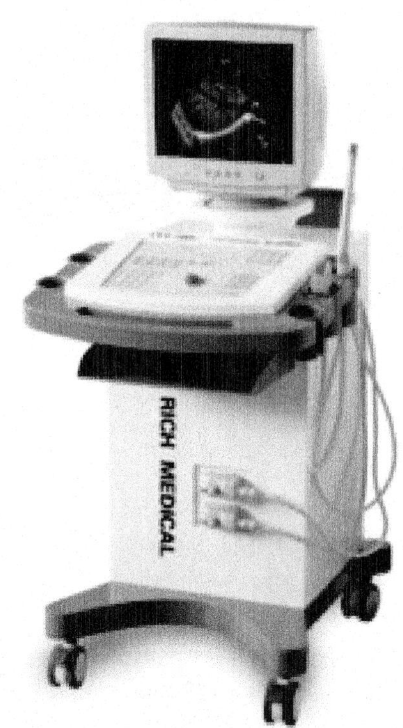

Figure 8. Handheld Ultrasound
Courtesy: www.ohgizmo.com

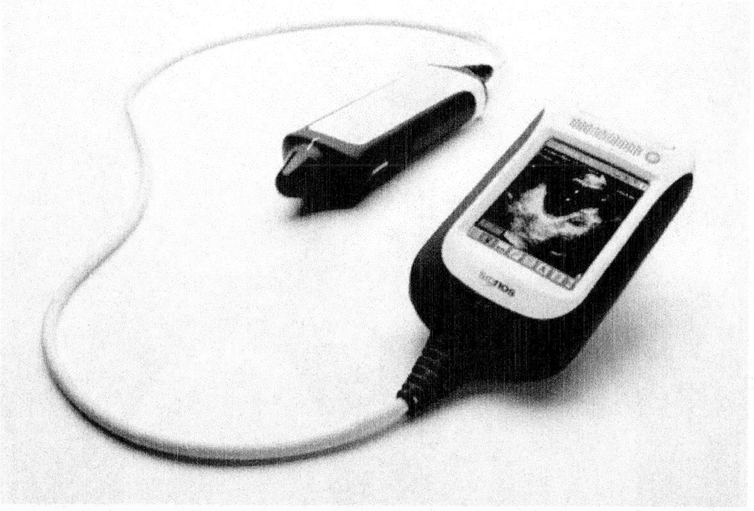

Figure 9. Computed Tomography
Courtesy: www.ecomagination.com

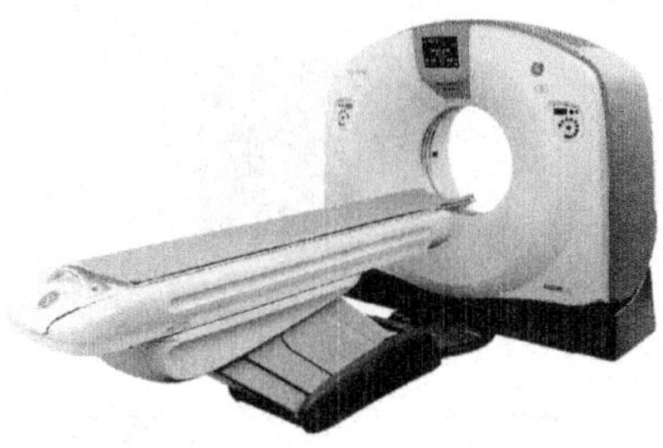

Figure 10. CT images
Courtesy: www.ecomagination.com

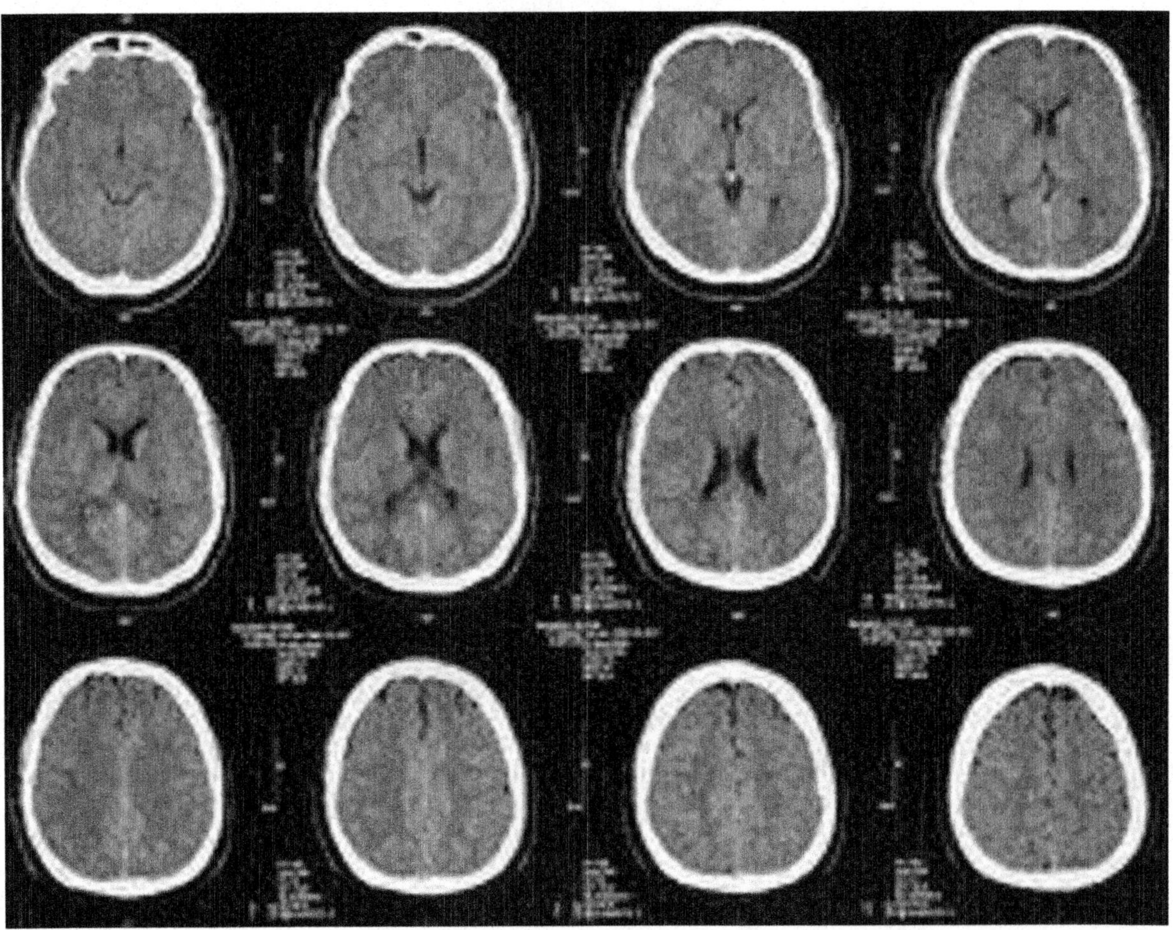

of images outside the region of interest. Due to its high contrast, tissues differing in physical density by less than 1% can be distinguished. However exposure to radiation in CT is more when compared to other techniques and has been a matter of concern from the initial days though there has been tremendous growth in the usage of the same in clinical settings.

Though images produced by CT are faithful, they are prone to following kinds of artifacts.

- **Noise:** Due to low signal to noise ratio, a grain on the image. This is usually seen during slice thickness.
- **Motion Artifacts:** Due to the movement of image being scanned, blurriness in the image. Its overcome by a technique called incompressible flow tomography.
- **Ring Artifact:** Due to defaults in detectors or miss-calibration of detectors, a ring is formed on the images.

Virtual Endoscopy

It's a technique where in hollow structures of the human body are viewed in three dimensions using high resolution imaging techniques and processing methods. This has happened due to advancement in processing helical tomographic data sets. These methods are non-invasive and have minimum patient preparation and reluctance. Virtual endoscopy is done to examine and evaluate the colon, bronchi, stomach, blood vessels, bladder, kidney, larynx, and paranasal sinuses. The important contribution of virtual endoscopy has been in screening cancer. The three dimensional virtual endoscopy assists the clinicians in determination of surgical approach.

Basically the data obtained from helical CT scanning has enabled virtual endoscopy and volume rendering. At the data processing side, there are two ways, volume and surface rendering which gives out the contours of the objects. At a clinical setting, virtual endoscopy will enhance preoperative planning and postoperative follow up even outside the clinical settings. A substantial research is being done in coming up with quicker and affordable methods of evaluation.

Fundus Camera

This technology is used by the optometrists, ophthalmologists and trained medical professionals to capture the images of inner parts of the eye (retina, optic disc, macula and posterior pole or fundus). This device is used for monitoring progression of the disease, diagnosis of the disease or screening programs and epidemiology. A notable advantage of the fundus photography is storage of the image for the future reference though the device has disadvantage of being heavier than the ophthalmoscope. Fundus camera is constructed on the principle, monocular indirect ophthalmoscopy giving a magnified view of the fundus. It has a zoom or auxiliary lenses from 15°, which provides 5x magnification, to 140° with a wide angle lens, which minifies the image by half (Figure 11).

There has been substantial advancement in automation the fundus camera's, enabling functionalities such as, auto focus, auto align and giving flexibility in data management. The instruments are network enabled (LAN), EMR integrated and integrated peripherals such as USB, Ethernet etc. In the recent advancements, at the patient side, the intensity of the flash has been lowered, blink detectors have been installed. Having been able to share the images in real time, clinicians can use to discuss the disease

Figure 11. Fundus Camera
Courtesy: http://en.wikipedia.org/wiki/Fundus_photography

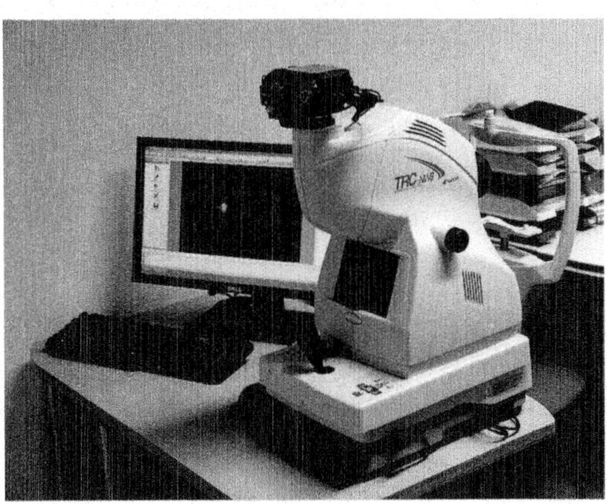

progress with the patients. There is also great potential for advancements in telemedicine using fundus photography.

Otoscope

An otoscope is a device used to view the ear canal and tympanic membrane and investigate the ear symptoms. Basically the device consists of a hand and a head. The head contains a light source and a detachable magnifying lens. The distal end of the otoscope has an attachment for disposable plastic ear specula. Commonly otoscope is used to detect otitis media and otitis externa, infection of the middle and outer parts of the ear, respectively (Figure 12).

Given the limitations in measurement of middle ear disorders due to their spatial insensitiveness, there is a scope for further advancements by integrating fiber optics and digital processing.

Electroencephalography (EEG)

This is used to record the electrical activity of the brain along the scalp. Voltage fluctuations happening in the brain due to current flowing within the neurons are recorded using EEG. Multiple electrodes are

Figure 12. Otoscope

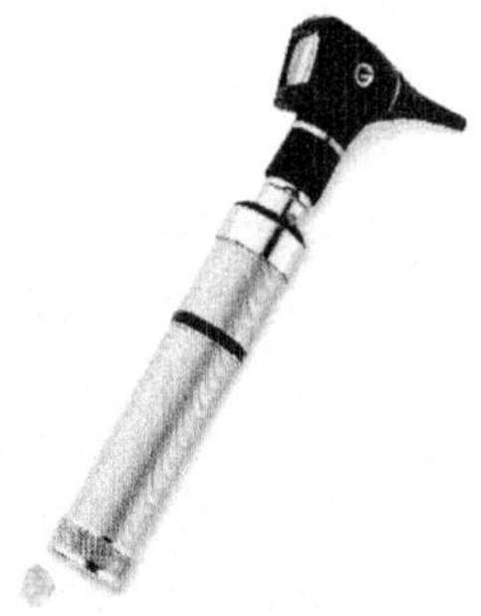

Figure 13. Placement of electrodes

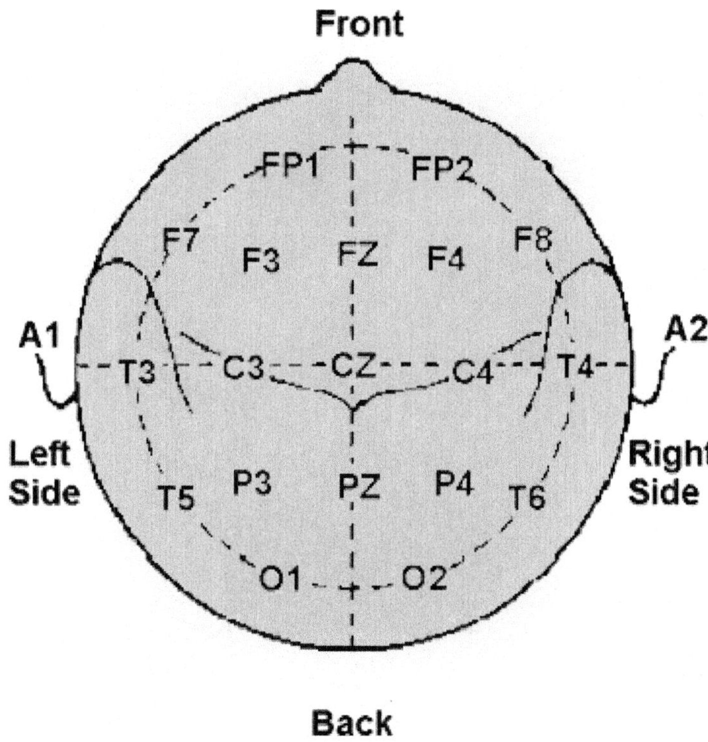

placed on the scalp mainly to diagnose the type of oscillations caused in the brain signals. EEG is used to diagnose epilepsy, sleep disorders, coma, encephalopathies, and brain death. It is also used to diagnose tumors, stroke and other focal brain disorders. Though with the advent of advanced technologies like MRI and CT the usage of EEG still remains to be valuable tool when there is a requirement of minute temporal resolutions. The application of EEG is mainly seen in cognitive science, cognitive psychology and psychophysiological research.

Scientists have been successful in coming up with a new concept called source localization, which enables to find out which part of the brain is communicating. Recent advancements in neuroscience with technical advancements in imaging have been able to specifically identify what part of the brain is performing which activity. Researchers have gone one step ahead in coming up with portable EEG which is affordable, accurate and does not need a human score.

Observation

Non-invasive diagnostic modalities have enormous potential to bring health care to the patient, and promote ongoing monitoring of their condition, which is particularly relevant in critical illness, or chronic diseases like diabetes where the underlying health condition may remain under treatment for extended periods of time. Advances in technology and reduction in costs have fostered increasing adoption and evolution of such technologies around the world. One can witness a dramatic change in the approach to biomedical instrumentation in the past decade, embracing advancements in digital signal and image processing, semiconductor technology, software engineering, telecom and internet infrastructure, etc.,

Figure 14. Advanced EEG device (headset)
Courtesy: www.kickstarter.com

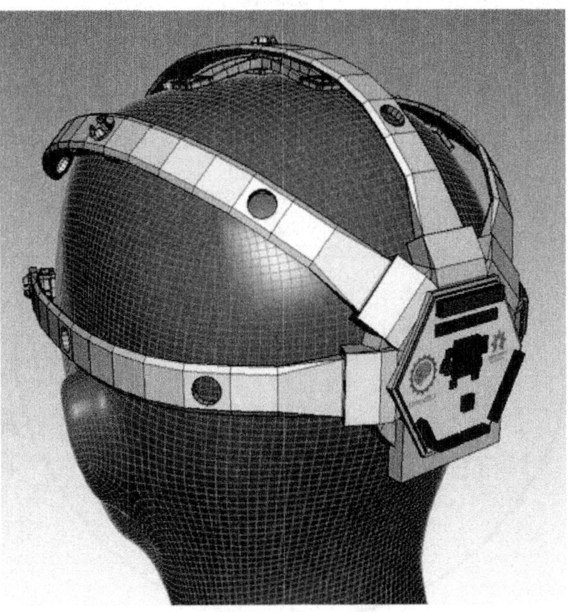

However, one can also sight that the advancement of biomedical equipment industry in adopting these technologies has been far behind in its pace compared to other domain such as banking, financial markets, entertainment, etc. Part of this reason is probably the risk associated in health care intervention, and hence the long, stringent process of clinical trials and certification that has to be achieved before releasing new innovations as products into the market. By transiting away from invasive, painful or inconvenient interventions in diagnostic measurements a significant jump in acceptability and willingness to participate in tests is observed in patients. However, in spite of devices becoming smaller, smarter, simpler and cheaper at the point of care, the primary consumers of devices penetration of devices are still predominantly in hospitals and not in clinics and homes. One of the reasons for this is perhaps the patient's psychology - more confidence in a doctor than themselves and the lack of priority for preventive care that can be practiced outside hospitals, in daily life(such as diet, exercise, work-life balance, etc.,). The directions of the impending paradigm shift that the non-invasive diagnostic technology can bring in the next decade seems to be in extending care from hospital to clinics and home, from palliative, curative to preventive, from cities to remote rural areas, from disease management to lifestyle management, extending care from the ill to the not yet born.

CONCLUSION

The chapter has dealt with various noninvasive techniques available as monitoring and diagnosis equipment's in healthcare. Non-invasive diagnostic modalities have enormous potential to bring health care to the patient, and promote ongoing monitoring of their condition, which is particularly relevant in critical illness, or chronic diseases like diabetes where the underlying health condition may remain under treatment for extended periods of time. Advances in technology and reduction in costs have fostered increasing adoption and evolution of such technologies around the world. The study has also showcased the advancements so far and the scope for further research in the noninvasive technologies to enable future enhancements in care.

REFERENCES

Barker & Badal. (2008). *Measurement of Dyshemoglobin and total Hemoglobin by pulse oximetry.* Wolters Kluwer Health | Lippincott Williams & Wilkins.

Brecht, Prough, Petrov, Petrova, Deyo, & Esenaliev. (2004). Accurate, Noninvasive measurement of total hemoglobin concentration with optoacoustic technique. In *Proceedings of the 26th Annual International Conference of the IEEE EMBS.* San Francisco, CA: IEEE.

Doshi, & Panditrao. (n.d.). Optical Sensor System for Hemoglobin Measurement. *International Journal of Computational Engineering Research, 3.*

Harder, & Boshkov. (n.d.). *The optimal Hematocrit.* Department of Pulmonary and Critical Care Medicine, Oregon Health and Sciences University.

Kaur, Kumar, Sardana, Bhatnagar, & Mehla. (n.d.). *Non Invasive Blood Glucose Measurement Using Optical Method: Feasibility Study And Design Issues.* Central Scientific Instruments Organization, Chandigarh (A Lab. of Council of Scientific and Industrial Research, New Delhi).

Ozaki. (n.d.). *Near-Infrared Spectroscopy—Its Versatility in Analytical Chemistry.* Department of Chemistry, School of Science and Technology, Kwansei Gakuin University.

Robinson, Eaton, Haaland, Koepp, Thomas, Stallard, & Robinson. (n.d.). *Noninvasive Glucose Monitoring in Diabetic Patients: A Preliminary Evaluation.* Academic Press.

Shinde. (n.d.). Non Invasive Blood Glucose Measurement using NIR technique based on occlusion spectroscopy. *International Journal of Engineering Science and Technology.*

KEY TERMS AND DEFINITIONS

Aggregated Computing: A comprehensive processing of all the functionalities as all in one module.

Aggregation of Demand: Total demand for a product and its services at a given economy and time.

Biomedical Sensing: Capturing the Information of vital parameters of the human body through sensors.

Continuum of Care: A concept involving in integrated system of care that guides and tracks the patient over the time.

Glyceamic Control: Typical level of blood sugar in a person having diabetes mellitus.

Non Invasive Medical Devices: Devices which operate without any contact to the mucosa or skin or internal body cavity.

Spectrophotometric: A method of measuring the intensity of light in a part of the spectrum.

Chapter 4
Healthcare Services for Nomadics through a Mobile Framework

Suama Hamunyela
Namibia University of Science and Technology, Namibia

Tiko Iyamu
Cape Peninsula University of Technology, South Africa

ABSTRACT

Many patients are often associated with various types of health related records, needing care and attentions. Healthcare system is intended for all that live in the country. Normally, there is spread of people across the geographical locations, of both the rural and urban communities. Even though the healthcare service is intended to spread across the country, the services are not always available as individuals require it. Hence, there is need for Mobility of healthcare services at both primary and secondary healthcare levels, particularly in the developing countries such as Namibia. In Namibia, the population is scantly spread far apart in the average of about 175 kilometres between major towns, necessitating movements of individuals and groups, particularly the old, poor, and nomadic people. The challenge is, healthcare records in the country are not centralised or virtualised, making accessibility into patients' records difficult or impossible. As a result, healthcare service delivering is challenged. This chapter explored the possibility healthcare services through virtualisation or centralisation as empowered by different translation of activities. The objectives of the study were to identify and discuss actors in the mobility of healthcare services. Mobility in this paper refers to the availability of services to the nomadic patients. The study employed the qualitative approach, within which data was gathered from primary healthcare services providers using open-ended questionnaires. The moments of Translation from the perspective of ANT was used a lens to analyse the data to examine and understand the power and factors which could influences mobility of healthcare service in Namibia.

DOI: 10.4018/978-1-4666-9446-0.ch004

1. INTRODUCTION

The Ministry of Health and Social Services (MoHSS) in Namibia is the leading organisation in Namibia when it comes to healthcare provision. It is mandated to provide an integrated, affordable, accessible, quality health and social welfare services, which is responsive to the needs of the Namibian population(MoHSS,2012) at healthcare facilities located at different levels of operandi (Hamunyela &Iyamu, 2013) of the health sector. Processes and activities at the MoHSS, are performed either on paper-based technology or HIS. This can be a huge setback for the services which the MoHSS provides to the communities in the country such as distribution of the HIV treatment and immunisation against contiguous decease's outbreaks. Worse, the manual approach significantly delays centralisation of processes and activities (Hamunyela & Iyamu, 2013). This indeed is dangerous to patient needs, particularly those who are of intensive and chronic nature and nomadic patients.

In addition, there is mobility of individuals and groups within a country. Hence, there is need for the inclination of centralizing healthcare services at both primary and secondary healthcare levels in developing and developed countries. In Namibia, the geographical spread of the population, the widely held image of the healthiness of people in rural area, different groups with needs for healthcare (the old, the poor, nomadic people est.) necessitates the mobility of healthcare services.

The movement and spread of the population in developing countries can impact healthcare service provision (Hjortdahl, 2007). To ensure effective healthcare services provision, states and healthcare organisations are engaged in transforming the industry. According to Sander Granlien and Hertzum (2012), to improve the quality and efficiency of healthcare many hospitals are involved in extensive efforts to substitute electronic patient records for paper records. Another effort that has been made by some organisations is the integration of health information systems to improve quality of healthcare service.

Also, the shift from curative to planning and preventing of disease outbreaks and control has significantly necessitated the need for Healthcare data management, efficient service delivery, healthcare information flows between health practitioners and patients, as well as information sharing between healthcare levels of operandi (Chaulagai, 2005). The mission of curative, preventing and disease control can only be made possible if the information of the whole population based is made available to policy makers, healthcare profession, administrators, donors and all healthcare organisations.

However, different categories of patients exist in the healthcare sector and the needs for healthcare services are diverse. There is the nomadic patient. This inflates the need to investigate different dimensions of healthcare service provisions processes in a country (HIS module 11). In Chang's (2011) argument, there is a scenario where the patient may visit a different healthcare organisation, either because the patient is dissatisfied with the treatment of his or her previous visit or the patient moves to a different location. Distinctively in this case is the mobility of healthcare services in Namibia.

Mobility in this paper refers to the state of easy accessibility of health services from any geographical location. The essentiality of mobility of healthcare is centred on factors such as portability, transferability and availability of healthcare information including real-time interaction between healthcare providers and the needing (Fardoun and Oadah, 2012). In healthcare, mobility is typically associated with mobile healthcare systems and applications, the use of health public kiosk, cellular phone devices, and other portable computing devices (Cisco, 2007), this paper argues that mobility can also be classified by the availability of healthcare services at different levels of healthcare operandi.

Mobility of healthcare services could be translated by various human actors (patients and healthcare workers), based on the different moments. Translation is a key tenet of actor network theory (Latour,

1991). In actor network theory (ANT), translation is influenced by interest of the actors (Iyamu, 2013). Translation takes place between the object and the actors it encounters as the initial program or script is altered through interaction.

ANT is popular for its ability to provide a rich and dynamic way of bringing together the socio technical and non-technical aspects of the organization (Wickramasinghe et al, 2011). In ANT, society and organisations are a formation of different agents, and the agents interact to form heterogeneous networks (Law, 1999; Tatnall & Gilding, 1999; Cresswell et al., 2010). Networks define, describe and provide substance to agents. ANT then, deeply question and provide retorts to the existence of strong and weak (thus power) networks.

The Namibian healthcare levels of operandi cover both rural and urban areas following the thirteen political and administrative regional demarcations of the country. As a developing country, majority of Namibians still resides in rural areas.

2. HEALTHCARE SERVICE

The healthcare sector in many countries consists of a large contingence of institutions and organisations, ranging from centres, small and medium to large and technologically advanced hospitals (Braa et al., 2007). The institutions are classified differently in many countries. In Namibia for example, the healthcare centres are classified according to geographical areas, namely, community (constituency) and district level, regional level and national level (Hamunyela & Iyamu, 2013). The levels of categories cover both rural and urban geographical locations. As in many developing countries, in Namibia, 58% of the population resides in rural areas while the remaining percentage resides in urban areas (NPC, 2012).

Due to the essentiality of healthcare, different studies have been conducted in pursuit to establish and describe health services to different healthcare seekers. Rygh and Hjortdahl (2007) drew their attention to Mobile health as an innovative to providing healthcare services to patients who reside in remote locations. The later stated that locality influences healthcare service delivery, therefore Mobile healthcare services are essential. This is affirmed by Faudoun and Oadah (2012) stating that, Mobile health greatly benefits patients who reside in remote areas.

Due to the geographical spread of citizens, Mobile healthcare is highly essential, however, challenges does exist. According to Rygh and Hjortdahls (2007), healthcare providers in rural areas face numerous challenges in providing coherent and integrated services as compared to those in urban areas, which results from lack of mobile healthcare facilities. Also, the approaches that are often used by primary healthcare service providers in the rural areas are primitive and obsolete (MoHSS, 2007). This also could be attributed to the fact the recipients of the services do question or protest the act by the service providers.

Mobility as emphasised by Faudoun and Oadah (2012) is that of mobile technologies in healthcare service, which is typically associated with the availability of healthcare services at different places, and same time; different places, and different times; and same time, and same place. Also electronic records via mobile health device are shared among healthcare providers across systems. It is assumed that, with the mobile health technologies, healthcare problems such as inadequacy of doctors and poor clinical examination as a result of insufficient skilled workers and scarcity of centre are eradicated (Narang, 2011). Since available healthcare providers can now remotely interact with patients and conduct analysis remotely.

M-health offers a variety of benefits to healthcare organisation, providers and patients. Most commonly discussed benefits of mobile health services are (Istepanian et al., 2004):

1. Timely access to patient record and or history from any given location.
2. **Diagnosing and Monitoring Patients Remotely:** Mobile health tools supported by different network platforms allows people from different locations to interact. For example, healthcare providers can monitor patient's health status. Via mobile technology diagnosis can be done.
3. **Improves Quality of Patient Care:** Patients can arrange appointment on the internet services or request for medical consultation via mobile device or more advanced, patients can be informed about their conditions and are psychologically closer to their doctors.
4. Increased empowerment and management of medical expertise especially in rural and under-served areas.

The need for accessibility and quality of health information particularly in developing countries such as Namibia necessitates refection and attention. Thus, there is need for investigation on the Mobility of services to improve delivering of healthcare. It has been empirically unveiled, it is important to have healthcare services at the communities' disposal, and at any location, as opposed to the difficulty of accessibility due distances. The investigation to ensure achieving this objective was carried through a study. The methodology that was applied in the study is explained next.

3. METHODOLOGY

A qualitative interpretive methodology was employed, using the three healthcare levels (national, district and community) of operandi in the country, Namibia. The methodology was adopted to explore and understand mobility of healthcare services at rural and urban areas and for the creation of healthcare knowledge in Namibia.

Questionnaires and interviews were used in this case to explore the formation and development of networks and examine the alliances built as the development progress. Up on completion of the questionnaire, follow up telephonic interviews were done to establish deeper understanding of the formation of networks and build of alliances. The two techniques are well established forms of data collection in social science studies. The following are identified actants in the mobility healthcare services:

We consider the MoHSS management, healthcare givers, patients, medical paper technology (heath passport) and medical ICT tools as actants in the mobility of healthcare services study. The most important point in the providing healthcare services is that, people (in this case patient) receive the most needed health service anywhere without being subjected to locations.

The research questions were: How do you (or your organisation) attend to patients who frequently travel from one place to another, in terms of their medical records?; What are some of the challenges that you normally encounter with travelling (who move from one place to the other without medical record) patients?; How do you think that these challenges can be addressed?; and how do you think they should be addressed?

The data analysis was carried out, using the moments of translation from the perspective of actor network theory (ANT). The approach was selected mainly because it allows us to examine the process of change, and the interaction that take place between actors which consists of both technical and non-technical. For example, occurs when actors start to define roles, distribute and redistribute roles and power, it help us to understand how alliances of technical and non-technical are formed.

Translation occurs when actors start to define roles, distribute and redistribute roles and power, describe a scenario to form alliances of technical and non-technical. Translation stage involves a process of change, which occur via four major moments. The ANT translation stage involves a process of change, which occur via four major moments: problematization, interessement, enrolment and mobilization. This occurs when actors start to define roles, distribute and redistribute roles and power, describe a scenario to form alliances of technical and non-technical.

The moments of translation elements can be summarised as follows: (i) Problematization stage reveals what necessitate the network formation. Uden & Francis (2011) elaborated that during problematisation, actors establish themselves as an obligatory passage point between them and the network for indispensability. (ii) Interessement: at this stage, actors consciously or unconsciously reveal their individual or groups interest on the item that has been problematized by the focal actor. (iii) Enrolment: process begins with a primary agent imposing their will on others for involvement to be successful; this act requires yielding from different actants. (iv) Mobilization: an enrolled actor speaks on behalf of the network, and tries to an interest to persuade others to partake in the activities of the network.

4. DATA ANALYSIS

As mention earlier in the methodology section, the analysis of the data was done, using the lens of actor network theory. The components of ANT that were followed include Actor, Network, and moments of translation.

It is clear from interview that healthcare givers are stationed at different levels of operant and that healthcare services are available to nomadic and in transit patients provided that they report to any health care centre. "There is a national policy on how to handle in transits patients". They are handled according to the national policy of in transit patients which stipulates the maximum duration of three months for one to be assisted as an in transit patients. Hence patients seeking for health services within three months or more are not denied access to treatment. Interviewees indicate that a letter or medical passports is required for treatment history and diagnosis done at previous consultations. Furthermore, crisis such as losing the medical passport or unable to present the health passport arises in this process; it does not hinder service provision. Rather a new medical passport is issued. Another source of information in this case and is a significant actant are the labels on the tablet containers.

Patients are attended to when seeking for health services at the centre, where a discussion (problematisation) between the patient and the healthcare takes place. It is procedural to bring along a medical passport when seeking for health services and routine for the healthcare giver to note in the health passport the diagnosis taken and prescriptions. Interactions between healthcare and patients can be classified as part of a durable network that exists to offer services. It is a durable network because a fixed health centre exists and there are actants stationed at each centre.

Currently there are no records readily available when attending to in transit patients except for the health pass port and the medication labels which might not be available at times or lost. For example HIV patients who have been under the care of private doctors and wish to move to state hospitals might not be attended to or attended to after a long time due to communication break. Most common challenges encounter by the healthcare givers are such as repetition of treatment course which are not effective, there are no records to show that the same treatment or test was given or done and not effective. One way to overcome these issues an Electronic Patient Monitoring System (EPMS) and Electronic Dispensary Tool (EDT) should be linked to all health facilities providing HIV care for patients to be helped without relying on hard copies for example.

4.1 Actor

The human actors in the healthcare sector includes healthcare needing people, healthcare professionals (Doctors and Nurses), and the government MoHSS. The non-human actors consists of processes, ICT artefacts and. Within the environment, different networks existed as at the time of this study. Some of the networks were nurses' professionals, urban patients, rural patients, and tribal patients.

Each of the actors existed for different interest, and could make a different, either as a receiver or provider of healthcare service. The different is based on the impact the actors have on each other. For example, the knowledge a professional acquired in the course of providing health service to a patient.

4.2 Actor-Network

Currently, there exist different networks to which the actors belong. The enrolment of actors in the different networks was influenced by their interests. As gathered from the participants in the study, the primary interest of the general actors were, to receive service from the practitioners, and to render service to the patients. These interests were however, influenced and manifested by other factors and interests, which included spoken language, culture, and accessibility.

Some of the patients could only enrol in the network where there preferred language was used as the medium of communication. Even though interpreters were readily available, they preferred to express themselves than the use of translation. Enrolment into a network by many patients in some parts of the country was influenced by their culture. According to some of the participants, their tradition does not allowed them to be treated by professional of opposite sex.

4.3 Moments of Translation

The moments which consist of four stages, namely problematisation, interessement, enrolment and mobilisation was employed in the analysis primarily to examine and understand the interactions which happen amongst the actors. This was to further understand the suitability and transformation of the current *status quo* to era of mobility or centralised of service within the healthcare environment.

4.4 Problemetisation

The activities of the healthcare sector were initiated, problematised through two primary channels, patient and the government. The patients problematise an activity through illnesses, which were often varied. While the other focal actor, the government does same, problematise its healthcare related activities through the Minister of the Ministry of Health and Social Services (MoHSS).

The patients or their representatives (guardian) report incidents of illness, including vehicle accident involving human at the nearest healthcare centre. The incidents were recorded by the front-office professional, who normally were the Nurses. The Nurses escalate the incidents to the appropriate or respective specialist for further and detailed attention. Another criterion that was used for the referral of patients was language, to enable communication and precise understanding between actors (patient and specialist). The Nurses does so, record and escalate incidents based on the power bestowed on them by the authority of the organisation, which comes from their qualification to practice.

The government problematises all initiatives relating healthcare in the country through the Minister of the MoHSS. The Minister further problematises the initiatives to heads of units and departments of agencies and organisation within the health sector, through workshops and strategic meetings. Unfortunately, the initiatives are not fit for the districts and rural communities, where they are considered to needed most e.g. Unavailability of medical reports 'breaks' the continuity of HIV care between health districts.

The overall problem is the provision of healthcare services to the nomadic patients of the country. The MoHSS aim to provide effective services to all patients regardless of their dwelling status are currently a challenge, as many of the patients are given too much responsibility in addition to their individual illness. In response to the need for a more effective health services, highly qualified and skilled workforce is enrolled in this activities. Furthermore, procedures to deliver or receive healthcare services are enforced (e.g. only registered nurses can attend to patients or patients should carry their healthcare passport in case looking for healthcare services). This in turn leads to the consideration of suitable healthcare provision, healthcare received and medical history for patients. For healthcare service innovation by the MoHSS, the problematisation proposed by the instigators is that to improve healthcare services to all patients including the nomadic patients, there must be service innovations that enable the desired outcomes. This is seen as an OPP by the MoHSS to remain a competent healthcare service provider in the country. In the case of the patients, they need to be certain that they will receive adequate services at any time anywhere. To fully understand the problematisation in any scenario, it is vital to identify stakeholders.

4.5 Interessemment

As earlier revealed in the analysis, the actors had different interests. The actors were categorised into two main groups, healthcare service recipients and providers, which consist of patients and professionals, respectively. The interests of these groups were diverse, even though the primary goal was healthcare services.

The interest of the healthcare recipients were influenced by factors such as locations, type of health related service that was required, and affordability of services. Proximity was a hindrance to many of the people who lived in the rural areas of the country. The healthcare facilities were far apart from each other. As a result, there were no many options to those who need services such as HIV patients, who needed to get their ARV medications from healthcare centre. Due to the fewness of the facilities, the common one was "General Practitioners". This made it difficult or impossible to access specialists and certain services.

The MoHSS for instance, interest concern its public mandate and social responsibility visible in different directorates and divisions that formed up the MoHSS. The MoHSS also has directorates and division managers in different roles that oversee the execution of duties (e.g. delivery of services), managing healthcare centres, recruit healthcare givers, procurement of necessary medications and other equipment's. These individuals set themselves up as the focal actors and as such, making rues for obligatory passage point.

The healthcare givers interests were of professional progress, income, status and job descriptions. Healthcare givers in service benefited differently during the course of their duties, depending on the location and the responsibilities that they were assigned. Some of the benefits included flexibility and shifts working hours, housing subsidy, and free medical aid. Also, exposure to different health related cases which in long term can be attributed to experience gained.

ICT artefacts were used differently in the healthcare organisations to support the delivery of services, such as diagnostics and documentation of individual and group records. The use of ICT artefacts were also based on the interest of the users. The interests were informed by their technical skill and know-how of the technologies, and what they needed them for. Another factor was whether the technologies were supported for use in the environment that they were deployed. This played a critical factor in individual and group interest to make use of available technologies for healthcare services in Namibia. As a result, many of the professional anchor their interests on paper-based processes, which they were more comfortable with in delivering services. Paper technology is crucial to nomadic patients thus; it is required for them to forward the healthcare passport to receive the necessary services.

4.6 Enrolment to the Network

This process begins with a primary agent (in this case the MoHSS management) imposing their will on others in attempt to achieve for common goal. This was mainly because of the significant of participation of all key stakeholders, which determines the success of failure of healthcare initiatives in Namibia. However, participation was always a challenge, as a result, definition of roles and responsibilities were seen as critical.

The ministry defines the regulations, roles and responsibilities to healthcare givers, and standards of service deliveries at public healthcare centres (MoHSS designs enrolment strategies). This process centred on negotiation and alignment of actants' interests within the different networks. The process was challenging in that it was always lengthy and difficult, and so many conflicts arose. The challenges were manifestation of the different cultural background, interests' focuses, as well as recording keeping. For example, some patients had relocated, and others had lost their health passport, and they needed medical attention. In such cases provision was made to create a new health passport for them through negotiation.

Even though health services were considered essential and critical, some patients would not enrol or reluctantly enrolled in the health related programs. This challenge was prevalence in the rural parts of the country. Many of the communities' members cited the same reason for their lack of participation in the health programs. Some of the reasons included accessibility, literacy, and affordability. For example, some of the participants in this study claimed that many of them are not literate enough to understand the messages which were used as medium of communication to them. Inscription occurs in this case in the sense that the primary interest of the MoHSS at different healthcare centres was to provide efficient services to all patients including the nomadic patients. Interest of all actants has been aligned and now there is a need to maintain the network. This results into a durable or not durable network.

Existence of conscious and unconscious networks of people, and their enrolments which were created overtime and space across the country signifies that there is need for durability and mobility of healthcare services. Thus, patients communicate their healthcare complains to healthcare givers, provide the healthcare passport if in possession, healthcare givers carry out the diagnosis process and offer prescriptions, again healthcare givers communicates the different cases encountered at reporting intervals to supervisors which in return reports to management (regional, district or national). Or though healthcare givers have power in durability of the network, MoHSS management have the most power to ensure the existence and the growth of the network.

4.7 Mobilisation

Due to the essentiality of health services in the country, it was vital for some actors from both MoHSS and the community to mobilise the healthcare service providers and recipients towards a common goal.

During mobilisation, some actors were assigned the role of new initiators by becoming delegates or spokesperson for the focal actor (Iyamu &Tatnall, 2011). In this case, hospital matrons, and supervisors at different healthcare centres tried to mobilise healthcare givers to actively participate in the network (carry out their duties). This resulted to a stability of the process of delivering healthcare services in some areas, particularly in the urban region such as Windhoek.

As a result of the stability through adequate services, more patients became spokespersons to different centres. The self-appointed spokespersons encouraged others with the same or different health issue to seek healthcare services from designated locations of their preference. Also, the altitude and tribal inclination were the others factors which influenced mobilisation and of patients. For example, some patients recommended others to visit or seek assistance from health centres where majority of the health professional were on their tribal origin and spoke the same language as them.

5. MOBILITY OF HEALTHCARE SERVICES IN NAMIBIA

People, technology and procedures are the actors in the process of healthcare service delivery. ANT's translation process that was followed in this study defines the formation of networks, which helped to identify the groupings and how they were created. The process starts with the main actor who defines the roles through problemitisation of the issue or item. This was done by localization of the issue, so as to foster relationship, and get more and regional actors to be interested, and partake in the initiative.

Although the employment of technical actants can be viewed as the consequences of the action of all actants to an extent, the ministry of health in this case has power to hire healthcare providers and extend the provision of services to all health service level of operation. This signifies authority to define procedures of service delivery e.g. change the national policy of the in transit patients or implement EPMS at health centres. By so doing, associations of technical and non-technical actants are strengthen.

Moreover, the mobility of healthcare services is enabled and constrained within network such as community by the actions of actors, which often based on individual or group knowledge. Mobilisation is necessary to educate and inform actants about the services. Patients need to know about their rights to health services at any location and the importance of a health passport.

A health passport, referral letter or medication container was issued to patients by medical personnel at different locations or health centres across the country. Thus, the patients present whenever they needed health related treatment anywhere in the country. Challenge of presenting the above is that they are vulnerable to loss or results to unclear information on the passport or letter. The consequence of such loss and unclear information make services complex and complicated to both healthcare service providers and the patients. Hence it is critical to enforce electronic systems, which allow access to patients' health related records from anywhere across the country, and on real-time.

6. CONCLUSION

This paper presents a critical analysis of the role and account of actors in the mobility of healthcare services in Namibia. The analysis is of vital important to the Namibia, and other countries which has similar setup and challenges, in that it unveiled issues that the State government and many healthcare professional are not aware of, take for granted.

In the past, and continuous (before this study), the state Government as in many developing continue to invest and focus on technical issues, which often become "white elephants" due to lack of usefulness. This paper revealed fundamental and primary issues, which makes technology useful and ease of use in the mobility of healthcare services across Namibia.

We consider the MoHSS management, healthcare givers, patients, medical paper technology (heath passport) and medical ICT tools as actants in the mobility of healthcare services study. The most important point in the providing healthcare services is that, people (in this case patient) receive the most needed health service anywhere without being subjected to locations.

The paper emphasises on the importance of relationships between the actors (health professional and patients), and as well the significance of networks in the mobility of healthcare services at different health operandis. As at the time of the study, patients in transit were handled in accordance to the national health policy as promulgated by the MoHSS. The paper revealed how healthcare service providers, through the use of spoken language and tribal origin, enable and at the same time constrain the services that they are supposed to render to the patients for better healthcare. These factors were often conscious, and sometimes unconsciously exhibited by the actors. However, little or nothing was known of the impact, the service providers of healthcare in Namibia.

REFERENCES

Braa, J., Hanseth, O., Heywood, A., Mohammed, W., & Shawn, B. (2007). Developing information systems in developing country: The flexible standards strategy. *MIS Quartely, 31*, 1–22.

Chang, P. (2011) Modeling the Management of Electronic Health Records in Healthcare Information Systems. *2011 International Conference on Cyber-Enabled Distributed Computing and Knowledge Discovery*. doi:10.1109/CyberC.2011.98

Chaulagai, C.N, Moyo, C.M, Koot, J., & Moyo, H.B. (2005). *Design and implementation of a health management in Malawi: issues inovation and results*. Oxford University Press in association with The London School of Hygiene and Tropical Medicine.

Cisco. (2007). *Mobility solution for healthcare: voice, text, images and information, delivered to the point of care*. Available at: http://www.cisco.com/web/strategy/docs/healthcare/07cs1084-MobForHC_062708.pdf

Creswell, K., Worth, A., & Sheikh, A. (2010). Actor-Network theory and its role in understanding the implementation of information technology developments in healthcare. *BMC Medical Informatics and Decision Making*, 10–67.

Hamunyela, S., & Iyamu, T. (2013). Readness Assessment model for the deployment of health information systems in the Namibian MoH. *International Federation for Information Processing, 12*[th] *Internation Conference on Social Implications of Computer in Developing countries*.

Istepanian, R. J., Jovanov, E., & Zhang, Y. T. (2004). Guest Editorial Introduction to the Specialon M-Health: Beyond Seamless Mobility and Global Wireless Health-Care Connectivity. *IEEE Transactions on Information Technology in Biomedicine, 8*(4), 405–414. doi:10.1109/TITB.2004.840019 PMID:15615031

Iyamu, T. (2010). Theoretical Analysis of the Implementation of Enterprise Architecture. *International Journal of Actor-Network Theory and Technological Innovation, 2*(3), 27–38.

Iyamu, T., & Tatnall, A. (2011). *The impact of netwrork of actors on the infomation technology. In Actor network theory and technology innovation: advancements and new concepts journal.* Hershey, PA: Information Science Reference.

Law, J. (1992). *Notes on the theory of the Actor Network: ordering, strategy and heterogeneity.* Available at: http://comp.lancs.ac.uk/sociology/soc054jl.html

MoHSS. (2012). *Integrated healthcare delivery the challenge and implementations.* Available at: http://www.healthnet.org.na/documents.html

Namibia, M. (2007). *Community-based healtcare policy.* Windhoek: MoHSS.

Narang, J. K. (2011). Quality of Healthcare Services in Rural India: The User Perspective. *VIKALPA*, 51-60.

NPC. (2012). *Namibia 2011 population and housing census.* Available at: www.npc.gov.na

Rygh, E. M., & Hjortdahl, P. H. (2007). Continuous and integrated health care services in rural areas. A literature study. The International Electronic Journal of Rural and Remote Health Research, Education Practice and Policy, 7(766), 1-10.

Sander Granlien, M., & Hertzum, M. (2012). Confirmatory factor analysis of service quality dimensions within mobile telephony industry in Ghana. *The Electronic Journal Information Systems Evaluation, 15*(2), pp197–pp227.

Sinha, R. K. (2010). Impact of Health Information Technology in Public Health. *Sri Lanka Journal of Bio-Medical Informatics, 1*(4), 223–236. doi:10.4038/sljbmi.v1i4.2239

Tatnall, A., & Burgess, S. (2002). Using Actor-Network to research the implementation of a B-B Portal for Regional SME in Melbourne. *15th Bled Electronic Commerce Conference.*

Uden, L., & Francis, J. (2011). *Service Innovation using Actor-Network theory. In Actor-network theory and technology innovation: advancements and new concepts journal, Advancements and new concepts journal.* Hershey, PA: Information Science Reference.

KEY TERMS AND DEFINITIONS

Actants: Technical and non-technical participants in a process or activity.

In-Transit Patient: The one who happen to obtain or needs medical attention, care while relocated.

Mobility of Healthcare: The state of easy accessibility of healthcare services from any geographical location.

Nomadic Patients: Patients belonging to the society that moves around in pursue of improved living conditions.

Chapter 5
An Investigation of the Role of Using IS/IT in the Delivery of Treatments for ADHD in University Students

Bader Binhadyan
RMIT University, Australia & Ministry of Education, Saudi Arabia

Nilmini Wickramasinghe
Deakin University & Epworth HealthCare, Melbourne, Australia

ABSTRACT

Over the last decade, the popularity of incorporating advances in information systems and information technology (IS/IT) has been steadily growing. IS/IT can improve the delivery for better intervention and treatment with many different mental illnesses; however, there appears to be great potential for IS/IT in the context of young adults with mental disorders such as Attention Deficit Hyperactivity Disorder (ADHD). ADHD affects approximately 11% of the university population; negatively impacting students' academic performance, study skills, and social life. The study design outlined in this paper suggests a possibility for the role of IS/IT in the delivery of treatments and management of ADHD in university students to be examined with the view to introduce IS/IT into the traditional treatment context. This research involves collecting data from psychologists in the form of semi-structured interviews and a grounded theory methodology using multiple cases is adopted.

INTRODUCTION

In recent years, Australia has become one of the leading countries in providing e-mental health services (Christensen & Petrie, 2013). Technology tools, such as the Internet and mobile devices, have the promise to improve mental health services especially by enabling early intervention and treatment for many people (Christensen, Griffiths, & Evans, 2002), especially young adults with mental disorders such as Attention Deficit Hyperactivity Disorder (ADHD).

DOI: 10.4018/978-1-4666-9446-0.ch005

Approximately 11% of students at university level have symptoms of ADHD (Dipeolu, 2010). These symptoms negatively impact academic performance (Heiligenstein, Greta Guenther Msn, Levy, Savino, & Fulwiler, 1999) and usually affect such students in terms of keeping up with their academic load and various aspects of social life (Barkley 1998; Quinn, 2001). Typically, individuals with ADHD are deficient in executive functions, such as Working Memory (WM) and planning (Barkley, 1997b) which is related to academic performance (Gropper & Tannock, 2009). ADHD often co-occurs with learning disabilities (LD) such as difficulty in organizing time, poor reading, writing or spelling skills, or completing tasks abilities (Mayes, Calhoun, & Crowell, 2000). Today, one of the most effective approaches to treat ADHD is the multimodal framework which includes: medication, education, therapy and coaching (Canadian Attention Deficit Hyperactivity Disorder Resource Alliance (CADDRA), 2011; Department of Human Services Victoria, n.d.).

The emphasis of this research design is on the non-pharmaceutical components of the multimodal framework: coaching, therapy and education. The role of IS/IT in each of these components is examined with the view to introduce IS/IT into the traditional treatment context. In addition, four cases are therefore chosen to represent the key treatment components; namely, case1:- coaching and Education (Swartz, Prevatt, & Proctor, 2005); case2:- Working Memory Training (WMT) therapy (Puffenberger, 2011); case3:- Cognitive Behavioural Therapy (CBT) (Ramsay, 2012); and case4:- Neurofeedback Therapy (De-identified patient data). Furthermore, the role of IS/IT in each of these cases will be examined. This research design does not involve gathering information from patients; it involves collecting data from psychologists in the form of semi-structured interviews and a grounded theory methodology using multiple cases is adopted. The main research question guiding this study is: How can an IT solution be designed to enable mental health providers to facilitate the delivery of treatments of ADHD?

RELATED LITERATURE

In this section, a brief background of the general use of IS/IT in healthcare is provided, followed by a definition of e-health and the general use of technology in mental health services and ADHD in particular. The last part of this section will point out the relevance of ADHD in university students and what current non-pharmaceutical treatments are used to treat and manage ADHD.

Background

The use of IS/IT in healthcare has the potential to assist developed and developing countries to solve many issues they are facing (Wickramasinghe, Geisler, & Schaffer, 2005), such as easy access to information and services, coping with changes in population health patterns and satisfaction and safety of stake holders. Healthcare is becoming technology-driven (Moumtzoglou, 2011) with the possibility of successful adoption of e-business in the form of e-health(Wickramasinghe, Geisler, et al., 2005). There is a wide range of e-health services (Eysenbach, 2001; Wickramasinghe, Fadlalla, Geisler, & Schaffer, 2005) and E-mental health is one such service.

Although the use of technologies in mental healthcare is relatively new, there are positive feelings in using technologies among different age groups for different mental illness preventions, treatments and management (Whittaker et al., 2012). Technology has the potential to improve efficiency, accessibility and the opportunities for early intervention and treatment of young adults (Anthony, Nagel, &

Goss, 2010; Christensen et al., 2002); especially in treating young adults with ADHD (Beck, Hanson, Puffenberger, Benninger, & Benninger, 2010).

Technological tools and methods, such as Internet-based interventions and mobile-based applications or Short Message Services (SMS) therapy are used for the treatment of people with mental illness like depression and anxiety (Whittaker et al., 2012). They also can target young adults seeking mental health attention (Christensen et al., 2002). The use of these types of technologies allowed Australia to be advanced in e-mental health services (Christensen & Petrie, 2013).

Australian E-Mental Health Development

The Australian government is investing heavily in e-mental health services because technology can assist in overcoming issues that are preventing young people from seeking mental health services and providers which create barriers to treatment. Problems include: lack of access to mental health services due to location, time or perhaps financial matters (Booth et al., 2004); stigma incurred by seeing a therapist (Burns, Davenport, Durkin, Luscombe, & Hickie, 2010; Christensen & Hickie, 2010); and therapist time and efficacy (Jorm, Wright, & Morgan, 2007). Reynolds, Griffiths, and Christensen (2011) argue that there are two types of e-mental health programs in Australia:

1. Information, support and assessment web sites including: informative website, diagnostics tools and screening methods;
2. Symptom prevention and management programs which are designed to treat or manage specific mental illness such as depression and anxiety.

The Australian Government has invested $70.4 million to date into developing and funding e-mental health services and telephone crisis assistance; also, the Australian Government will invest a further $110.4 million in the next four years targeting young adults (Australian Government, 2012). In addition, an estimate conducted between 2012 - 2013 showed that 96.5% of 15- to 24-year olds use the Internet in Australia (Australian Bureau of Statistics, 2014). By reviewing the list of the online or telephone services that were provided in the E-Mental Health Strategy for Australia documents (Australian Government, 2012), the majority of e-mental health programs are targeting illnesses related to depression, anxiety and suicidal thoughts. Although approximately only one in ten young Australians suffer from ADHD (The Royal Australian College of Physicians, 2009), this commitment to the adoption of technology in Australia makes the country a potentially rich site in which to consider possibilities.

ADHD

ADHD is one of the most common childhood behavioral disorders and can continue through adolescence and adulthood(Fischer, Barkley, Edelbrock, & Smallish, 1990), with between 5% and 10% of the childhood population having ADHD (The Royal Australian College of Physicians, 2009). Barkley (1998) argues that the symptoms of children with ADHD are usually hyperactivity, inattention, daydreaming, and impulsiveness. Some of these symptoms will vary from one child to another (Barkley 1998).

ADHD in young adults causes attention difficulties and emotional instability which affects their life outcomes and results in underachievement (Wallace, Winsler, & NeSmith, 1999). They are at greater risk of developing anxiety, depression (Heiligenstein & Keeling, 1995), learning disabilities (Wender,

Wolf, & Wasserstein, 2001) and deficits in executive functions, such as WM and planning (Barkley, 1997a). ADHD is estimated to affect approximately 11% of university populations and the majority of these students will face academic difficulties and perhaps will not complete their degree (Dipeolu, 2010; Grenwald-Mayes, 2001).Gropper and Tannock (2009) argue that there is a relationship between WM and academic performance in university students with ADHD also.

Studies have indicated that there is a relationship between ADHD symptoms and university students' academic underperformance (Heiligenstein et al., 1999) . Fewer ADHD students complete their degree than non-ADHD students (Barkley, 2006; Barkley, Murphy, & Fischer, 2008). There are issues that university students with ADHD face during their studies (Quinn et al., 2003) such as finding university academic style and social life overwhelming and hard to adjust to which may result in dropping out (Barkley 1998).

Often university students with ADHD are lower in function on a number of academic variables compared to their peers (Heiligenstein et al., 1999). These include: study skills, note taking, summarizing, and organizing (Mannuzza, Klein, Bessler, Malloy, & LaPadula, 1998). These academic variables craft common academic behavioural aspects; namely, higher rates of subject failure (Grenwald-Mayes, 2001), Lower Grade Point Averages (Murphy, Barkley, & Bush, 2002), and/or low class attendance (Wolf, 2001). Furthermore, anxiety, depression and low motivation are commonly found in university students with ADHD (Meaux, Green, & Broussard, 2009).

ADHD Treatment and Management

Department of Human Services Victoria (n.d.) and the Canadian Attention Deficit Hyperactivity Disorder Resource Alliance (CADDRA) (2011) state one of the most effective approaches to treat ADHD is the multimodal framework Figure 1. This framework contains multiple components that best work together to support each other. This includes: medication, education, therapy, and coaching. The Therapy methods include: CBT (Safren et al., 2005), Neurofeedback therapy (Lansbergen, van Dongen-Boomsma, Buitelaar, & Slaats-Willemse, 2011) and WMT (Westerberg et al., 2007). Coaching is effective for adults with ADHD (Tuckman, 2009).

Therapies that have been found useful for treating ADHD in adults include CBT (Ramsay, 2012), Neurofeedback Therapy (Gevensleben et al., 2009) and WMT (Klingberg et al., 2005).

- CBT "refers to the pragmatic combination of concepts and techniques from cognitive and behavioural therapies common in clinical practice." (Kaltenthaler et al., 2006, p. vii);
- Neurofeedback Therapy appears to be a promising alternative or additional treatment without reported adverse effects (Arns, Gunkelman, Breteler, & Spronk, 2008; Gevensleben et al., 2009). Neurofeedback training involves the self-regulation of ongoing neuronal oscillations which are recorded by Electroencephalography (EEG), in one or more frequency bands by visual or auditory feedback, aimed at normalizing and/or self-regulating brain activity (Lansbergen et al., 2011).
- WMT aims to improve an individual's working memory. This includes algorithm, non-algorithm or both computerized programs that automatically adjust the training difficulties based on the individual's answers (Klingberg et al., 2005).

Figure 1. The Multimodal framework
(Canadian Attention Deficit Hyperactivity Disorder Resource Alliance (CADDRA), 2011; Department of Human Services Victoria, n.d.)

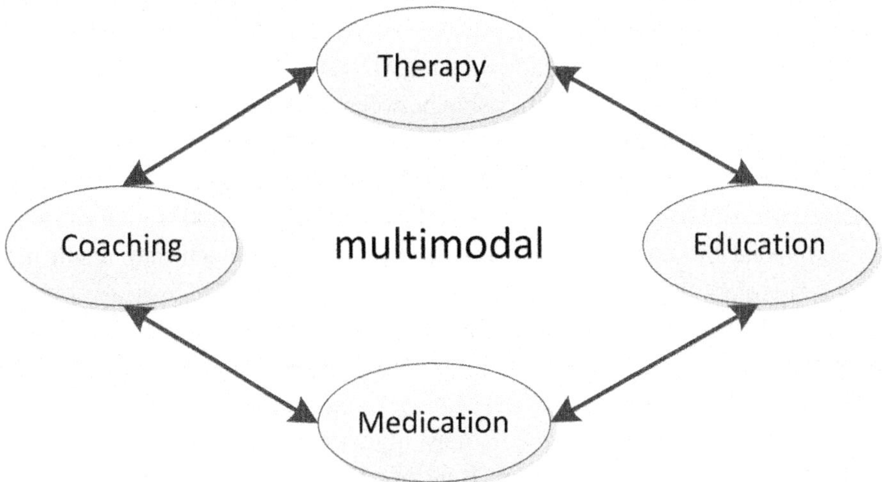

Education includes information on intervention related to educational accommodations, support, and school management (Wilens et al., 2008).

Coaching which includes improving time management, studies, and social skills at university (Swartz et al., 2005).

Technology Tools in the Multimodal Framework

This research will look at each one of the treatment options: therapy, education, and coaching. The study is designed to explore and to investigate the use of technology in the delivery of the treatment of ADHD in university students. The Multimodal framework is adapted to see where IS/IT is used or where it can be introduced. In addition, some of the technology tools that have been found in the literature and previous studies are listed in Table 1.

Table 1. Tools used in the multimodal framework

Treatment	Tool	References
Therapy	Neurofeedback Therapy CBT WMT	(Arns, de Ridder, Strehl, Breteler, & Coenen, 2009) (Wilens et al., 1999) (Klingberg et al., 2005)
Education	Informative Website and Social media	(Canadian Attention Deficit Hyperactivity Disorder Resource Alliance (CADDRA), 2011)
Coaching	Smartphone / SMS reminder Alarm/computerized reminders Email coaching/Time management	(Prevatt, Lampropoulos, Bowles, & Garrett, 2011)

RESEARCH DESIGN FRAMEWORK

The research design framework (Figure 2) is to guide the investigation in using the technology in treating and managing ADHD symptoms, and investigating whether these technologies have a positive impact on the academic performance of university students with ADHD.

METHODOLOGY

Choosing the suitable research method can sometimes be a challenge for academic researchers (Yin, 2002). Because this area of study has not been explored previously and the research questions do not have defined characteristics, a qualitative research method is the most suitable method and case studies and grounded theory are used as the framework for data collection and analysis. Therefore, this research design will use multiple case studies and grounded theory methodologies

Case Study

Case studies are a tool of investigation found in numerous fields, especially evaluation, in which the researcher develops an in-depth analysis of a case (Creswell, 2013). According to Stake (1995), there are three types of case study research: intrinsic, instrumental, and collective case studies. To gain more insight and knowledge into this research topic, collective case studies have been chosen.

They are also called multiple-case design (Yin, 2009). Collective studies study in depth more than one case in one overall research study and are usually designed for the purpose of comparison (Yin, 2009). Soy (1997) mentions that when multiple cases are adopted in the research; each case should be treated as a single case and then each case's conclusions could be used as data contribution to the whole study. Lapan, Quartaroli, and Riemer (2011) argue that all the case studies conducted in the research should share the common characteristics. Case studies typically combine data collection methods such as interviews and focus groups (Eisenhardt, 1989).

There are advantages to using collective case studies as comparative type of studies can be conducted in which a number of cases are compared for similarities and differences. However, the depth of the analysis will have to be sacrificed due to the breadth of analysis (Johnson & Christensen, 2008).

This research design uses the 8 steps recommended by Eisenhardt (1989) as follows:

- Getting Started
- Selecting Cases
- Crafting Instruments and Protocols
- Entering the Field
- Analyzing Data
- Shaping Hypotheses
- Enfolding Literature
- Reaching Closure/recommendations.

Figure 2. Proposed framework of the use of technology in ADHD

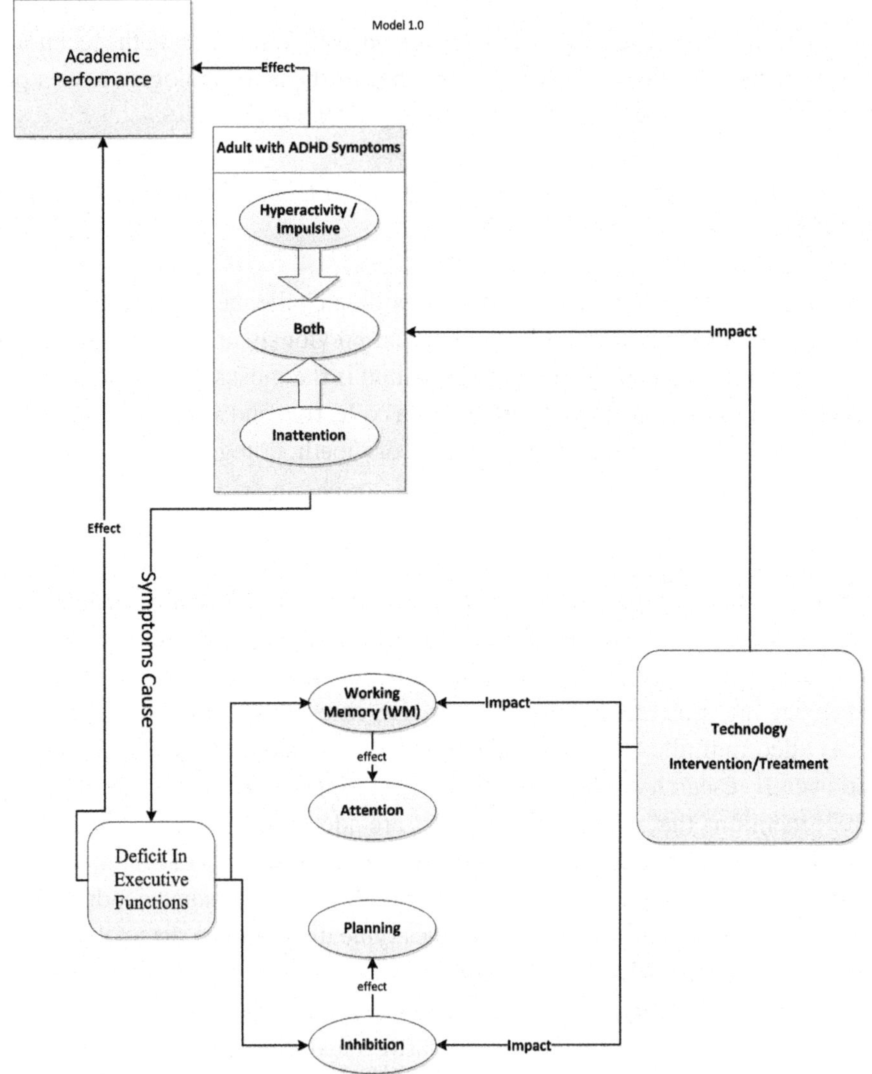

Grounded Theory Methodology

Grounded theory has been used in health informatics since its inception, and grounded theory has been found effective in pointing out and describing the impact of Health information systems and their associated devices where an area has not been studied or is not easily described by quantitative approaches (Cummings & Borycki, 2011). In addition, Cummings and Borycki (2011) cite that grounded theory has been viewed as a powerful tool when it comes to a development of health informatics' frameworks and/or applications.

Grounded theory, like other forms of qualitative research methods, has key concepts which differentiate this methodology from others.

The research will follow the systematic design in grounded theory focusing on the use of the data analysis steps of open, axial and selective coding,

- **Open Coding:** Also known as initial coding, is the first step of data analysis which is identifying important words or groups of words in the data collected and then labelling them accordingly. Open coding is a process of reducing the data to a small set of themes that appear to describe the phenomenon under investigation (Glaser & Strauss, 1967);
- **Axial Coding:** This process facilitates building connections within categories;
- **Selective Coding:** The process of selecting and identifying the core category and systematically relating it to other categories.
- Memos.

RESEARCH DESIGN

There are steps and processes that have been developed using a combination of those two methodologies to illustrate the research design (Figure 3). In this research design, two case study steps such as getting started and selecting case studies will be combined into one process. The research question is created to guide this paper, and avoid any unwanted data. Based on the research question, priori constructs were explored to assist in further measurement.

Four case studies will be selected with each representing an element of the multimodal frame or more. Case studies will be reviewed and notes and comments will be stored in the memos process.

Four case studies are chosen to represent key components of the multimodal framework. These case studies are shown in Table 2.

Writing Memos

Memos are written records of thoughts and ideas during the process of undertaking the grounded theory studies; they differ in intensity, coherence, subject, theoretical content and usefulness to the finished product. It is highly recommended that the memo be kept until the end of the research and never thrown away. In this research, writing a memo is an important process that overlaps and affects every single step and element of this research. It will start from developing the research questions to enclosing the literature review.

Data Collection

Both case studies and grounded theory share the same concept of data collection and analysis overlap and research can go back and forth until the main theory emerges.

Crafting Instruments and Protocols

For this research, between 8 and 12 registered psychologists will be recruited to participate. The targeted participants will be divided in four groups equally. Each group will be allocated to a case study. The

Figure 3. Process of Building the Research
Adapted from (Birks and Mills 2010, DiCicco-Bloom and Crabtree 2006, Eisenhardt 1989, Fernández 2004)

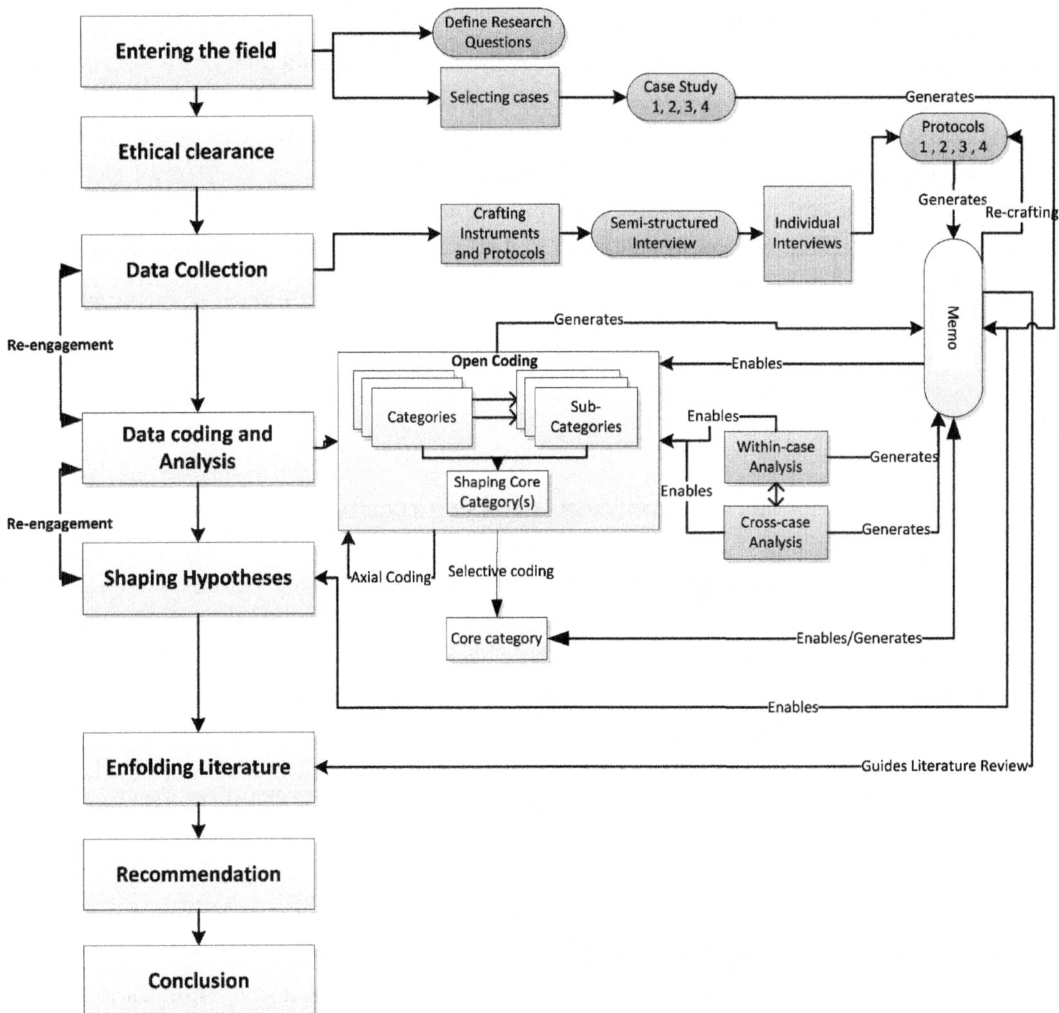

Table 2. 4 Selected case studies

Case Study	Treatment	Tool	Brief
1	Coaching Education	Coaching Education	Swartz et al. (2005) applied face2face coaching and education techniques to manage a university student's ADHD symptoms in the UK.
2	Therapy	WMT	Puffenberger (2011) explored WMT training in individuals with Attention-Deficit/Hyperactivity Disorder to how effective this treatment is.
3	Therapy	CBT	Ramsay (2012) used traditional CBT on one of the his patients to help him reduce his ADHD symptoms.
4	Therapy	Neurofeedback Therapy	Neurofeedback Therapy is a recognized tool to treat ADHD (Wang & Hsieh, 2013). This case study will be based on an unpublished case from a clinic in Melbourne, Australia, where Neurofeedback therapy was used in the treatment of ADHD in a university student.

participants, registered psychologists, will be selected based on four dimensions: educational level, years of experience, specialization in ADHD and offering Internet technology as a treatment tool.

Thus, psychologists will be chosen who are:

- Specialized in treating/preventing adults with ADHD;
- Have a minimum of 10 years of experience;
- Offer at least one of Internet technologies to deliver his/her services. i.e. Skype, Email, SMS;
- Have used at least one of the following tools which will identify which case they will fall into:
  - Coaching/Education;
  - WMT;
  - CBT (CBT);
  - Neurofeedback Therapy.

The participants will be reached via email or mail requesting participation in the research. In addition, a brief introduction of the purpose of the research as well as its scope and objectives will be enclosed. With regard to Individual Semi-structured interviews, the participants will be requested to take part in the study only after they provide their consent. This can be delivered to the researcher in two ways: e-mailing back a signed form or replying via e-mail to an invitation to participate by stating in the message that "The consent form was read and agreed to" (Meho, 2006).

The participants will be interviewed individually on a face to face basis as a primary tool of data collection; the secondary tool will be using an online video conference; Skype, for example, if the location of the participant is outside Melbourne. Other data collection option tools will be considered such as e-mail or phone interviews or a video conference (Skype).

The individual semi-structured interview's protocol will be developed, which will mainly be focused on their perspective of the non-medication therapy that was introduced in the case studies and IS/IT involvement in the Multimodal Figure 2. The interview will also include the participants' professions, years of experiences, number of patients with ADHD, and educational level.

Coding and Analysis of Data

Coding is the process of naming or labeling data, categories, and properties (Cummings & Borycki, 2011). In coding analysis, the researcher moves back and forth from data collection and coding and analysis; this process will continue until a main theory starts to take shape. The data is analysed by within-case analysis and later cross-case analysis.

- **Open Coding:** The data collected will be divided into segments and then examined for common aspects that reflect categories or themes. After categorizing the data, extra examination of properties that will develop subcategories and based on common character has to be conducted.

For instance, the important words or group of words data collected will be divided into categories; later, with more depth analysis, these will create sub categories accordingly. From these categories and their subs, the Axial coding will be initiated.

- **Axial Coding:** Identifying and improving relationships between the open coding's categories and sub-categories. A core category will start to develop or take shape.
- **Selective Coding:** Selecting and identifying the core category and systematically relating it to other categories will occur in this level. The relationship will be validated and the categories will be refined. Most likely all the findings which will help in shaping the theory will occur in this stage.

Shaping Hypotheses

In this level the hypotheses will be compared to the four cases, which will improve the quality of the outcomes of this research.

Enfolding Literature

In this level, the findings will be compared with similar and conflicting literatures.

Recommendation

Based on the outcomes of the data analysis and findings and the literature, a recommendation will be created.

LIMITATIONS AND RISKS

This research will be limited to Australia and the participants will be asked only about the use of technology in treating ADHD in university students.

Participants' location will be considered as risks which might affect the data collection if the participant lives or works outside Melbourne and is not able to use video conference tools.

Discussion

This research aims to explore how psychologists think of the use of technology in the delivery of treatment and management of ADHD in university students. It will discover how these professionals will use such IS/IT in their routine treatment or management. The outcomes will contribute to Australian e-mental health strategy and programs.

On a micro level, this research will be seen in three different areas. These include: human resources, mental healthcare cost for the Australian economy, general mental health and wellbeing for university students with ADHD, and Australia's e-mental health program.

As mentioned earlier, university students are unlikely to complete their degree compared to their peers; dropping out or failing to complete a university degree is a waste of resources. "In this respect, a key area of economic and social policy should be to ensure all young people have the capacity to contribute to the economy in the future." (Lahey, 2003, p. 4). There are a number of challenges Australia is going to face in the next ten years. Firstly, to support the strong and growing economy is to have an adequate number of human resources to participate in the workforce (Lahey, 2003). These individuals have to be skilled and have the capability to be efficient and effective to their society. By increasing the access to and improving the delivery of mental health services that will assist university students with ADHD, e-mental health services will reduce the risk of these economic challenges that Australia might face.

Much of Australian universities' direct revenue comes from international students. These students comprise approximately 24% of the total university student population (Khawaja & Dempsey, 2008) and they generated revenue of $3.892 billion in 2011 as reported by 37 Australian Universities (O'Brien, 2011). Therefore, international students with ADHD who will drop out or fail to complete their degree, will be considered an instant loss of revenue.

By improving the accessibility, it will reduce the demand on clinics by allowing individuals with mild to moderate mental health issues to seek assessment online. This will increase the opportunity and the availability of traditional face to face assessment for people who have complex mental health issues. Christensen et al. (2009) argued that e-mental health services will provide first contact with mental health providers without the need to contact the general practitioners (GP), or as they were called 'gatekeeper'. In fact, it will reduce the overall cost and workload on clinics (Christensen & Hickie, 2010).

With all the benefits that e-mental health services provide, there is the possibility to improve the Medicare-rebated psychological services. In Australia, for any individual with assessed mental disorder to receive help under Medicare, she/he must be referred by a GP (Australian Psychological Society, n d). E-mental health service can improve the delivery of this process by providing online forms or email. It does not have to be to every single case but can be organized for people who are known to the GP or have a long history of mental disorder. This will also reduce the cost of visiting a GP.

IS/IT will not only allow the mental health services to be accessible for people in rural areas in Australia (Wickramasinghe & Misra, 2004), IS/IT will also minimize the financial barriers that prevent individuals accessing mental health services (Christensen & Hickie, 2010). To date, most of the E-mental health programs in Australia are provided free of charge to allow young adults to use most of the mental health services.

The outcome of this research will not only help such students to successfully complete their degree, but it will also assist them with their general happiness, mental health and wellbeing and sense of achievement. Students with ADHD might ultimately feel improved self-worth when they see technology helps them to improve their study skills and their ADHD symptoms. This research outcome will also provide solutions and recommendations to increase the delivery and improve accessibility of treatment and management for ADHD in university students.

This research will contribute to the development of an Australian e-mental health program, which will help to cover a broad area in mental health disorders and services and provide high quality outcomes that will assist both university students with ADHD and mental health providers.

CONCLUSION

This research in progress has served to investigate the possibilities for incorporating IS/IT into the treatment and management of ADHD in university students and assist such students in their studies. In particular, it suggests that such technology solutions can enable ADHD students to enjoy better outcomes at university and also better manage their ADHD.

Given the increasing costs of healthcare and tertiary education, solutions that aim to support successful outcomes at universities as well as better healthcare outcomes are prudent and should be further investigated. Australia has become one of the leading countries in providing e-mental health services (Christensen & Petrie, 2013). This study serves to leverage this and specifically investigate the potential for e-mental health in the context of ADHD. Currently, the Australian government aims to develop a mature e-mental healthcare program by 2016; therefore, this research serves to significantly contribute to this development. Moreover, it provides high quality outcomes that will facilitate the use of IS/IT in the treatment of ADHD in university students and will assist these students to succeed in their studies. This research contributes to both practices; i.e., e-mental health practice in Australia as well as serving to extend theories regarding e-health and e-mental health.

REFERENCES

Anthony, K., Nagel, D. M., & Goss, S. (2010). *The use of technology in mental health: Applications, ethics and practice*. Charles C Thomas Pub Limited.

Arns, M., de Ridder, S., Strehl, U., Breteler, M., & Coenen, A. (2009). Efficacy of neurofeedback treatment in ADHD: the effects on inattention, impulsivity and hyperactivity: a meta-analysis. *Clinical EEG and Neuroscience, 40*(3), 180–189. doi:10.1177/155005940904000311 PMID:19715181

Arns, M., Gunkelman, J., Breteler, M., & Spronk, D. (2008). EEG phenotypes predict treatment outcome to stimulants in children with ADHD. *Journal of Integrative Neuroscience, 7*(03), 421–438. doi:10.1142/S0219635208001897 PMID:18988300

Australian Bureau of Statistics. (2014). *Personal internet use. 8146.0 - Household Use of Information Technology, Australia, 2012-13*. Retrieved from http://www.abs.gov.au/ausstats/abs@.nsf/Lookup/8146.0Chapter32012-13

Australian Govermment. (2012). *E-mental health strategy for Australia*. Retrieved from http://www.health.gov.au/internet/main/publishing.nsf/Content/7C7B0BFEB985D0EBCA257BF0001BB0A6/$File/emstrat.pdf

Australian Psychological Society. (n.d.). *Australian Psychological Society: Medicare and psychology*. Retrieved from http://www.psychology.org.au/medicare/

Barkley, R. A. (1997a). Behavioral inhibition, sustained attention, and executive functions: Constructing a unifying theory of ADHD. *Psychological Bulletin, 121*(1), 65–94. doi:10.1037/0033-2909.121.1.65 PMID:9000892

Barkley, R. A. (1998). *Attention deficit hyperactivity disorder: A handbook for diagnosis and treatment* (2nd ed.). New York: Guilford.

Barkley, R. A. (2006). *Attention-deficit hyperactivity disorder: A handbook for diagnosis and treatment* (3rd ed.). New York: Guilford.

Barkley, R. A., Murphy, K. R., & Fischer, M. (2008). *ADHD in adults: What the science says*. New York: Guilford.

Barkley, R. A. X. (1997b). *Attention-deficit Hyperactivity Disorder and the Nature of Self-control*. The Guilford Press.

Beck, S. J., Hanson, C. A., Puffenberger, S. S., Benninger, K. L., & Benninger, W. B. (2010). A controlled trial of working memory training for children and adolescents with ADHD. *Journal of Clinical Child and Adolescent Psychology*, *39*(6), 825–836. doi:10.1080/15374416.2010.517162 PMID:21058129

Booth, M. L., Bernard, D., Quine, S., Kang, M. S., Usherwood, T., Alperstein, G., & Bennett, D. L. (2004). Access to health care among Australian adolescents young people's perspectives and their sociodemographic distribution. *The Journal of Adolescent Health*, *34*(1), 97–103. doi:10.1016/S1054-139X(03)00304-5 PMID:14706412

Burns, J. M., Davenport, T. A., Durkin, L. A., Luscombe, G. M., & Hickie, I. B. (2010). The internet as a setting for mental health service utilisation by young people. *The Medical Journal of Australia*, *192*(11), S22. PMID:20528703

Canadian Attention Deficit Hyperactivity Disorder Resource Alliance (CADDRA). (2011). *Canadian ADHD Practice Guidelines* (3rd ed.). Toronto, Canada: CADDRA.

Christensen, H., Griffiths, K. M., & Evans, K. (2002). e-Mental health in Australia: Implications of the Internet and related technologies for policy. Canberra: Commonwealth Department of Health and Ageing Canberra.

Christensen, H., & Hickie, I. B. (2010). E-mental health: A new era in delivery of mental health services. *The Medical Journal of Australia*, *192*(11), S2. PMID:20528702

Christensen, H., & Petrie, K. (2013). Information technology as the key to accelerating advances in mental health care. *The Australian and New Zealand Journal of Psychiatry*, *47*(2), 114–116. doi:10.1177/0004867412471088 PMID:23382508

Christensen, H., Proudfoot, J., Andrews, G., Klein, B., Kavanagh, D., O'Neil, D., . . . Graham, K. (2009). *E-mental health: a 2020 vision and strategy for Australia*. Academic Press.

Creswell, J. W. (2013). *Research design: Qualitative, quantitative, and mixed methods approaches* (4th ed.). London: Sage Publications, Incorporated.

Cummings, E., & Borycki, E. M. (2011). *Grounded Theory Evolution and Its Application in Health Informatics*. Paper presented at the ITCH.

Department of Human Services Victoria. (n.d.). *Attention deficit hyperactivity disorder - adults*. Retrieved from http://www.betterhealth.vic.gov.au/bhcv2/bhcarticles.nsf/pages/Attention_deficit_hyperactivity_disorder_and_adults#

Depeoulu, A. O. (2010). College Students With ADHD: Prescriptive Concepts for Best Practices in Career Development. *Journal of Career Development*.

Eisenhardt, K. M. (1989). Building theories from case study research. *Academy of Management Review*, *14*(4), 532–550.

Eysenbach, G. (2001). What is e-health? *Journal of Medical Internet Research*, *3*(2), e20. doi:10.2196/jmir.3.2.e20 PMID:11720962

Fischer, M., Barkley, R. A., Edelbrock, C. S., & Smallish, L. (1990). The adolescent outcome of hyperactive children diagnosed by research criteria: II. Academic, attentional, and neuropsychological status. *Journal of Consulting and Clinical Psychology, 58*(5), 580–588. doi:10.1037/0022-006X.58.5.580 PMID:2254504

Gevensleben, H., Holl, B., Albrecht, B., Vogel, C., Schlamp, D., Kratz, O., & Heinrich, H. et al. (2009). Is neurofeedback an efficacious treatment for ADHD? A randomised controlled clinical trial. *Journal of Child Psychology and Psychiatry, and Allied Disciplines, 50*(7), 780–789. doi:10.1111/j.1469-7610.2008.02033.x PMID:19207632

Glaser, B., & Strauss, A. (1967). *The discovery of grounded theory: strategies for qualitative research.* New York: Aldine.

Grenwald-Mayes, G. (2001). Relationship between current quality of life and family of origin dynamics for college students with attention-deficit/hyperactivity disorder. *Journal of Attention Disorders, 5*(4), 211–222. doi:10.1177/108705470100500403 PMID:11967477

Gropper, R. J., & Tannock, R. (2009). A pilot study of working memory and academic achievement in college students with ADHD. *Journal of Attention Disorders, 12*(6), 574–581. doi:10.1177/1087054708320390 PMID:19380519

Heiligenstein, E., Greta Guenther Msn, M. S., Levy, A., Savino, F. P., & Fulwiler, J. P. (1999). Psychological and academic functioning in college students with attention deficit hyperactivity disorder. *Journal of American College Health, 47*(4), 181–185. doi:10.1080/07448489909595644 PMID:9919849

Heiligenstein, E., & Keeling, R. P. (1995). Presentation of unrecognized attention deficit hyperactivity disorder in college students. *Journal of American College Health, 43*(5), 226–228. doi:10.1080/07448 481.1995.9940481 PMID:7499637

Johnson, B., & Christensen, L. (2008). *Qualitative Research Educational research: Quantitative, qualitative, and mixed approaches* (3rd ed.). London: Sage.

Jorm, A. F., Wright, A., & Morgan, A. J. (2007). Where to seek help for a mental disorder? *The Medical Journal of Australia, 187*(10), 556–560. PMID:18021042

Kaltenthaler, E., Brazier, J., De Nigris, E., Tumur, I., Ferriter, M., Beverley, C., & Sutcliffe, P. A. et al. (2006). Computerised cognitive behaviour therapy for depression and anxiety update: A systematic review and economic evaluation. *Health Technology Assessment, 10*(33), 1–186. doi:10.3310/hta10330 PMID:16959169

Khawaja, N. G., & Dempsey, J. (2008). A comparison of international and domestic tertiary students in Australia. *Australian Journal of Guidance & Counselling, 18*(1), 30–46. doi:10.1375/ajgc.18.1.30

Klingberg, T., Fernell, E., Olesen, P. J., Johnson, M., Gustafsson, P., Dahlström, K., & Westerberg, H. et al. (2005). Computerized training of working memory in children with ADHD-A randomized, controlled trial. *Journal of the American Academy of Child and Adolescent Psychiatry, 44*(2), 177–186. doi:10.1097/00004583-200502000-00010 PMID:15689731

Lahey, K. (2003). *The cost of dropping out: The economic impact of early school leaving.* Australia: Business Council of Australia.

Lansbergen, M., van Dongen-Boomsma, M., Buitelaar, J., & Slaats-Willemse, D. (2011). ADHD and EEG-neurofeedback: A double-blind randomized placebo-controlled feasibility study. *Journal of Neural Transmission, 118*(2), 275–284. doi:10.1007/s00702-010-0524-2 PMID:21165661

Lapan, S. D., Quartaroli, M. T., & Riemer, F. J. (2011). *Qualitative research: An introduction to methods and designs* (Vol. 37). Wiley.com.

Mannuzza, S., Klein, R. G., Bessler, A., Malloy, P., & LaPadula, M. (1998). Adult psychiatric status of hyperactive boys grown up. *The American Journal of Psychiatry, 155*(4), 493–498. doi:10.1176/ajp.155.4.493 PMID:9545994

Mayes, S. D., Calhoun, S. L., & Crowell, E. W. (2000). Learning Disabilities and ADHD Overlapping Spectrum Disorders. *Journal of Learning Disabilities, 33*(5), 417–424. doi:10.1177/002221940003300502 PMID:15495544

Meaux, J. B., Green, A., & Broussard, L. (2009). ADHD in the college student: A block in the road. *Journal of Psychiatric and Mental Health Nursing, 16*(3), 248–256. doi:10.1111/j.1365-2850.2008.01349.x PMID:19291153

Meho, L. I. (2006). E-mail interviewing in qualitative research: A methodological discussion. *Journal of the American Society for Information Science and Technology, 57*(10), 1284–1295. doi:10.1002/asi.20416

Moumtzoglou, A. (2011). E-Health: A Bridge to People-Centered Health Care. *E-health Systems Quality and Reliability: Models and Standards, 47.*

Murphy, K. R., Barkley, R. A., & Bush, T. (2002). Young adults with attention deficit hyperactivity disorder: Subtype differences in comorbidity, educational, and clinical history. *The Journal of Nervous and Mental Disease, 190*(3), 147–157. doi:10.1097/00005053-200203000-00003 PMID:11923649

O'Brien, J. (2011). *Revenue up despite drop-off in international students.* Retrieved from http://www-public.jcu.edu.au/news/current/JCU_101879

Prevatt, F., Lampropoulos, G. K., Bowles, V., & Garrett, L. (2011). The use of between session assignments in ADHD coaching with college students. *Journal of Attention Disorders, 15*(1), 18–27. doi:10.1177/1087054709356181 PMID:20019381

Puffenberger, S. S. (2011). *The Efficacy of Working Memory Training for Children and Adolescents with Attention-Deficit/Hyperactivity Disorder-Combined type compared to Children and Adolescents with Attention-Deficit/Hyperactivity Disorder-Primarily Inattentive type.* Ohio State University.

Quinn, J. A., Reardon, D. A., Friedman, A. H., Rich, J. N., Sampson, J. H., & Provenzale, J. M. et al.. (2003). Phase II trial of temozolomide in patients with progressive low-grade glioma. *Journal of Clinical Oncology, 21*(4), 646–651. doi:10.1200/JCO.2003.01.009 PMID:12586801

Quinn, P. O. (2001). *ADD and the college student: A guide for high school and college students with attention deficit disorde.* Washington, DC: Magination Press.

Ramsay, J. R. (2012). "Without a Net" CBT Without Medications for an Adult With ADHD. *Clinical Case Studies*, *11*(1), 48–65. doi:10.1177/1534650112440741

Reynolds, J., Griffiths, K., & Christensen, H. (2011). Anxiety and depression-online resources and management tools. *Australian Family Physician*, *40*(6), 382. PMID:21655483

Safren, S. A., Otto, M. W., Sprich, S., Winett, C. L., Wilens, T. E., & Biederman, J. (2005). Cognitive-behavioral therapy for ADHD in medication-treated adults with continued symptoms. *Behaviour Research and Therapy*, *43*(7), 831–842. doi:10.1016/j.brat.2004.07.001 PMID:15896281

Soy, S. (1997). *The case study as a research method: Uses and users of Information–LIS 391D*. Unpublished.

Stake, R. E. (1995). *The art of case study research*. Academic Press.

Swartz, S. L., Prevatt, F., & Proctor, B. E. (2005). A coaching intervention for college students with Attention Deficit/Hyperactivity Disorder. *Psychology in the Schools*, *42*(6), 647–656. doi:10.1002/pits.20101

The Royal Australian College of Physicians. (2009). *Australian Guidelines on Attention Deficit Hyperactivity Disorder (ADHD) (draft)*. Canberra, NH: MRC.

Tuckman, A. (2009). *More attention, less deficit success strategies for adults with ADHD*. Plantation, FL: Specialty Press.

Wallace, B. A., & Winsler, A., & NeSmith, P. (1999). Factors Associated with Success for College Students with ADHD: Are Standard Accommodations Helping? Wang, J.-R., & Hsieh, S. (2013). Neurofeedback training improves attention and working memory performance. *Clinical Neurophysiology*.

Wender, P. H., Wolf, L. E., & Wasserstein, J. (2001). Adults with ADHD. *Annals of the New York Academy of Sciences*, *931*(1), 1–16. doi:10.1111/j.1749-6632.2001.tb05770.x PMID:11462736

Westerberg, H., Jacobaeus, H., Hirvikoski, T., Clevberger, P., Östensson, M.-L., Bartfai, A., & Klingberg, T. (2007). Computerized working memory training after stroke-A pilot study. *Brain Injury: [BI]*, *21*(1), 21–29. doi:10.1080/02699050601148726 PMID:17364516

Whittaker, R., Merry, S., Stasiak, K., McDowell, H., Doherty, I., Shepherd, M., & Rodgers, A. et al. (2012). MEMO—A mobile phone depression prevention intervention for adolescents: Development process and postprogram findings on acceptability from a randomized controlled trial. *Journal of Medical Internet Research*, *14*(1), e13. doi:10.2196/jmir.1857 PMID:22278284

Wickramasinghe, N., Geisler, E., & Schaffer, J. (2005). *Assessing e-health. E-Health Systems Diffusion and Use: The Innovation, the User and the USE IT model*. Hershey, PA: Idea Group.

Wickramasinghe, N., & Misra, S. K. (2004). A wireless trust model for healthcare. *International Journal of Electronic Healthcare*, *1*(1), 60–77. doi:10.1504/IJEH.2004.004658 PMID:18048204

Wickramasinghe, N. S., Fadlalla, A. M. A., Geisler, E., & Schaffer, J. L. (2005). A framework for assessing e-health preparedness. *International Journal of Electronic Healthcare*, *1*(3), 316–334. doi:10.1504/IJEH.2005.006478 PMID:18048213

Wilens, T. E., Adler, L. A., Adams, J., Sgambati, S., Rotrosen, J., Sawtelle, R., & Fusillo, S. et al. (2008). Misuse and diversion of stimulants prescribed for ADHD: A systematic review of the literature. *Journal of the American Academy of Child and Adolescent Psychiatry, 47*(1), 21–31. doi:10.1097/chi.0b013e31815a56f1 PMID:18174822

Wilens, T. E., McDermott, S. P., Biederman, J., Abrantes, A., Hahesy, A., & Spencer, T. J. (1999). Cognitive therapy in the treatment of adults with ADHD: A systematic chart review of 26 cases. *Journal of Cognitive Psychotherapy, 13*(3), 215–226.

Wolf, L. E. (2001). College students with ADHD and other hidden disabilities. *Annals of the New York Academy of Sciences, 931*(1), 385–395. doi:10.1111/j.1749-6632.2001.tb05792.x PMID:11462755

Yin, R. K. (2002). *Case Study Research: Design and Methods*. SAGE Publications.

Yin, R. K. (2009). *Case study research: Design and methods* (Vol. 5). Sage.

KEY TERMS AND DEFINITIONS

Complementary and Alternative Medicine (CAM): CAM refers to a broad set of healthcare practices that are not part of a country's dominant healthcare system. They are used interchangeably with the main healthcare system medicine in some country. For example, acupuncture is used to help easing side effects of cancer treatment.

Cupping: Cupping therapy dates back to ancient Egyptian, Chinese, and Middle Eastern cultures. This treatment creates a local suction on the skin. Practitioners believe this mobilizes blood flow in order to promote healing. Suction is created using heat (fire) or mechanical devices (hand or electrical pumps).

Electronic Medical Record (EMR): An EMR is a digital version of a paper chart that contains all of a patient's medical history from one practice. An EMR is mostly used by providers for diagnosis and treatment.

Inquiring Systems: Charles West Churchman defines inquiry as an activity that produces knowledge. He examines the epistemologies of five schools of philosophy from the perspective of general systems theory, asking the question as to whether each is suitable as the basis for the design of computer-based "inquiring systems." He describes five inquiring systems which later helped form the basis for the design of knowledge management systems and Information System.

Moxibustion: A Chinese medicine therapy using moxa made from dried mugwort (Artemisia argyi - an herbaceous perennial plant with a creeping rhizome). Suppliers usually age the mugwort and grind it up to a fluff. Practitioners burn the fluff or process it further into a cigar-shaped stick. They can use it indirectly, with acupuncture needles, or burn it on the patient's skin.

Qigong: An ancient Chinese health care system that integrates physical postures, breathing techniques and focused intention. Qigong practice typically involves moving meditation, coordinating slow flowing movement, deep rhythmic breathing, and calm meditative state of mind.

Tuina (Chinese Remedial Massage): Tui Na uses rhythmic compression along energy channels of the body, as well as a variety of techniques that manipulate and lubricate the joints. The practitioner may brush, knead, roll/press and rub the areas of the joints.

Chapter 6
Radio Frequency Identification Technology in an Australian Regional Hospital:
An Innovation Translation Experience with ANT

Chandana Unnithan
Victoria University, Australia

Arthur Tatnall
Victoria University, Australia

ABSTRACT

Australian hospitals had begun exploring Radio Frequency Identification, a wireless automatic identification and data capture technology for improving the quality of their services towards the end of 2000s. After many an unsuccessful pilots, a breakthrough for large hospitals came in 2010, with a key learning rendered by a large regional hospital that not only experimented with the technology, but also have made it all pervasive in their operations. In this chapter, we present the case study, through an innovation translation perspective, focusing on the socio-technical factors captured through elements of Actor-Network Theory.

INTRODUCTION

Healthcare has become a large part of expenditure in Australia, as in the case with many economies (Wamba, Anand & Carter, 2013). Using the Organisation for Economic Co-operation and Development's (OECD) methods, in 2011–12, Australia's health expenditure to GDP ratio was marginally above average compared with other OECD countries (AIHW, 2014). In 2010, the overall private and public spending on health was estimated at about 10% of the country's GDP or approximately about A\$ 65,000 million in annual spending (GS1-Australia, 2010). In 2011-12, A\$ 140.2 billion was spent on health, which is

DOI: 10.4018/978-1-4666-9446-0.ch006

approximately 1.7 times higher in real terms (inflation adjusted) than in 2001-02 or expenditure has increased from A\$ 4,276 per person in 2001-02 to A\$ 6,230 in 2011-12 (AIHW, 2014).

Amongst the main stakeholders in Healthcare are large hospitals, which are trying to influence policies and governments to leverage the effective use of Information Communication Technologies (ICTs) to enable better quality of service (Payton et al, 2011). In the last decade, radio frequency identification (RFID) technology has captured the interest of hospitals worldwide (Ngai et al., 2009, Oztekin et al, 2010). Considered as a non-disruptive, open innovation, it is a technology that enables wireless automatic identification and data capture (Fosso Wamba et al., 2008, Foss Wamba, 2011).

RFID offers an improved means of reducing errors in patient care, such as adverse drug effects, allergies, patient–medication mismatches and medication dosage errors (Tu et al., 2009). Conversely, it promotes better management of critical healthcare assets (e.g., infusion pumps, wheelchairs) by enabling real-time identification, tracking and tracing (Bendavid et al., 2010). The capabilities of RFID technology have resulted in its potential to create value in health care (Dominguez-Péry et al., 2011). For example, (Najera et al., 2011) purports that the technology can enable healthcare stakeholders to monitor all steps related to the patient blood collection and transfusion process. This may include the identification of blood bags at the collection point, the tracking and tracing of products from the collection point to the hospital, and blood transfusion to a dedicated patient.

The value of RFID in the market rose from US\$ 5.63 billion in 2010, to almost US\$ 5.84 billion in 2011 (Das and Harrop, 2011). According to Pleshek (2011), there were approximately 150 million RFID tags in use within healthcare worldwide. It is no doubt, evident that the technology has high operational efficiencies and strategic potential in healthcare for improvement of quality services. A research conducted by Fosso Wamba et al (2013) found that the highest number of published research focuses on the technology issues of implementing RFID in hospitals (39.27%) . The research also found that organisational issues, focused on finance, was 37.24%, followed by data management, security and privacy issues that constituted 23.48%. These results are indicative of the fact that the focus is still remaining on the technical issues regarding RFID implementation, even in the year 2013.

Technical issues in implementing RFID had remained the main focus in many Australian hospitals (Unnithan and Tatnall, 2014). While adoption of this mobile technology has been investigated over a decade in hospitals (Coustasse et al., 2013), the focus is on using economic models (Yao, Chu and Li (2012) that try to explore the cost-benefits of the technology in relation to its rate of adoption. Conversely, RFID had only begun to be explored in Australian hospitals (Chowdhry & Khosla, 2007) since 2006, typically with vendor driven implementations that suited the cost-benefit analysis of hospitals (Chen, Wu, Su, & Yang, 2008; Unnithan and Tatnall, 2014).

In this chapter, we present the experience of a regional hospital in Australia, which focused on visualizing socio-technical factors that seem germane for the effective translation of RFID into hospital operations, through elements of Actor-Network Theory (ANT). This hospital has successfully jump-started the innovation translation of RFID in the regional public hospitals, while many pilots had been rendered unsuccessful.

HEALTHCARE CONTEXT IN AUSTRALIA

Prior to 2001, Australian health context was slow in adopting technologies in hospitals (Whetton, 2005; Duckett, 2007). As technologies had evolved over decades with patchy funding from government, hospitals had legacy systems that did not integrate or rather 'talk to each other'. It was in the decade 2001-2010 that technology refreshments had begun to occur in earnest, with the imminent national health records system (Muhammed, Teo & Wickramasinghe, 2012). Towards 2010, with the joint efforts of organisations such as Health Informatics Society of Australia (HISA, 2014), National E-health Transition Authority of Australia (NeHTA, 2014) and the Australasian College of Health Informatics (ACHI, 2014), hospitals in Australia had begun ardently testing and deploying technologies that would improve their quality of services to patients.

As Ho (2012) indicated, the demand for increased access to high-quality health care, an ageing population, shortage of clinicians in the regional areas, and increasing budgetary pressures have an impact on regional hospitals in particular. Two of the largest issues these hospitals face are enhancing worker productivity and reducing human error (Ho, 2012).

RFID IN AUSTRALIAN HOSPITALS

In Australia, health care is heavily affected by privacy regulations (Privacy Act of Australia 1988; Privacy.Gov 2013). While privacy and legal procedures do receive attention in many nations (for example, Fisher & Monahan point out that HIPAA significantly affects technology implementation, as well as health sector compliance in the USA), in Australia, the Privacy Act is more formidable (Privacy Act of Australia 1988, 2013). Often it is so doctrinaire that any data regarding an adult patient is not even provided to parents, unless they are named as carers, and if the patients are unable to handle themselves. This poses significant difficulties in emergencies, when an adult may be in perfectly good health, but not in a capacity to care about himself or herself at the time. Yet, the details of a condition may not even be immediately revealed to close relations (Duckett & Wilcox 2011).

In such restrictive conditions affecting the health sector, a piece of technology, such as RFID with its surveillance potential, was unacceptable in its original form to Australian hospitals. They had to be compliant with the existing privacy laws and standards. If not, perhaps similar to the USA (Fisher & Monahan 2008), organisations such as the nurse's union would have taken action and protested over the surveillance of people. Additional to this problem is the privacy of patients or individuals who may be moved using a wheelchair tagged by RFID.

The health care sector in Australia has received much attention from the government from the beginning of 2000s (Crompton 2002), when subsequent Productivity Commission (2005, 2006) reports recommended significant introductions of technologies in hospitals to improve processes. The National Health and Reforms Commission (2009) argued in favour of introducing technologies to improve efficiencies in the health sector. Novak and Judah (2011) suggest that the agenda for boosting productivity in the health sector is in progress. However, it may be noted that in the process of implementing technology agendas, state governments have to implement the policies and reforms enacted by the federal parliament (Gabbitas & Jeffs 2007; Goss 2008). In this continuum, many experiments occur. Often there are significant failures of implemented systems (Ducket & Willcox 2011). For example, the state of Victoria (Hopewell 2012) experimented with the HealthSmart system for refreshing technologies in hospitals; this was eventually cancelled being out of scope and overbudget. In the process, many new technologies were introduced, causing a lack of interoperability with existing systems and adding new ones (Dunlevy 2013).

RFID, as an innovation, was still being trialled towards the end of the 2000s, and was not yet fully accepted as a standard way of asset-tracking in hospitals. As Australian hospitals were on the pathway to e-health records at a national level, many large hospitals paused their proposed systems implementation projects, including RFID (Duckett & Wilcox 2011). An early report of RFID-enabled functions in Australia by Bacheldor (2006), reported that the Rockhampton Base Hospital in Queensland, Australia, used RFID to improve nurse safety in mental health ward buildings. Specifically, nurses in the hospital's mental health ward were using 'alarm cards, which combined a long-range wireless duress transmitter, a photo ID and proximity access control in one credit-card size device. The duress transmitter featured a battery-powered RFID tag. Any nurses in danger or in need of assistance pushed a button built into the back of the card, causing the transmitter to send a signal to an RFID reader, alerting co-workers. To make the process convenient, nurses received the cards when they signed in at the beginning of their shifts; the tag's unique ID numbers correlate in a database with the nurses' names and photos.

Chowdhury and Khosla (2007) provided an overview of the main components of an RFID-based patient management system, based on a model built for hospitals in Australian context. They argued that hospitals could track patients accurately and efficiently, improve the safety of clients by capturing basic data such as drug allergies, and prevent and reduce medical errors, as well as build a more collaborative environment with varied departments such as wards, medication and payments. Many pilot implementations, such as those at RMH and Barwon Health in Victoria (and others in Western Australia and Queensland) were introduced for not only asset-tracking but also patient tracking (infants, geriatrics & mentally disabled). However, most of these pilots did not result in full-scale implementation, or implementation was restricted to certain critical-care areas (Chowdhry & Khosla 2007).

Royal Adelaide Hospital in South Australia partnered with technology specialist Visionstream to deploy an integrated wireless network that combines tagging and tracking functionality to manage patient intake and care, as well as track availability of health care equipment throughout the hospital. The project is designed in conjunction with the South Australian government's new model of health care, which focuses on using technology to enable safe care solutions, reducing time spent on administration and increasing clinician-patient time (RFID 2012).

INNOVATION TRANSLATION AND ANT

In a systematics review of literature from 2002-2012, there was a gap that existed regarding socio-technical issues that impeded the successful translation of RFID into hospitals. Seminal work of academics as they reviewed RFID in the decade (Fisher & Monahan 2008; Roark & Miguel 2006; Hoskins 2006; Yao et al., 2012; Coustasse et al., 2013) pointed to mainly technical and economic issues relating to RFID, de-emphasising social and legal issues. Despite Australian hospitals piloting the technology towards the end of the decade, unsuccessful and abandoned examples persisted. Overall, research was still emerging regarding socio-technical issues in RFID adoption, even in 2013. RFID in Australia not only needed to be adopted widely, combatting all the interoperability and privacy issues, but also needed to be customised into this context, to be widely accepted. Rather, it was an innovation in the health sector that needed to 'translate' or become part of the context. Set in this premise, we explored the conceptual framework of 'innovation translation'.

Table 1. Questions for Moments of Translation

1.	**Problematisation:** What are the benefits defined by actors while introducing RFID? What are the roles of actors? What is the obligatory passage point?
2.	**Interessement:** How did the champions of RFID negotiate with other actors to establish and extend their network? How did they get others interested?
3.	**Enrolment:** Did key actors coerce, influence or impose on others to enrol them into the network of RFID acceptance?
4.	**Mobilisation:** Has the RFID solution/s gained wider acceptance? How was this achieved?

Callon (1986:196) outlined this novel approach to the study of power, the 'sociology of translation' using four moments of translation. We drew from this seminal work to build the conceptual framework, described as follows.

Moment 1: *Problematisation* is where key actors define the issues that RFID proposes to address in the hospital and their roles. The issue being addressed is 'translated' in terms of solutions offered by all actors, who then attempt to establish themselves as an 'obligatory passage point' (OPP) (Callon 1986), which must be negotiated as part of the solution. In other words, Callon (1986) refers to an OPP that has to occur for all the actors to satisfy the interests attributed to them by the focal actor. In this situation, we identified the actors, the issues they define and their defined roles. The idea of this *moment* is to foster relationships, to allocate or reallocate power between actors.

Moment 2: *Interessement* is whereby the actors defined in Moment one impose the identities and roles defined on other actors, thus building a network of relationships where all actors become involved. In this context, we studied how the champions or key actors negotiate with others in the network. *Interessement* is the set of actions by which an entity attempts to impose and stabilise the identities of actors in the same network for problematisation (Callon 1986). It involves a process of convincing other actors to accept the solution proposed. The actors are engaged in the process of confirming the OPP.

Moment 3: *Enrolment* occurs after the success of Moment 2, when a process of coercion, seduction and consent leads to the establishment of stable alliances. In this situation, we studied how the actors enrolled others into accepting the solution of RFID. More specifically, did they coerce, impose or influence others into enrolment? *Enrolment* involves consolidation of alliances through negotiations. It is the successful outcome of the first two moments.

Moment 4: *Mobilisation* occurs when the solution gains wider acceptance. In this situation, RFID gains wider acceptance as a solution for the proposed reason, within the hospital context. We investigated if this has occurred and how. *Mobilisation* of allies is a set of methods used to represent the group effectively or in other words 'who speaks for whom'? (Callon 1986) While some actors are used as initiators, others become spokespersons. This moment leads to stabilisation of the network. The questions we posed for eliciting the answers posed by these moments were as shown in Table 1.

The process of translation through the four moments may also be called a process of negotiation (Muhammad, Moghimi, Taylor, Redley, Nguyen, Stein, Kent, Botti & Wickramasinghe 2013). We considered a novel approach of visualising the data through a lens informed by ANT. Specifically, the

Table 2. ANT Depiction of Actors (Human and Non-Human) and Case Site

Actors/ Blackboxes	Name	Details (Non-Human Actors Have Been Given a Voice by a Human Actor)
Blackboxes	Regional hospital	The site where RFID entered into the context and has propagated successfully
	New Site	The new site of the regional hospital under construction
Non-Human Actors	DHS (Department of Health Services)	The external entity, which funded RFID implementation via a grant
	Symposium article	Voiced by CIO (Past)
	RFID tags/equipment, external entity (includes temperature tags)	Voiced by CIO (past and present)
	RFID results	Voiced by CIO (Current)
	RFID maps	Voiced by CIO (Current)
Considered Non-Human Actors	Nursing staff/orderlies	Voiced/represented by CIO in the focus group
	Pathology Food Services Engineering ICU OHS Infection Control	Voiced and represented by CIO (1) and CIO (2), Deputy Pharmacist
Human Actors	CIO (1) (The Champion)	The CIO is overall in-charge of all technology-based strategic decisions and drove the cause of RFID; the Godfather of RFID, who launched its career
	CIO (2) (reigning champion or current CIO—named as CIO)	This CIO was earlier the deputy head of ICT, second in command to the CIO; he is currently the CIO and also the champion of RFID who coaxed all the departments into trialling RFID and was successful
	Deputy Pharmacist	Deputy Head of Pharmacy Operation who drove RFID pioneering and propagation in the focus group
	Simpkin House Head	Voiced by the CIO in the focus group—followed up for confirmation by the Cameo
	Cameos (Researchers)	Researchers conducted direct interviews and focus group through a moderator, who then becomes the voice of cameos.

presentation of interplay between all the factors (actors), while the solution of RFID as a technology was being considered and deployed, could be visualised better using elements of the ANT lens.

Actor-Network Theory (ANT), which was developed in 1980s by Bruno Latour (1986), and Law and Callon (1988), is an attempt to give voice to technical artefacts; they viewed that both social and technical determinism as flawed. ANT offers an advantage over other theories in that it does not have a dividing line between human and non-human entities nor an 'essence' attributed to either (Tatnall 2011). ANT has been applied to implementing and adopting different health care innovation studies (Berg 2001; Hall 2005; Bossen 2007; Cresswell, Worth & Sheikh 2010; Wickramasinghe, Bali, Tatnall, 2012; Muhmmed, Zwicker, Wickramasinghe, 2013).

The use of Actor–Network Theoretical conceptions has been used as a framework in narrating this case study. ANT uses the elements of blackboxes (or hospital/site in this instance), actors (human and non-human stakeholders), their relevant roles and the interplay between them, as the innovation (RFID) translates into the context of the hospital. In this case, RFID itself is considered the key actor (non-human) in this hospital. It debuts as an innovation, translates or 'integrates' itself into the context while re-negotiates the existing network of relationships within the hospital and establishes/sustains its presence, while evolving and emerging as a 'Star' that holds much promise in the future. In other words, RFID technology entered the hospital (blackbox) as a key non-human actor and retained a position while enabling varied networks. In the continuum, it translated or integrated into this blackbox (hospital), transitioning into a more influential actor who has now become the 'Superstar', as it has been accepted as the 'key technology' for the new regional site.

CONTEXT AND PRECIS

The regional hospital in this research is situated in Victoria, in Australia, with more than 3,400 staff and 653 beds. It treats more than 37,000 in-patients annually; deals with more than 45,000 emergency cases and approximately 1,200 births annually. A 60-bed rehabilitation unit, eight-bed intensive care unit and five operating theatres complement the services, where almost 10,000 surgical procedures are performed annually. The organisation provides services in emergency, maternity, women's health, medical imaging, pathology, rehabilitation, community services, residential aged-care, psychiatric care, community dental, hospice, palliative care, cardiology, cancer services and renal dialysis.

In July 2010, the hospital began to roll out a Wi-Fi-based solution to manage the flow of patients through its surgical wards (Friedlos 2010). In 2011, it expanded the use of the system to include the temperature monitoring of pharmaceuticals and blood supplies, and a staff safety system for doctors and nurses. The system operates on a standard Wi-Fi network and utilises RFID tags and Real Time Location Systems (RTLS) software, as the hospital received funding to install Wi-Fi in its surgical theatre. Initially, the hospital wanted to obtain better real-time data regarding theatre and staff utilisation in its perioperative suite, which handles up to 10,000 surgical procedures annually. Upon arrival in the surgical theatre, orthopaedic patients are given a tag that provides information on the patients' location and movements, thereby enabling staff members to ensure that scheduled procedures start on time and that patients receive proper care.

The system collects data as it follows a patient's journey through theatre, from the admissions area to the waiting area to the theatre complex and the anaesthetic bay. This allows for business decisions to be merged into the complex flow of staff and resources to the perioperative suite. It was expected that the hospital would be able to process patients through the surgery more efficiently and use resources better. The system operates on the hospital's existing unified wireless network with access points throughout the hospital that act as RFID interrogators. This aspect resulted in a lower total cost of ownership for the hospital. The system utilises active tags, which are 802.11-compliant and operate at 2.4 GHz. Information is transmitted from the tags across the Wi-Fi network to MobileView software from AeroScout, which can be accessed by all employees on any computer monitor (Friedlos, 2010)

This regional hospital effectively gathered market information from the cases of failures in RFID implementation, while the technology was still evolving. In 2010, medical grade tags had evolved and technology costs had become lower. However, within the Australian health sector, interoperability issues and the strong resistance from hospital staff (particularly orderlies and nurses) was still impeding the innovation translation of this technology. It was at this time, the first author (and primary researcher) had met with the CIO of the hospital. A data collection ensued over a 2 year period with unstructured interviews including 2 CIOs, who succeeded each other (and worked together), and the department representatives in a focus group facilitated by a moderator.

FINDINGS AND DISCUSSION

Problematisation

We analysed the findings using the questions as follows:

What are the benefits perceived to be achieved by key actors while introducing RFID? What are the roles of the actors? What is the Obligatory Passage Point?

The case of RFID was introduced into this hospital via a pilot in 2010. However, a full-scale RFID implementation in the theatres/emergency area did not occur. The rationale is evident from the following excerpt:

HealthSmart in Victoria did not approve to send HL7 messages to iPM to enter data into the PAS in real time, and therefore, the project was abandoned, as efficiency was minimal. A nurse had to still physically enter details and be present throughout the patient journey, in addition to using the RFID system…The nurses accepted it at the beginning but—after six months they said, 'you've had a good trial, we don't need to do this any more, use the tags for something else', which is what we did, we just repurposed them and used them for something else, they weren't lost or anything…

Further probes into the situation revealed that RFID tags were repurposed for the ICU and related areas. Specifically, the initial problem was 'tracking the patient journey' in the orthopaedic surgeries. The problem owners were nurses. In the re-problematisation, the problem was owned by the ICU department, driven by nurses as the head of the department. Although it is a different department, nurse remained the problem owner. The solution owner did not change in this case; RFID was simply re-purposed. The problem was to track assets in the ICU using RFID (the OPP):

Asset management and some of them have actually gone up to the ICU for the bed tracking… …high-value assets are tracked…Computers on wheels, ICU beds, emergency resuscitation equipment—it all came back from the fact that after Emergency Dept had their little rework last year, there was a $30,000 piece of equipment that no one could find anywhere—it had been submerged somewhere during the refit.

Clearly, a *re-problematisation* moment was visible. The benefits of RFID were realised not only by nurses who recommended that it be repurposed (almost six months after the trial), but ICU staff also accepted it. Two different departments—namely OHS and Infection Control—had to be involved in the trial, as it was a requirement. Thus, the tracking of equipment using RFID passed the OPP with a set of new actors. Then we discovered that RFID had taken another role in the hospital. Accidentally, a new form of tags—namely temperature tags that could monitor the temperature of equipment such as fridges—came into the hospital.

The supplier gave it to us…threw a box of temperature tags…said 'here have temperature tag to play with as well'…Well, once we got it and put it in the first fridge and found the fridge was faulty…results of this simple exercise was brilliant. We then went to Pharmacy and said 'would you like to be able to give a five-minute result on all your fridges?' and they said, 'yes, thank you'

The CIO and his team had taken the temperature tags concept to Pharmacy for a trial, outlining its benefits.

CIO: *… RFID tags to all pharmacy fridges were deployed. Data was logged in real time at five-minute intervals, which then set alarms to notify the Pharmacy when temperature varied outside a pre-set range. This data was then used to identify fault fridges. This project was successful.*

Pharmacist: *Wi-Fi gave us ability to set alarms, ability to have real-time monitoring…saved us at least a couple of hours a work week. Now, we get reports once a week and look at them, but if we get any alarms, basically we follow them up.*

There is a new problematisation moment visible here. Obviously, the two key actors here are the CIO and head of Pharmacy, who saw a clear benefit in the temperature tags. The Pharmacy decided to take up the trial, which was successful, and it decided to implement temperature tagging using RFID, which herein is the OPP. Problematisation was initiated by the CIO here and driven by Pharmacy (users), and the OPP was to use the RFID temperature tags to monitor temperatures.

Then we chanced upon the fact that 'staff tagging' had occurred to monitor staff duress in the high-care and mental health facility of the hospital. Upon exploring this further, we became aware that it was introduced by customising the regular RFID tracking tags that were used for patients and equipment, and were worn by staff. Thus, another problematisation moment was revealed. The key actors for problematisation were the OHS and ICT departments:

The OHS department had an audit…they needed a solution for managing staff duress. And there was also an incident. A theatre cleaner had a heart attach in the middle of the night and no one came running. So before he came back to work as part of his OH&S plan, they needed a process to be able to prevent further recurrence of being isolated.

It was evident that the problematisation occurred with the key actors planning to use RFID tags for staff in high-care facilities in order to reduce staff duress and isolation. The staff tagging using wearable RFID tags were fitted with a button that could trigger alarms elsewhere (the OPP). The problematisation moments continued to re-occur throughout the year.

Interessement

How did the champions of RFID negotiate with other actors to establish and extend their network? How did they get others interested?

It appeared that there was an interest among theatre nurses in a white paper from the US that discussed surgeons causing the delay in attending to patients from surgery by tracking the patient journey using RFID. The CIO indicated that in Australia, to track delays in attending to patients, the situation had to be handled differently. Specifically, if surgeons felt that their productivity was being tracked, that would raise privacy issues, and unions would also enter the fray. The following excerpt is relevant.

CIO: *... you can't tell surgeons they're the delay, so they ended up putting a big display board up, which tracked the patients through and after...so the surgeons could sit there and say, 'Hmm, there's a patient there waiting, and they're waiting for me—maybe I should be doing something, yes'. If someone is sat in the holding bay for a period of time...or say 10 patients are in the holding bay, alarms could be set up.*

The nurses who went into RFID tracking became interested by the white paper, which could monitor clinician productivity. Conversely, clinicians in Australia, who could not be tracked or monitored by law, were implicitly driven into interessement, as they could visualise the patients in the waiting bay. The CIO and the ICT department were consulted on this, and they felt that that they could improve efficiencies by facilitating RFID deployment. Thus, the ICT area became interested.

At another time, the conversation with the CIO revealed how the ICU became really interested in RFID tagging:

The biomedical people, we'd given them a little taste...tracked a few of their fusion pumps. When they go to do a service on the fusion pumps it can take them three and a half to four weeks to locate them all—they loved the fact that they can press a button and at least find four of them in a minute and a half. So they're quite happy to go down the 'yes let's tag everything' path because it saves them a lot of time. And we use the simplest interface—just have a webpage that shows you a picture of where they are ...

Thus, RFID was able to capture the attention and interest of related areas of emergency, namely ICU and wards. The champions of RFID were the CIO, his team and the pharmacist. The success of the Pharmacy area was shown to Pathology, which then became interested. In this case, it is the user (pharmacist, regarded in this investigation as clinical staff or equivalent to nurses).

CIO: *We mentioned the success of Pharmacy to Pathology. They decided to install tags for fridges, including sub-zero freezers.*

Subsequently, Food Services began using temperature tags for monitoring cabinet temperatures...it worked too.

Engineering...once they saw it in place and saw the results, they thought 'this is a good idea, we'll buy some of them ourselves'

Thus, it can be seen that multiple departments—Pharmacy, Pathology and Food Services—became interested in the concept, influenced initially by Pharmacy and enabled by the CIO/ICT department. The important fact is that each department saw the results from the earlier departments and subsequently decided to 'go for it'. The ICT department had been the champion, although it had worked indirectly. It was the actual users of the system who propagated and got others interested.

Subsequently, the OHS area was looking for options and negotiated the new tagging with the ICT department. The following quotations revealed that the actual users became interested through the negotiation of the ICT and OHS people. The key element in this conversation was that the CIO was influenced by the residential manager of nursing facilities to push the concept of duress alarms. This residential manager was also a nurse.

CIO: *The earlier residential manager of nursing facilities was pushing the concept of duress alarms at some stage…and here was an option, it works better.*

Subsequently, there was a question raised from the nursing staff about the use of RFID in staff tracking, when the CIO realised that they had the back end for RFID already, so they could make use of it. This resulted in three levels of tracking in high-care facility—namely Wi-Fi tracking, ward tracking as patients move in and out, and room tracking for accurate location. As they already had the RFID tags and Wi-Fi, they therefore had a roaming duress alarm that covered 2–3 areas with just one staff member.

CIO: *… the theatre cleaner had a heart attack and was on the job, and it was a couple of hours before anybody found him. He was quite happy, he was fine, but now he has a tag.*

More important was the fact that nurses recommended it and the staff user became interested because it assisted him to call for help when needed. He felt safe with an RFID tag.

Thus, the interessement was initiated by a nurse and always enabled by the CIO/ICT taking a supportive role; however, being proactive. While the nurses were able to get all other user groups convinced, the CIO/ICT department was also able to convince the pharmacist initially for a different type of tag to monitor temperatures. The pharmacist was also considered a key 'clinical' person in the hospital in charge of trauma fridges, emergency blood etc. Through this person, other related departments, such as Pathology, Food Services and Engineering, became interested. From another viewpoint, the interessement was really through the influence and propagation of nurses, who were also convinced about patient and clinician safety, using duress alarms. Here again, the nurse was the pivotal element in getting all others interested.

Enrolment

Did key actors coerce, influence or impose on others to enrol them into the network of acceptance?

The nurses influenced the decision of enrolment on the ICT department, theatres, nurses and clinicians. The theatre nurses were then responsible for word-of-mouth propagation to the ICU and wards, while the ICT department influenced the BioMed department. Regardless of the influence, it was an important finding that the key actors managed to influence and enrol everyone concerned into the network of acceptance. Specifically, the nurses and orderlies had transformed into the role of influencers for RFID. This transformation was empowering for the actual users of the system, who then continued to propagate it.

The key actors in the second part of the propagation of RFID were the ICT department and the pharmacist. These actors influenced other departments, namely Pathology, Food Services and Engineering, which enrolled into the network of acceptance. The enrolment was assisted by the fact that there was proof or evidence of success available to them, in addition to the word-of-mouth propagation.

CIO: *Pathology followed on from Pharmacy and then in Food Services, we just sort of gave them to them and they said, 'Yes we'll have that' because I had shown the some of the results coming out of Pharmacy.*

… Engineering…were the hardest but once they saw it in place and saw the results, they thought. 'this is a good idea, we'll buy some of them ourselves'…Engineering…have jumped on board…They use them when people complain about air-conditioning, because you can put a tag there and within 24 hours they have a complete history of the temperature within that location.

If it is a the ED trauma fridge—it sends to the Pharmacy alert staff that this alert has been triggered, as well as sending to the ED shift manager, so not only the Pharmacy manager knows about it but the shift manager knows about it and can do something about it, probably before the pharmacy guy can ring the phone and say, 'what's wrong'?

It was evident that not only did the ICT people influence the decision, but the interlinked roles of Pharmacy and emergency nurses being linked together also affected the enrolment process. In an emergency, if blood is required in the operating theatres, the nurse calls for it by connecting to Pathology and Pharmacy (where blood is stored). Keeping the temperature of the fridges correct is a requirement for emergency blood bottles kept in the fridges.

When it came to Food Services and Engineering, it was more the convenience and efficiency gains that drove the enrolment. While Food Services wanted to gain efficiencies through less wastage of food, particularly when it was needed, Engineering was driven by an OHS audit. The OHS area was already in the milieu, having been involved with the first RFID-tracking enrolment. They were looking into maintaining 'location temperatures', and with the RFID tracking of temperature, it was possible to determine whether there was a problem with the equipment, or whether a fan was not working. Thus, four different areas were enrolled based on other departmental experiences.

It was also revealed that the key champions of RFID in the hospital sought a solution that was then recommended by nurses and given to them by the ICT department. The process of enrolment here was through continuous negotiations and influence. The enrolment process was successful, as the key actors were able to influence others into the network of acceptance. It is interesting to note that RFID itself, as a non-human actor, influenced the enrolment decisions.

CIO: *In high-care facilities—their existing duress system…basically a buzzer…makes a horrible noise… that upsets all the patients, so the patients come to see what the noise is and the incident increases. Whereas with the RFID version—they get Jamaica (software) on their phones and it tells them where to go to…basically it tells everybody that you need to know about it exactly where the staff member is when the button is pushed and it continues to track the button until that incident has ceased.*

In summary, the enrolment occurred smoothly, as it propagated through nurses in the first place. In this case, although the ICT/CIO was a strong champion of RFID, he never pushed the technology directly. Rather, he enlisted the nurses and pharmacist, who then propagated the cause of RFID throughout the entire hospital. One important aspect is clear; the nurse was the strongest influencer, or 'the voice', that everyone listened to. The ICT department had succeeded only when it made the nurses the mouthpiece for the cause.

Mobilisation

Has the solution gained wider acceptance? How was this achieved?

It was evident that RFID had already propagated into the hospital widely through the initial involvement of nurses, the OHS department and Infection Control, and supported by the ICT department. By involving a wider set of key actors, including strategists, technologists, medical staff (nurses, orderlies, clinicians), administrative and operations people (OHS, Infection Control), the solution was rapidly gaining a wider audience.

It was evident that the RFID solution was rapidly gaining wider acceptance. The take-up of temperature tags had proliferated into other areas of the hospital; two other departments were considering RFID as a solution for completely different purposes with temperature tagging. Indeed, mobilisation had occurred with temperature RFID tags as also reflected in the CIOs statements.

CIO: ... *So it's expanding—so there's the theatre, there's another facility where there is just one staff member looking after low-care patients that are on their way home basically or going to go into surgery first thing in the morning, there's all of the food service people who work after hours, and it's just been expanded again—there's a ward that only has one staff member over night so that means a tag. We now also have the roaming duress alarm for staff involved in another facility, under maternity. A lot of young mothers come up here to deliver without telling their husbands in Melbourne for particular reasons that they're delivering up here, and the husband usually if he finds out…storms into the place. The reason is usually that there is an intervention order…so staff have to say 'go away'. For instances such as this, staff may be working out of hours…they use a roaming tag…*

Further, RFID had proved itself as a solution that fits in, integrates and is versatile. Minimal training was provided, but users (medical staff including nurses, orderlies, clinicians and administrative staff) did not need much training. The tracking used a web-based system and the tags were wearable and anonymous. Specifically, an RFID tag only had a number and was wearable around the neck. It only traced the person who was wearing it as the number on the day. When the day was over, the tags were returned, and the person could no longer be tracked. No individual names or persons could be stalked using the tags unless they chose to wear it for specific purposes within the hospital. For example, a person working in mental health facilities or a clinician in a highly sensitive area felt safer with a tag that could help him or her find assistance quickly. It was clear that mobilisation had occurred as the solution gained wider acceptance in the CIO's words.

CIO: *It's certainly in our specifications…We'll have the Wi-Fi system set up six months before if we can. And the equipment won't leave the loading bay until it is tagged and on the database…basically the tag will become ubiquitous across the entire hospital, and it's engineered at construction. And with the new electronic patient record, it fits in very—it's one arm of the new patient record—you need to have some form of patient tracking, so the only way to do that is with RFID.*

RFID as a solution assumed many forms, permeated into many departments and completed all moments of translation. The network of acceptance is now stabilised, as the hospital is planning to integrate RFID from the ground level into the architecture of the new building, and also with the e-health records' implementation. RFID has translated into the context of this hospital completely through all moments of translation. The acceptance of the solution across the hospital gained impetus from the onset, as the key users (nurses) recommended it to others. In addition, as the technology itself had advanced in 2010, there were other uses, such as tracking temperature movements, which helped the hospital's major departments, including Pharmacy, Pathology, Food Services and Engineering.

As this hospital had begun with the Wi-Fi infrastructure, it had the advantage of better accuracy in tracking and linking all departments. Conversely, they were also completing the e-health records implementation as recommended by the national government. At the onset, there was support from the government for implementing the technology within the emergency area, which is regarded as a crucial point for any technology take-up. Specifically, if the solution worked in emergency, most medical staff would accept the solution. In this case, that was indeed the experience.

Nurses, who are the key users of the system, instilled confidence in this technology to all other users within the hospital. Thus, it penetrated through to the ICU, wards and related areas. Conversely, the OHS and Infection Control, who were administratively involved with the implementation, also found different uses for RFID, as they were linked in from the beginning. While the nurses recommended and influenced its translation, the ICT department facilitated it.

Conversely, the new avatar of temperature tags that were incidentally left by the technology vendor implicitly found its way into other departments. OHS, which was seeking a solution to address staff duress subsequent to an audit, found a different use to RFID tags (i.e., to assist staff in duress situations by triggering alarms using a tag). A wearable tag is attached with a button that helped lodge the call for assistance without making a noise, which could upset the patients. This aspect of RFID made it beneficial to improve the quality of work processes within the hospital and made it popular among the staff.

Nurses did not find the process as a work intensification, as RFID was originally recommended by them and was well integrated into the hospital systems. Clinicians did not consider it a surveillance technology for monitoring their productivity, as the technology was used to track the patient journey rather than them. Patients in the waiting bay were tracked, and a screen indicated the number of people in the bay. If there was overcrowding in the waiting bay, clinicians could visualise it on the screen, which alerted them to their own duties without ordering them. This subtle persuasion helped to improve the quality of care.

Overall, the medical staff accepted the technology as a helpful solution for improving their workflows. Conversely, the enhancements over the past few years had improved the use of technology and its initial hiccups, making it conducive for hospitals as well. For example, the Wi-Fi infrastructure-based location helped remove additional tracking equipment, and it improved the accuracy of the location. The problematisation moment flowed into a 'closing the loop' each time, with the moment being completed through interessement, enrolment of actors and mobilisation.

By involving all key users of the technology, not only did RFID translate well into the hospital, but it is also gaining wider acceptance. Medical staff who were tagged with an RFID tag felt safer in high-care and certain areas where their safety was under threat. Clinicians did not feel monitored (which would have been against the privacy law in Australia), as they were not tagged. Rather, patients in the bay on a monitor indicated indirectly to them that their attention was needed. The hospital had thus found a way around the privacy implications in Australia. Further, by making the paramedical and other staff feel safer (rather than being monitored), they also worked around the potential union problems that could have emerged. The success of this hospital is the way in which RFID was introduced, negotiated through users and translated indirectly, thereby realising its versatility.

From the perspective of Innovation Translation and ANT, tokens exchanged between nurses, orderlies, clinicians, department heads and the ICT remained positive, resulting in the successful translation of RFID. The Emergency Department had the highest power in relation to implementation of RFID technology. Confirming the literature, the ED is the area where RFID technology has the largest effect. Having a strong network relationship with nurses, clinicians and orderlies across all departments, the positive exchange of tokens was done with ease. In this case, the ICT department played a supportive, facilitating role, and an evidence-based coaxing strategy to implement the technology. In addition to all nurses and clinicians being aware of the use of RFID (being initiated by them), the ICT department was also conversant with the health and hospitals sector for many years. The confidence of the varied department heads in the suggestions made for RFID implementation by the ICT regarding temperature tags were taken positively because there was evidence supporting it that was visible almost immediately. The positive exchange of tokens between medical staff (nurses, clinicians, orderlies) and IT staff resulted in correct punctualisation. The web of relationships is invisible but strong in enabling the translation of RFID.

EMERGING THEMES FROM THE MOMENTS OF TRANSLATION

Theme 1: The key to innovation translation in the health context is its introduction and involvement by influential caregivers.

In Innovation Translation theory (Callon 1986; Tatnall 2011,), problematisation is a key moment where a group of one or more key actors attempts to define the nature of the problem and the roles of other actors. This is done in such a way that the key actors are seen as indispensible to solving the problem. The problem is often refined by the terms of solutions offered by these key actors. To pass through the OPP, all actors need to accept a set of specific assumptions and ways of operation specified by the assorted engineers. If this occurs, a stable network of relationships will result (Callon 1986).

Although RFID was imposed by the CIO and his ICT department, the RFID solution was initiated via the orthopaedics department, which had successfully applied for a grant from the Department of Health Services to track the patient journey into operating theatres. The caregivers (nurses) had the solution in mind for enhancing the quality of care rendered to patients. For operational reasons relating to the PMS, they could not continue the adoption of technology at the time. However, the nurses influenced the decision to pass on the RFID tags to the ICU for asset-tracking, which did not require the use of PMS. It should be noted that the decision to deploy and repurpose was initiated and influenced by caregivers in this context. Further, the ICT and other administrative departments were facilitating the technology by demonstrating it and on the recommendation of nurses. This supportive attitude to caregivers also helped the permeation of the technology in the hospital.

As a result, this hospital site is progressing rapidly towards the adoption of RFID more completely, rather than as a sporadic deployment within some areas.

Theme 2: Innovation translation in hospitals occurs through persuasive champions who understand the context of care.

Innovation Translation theory purports 'interessement', which is a series of processes which attempt to impose identities and roles defined in the problematisation, on other actors. This process means interesting another participant by coming between the proposed technology and the actor. According to Law (1986), the 'enrollers' attempt to lock the other actors into roles proposed for them. Gradually existing networks are dissolved and replaced with networks created by the enrollers.

This hospital revealed the success of champions and the persuasive power. CIO (1), who was the champion of the technology in the hospital, did not introduce it himself or impose it on the hospital. Nonetheless, the CIO and the ICT department were not only aware, but also championed the technology by providing the results of the successful deployment to other departments sequentially. One success followed the other due to the subtle persuasive skills of the champions—namely the CIO and ICT staff in this hospital.

The ANT purports tokens, which are successful outcomes or functions of actors that are passed on to other actors within the network. When the token is increasingly transmitted, it becomes increasingly punctualised and reified. The results of successful implementation and improvement in the workflow were passed on as a token to other departments by the champions. These tokens resulted in increased punctualisation. The ANT also suggested that an incorrect passage of token could break down the social network. The nurses correctly passed on word-of-mouth recommendations as well as actual results through the ICT department to other actors in the network, which in turn stabilised the network.

Theme 3: The strength of innovation translation in hospitals is in number of caregivers enrolled in the network.

In the Actor–Network Theory (Latour 1986) purported that:

Power vested in a person or technology does not automatically confer the ability to change or cause change in a context. Potential adopters need to be persuaded to adopt a technology. The more the number of people willing to adopt in the situation, the better is the proposed adoption.

Conversely, as McMaster, Vidgen & Wastell (1997) pointed out, innovations do not wait passively to be invented or discovered, but are created from chains of weaker or stronger human and non-human associations. Each actor enrolled in the translation influences the innovation to shape it into the ultimate form, which is adopted in the blackbox. The ANT purported that a network of materially heterogeneous actors that is achieved by a great deal of work that both shapes those varied social and non-social elements and disciplines them so they work together is necessary for successful technology adoption.

The initial network was formed 'circumstantially' by a set of actors influential actors who were enrolled selectively in the context. From this network, a set of coaxing relationships ensued into other departments, via the ICT department. These coaxing relationships ultimately resulted in a harmonious heterogeneous networks and successful translation of the technology. The key to innovation translation is the creation of a powerful consortium of actors to carry it through and the ability of those involved to construct the necessary alliances amongst other actors (McMaster, et al., 1997).

From the view point of innovation translation, if interessement is successful, enrolment will follow through a process of coercion, seduction or consent (Grint & Woolgar 1997), leading to establishment of a stable network of alliances. However, enrolment involves more than one actor to impose their will on others, and others do need to yield (Singleton & Michael 1993).

The champion of RFID, namely the CIO was able to enrol 4–5 departments of care-givers beginning with nurses. It would be correct to suggest that enrolment occurred initially through the consent/persuasion of nurses; and other departments through 'seduction' where the participants yielded willingly. The strength increased in numbers as the number of participants rose. As reflected in this voice: 'basically RFID will become ubiquitous across the entire hospital, and it's engineered at construction'.

Innovation translation theory also purport the concept of mobilisation when the proposed solution gains wider acceptance and even larger network of absent entities is created through some actors acting as spokespeople for others, mobilisation is said to have occurred. The champions continue to propagate RFID to other areas such as 'high and low care'—where a new adaptation of the technology is being initiated for 'duress alarms'.

Theme 4: Technologies had to be customised before being adapted into the health context.

Innovation Translation theory suggests that innovations have to be customised before being translated into any context. RFID tags were accepted into the pilot only after validation by Infection Control and OHS departments of the hospital, as being medical grade—customised to the context for tracking. The 'incidental RFID tags' supplied in addition to the original customised RFID tags, resulted in a set of new functions for RFID. This had resulted in the technology being translated into the context faster.

Technology had to be customised to fit the perceptions of the caregivers (users) before being adopted into the context. Specifically, the caregivers had to be satisfied that the technology will enhance their workflows and empower them with the ability to provide better care, with efficiency. As endorsed by, only real results from implementation as a token passed on successfully in the network, could effectively help in successful adoption of the technology.

From the emerging themes it is clear that in health care, as against other regular businesses, technology adoption is not based on a business case acceptance. The context of health care makes it unique in that the current processes cannot be disrupted as it involves human life. Strategists and technologists may be able to build a business case and deploy it successfully after a pilot in other businesses. However, in hospitals, the acceptance of a technology would depend on caregivers. The involvement of caregivers or frontline medical staff, who may initiate and propagate the technology is a necessity in this complex and dynamic environment.

Any technology that is deployed in hospitals is best adopted when initiated by a caregiver. Familiarity of the technology within the context by caregivers is also a necessity, before it can be considered for deployment. The rationale is that in the context of saving human life or patient care, no mistakes can be made by technology. In other words, technology and human beings are considered equal in the context— no mistakes can be made by both, which may affect lives. In such complex environment, technology adoption can only occur if customised to suit the needs of caregivers and their perceptions of care, as technology can only help extend the quality of care.

In this first successful case of RFID translation in Australian hospitals, a large hospital in the regional area of the State of Victoria had implemented it. The users and all supportive administrative departments were involved in the design and implementation of this technology in the emergency areas. Beginning with tracking patient journey into theatres and then wards, the technology permeated to all across the hospital. Nurses recommended it, clinicians accepted it as it impacted their moral conscience indirectly, and all users accepted the recommendations of key users—the nurses. The technology was negotiated in a different format by key departments, with the ICT department supporting its promulgation. It had to be noted that unlike a large hospital in the State of New South Wales, the State of Victoria had additional hurdles in terms of ethics to cope with, where RFID technology was implemented. There are

State imposed regulations such as an additional check on the privacy issues touched by this technology, which had the potential to permeate everywhere.

Although many technology vendors had attempted to push technologies in Australian hospitals, the success of this hospital indicates that key in translation of the technology smoothly was the social factors (users of the technology). This highly ignored or dismissed factors are pivotal in the translation of RFID in Australian hospitals. Social factors include users of the technology (mainly nurses, Patient Care Orderlies or Patient Care Assistants or simply Orderlies) as well as the Champions (namely IT department and other administrative areas) of the technology, who understand the context of care and legal issues associated with technology implementation that may be specific to Australian hospitals.

KEY LEARNING

The first factor that emerged was timing of introduction of RFID into the hospital. RFID did translate well into the hospital because the *timing* was indeed *appropriate* by the time of implementation in this environment. It was already 2010 when RFID had evolved as a technology. Hospital grade tags were already in the market and the technology standards had stabilised. Australia was rapidly transitioning into e-health records systems and many hospitals had refreshed their existing legacy systems with the help of national and State level government grants. The timing being a factor also involved infrastructure issues before Wi-Fi had become common as well as handheld devices that could be used for tracking. As the nation is gearing up for e-health record systems, having technology refreshments in all hospitals nationwide, enabled by Wi-Fi and handheld devices; RFID will emerge as a versatile technology.

The biggest influencing factor was the actor-network relationships between caregivers in hospitals. The findings reveal that the negotiation and network of relationships between the users are pivotal in promulgating the technology. The network of actors in hospitals are complex. Nurses and orderlies are the life of hospital operations. They are the key social actors (factors) who impacted the translation of any technology in the system. These factors need to be involved at the onset as any introduction of technologies impact their workflows. If the users were able to negotiate changes in the workflow successfully, that would enable translation of the technology into the milieu.

In this case, the negotiations between nurses and other medical staff were facilitated by the champions. The hospital champions also considered the privacy regulations of the Australian environment, and successfully worked around them such that the technology did not alter the workflows of medical staff. As a result, there was successful negotiation/interaction between all the social factors (actors) and also the non-human actor, namely RFID technology. Clearly, there are significant indictors that the socio-technical factors do impact the successful translation of RFID technology in the Australian context.

More significantly, the findings reveal that there is a complex, yet silent web of relationships between the key actors in hospitals, in relation to promoting RFID technology. In this case, the nurse–nurse, nurse–clinician and nurse–ICT relationships, which are not clearly visible at the onset, is indeed the most powerful social factor for RFID implementation. The findings indicate that a nurse-led approach would work for RFID implementation, as they are listened to by all actors. While the ICT department feels imposed upon by medical directors, if the nurse is the person raising the issue, they will accept take it on board and enable it. Doctors do not question nurses neither do the patient care orderlies. Nurse happens to be the *lynchpin* in Australian hospitals.

While most people say that technology needs to be clinician led, it needs to be translated into context by the key actors (or social factors), namely the nurses. A doctor may be listened to initially for reasons of obtaining a funding, but ICT department may not be really happy about the situation, as reflected in the comments. However, if the nurse is leading an issue and taking it up to the ICT department, it usually is taken on board and given sufficient consideration or immediate attention. Conversely, the nurses always seem to have 'one voice' no matter which department they are based in. None of the nurses seem to contradict any others. In terms of ANT, the nurse becomes the pivotal actor, who can stabilise the network and enable all other actors to pass through the OPP.

Amongst the factors that emerged is the dynamic nature of the technology itself that helped it emerge as the superstar. RFID was already an accepted technology in many industry sectors although it is relatively new to hospitals. From tracking assets to patients using location tracking ability, it evolved into 'monitoring temperatures' for fridges and spaces. In hospitals, refrigeration is indeed a key element that supports quality of services. Keeping blood and life support medicines in certain temperatures is critical to emergencies. This was enabled through temperature monitoring tags—an evolution of the technology towards 2010. The technology presented a solution as an alarm device, that is non-interventional in high-care facilities within hospitals. An alarm device, if pressed made a buzzing noise, which could adversely affect patients. An RFID tag worn with a button to be pressed, reported the staff in need request as a 'call for help' silently. The staff member in need was tracked without upsetting the rest of the patients in the hospitals. The technology thus integrated itself into the environment, being supportive, yet evolving in its uses.

The versatility of RFID technology, as visible in the case with regular and temperature tags, helped its propagation. In summary, RFID has evolved as a technology, it has become versatile in a way that it can be worn by people, embedded into equipment or tagged for tracking assets. These forms of tracking are now accepted by Australian hospitals and are slowly being trialled. While the technology itself has now progressed to the level of bio-degradable RFID tags used in Oncology (Yang & Halvorsen 2010), in the US, Australia has still a long way before the technology is permeated and accepted in healthcare completely. Nonetheless, the encounters of RFID technology with its users have instilled a level of confidence in its technical location tracking ability, enabling its successful translation into Australian hospitals.

LIMITATIONS

This chapter is focused on one regional hospital in Australia and captures a view of a decade. While it is still the single successful case in Australia, as the technology evolves and becomes part of the fabric in Australia, the findings and recommendations may eventually need to be revisited. A generalisation is not possible, although the case provides very good indication on what is relevant in the Australian hospitals in relation to RFID technology translation.

CONTRIBUTIONS

As pointed out when answering the research questions, the key contribution of this research thesis is for Australian hospitals which are considering or have been unsuccessful in RFID technology implementation thus far. RFID is still considered an innovation for Australian hospitals, and to an extent an intrusion to existing workflows, due to the existing privacy controlled environment. In such an environment, the users of the system—mainly nurses, orderlies need to accept and propagate the technology—so that it can successfully translate realising its potential to improve efficiency of workflows and effectively, improving quality of care.

The chapter would help hospital administrators and decision-makers to better understand the factors that make RFID implementation more difficult, in particular, convincing hospitals to use it to the fullest ability. The successful case revealed that the dynamic versatile nature of the technology where it can be integrated well with the support of users. The socio-technical factors, or interaction between the technology and the users became positive as the findings revealed.

Implementing innovative technologies is not a concept that is unfamiliar in any industry sector. As against other industry sectors such as retail or manufacturing supply chains, where RFID has been deployed over the last decade for tracking based on location, health sector is different. Initially, RFID as a technology was not accepted because of potential apprehensions regarding its interference with medical equipment. This was addressed easily as the technology evolved. Over the past decade, there was much research and implementation of this technology in hospitals all over the world. However in Australia, it is still a nascent technology for the hospitals.

The unique proposition in Australian hospitals is the current transition into e-health records and moving away from the legacy systems. This transition preordained that many legacy systems needed to co-exist until all health-related systems are linked and updated over time. In the milieu, RFID was thrown in as an innovation which was seen more as another piece of technology, although useful, but creating further upheaval within frenzied hospitals. In addition, Australian hospital sector and the environment is privacy regulated by law, and culturally, this has had a significant impact of introducing any new technology that is interventional. While the technology was meant to only locate equipment initially, the potential of location tracking with patients and staff made it susceptible to reluctant acceptance.

The views in academic literature were mainly from the USA, where the privacy regulation and the environment of hospitals is quite different. In the Australian context, RFID was still a new concept being accepted or rather translating slowly into the environment. The socio-technical aspects of translation have been rather ignored largely in terms of this technology. In the Australian context in particular, while there are RFID implementation models being constructed, studies that elicited factors that contributed to successful translation are still to emerge (at the time of this thesis submission). Therefore, the main contribution of this chapter is that it studied the process of translation (or negotiation) as RFID translates into the hospital and elicited success factors.

The theory framework of Innovation Translation was confirmed using the data analysis and moments of translation. There are 'problematisation' moments that occurred and went through *interessement, enrolment and mobilisation* sequentially. Here is an indication of successful translation of the technology. In addition, the conceptual framework presented with the ANT lens strengthens the ability of Innovation Translation theory to recommend future strategies for successful translation of technology.

Moreover, the contributions in this chapter reflects real-life experiences and successes where the key learning could be used for better translation of RFID in Australian hospitals. The successful translation as reported in subsequent publication that arose from the thesis is a good vaulting point for other hospitals that are considering RFID implementation. It is clear that making nurses the 'mouth piece' for the technology, and enabling it from ICT department (indirectly), is the best way to realise the benefits from this powerful technology. Industry expert validation is also supportive of this view, and in particular that nurses are the lynchpin in Australian hospitals.

The chapter also brought out the views from ICT department view (including implementation managers, CIO, consultant) and from clinician viewpoint (nurses, orderlies). These different perspectives that form the foundation of the web of network relationships that need to be stabilised for successfully translating the technology into Australian hospitals becomes apparent to hospital decision-makers. In turn, it helps them to better understand the process of successful translation and enable the process. For Australian hospitals, practitioners and technology vendors, the insights from this chapter is a start off point for incorporating better implementation processes within their own area. For academia, there is scope for study using ANT in the health sector, with a focus on Australian context.

REFERENCES

ACHI. (2014). *Australasian College of Health Informatics*. Retrieved from http://www.achi.org.au

AIHW. (2014). Australian Institute of Human Welfare, Australian Hospital Statistics report 2013-14, Australia. AIHW.

Bacheldor, B. (2006). RFID Fills Security Gap at Psychiatric Ward. *RFID Journal*. Retrieved October 24, 2007 from http://www.rfidjournal.com/article/articleview/2750/1/1

Bendavid, Y., Boeck, H., & Philippe, R. (2010). Redesigning the replenishment process of medical supplies in hospitals with RFID. *Business Process Management Journal, 16*(6), 991–1013.

Berg, M. (2001). Implementing information systems in health care organizations: Myths and challenges. *International Journal of Medical Informatics, 64*(2–3), 143–156. doi:10.1016/S1386-5056(01)00200-3 PMID:11734382

Bossen, C. (2007). Test the artefact – develop the organization: The implementation of an electronic medication plan. *International Journal of Medical Informatics, 76*(1), 13–21. doi:10.1016/j.ijmedinf.2006.01.001 PMID:16455299

Callon, M. (1986). Some elements of a sociology of translation: domestication of the scallops and the fishermen of St Brieuc Bay. In *J. Law, Power, action and belief: a new sociology of knowledge?* (pp. 196–223). London: Routledge.

Chen, C.C., Wu, J., Su, Y.S., & Yang, S.C. (2008). Key drivers for the continued use of RFID technology in the emergency room. *Management Research News, 31*(4), 273–288.

Chowdhury, B., & Khosla, R. (2007, July). RFID based Real Time Patient Management System. Computer and Information Science, 363–368.

Coustasse, A., Tomblin, S., & Slack, C. (2013). A review of Radio Frequency Identification Technologies and Impacts on the Hospital Supply Chain: 2002-2012. In *Proceedings of Academic and Business Research Institute (AABRI) International Conference*. MMM Track.

Cresswell, K. M., Worth, A., & Sheikh, A. (2010). Actor-network theory and its role in understanding the implementation of information technology developments in healthcare. *BMC Medical Informatics and Decision Making, 10*(1), 67. doi:10.1186/1472-6947-10-67 PMID:21040575

Crompton, M. (2002). *Privacy, Technology and the Healthcare Sector, Federal Privacy Commissioner Report*. Paper presented at the Australian Financial Review—4th Annual Health Congress, Sydney, Australia.

Dominguez-Pery, C., Ageron, B., & Neubert, G. (2013). A service science framework to enhance value creation in service innovation projects - An RFID case study. *International Journal of Production Economics, 141*(2), 440–451. doi:10.1016/j.ijpe.2011.12.026

Duckett, S. J. (2007). *The Australian Health Care System* (3rd ed.). Australia: Oxford University Press.

Duckett, S. J., & Willcox, S. (2011). *The Australian health care system* (4th ed.). Melbourne: Oxford University Press.

Dunlevy, S. (2013). *Outrage as eHealth record sign-up squads hit Australian hospital patients in bid to boost numbers*. News.com.au. Retrieved April 30 2013 from http://www.news.com.au/national-news/ outrage-as-ehealth-record-sign-up-squads-hit-australian-hospital-patients-in-bid-to-boost-numbers/ story-fncynjr2-1226619874616

Fisher, J. A., & Monahan, T. (2008). Tracking the social dimensions of RFID systems in hospitals. *International Journal of Medical Informatics, 77*(3), 176–183. doi:10.1016/j.ijmedinf.2007.04.010 PMID:17544841

Fosso Wamba, S. (2011). Positioning RFID technology into the innovation theorylandscape: A multidimensional perspective integrating case study approach. In *Proceedings of the 15th Pacific Asia Conference on Information systems (PACIS)*. Brisbane, Australia: PACIS.

Fosso Wamba, S., Anand, A., & Carter, L. (2013). A literature review of RFID-enabled healthcare applications and issues. *International Journal of Information Management, 33*(5), 875–891. doi:10.1016/j. ijinfomgt.2013.07.005

Fosso Wamba, S., Lefebvre, L. A., Bendavid, Y., & Lefebvre, E. (2008). Exploring the impact of RFID technology and the EPC network on mobile B2B eCommerce: A case study in the retail industry. *International Journal of Production Economics, 112*(2), 614–629. doi:10.1016/j.ijpe.2007.05.010

Friedlos, D. (2010, December). Australia's Bendigo Health Improves Efficiency Through RFID. *RFID Journal*.

GS1-Australia. (2010). *Healthcare Industry Report*. Author.

Gabbitas, O., & Jeffs, C. (2007). *Assessing productivity in the delivery of health systems in Australia: some experimental estimates*. Paper presented to the ABS-PC Productivity Perspectives 2007 Conference. Retrieved from http://www.pc.gov.au/research/conference-papers/health-service-productivity

Goss, J. (2008). *Projection of Australian health care expenditure by disease, 2003–2033, Cat. No. HWE 43*. Canberra: Australian Institute of Health and Welfare.

Grint, K., & Woolgar, S. (1997). *The machine at work- technology, work and organisation*. Cambridge: Polity Press.

Hall, E. (2005). The 'geneticisation' of heart disease: A network analysis of the production of new genetic knowledge. *Social Science & Medicine, 60*(12), 2673–2683. doi:10.1016/j.socscimed.2004.11.024 PMID:15820579

Health and Hospitals Reform Commission. (2009). *A healthier future for all Australians: Final Report.* Canberra: Commonwealth of Australia. doi:10.4018/978-1-60960-197-3.ch004

HISA. (2014). *Health Informatics Society of Australia.* Retrieved from http://www.hisa.org.au

Ho, G. (2012, April 27). *Can technology help overcome Australia's healthcare challenges?* Australian Broadcasting Corporation (ABC) - Technology and Games.

Hoskins, R. (2006). *InfoLogix Announces HealthTrax RFID Asset Tracking Software for Hospital Mobile Assets Management.* Retrieved 12 February 2006 from http://www.bbwexchange.com/pubs/2006/02/11/page1395-98309.asp

Latour, B. (1986). Article. In J. Law (Ed.), The power of association, Power, Action and Belief – a new Sociology of Knowledge, Sociological Review Monograph 32 (pp. 264–280). London: Routledge and Kegan Paul.

Law, J., & Callon, M. (1988). Engineering and Sociology in a Military Aircraft project: A network analysis of Technological Change. *Social Problems, 35*(3), 284–297. doi:10.2307/800623

McMaster, T., Vidgen, R. T., & Wastell, D. G. (1997). *Towards an understanding of technology in transition - Two conflicting theories.* Paper presented at Information Systems research in Scandinavia, IRIS20 Conference, Hanko, Norway.

Muhammad, I., Moghimi, F. H., Taylor, N. J., Redley, B., Nguyen, L., Stein, M., & Wickramasinghe, N. et al. (2013). Using ANT to uncover the full potential of an intelligent operational planning and support tool (IOPST) for acute healthcare contexts. *International Journal of Actor-Network Theory and Technological Innovation, 5*(2), 29–49. doi:10.4018/jantti.2013040103

Muhammed, I., Teoh, S., & Wickramasinghe, N. (2012). Why Using Actor Network Theory (ANT) Can Help to Understand the Personally Controlled Electronic Health Record (PCEHR) in Australia. *International Journal of Actor-Network Theory and Technological Innovation, 4*(2), 44–60. doi:10.4018/jantti.2012040105

Muhmmed, I., Zwicker, M., & Wickramasinghe, N. (2013). How Using ANT Can Assist to Understand Key Issues for Successful e-Health Solutions. *International Journal of Actor-Network Theory and Technological Innovation, 5*(3), 1–17.

Najera, P., Lopez, J., & Roman, R. (2011). Real-time location and inpatient care systems based on passive RFID. *Journal of Network and Computer Applications, 34*(3), 980–989. doi:10.1016/j.jnca.2010.04.011

NEHTA. (2014). *National E-Health Transition Authority of Australia.* Retrieved from http://www.nehta.gov.au

Ngai, E. W. T., Moon, K. K. L., Riggins, F. J., & Yi, C. Y. (2008). RFID research: An academic literature review (1995–2005) and future research directions. *International Journal of Production Economics, 112*(2), 510–520. doi:10.1016/j.ijpe.2007.05.004

Ngai, E. W. T., Poon, J. K. L., Suk, F. F. C., & Ng, C. C. (2009). Design of an RFID-based Healthcare Management System using an Information System Design Theory. *Information Systems Frontiers, 11*(4), 405–417. doi:10.1007/s10796-009-9154-3

Novak, J., & Judah, A. (2011). *Towards a health productivity reform agenda for Australia*. South Melbourne: Australian Centre for Health Research.

Oztekin, A., Foad, M. P., Delen, D., & Swim, L. K. (2010). An RFID network design methodology for asset tracking in healthcare. *Decision Support Systems, 49*(1), 100–109. doi:10.1016/j.dss.2010.01.007

Payton, F. C., Pare, G., LeRouge, C., & Reddy, M. (2011). Health care IT: Process, people, patients and interdisciplinary considerations. *Journal of the Association for Information Systems, 12*(2), i–xiii.

Privacy Act of Australia. (1988). Retrieved from http://www.privacy.gov.au/law/act

Privacy.Gov. (2013). *State and Territory Laws*. Office of the Australian Privacy Commissioner, Australia. Retrieved from http://www.privacy.gov.au/law/states

Productivity Commission. (2005). *Impacts of advances in medical technology in Australia*. Productivity Commission Research Report. Retrieved from http://www.pc.gov.au/study/medicaltechnology/finalreport/medicaltechnology.pdf

Productivity Commission (2006). *Potential benefits of the National Reform Agenda, Report to the Council of Australian Governments*. Canberra: Commonwealth of Australia.

Roark, D. C., & Miguel, K. (2006). Bar coding's replacement? *Nursing Management, 37*(2), 29–31. doi:10.1097/00006247-200602000-00009 PMID:16452888

Singleton, V., & Michael, M. (1993). Actor-Networks and Ambivalence: General practitioners in the UK Cervical Screening Programme. *Social Studies of Science, 23*(2), 227–264. doi:10.1177/030631293023002001

Tatnall, A. (2011). Innovation Translation, Innovation Diffusion, and the Technology Acceptance Model: Comparing three different approaches to Theorising Technological Innovation. In *Actor–Network Theory and Technology Innovation: Advancements and New Concepts*. IGI Global.

Tu, Y. J., Zhou, W., & Piramuthu, S. (2009). Identifying RFID-embedded objects in pervasive healthcare applications. *Decision Support Systems, 46*(2), 586–593. doi:10.1016/j.dss.2008.10.001

Unnithan C, Tatnall A (2014). Actor-Network Theory (ANT) based visualisation of Socio-Technical Facets of RFID Technology Translation: An Australian Hospital Scenario. *International Journal of Actor-Network Theory and Technology Innovation, 2*(2).

Whetton, S. (2005). *Health Informatics*. Australia: Oxford University Press.

Wickramasinghe, N., Bali, R., & Tatnall, A. (2012). A Manifesto for e-health Success- The Key Role for ANT. *International Journal of Actor-Network Theory and Technological Innovation, 4*(3), 24–35. doi:10.4018/jantti.2012070103

Yang, B., & Halvorsen, P. (2010). *Use of RFID to enhance the patient experience, increase safety and eliminate treatment errors, RFID in Oncology Clinics*. White Paper. Alliance Oncology.

Yao, W., Chu, C.-H., & Li, Z. (2012). The Adoption and Implementation of RFID technologies in Healthcare: A literature review. *Journal of Medical Systems*, *36*(6), 3507–3525. doi:10.1007/s10916-011-9789-8 PMID:22009254

Yen Y, Lo N, Wu T (2012). *Two RFID based solutions for secure inpatient medication.* Academic Press.

Yu, Y. C. Y., Hou, T. W. T., & Chiang, T. C. T. (2012). Low cost RFID real lightweight binding proof protocol for medication errors and patient safety. *Journal of Medical Systems*, *36*(2), 823–828. doi:10.1007/s10916-010-9546-4 PMID:20703651

KEY TERMS AND DEFINITIONS

Blood Cooler: Devices for keeping the blood cooled in hospitals.

BPM: Business Process Management (BPM) is the method of managing the redesign and redeployment of business processes within a given situation and organisation.

BPR: Business Process Redesign (BPR) is a process for assessing performance issues of a particular process and conducting radical redesign to the process, by redesigning the process itself and systems, policies or organisational structures.

Catheter: A thin tube used for medical purposes.

Defibrillator: Electric Shock Machine.

ED: Emergency Department.

Exciters: A device that uniquely extends the Real Time Location System of AeroScout, to provide robust and immediate Wi-Fi RFID tag detection capabilities. For example, the Exciter triggers AeroScout's RFID tags as they pass through a choke-point to transmit a message that is received by a standard Wi-Fi Access Point or AeroScout Location Receiver. This provides instant knowledge that a tagged asset or person passed through a gate, doorway or some other tightly defined area.

Implants: Something that is inserted into a human body during surgery.

Pacemaker: A device that regulates heartbeat.

PMS: Patient Management Systems.

Chapter 7
Introducing Mobile Device for Health Services:
The Semantics of Language Translation

Phathutshedzo Nemutanzhela
Namibia University of Technology, Namibia

Tiko Iyamu
Cape Peninsula University of Technology, South Africa

ABSTRACT

On one hand, healthcare has taken the centre stage of attention in recent years, due to many more activities of both natural and manmade. On another hand, the use of mobile technologies is increasingly growing across the world, particularly in developing countries. Mobile devices, including phones and computers are becoming significant ICT tools for many activities and process of healthcare service delivery in both urban and rural areas, by organisations and individuals, literates and educated. Also, both businesses (organisations) and individuals are involved in the delivering and accessibility (recipient) of healthcare services at different levels and locations. The nature of the diverse tribes and languages within some developing countries make it difficult to deliver or receive the services which are provided by some Healthcare organisations. This is so because particular language, such as English, as in the case of South Africa, is often used for communication. Even though majority of the citizens make use of Mobile devices (such as cellular phones), the media of communication exchange is English language. Due to the sensitivity, confidentiality, and private nature of healthcare information and services, a one-on-one and the use of language which the patient is comfortable with is critical. Otherwise, the services and objectives of the healthcare organisations continue to be challenged. As such, there is need to address the semantics of language through the use of electronic devices for healthcare services.

1. INTRODUCTION

In 2012, the World Health Organisation noted that countries, particularly in the Africa continent, will not develop economically and socially without substantial improvements in the health of their people. The

DOI: 10.4018/978-1-4666-9446-0.ch007

economic shifts of the past few years have further contracted economic growth worldwide and affected developing countries unduly, for example. If anything positive can be said about the global recession, it is that it more deeply binds the fate of nations together and provides momentum for new and systemic approaches to persistent cross-border challenges.

According to Wu & Hall (2012), it will take an unprecedented transformation to reverse the tide of failing health systems, particularly in light of shrinking resources that must now be used more efficiently. Fortunately, support is increasingly available through a set of breakthrough tools known as e-Health, commonly understood to be the innovative application of emerging information and communications technology in health systems. E-Health includes a broad range of implements, such as electronic health records, information gathering software, mobile devices, e-learning tools and horizon technologies that defy human imagination. Combined, these tools can narrow health disparities, equip health care providers and enable immense leaps in quality of care. For example, Linton (2010) argued that a nurse in a remote village can now access now access information through her laptop and mobile phone on the world's best treatments, previously only available to the rich and privileged, and can track and treat her patients using longitudinal electronic health records. It is argued in many quarters that the e-Health Portals makes healthcare and information more accessible with the end goal of improving patient care and the health status of all. "The use of technology to ultimately improve patient outcomes is not going away" (Bingman, 2001).

However, most of the areas that require the use of mobile devices are those that are at the rural areas where the language that is used as a media of exchange through these devices is not necessarily the same as their first language, and many of them are not fluent in the use. Therefore, this brings a gap that need to be addressed to make sure that a better healthcare service is rendered to everyone irrespective of where they stay and which language they use. This article therefore focuses its discussion on how to provide mechanism which could be used to synchronise healthcare data and services across the geographical locations of the country, and the translation of spoken language from local dialect to English through coding and decoding synchronised data, using mobile devices. Thus, the provision of healthcare services can be improved in countries, such as South Africa.

The focal question which this article discusses is, how can we address semantics of language translation on mobile devices to better the services of healthcare organisations? The article presents a prototype, which can guide the development of mobile application for the improvement of healthcare service delivery. This is to improve, by means of information, the capacity for the surveillance of, and rapid response to disease and public health emergencies for a wider coverage of citizens speaking different languages.

2. LITERATURE REVIEW

The need and use of Information and Communication Technology (ICT) has increased rapidly in recent years. It is difficult to find an area of businesses, organisations included, or individual life that doesn't imbibe the service of ICT, in respective of the perspective. Rouse (2005) argued that ICT is an umbrella term that includes any communication device or application, which encompasses different technologies, such as radio, television, cellular phones, and computer network, hardware, software, satellite systems and medical technologies for healthcare services.

Healthcare focuses on diagnosis, such as treatment, and prevention of disease, illness, injury, and other physical and mental impairments in humans, which relies on technologies. Health care is delivered by practitioners in medicine, chiropractic, dentistry, nursing, pharmacy, allied health, and other care providers. It refers to the work done in providing primary care, secondary care and tertiary care, as well as in public health (WHO, 2012).

Among other things, ICT has drastically improved communications, as well reduce distances in terms making the separation of logical and physical data to be available at real-time. Other examples are videoconferencing and distance learning. In short, ICT is a way to communicate and share our information using advance technology which may make it able to communicate or share with people in distance. Bayo-Moriones, Billon & Lera-Lopez, (2013), showed through a table that communication improvement leads to better operational performance. According to (Eysenbach, 2009) the rise in adoption of mobile phones and the Internet, in both industrialized and developing countries, has provided additional opportunities in e-health which is engaging large groups of people to perform a task. Mobile phones hold particular promise for this type of opportunity because they can be used as point-of-care devices, function in remote locations, and are readily carried and used at any time (Waegemann, 2010).

Even though ICT provide the platform, tools and artefacts to enable and support many processes and activities, such as communication and information sharing, different individuals and groups apply ITC artefacts in various ways. The application of ICT is often based on know-how and interest. Ballon & Van Heesvelde, (2010) be argued that many ICT platforms fulfil several or all of these functions, instead of being limited to one of them. However, the interest of individuals and groups are sometimes, impossible or difficult to fulfil. For example, not all African languages could be translated using the mobile devices. This makes it difficult for some services such as the Healthcare to be carried out in some areas of need. According to Daigle et al., (2011), not all non-English speaking people speak the same language. Therefore, this causes barriers, which can cause delays in real-time communications.

In order to provide holistic care there is a need to develop integrated approaches to health and social care delivery. Policymakers have realised that e-Health initiatives can help promote information sharing. ICT makes it possible for those delivering health and social care to exchange patient data without being constrained by time and distance (King, et al., 2012). E-health is defined as the application of Internet and other related technologies in the healthcare industry to improve the access, efficiency, effectiveness, and quality of clinical and business processes utilized by healthcare organizations, practitioners, patients, and consumers in an effort to improve the health status of patients (Marconi, 2002). According to the European Coordination Committee of the Radiological, Electro medical and (COCIR, 2010), E-Health describes the application of information and communications technologies across the whole range of functions that affect the health sector.

3. THEORETICALLY UNDERPINNING THE DISCUSSION

The discussion is how to improve upon the services of healthcare in wake of semantic of languages by recipient and providers of healthcare. This involves elements of existing of actors in their different roles and capacities; power and cultural relationships; and diffusing the innovation of semantic of language through mobile devices. Thus, we explored, for better understanding, through the lenses of moments of translation and Time from the perspectives of Actor network theory (ANT) and Diffusion of Innovation (DoI), respectively.

Actor network theory (ANT) focuses human and non-human actors, and their heterogeneity (Callon & Bruno (1981). In this context of this article, we employ the moments of transaltions, from the perspective ANT, to examine how networks of both reciepents and recipient of healthcare are created and maintained. The networks inturns enable and at the same time constrain how technology could be used to diffused to delivering of healthcare services overtime and geographical space. The theory of diffusion of innovation has been widely applied in disciplines such as education, sociology, communication, agriculture, marketing, and information technology (Rogers, 1995; Karahanna, Straub & Chervany (1999); Agarwal, Sambamurthy & Stair (2000). In the context of the theory, innovation is "an idea, practice, or object that is perceived as new by an individual or another unit of adoption" (Rogers, 1995, p. 11). Diffusion, on the other hand, is "the process by which an innovation is communicated through certain channels over time among the members of a social system" (Rogers, 1995, p. 5). Thus, the DoI theory argues that "potential users make decisions to adopt or reject an innovation based on beliefs that they form about the innovation" (Agarwal, 2000, p.90).

Callon (1986) defined 4 moments of translation, which are briefly described as follows:

1. **Problematisation:** This is the first stage of the moments of translation. According to Iyamu and Tatnall (2009: 30) this is the stage where an actor defines issues for a network, in his or her own terms. The new initiative is left for the network to find a solution.
2. **Interessement:** other actors in the network shows interests in the new initiative that was defined for them.
3. **Enrollment:** Actors accept the roles that have been defined for them during as they show interest in the new initiative. According to Iyamu and Tatnall (2009:30) ANT proposes that enrolling allies creates aligned interests and the translation of these interests must be such that participation will lead to the network's maintenance. Enrolment can be seen as a successful outcome of the problematisation and the interessement processes.
4. Mobilisation of allies.

The last stage is Mobilisation and it involves the buy-in of actors into the new initiative. This buy-in is carried out by new actors as they become the new spokespersons of the initiative. According to Iyamu (2011, 30) the network starts to operate in a target-oriented manner to implement the solution proposed, and grows as actors become mobilised to act as secondary focal actors.

Diffusion of Innovation: Innovation-Decision Process

According to Rogers (2003), the Innovation-decision process involves five steps. As shown in Figure 1, the process include: (1) knowledge, (2) persuasion, (3) decision, (4) implementation, and (5) confirmation. These stages typically follow each other in a time-ordered manner. The stages are briefly described below

- **Knowledge:** The innovation-decision process starts with the knowledge stage. In this step, an individual learns about the existence of innovation and seeks information about the innovation. What? How? and Why? are the critical questions in the knowledge phase. During this phase, the individual attempts to determine "what the innovation is and how and why it works" (Rogers, 2003, p. 21).
- **Persuasion:** The persuasion step occurs when the individual has a negative or positive attitude toward the innovation, but "the formation of a favorable or unfavorable attitude toward an innovation does not always lead directly or indirectly to an adoption or rejection" (Rogers, 2003, p. 176).

Figure 1. The Innovation-decision process

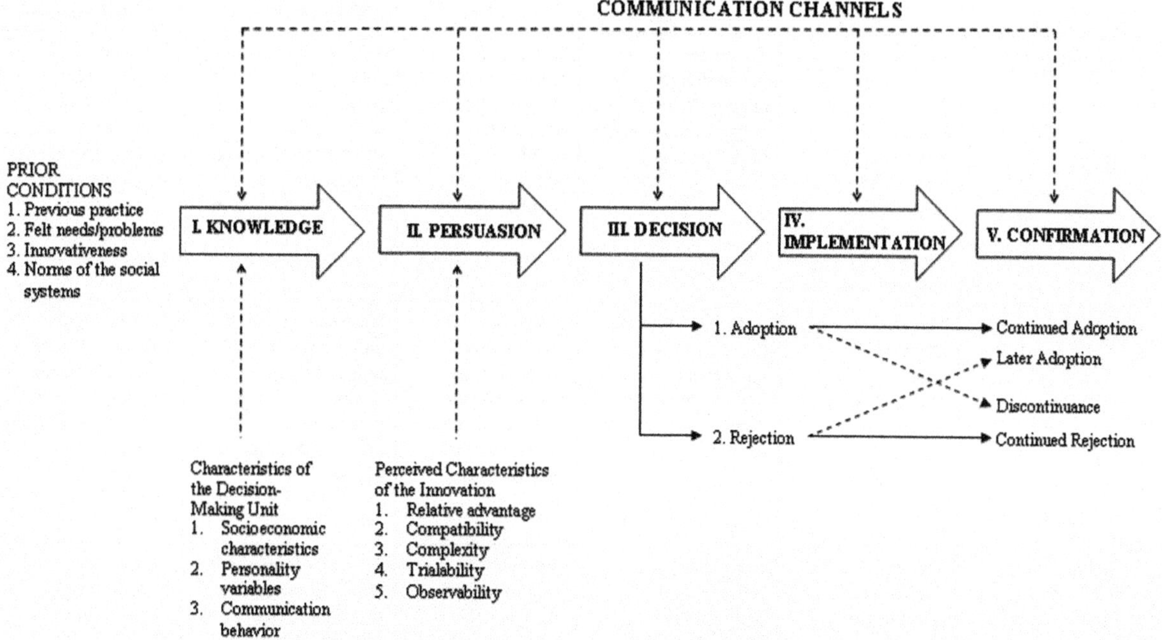

Observability will allow organisation and patients to observe how innovation works as this will give a positive impact on the users' attitude toward the system and intention to use the system.

- **Decision:** At the decision stage in the innovation-decision process, the individual chooses to adopt or reject the innovation. While adoption refers to "full use of an innovation as the best course of action available," rejection means "not to adopt an innovation" (Rogers, 2003, p. 177).
- **Implementation:** At the implementation stage, an innovation is put into practice. However, an innovation brings the newness in which "some degree of uncertainty is involved in diffusion" (p. 6). Uncertainty about the outcomes of the innovation still can be a problem at this stage.
- **Confirmation:** The innovation-decision already has been made, but at the confirmation stage the individual looks for support for his or her decision. According to (Rogers, 2003) this decision can be reversed if the individual is "exposed to conflicting messages about the innovation" (p. 189).

4. MOBILE DEVICE FOR HEALTH SERVICES: UNDERSTANDIGN THE SEMANTIC OF LANGUAGE TRANSLATION

Semantics of language is often referred to the study of the meanings of words and sentences. The Semantics of language is very critical in communication, particularly with the illiterates and people in the rural areas. Also, it Semantics of language is significant in terms of how technologies are used for communication purposes. As shown in Table 1, ANT and DoI were employed as lenses to examine how the semantics of language could be addressed through mobile application. This was done by understanding factors, such as, how network of the communities (service providers and recipients) are created, and the communication evolves. The figure should be read with the text so as to gain better understanding.

Table 1. Formation of Networks and Communication

	Knowledge	Persuasion	Decision	Implementation	Confirmation
Problematisation	Healthcare services are problematized based on the knowledge to understand what is needed and required by either the provider or recipient or both.	To initiate persuasion to receive or provide healthcare service, the language of interaction is critical.	The decision to initiate interaction towards receiving or providing healthcare service is influenced by spoken language and understanding of the semantics.	The use of technology such as mobile devices for translation of the semantics of spoken language can be initiated by any actor, for negotiation.	Conscious and unconscious acceptance by both the service providers and recipients, of the norm in facility that they make use of.
Interessment	The providers and recipient require degree of knowledge in order to show interest in healthcare services in the various communities.	Some of the factors that informs interest and persuasion include language of communication, type of services	Individual and group interest spurs the type of the decision that they make to access and how they access the facilities.	Healthcare services are of interest to all human beings. What is more significant is how the services are provided and accessed.	Translation of language and the semantics through cellular phone will affirm accessibility of healthcare services.
Enrolment	The recipients are selective, as informed by culture and language, on the facilities that they do access for healthcare services.	Both service providers and recipients at one point or the other influences each other in carrying duties and receiving services, respectively.	Activities in each of facilities influence the accessibility by the communities.	The use of mobile phone, through translation, to improve interaction between service providers and recipients, to increase accessibility.	This is valued or measured based on the number of recipients who access the facilities.
Mobilisation	The recipients encourage and discourage others from accessing health facilities based on factors, such as culture and spoken language.	Individuals and groups motivate others is based on interaction with the service providers and how they access health facilities.	Individual experience influence the decision to encourage or discourage others to access the health facilities.	Common and understanding of language semantics for self-motivation and to encourage others	Increase in accessibility of health facilities.

1. **Establishment of Initiative:** Healthcare services are initiated by either the recipient or providers. It is often planned when it is initiated by the providers, sometimes, informed by strategy. From the recipients' perspective, it is not always planned, except for purpose of routine check-up.

2. **Awareness and Attention:** Many of the recipients of healthcare are sometimes hesitant to visit the facilities mainly because of the language barrier. They often feel that they cannot express themselves in the language of their first choice, and therefore limit their interactions with the healthcare service providers. The challenges with spoken language has come a long way, and remain as at today. In Chomsky (1975), the author argued that as follows: "Language is a mirror of mind in a deep and significant sense. It is a product of human intelligence".

In respective of the spoken language, both providers and recipients of healthcare are interested in the use of mobile devices. Joe (2010) define mobile devices to be the sorts of things you might expect such as iPhones, BlackBerry devices, Android phones, Windows Mobile devices, etc. -- pocket size devices that can access the Internet via WiFi, cellular/3G, he further stretch the definition to include traditional laptops and tablet computers such as the iPad and maybe even conventional cell phones, thumb drives, etc.

3. **Roles and Responsibilities:** To offer and receive services and care at health facilities requires participation by both the provider and recipient, are roles and responsibilities that must be voluntarily mandatory carried out by the actors. The participation is as a result of interaction between the actors. However, the actors' spoken language is not always the same due to the numerous languages in South Africa. This has impact on the services, at the detriment of the recipient. According to Gleitman and Papafragou (2012), the limits of my language are the limits of my world and The fact of the matter is that the 'real world' is to a large extent unconsciously built upon the language habits of the group different communities of humans, speaking different languages, would think differently to just the extent that their languages differ from one another.

4. **Gratification and Revolt:** Both the providers and recipient mobilises for and against healthcare services, at different facilities. On one hand, some of the recipient voluntarily becomes spokespersons to encourage others in the community to make use of the facility where they find convenient in the use of language, without interpreter. Otherwise, they discourage others from visiting the facility. Also, some of the service providers, such as nurses and doctors represent the facilities in the manner that attract the recipient. This is sometimes done through proactive learning of the common and frequent spoken language in the community where they practice their trade. This they do by focusing on the semantic of the language spoken by the community.

The Innovation decision process is characterized by a process that occurs while individuals participate in a series of actions related to decisions (Rogers, 1995:162).

Knowledge occurs when individuals are aware of the Innovation and gain understanding of its functions.

Persuasion – this is when individuals or decision-making units exhibit favourable or unfavourable behaviour toward the innovation. Attitudes and behaviour usually occurs through personal and group channels and becomes more important in an attempt to change the stance in order to accommodate how healthcare services are provided to the community.

Decision indicates when the individual or unit decides to adopt or reject the Innovation. Based on individual and group knowledge that were acquired during persuasion, decisions are of subjective. The decisions are attributed to subjective characteristics primarily because they can be viewed differently depending on individual and group perceptions.

Implementation occurs when the individual or unit decides to use the Innovation. New opportunities emerge in the facilities as a result of converging new technologies, such as mobile phone which can cause sudden changes in the services are provided. Stability is threatened when cultural boundaries and language diverse merge.

Confirmation occurs when decision makers confirm or reject their decision to adopt the Innovation (Rogers, 1995:162). An innovation, using mobile phone for translation of language semantic will create new value. The service providers do required the innovation in order to improve delivering of healthcare to the communities.

5. MOBILE DEVICE FOR THE TRANSLATION OF LANGUAGE SEMANTIC

Based on the discussion above, a mobile application to translate language semantic is recommended for development, as well further study. We therefore present a prototype for the application, which could be used to Test, Evaluate and Assess the translation of language semantic. A prototype is an early sample or model built to test a concept or process or to act as a thing to be replicated or learned from. It is a term used in a variety of contexts, including semantics, design, electronics, and software programming. As presented in Figure 2, a prototype is designed to test and trial a new design to enhance precision by system analysts and users. Prototyping serves to provide specifications for a real, working system rather than a theoretical one (PC Magazine, 2012). Prototyping involves producing early working versions ('prototypes') of the future application system and experimenting with them (Lichter, Schneider-Hufschmidt & Zullighoven, 1994).

Figure 2. Prototype: Application Development

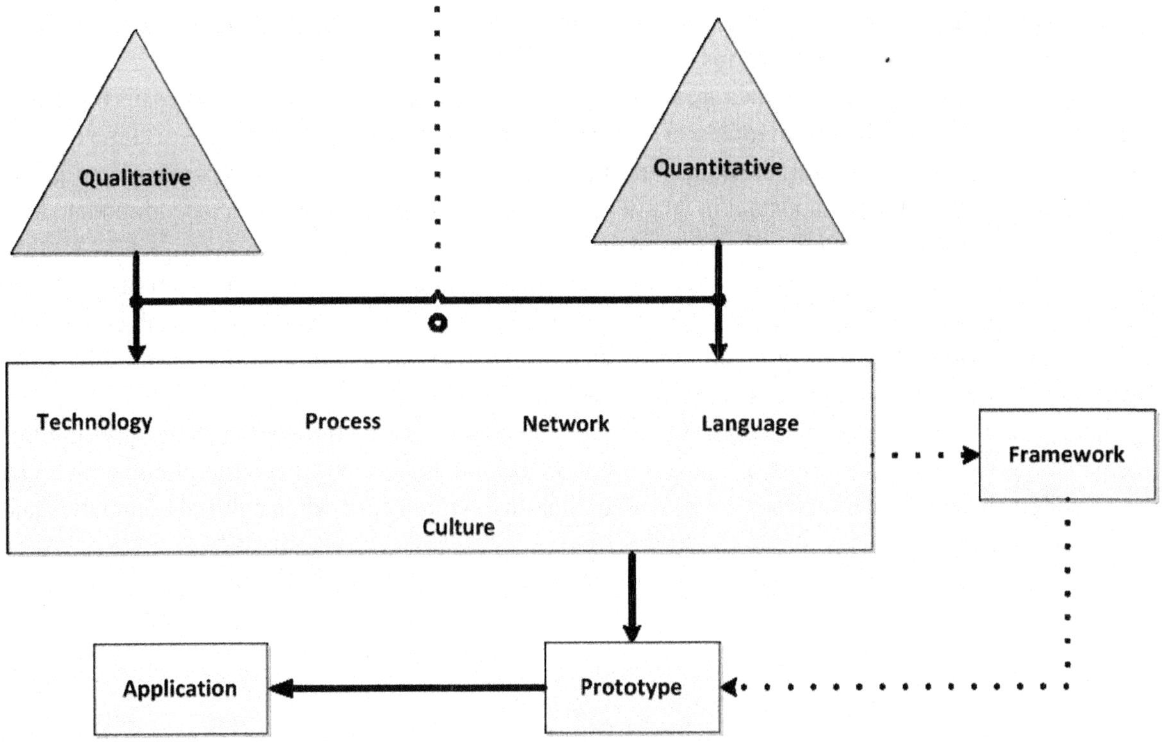

Development and Test

Development it's the actual design and building of the application that will be used to translate language semantics of the mobile devices used for e-health. The definition of testing according to the ANSI/IEEE 1059 standard is that testing is the process of analysing a software item to detect the differences between existing and required conditions (that is defects/errors/bugs) and to evaluate the features of the software item. The is a need to test the prototype before taking it to the user for all errors and make sure its bug free do to the sensitivity of data that will be used.

Evaluation and Assessment

According to Gagne, Bridges, & Wagne (1998), assessment is defined as data-gathering strategies, analyses, and reporting processes that provide information that can be used to determine whether or not intended outcomes are being achieved. Evaluation uses assessment information to support decisions on maintaining, changing, or discarding instructional or programmatic practices (Hanson & Price, 1992). These strategies can inform many factors, such (i) the nature and extent of learning; (ii) facilitate curricular decision making; (iii) correspondence between learning and the aims and objectives of teaching; and (iv) the relationship between learning and the environments in which learning takes place (Satterly, 1989).

6. CONCLUSION

This paper presents a foundation for further research into development of a mobile application for the translation of semantics of language. This is to foster relationship between healthcare service providers and recipients, thereby improving service delivering. Also, it will improve, by means of information, the capacity for the surveillance of, and rapid response to disease and public health emergencies for a wider coverage of citizens speaking different languages. The mobile health application is to improve the access, efficiency, effectiveness, and quality of clinical and business processes utilized by healthcare organizations, practitioners, patients, and consumers in an effort to improve the health status of patients.

REFERENCES

Agarwal, R., Sambamurthy, V., & Stair, R. (2000). The evolving relationship between general and specific computer efficacy: An empirical assessment. *Information Systems Research, 11*(4), 418–430. doi:10.1287/isre.11.4.418.11876

Agarwal. (2000). Individual Acceptance of Information technologies. *Educational Technology Research and Development, 40*, 90-102.

Anderson, J., & Gerbing, D. (1988). Structual equation modelling in practice: A review and recommended two-step approach. *Psychological Bulletin, 103*(3), 411–423. doi:10.1037/0033-2909.103.3.411

Ballon, P., & Van Heesvelde, E. (2010, August). Platform types and regulatory concerns in European ICT markets. *TPRC.*

Bayo-Moriones, A., Billon, M., & Lera-Lopez, F. (2013). Perceived performance effects of ICT in manufacturing SMEs. *Industrial Management & Data Systems, 113*(1), 117–135. doi:10.1108/02635571311289700

Bingman, K. (2001). E-Health Solutions Series. *Cerner 2001.*

Callon, M. (1986). Some Elements of a Sociology of Translation: Domestication of the Scallops and the Fishermen of St Brieuc Bay. In *Power, Action and Belief: A New Sociology of Knowledge.* London: Routledge & Kegan Paul.

Callon, M., & Bruno, L. (1981). Unscrewing the Big Leviathan: How ActorsMacro-Structure Reality and How Sociologists Help Them Do So. In K. Knorr-Cetina & A. V. Cicourel (Eds.), *Advances in Social Theory and Methodology: Toward an Integration of Micro- and Macro-Sociologies.* Boston: Routledge & Kegan Paul.

Chomsky, N. (1975). *Reflections on Language, (A good non-technical review of the extended standard theory and various philosophical issues related to generative grammar.).* New York: Pantheon.

COCIR. (2010). *The European Coordination Committee of the Radiological, Electro medical and Healthcare IT Industry: Glossary of Terms.* COCIR. Retrieved from http://www.cocir.org/uploads/documents/-883-

Crang, M. (1997). Analyzing qualitative material. Longman.

Daigle, M., Roychoudhury, I., Narasimhan, S., Saha, S., Saha, B., & Goebel, K. (2011). Investigating the effect of damage progression model choice on prognostics performance. In *Proceedings of the annual conference of the prognostics and health management society 2011* (pp. 323-333). Academic Press.

Denzin, & Lincoln. (2000). *Handbook of Qualitative Research.* London: Sage Publications.

Diffusion of innovations. (1995). New York: Free Press.

Dow, S., Heddleston, K., & Klemmer, S. (2009). The Efficacy of Prototyping Under Time Constraints. In *Proceeding of ACM Conf. on Creativity and Cognition.* ACM. doi:10.1145/1640233.1640260

Eysenbach, G. (2009). Infodemiology and infoveillance: Framework for an emerging set of public health informatics methods to analyze search, communication and publication behavior on the Internet. *Journal of Medical Internet Research, 11*(1), e11. doi:10.2196/jmir.1157 PMID:19329408

Gagne, R., Bridges, L., & Wagne, W. (1998). *Principles of Instructional Design.* Orlando, FL: Holt, Rinehart and Winston, Inc.

Gleitman, L., & Papafragou, A. (2012). New perspectives on language and thought. In K. Holyoak & R. Morrison (Eds.), *Cambridge Handbook of Thinking and Reasoning* (2nd ed.). New York: Oxford University Press. doi:10.1093/oxfordhb/9780199734689.013.0028

Hanson, G., & Price, B. (1992). Academic Program Review. In M. A. Wjitley, J. D. Porter, & R. H. Fenske (Eds.), *The Primer for Institutional Research.* Tallahassee, FL: Association for Institutional Research.

Iyamu, T. (2011). Institutionalisation of the enterprise architecture: The actor-network perspective. *International Journal of Actor-Network Theory and Technological Innovation, 3*(1), 27–38. doi:10.4018/jantti.2011010103

Iyamu, T., & Tatnall, A. (2009). *An actor-network analysis of a case of development and implementation of IT strategy*. Paper presented at the Information systems conference. Retrieved doi:10.4018/jantti.2009062303

Joe. (2010). Securing Mobile Devices! *Security Professionals 2011 Preconference Seminar*.

Karahanna, E., Straub, D., & Chervany, N. (1999). *Information technology adoption across time: A cross-sectional comparison of pre-adoption and post-adoption beliefs*. MIS Quarterly.

King, G., O'Donnell, C., Boddy, D., Smith, F., Heaney, D., & Mair, F. (2012). Boundaries and e-health implementation in health and social care. *BMC Medical Informatics and Decision Making, 12*(100).

Kvale, S. (1996). *Interviews: An introduction to qualitative research interviewing*. London, UK: Sage.

Kvale, S. (2007). *Doing interviews*. Thousand Oaks, CA: Sage.

Lichter, H., Schneider-Hufschmidt, M., & Zullighoven, H. (1994). Prototyping in Industrial Software Projects: Bridging the Gap between Theory and Practice. *IEEE Transactions on Software Engineering, 20*(11), 11,825–842. doi:10.1109/32.368126

Linton, N. (2010). *Connecting: the use of information and communication technologies by older adults in a retirement community*. Academic Press.

Magazine, P. (2012, May 3). Prototyping Definition. *PC Magazine*.

Marconi, J. (2002, May). E-Health: Navigating the Internet for Health Information Healthcare. Advocacy White Paper. *Healthcare Information and Management Systems Society*.

Myers. (2002). Qualitative research and the generalizability question: Standing firm with Proteus. *The Qualitative Report, 4*(3/4). Retrieved from http://www.nova.edu/ssss/QR/QR4-3/myers.html

Pilot, D., & Beck, C. (2014). *Study Guide for Essentials of Nursing Research: Appraising Evidence for Nursing Practice* (8th ed.). Philadelphia: Lippincott Williams & Wilkins.

Rogers, E. (1995). *Diffusion of innovations* (4th ed.). New York: Free Press.

Rogers, E. (2003). *Diffusion of innovations* (5th ed.). New York: Free Press.

Rouse, M. (2005). *ICT (information and communications technology - or technologies)*. Retrieved from http://searchcio-midmarket.techtarget.com/definition/ICT

Satterly, D. (1989). *Assessment in schools*. Oxford, UK: Basil Blackwell Ltd.

Shaughnessy, J., Zechmeister, E., & Jeanne, Z. (2011). *Research methods in psychology* (9th ed.). McGraw Hill.

State of Illinois. (2009). *Department of Central Management Services Bureau of Communication and Computer Services Effective October 01, 2009Version 1*. Author.

Waegemann, C. (2010). mHealth: The next generation of telemedicine?. *Telemedicine Journal and e-Health, 16*(1), 23–25. doi:10.1089/tmj.2010.9990 PMID:20070168

Welman, J., & Kruger, S. (2001). Research Methodology: for the Business and administrative sciences (2nd Ed.). Oxford University Press.

World Health Organisation. (2012). *Health systems*. Geneva: WHO.

Wu, S., & Hall, F. (2012). A Panel Analysis of the Strategic Association between Information and Communication Technology and Public Health Delivery. Journal of Medical Research, 14(5).

Yin. (2009). *Case Study Research: Design and Methods*. SAGE.

Chapter 8
An Analysis on the Utilisation of Health Information Technology to Support Clinical Operation of Chinese Medicine

Catherine Han-Lin
Deakin University, Melbourne, Australia

Siddhi Pittayachawan
RMIT University, Melbourne, Australia

Angela Wei Hong Yang
RMIT University, Melbourne, Australia

Nilmini Wickramasinghe
*Deakin University & Epworth HealthCare,
Melbourne, Australia*

ABSTRACT

Chinese Medicine (CM) has become increasingly demanding globally. Recent World Health Organisation traditional and complementary medicine strategy of integrating CM to Western Medicine (WM) indicates that it is crucial that CM developments have strong literature, scientific, and evidence-based medical approval and support. To achieve this, there is a need to form a synthesis foundation or platform for future studies. This chapter serves to discover this synthesis that is suitable for CM by discussing the basics of inquiring and Knowledge Management (KM) systems. It suggests that CM should follow a combination of Hegelian and Kantian inquiring systems with the support of Singerian and Leibnizian inquiring systems and KM features. This proposed synthesis is one of the first, if not the first study to apply Churchman's inquiring systems into the context of CM and differentiate them from WM.

INTRODUCTION

Information Systems/Information Technology (IS/IT) have been adopted in healthcare to facilitate superior service and delivery to patients (Lin et al., 2013, 2014c; Wickramasinghe, 2013). Examples of this can be seen in hospitals and clinics daily operations, such as ambulatory blood pressure measurement using automated devices which is now considered a more sensitive predictor of cardiovascular outcome than

DOI: 10.4018/978-1-4666-9446-0.ch008

conventional measurement (O'Brien et al., 2000). In other cases, doctors use telemedicine equipment like Tele-radiology and Tele-surgery to diagnose and treat patients (Hojabri & Manafi, 2012). Using IS/IT to assist doctors, specialists, and nurses in decision making can also be found in various hospital divisions. One good example of a decision support system (DSS) is linking characteristics of patients with chest pain to software algorithms recommending specific action (Ferlie et al., 2012). Technology has taken healthcare to a digital era and it is likely and will continually service healthcare with advanced technology (Lin et al., 2013, 2014c; Wickramasinghe et al., 2005). However, there is little IS/IT utilisation in complementary and alternative medicine (CAM) practice (Lin et al., 2013, 2014c). Therefore, we look into one of the CAM - Chinese medicine (CM) practice. The analysis of CM clinical operation activities can help identifying suitable IS/IT involvements and solutions.

The chapter is organised in the following sections: firstly, brief background information about current international CM practice is introduced; its position in world healthcare; why CM is important and hence proper IS/IT system should be studied and implemented. Secondly, typical CM clinic daily operations, activities, processes are identified and analysed. Thirdly, a new and suitable synthesis is suggested for CM developments. Fourthly, based on the proposed theory, possible and suitable IS/IT involvements and solutions are listed. Finally, this chapter concludes with the summary of contributions.

BACKGROUND

There are about 80% of the world population use CAM treatments (WHO, 2013). In Australia the number of people using CAM is rising. Research shows that the number of visits to CAM practitioners by adult Australians in year 2004 to 2005 reached 69.2 million, while the number of visits to primary care or general practice (GP) was 69.3 million in the same year (Xue et al. 2007). CM is one of the most popular CAM practices today (Lukman et al. 2007). There are 4,157 registered acupuncturists in Australia (CMBA, 2014) and more than 10 million visits to acupuncturists every year (Xue et al., 2008). CM is considered by many patients to have fewer side effects; more effective treatment to the root of the disease; and is good for the overall health of patients (Chi, 1994). Unlike western medicine (WM), CM's unique methods of diagnosis (combine inspection, auscultation and olfaction, inquiring, and palpation in every diagnosis) give each patient individualised treatment (Chi, 1994). This approach, to some patients, is a benefit and an advantage.

CM Strategic Movements

The World Health Organisation (WHO) summarised its traditional and complementary medicine (T&CM) strategy 2014 to 2023 (updated from strategy 2002–2005) in three areas: 1) a knowledge base to allow T&CM (including CM) to be managed actively through appropriate national policies that understand and recognise the role and potential of T&CM; 2) ensure quality assurance, safety, proper use and effectiveness of T&CM by regulating products, practices and practitioners through education and training, skills development, services and therapies; and 3) promote universal health coverage by integrating T&CM services into health service delivery and self-health care (WHO, 2013).

Countries around the world are making efforts to implement WHO's T&CM strategy at their own pace. In Canada, a comprehensive regulatory framework was introduced to CM. Policy, regulation, and guidelines were developed for CM practitioners to follow (WHO, 2013). In United States, the National

Figure 1. CM & WM integration map
(Adopted from Lin et al., 2014a) Source: ECIS 2014

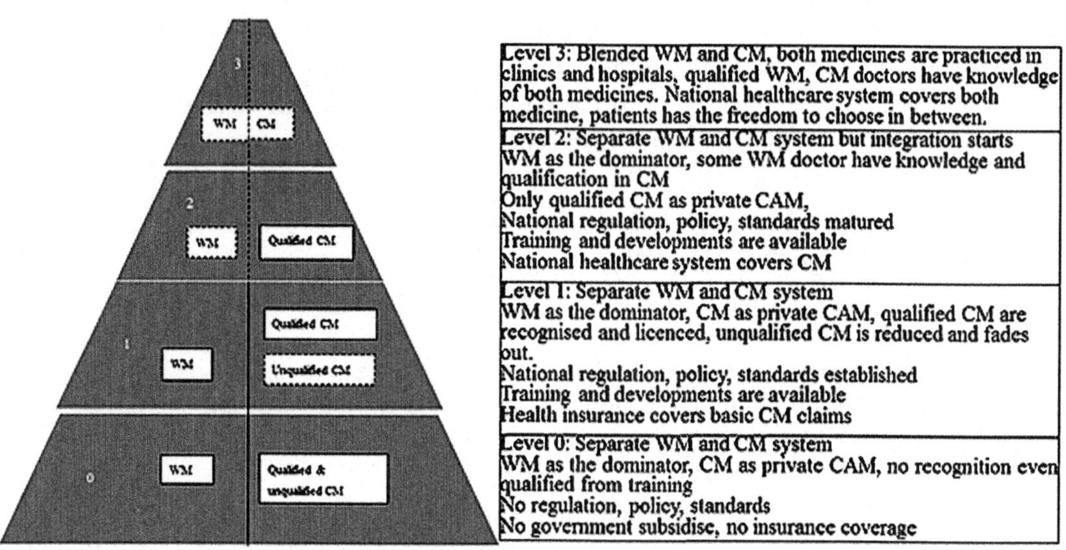

Level 3: Blended WM and CM, both medicines are practiced in clinics and hospitals, qualified WM, CM doctors have knowledge of both medicines. National healthcare system covers both medicine, patients has the freedom to choose in between.

Level 2: Separate WM and CM system but integration starts WM as the dominator, some WM doctor have knowledge and qualification in CM
Only qualified CM as private CAM,
National regulation, policy, standards matured
Training and developments are available
National healthcare system covers CM

Level 1: Separate WM and CM system
WM as the dominator, CM as private CAM, qualified CM are recognised and licenced, unqualified CM is reduced and fades out.
National regulation, policy, standards established
Training and developments are available
Health insurance covers basic CM claims

Level 0: Separate WM and CM system
WM as the dominator, CM as private CAM, no recognition even qualified from training
No regulation, policy, standards
No government subsidise, no insurance coverage

council for certification of acupuncture and Oriental Medicine developed assessment guidelines and examinations for acupuncturists and CM herbalists (Boodeker & Kronenberg, 2002). In Switzerland, CM is covered by the nation's compulsory health insurance program announced by the Federal Department of Home Affairs in 1998 (WHO, 2013). To assist CM strategic movement, it is helpful to identify and illustrate the different stages of CM and WM integrations. Figure 1 demonstrates these stages and it can also be used as a road map for implementation design, progress and updates.

Stage three in Figure 1 has the highest integration between CM and WM. It is also WHO's vision and goal that is to have a blended system which takes the best of each and compensates for the potential weaknesses in each (WHO, 2013). However, to date, this stage can be only seen in China.

CM and WM in China

As the birth country of CM, this traditional medicine has dominated the country's health system for thousands of years until the Opium war (Chi, 1994). Western power and invasion shook the Chinese self-confidence as well as CM. Reformers at the time turned to science as the salvation for China and considered WM as part of the new western science wonders. Supported by scientific evidence, WM was considered to be more advanced than CM (Chi, 1994). Chinese experienced and compared the treatment of both medicine types and they gradually shifted their preference to WM. The study of Chi (1994) suggested when WM was introduced to the majority of Chinese, advanced transportation and trade supported adequate supply of drugs and equipment which helped the sustainability of WM in China. CM lost its dominance from the early twentieth century until recently when large Chinese civilisations acknowledged the importance and necessity of modernisation (Chi, 1994). In this process, some intellectuals and key government officials believed that adopting various levels of western science should be accompanied by perfecting traditional Chinese culture. They proposed that CM must learn from WM to gain scientific knowledge, evidence and approval; on the other hand WM must study the popular and widespread spirit of CM (Chi, 1994). Today, China is the only country in the world which has the two medicine types practised alongside each other at every level of the healthcare services (Hesketh & Zhu, 1997). Almost 95% of general hospitals where WM is practised include CM departments and provide CM services to patients. Hesketh and Zhu (1997) reported that 40% of the prescriptions from WM hospitals are CM and equally 40% WM prescriptions are from CM hospitals and clinics. All WM schools devote around 15% of curriculum time to CM; similarly CM students must undertake some compulsory courses from WM (Hesketh & Zhu, 1997). In China, WM is seen as more effective in acute situations or where the aetiology is known, while CM is more effective for immune conditions, chronic illness and where the aetiology is unknown (Hesketh & Zhu, 1997).

CM in Australia

Australia has achieved some of the most impressive outcomes in implementing the WHO's strategies (CMBA, 2014). They are highlighted below:

- The CM profession is now included in the National Registration and Accreditation Scheme (NRAS). National registration of practitioners, acupuncturists, and dispensers of Chinese herbal medicine commenced on the 1st July, 2012 (CMBA, 2014).
- Policies, registration guidelines, codes and standards were created and published to assist the CM profession.
- CM undergraduate and postgraduate courses are offered in Australian tertiary education system.
- Accreditation standards and processes for consultation were developed by the Australian Health Practitioner Regulation Agency (AHPRA) and Chinese Medicine Board of Australia (CMBA) (CMBA, 2014).
- CMBA website is created which enables online service delivery and communication. Chinese Medicine Portal (CMP) is created and serves as an online CM knowledge pool where information and clinical data can be retrieved and accessed (Yang et al. 2009).
- AHPRA will directly allocate cost funding to CMBA to assist various activities undertaken by the agreement and strategies (CMBA, 2014).

Despite these remarkable achievements, our analysis suggests that much work and attention is needed for integrating CM into the Australian health care service delivery and self-health care. Therefore, CM and WM integration in Australia is at stage one (Lin et al. 2013, 2014a). CM authorities and individuals are working towards stage two where only qualified CM physicians are allowed in clinics and WM doctors are trained and have basic knowledge of CM. The two systems are still separate but more overlap and cross over occurs with more referrals and co-workers (CMBA, 2014).

CM PRACTICE AND ITS CLINICAL ACTIVITIES

CM is a system of primary health care that works holistically to maintain or restore balance, harmony and order in human bodies. CM philosophy is based on the Yin/Yang principle of balancing and harmonising conditions within the body (Hsu, 2001, Liao, 2011; Wang et al., 1999; Xue and O'Brien, 2003). The origins of CM go back thousands of years, and work with the philosophy that balanced and

Table 1. CM Five elements

Elements	Zang Organs	Fu Organs	Sense Organs	Body Tissues	Passions	Fluids	Pulses
Earth	Spleen	Stomach	Lips	Muscles	Thought/Anxiety	Saliva	Moderate
Fire	Heart	Small intestine	Tongue	Vessels	Joy	Sweat	Surging
Metal	Lung	Large intestine	Nose	Skin and hair	Sorrow	Nasal discharge	Floating
Water	Kidney	Urinary bladder	Ears	Bones	Fear/Fright	Spittle	Deep
Wood	Liver	Gallbladder	Eyes	Tendons	Anger	Tears	Taut

(Adopted from Liu & Liu 2009 p 23)

free-flowing Qi (energy) results in health, while stagnant or imbalanced Qi leads to disease. According to these philosophies, life energy is rhythmically channelled through a network of mutual influences between the five elements and the corresponding organs of the human body (Huang & Chen, 2007; Liu & Liu, 2009; Zhao et al., 1994). Table 1 summarises the key aspects of CM.

CM Diagnosis and Treatments

CM practitioners use four diagnosis methods: inspection, auscultation and olfaction, inquiring, and palpation (Huang & Chen 2007; Zhao et al., 1994). Inspection begins with the physician understanding and predicting the pathological changes of internal organs by observing abnormal changes in the patient's vitality, colour, appearance, secretions, and excretions (Huang & Chen 2007). Auscultation and olfaction involve listening and smelling. The physician listens to the patient's voice, breathing, coughing, and sounds emanating from the internal organs. Ear and stethoscope may also be applied in this process. A patient's "stinky" smell, for example, usually indicates heat syndromes while foul and sour smell implies retention of food (Huang & Chen 2007). Inquiring means the physician asking the patient about his/her condition such as chills, fever, perspiration, appetite, thirst, and pain, Huang and Chen (2007) explain. In palpation, the physician would put his/her first three fingers on the radial artery of a patient's wrist. A trained and skilled physician can detect over 30 different pulse qualities (e.g. floating, sunken, weak, and bounding) on each of the 12 pulses (Zhu & Wang 2011). The pulse qualities help the physician to identify the condition of the related organs. These four approaches are used in combination in every diagnosis and cannot be separated or omitted (Zhu & Wang 2011). A correct diagnosis can only be made based on a comprehensive and systematic analysis of a patient's condition at the point of care. This explains why CM diagnosis and treatments are different for the same patient and disease at different times (Kaptchuk, 2000; Lin et al., 2013, 2014c). CM physician's expert knowledge and comprehensive analysis of each patient's unique health condition is a key which differentiates between the two types of medicinal practices.

CM treatments can be a combination of the following: herbs (including leaves, seeds, roots, flowers, fruits, minerals and animal products); acupuncture, moxibustion, tuina (Chinese remedial massage), cupping, qigong and diet therapy (Xue & O'Brien 2003). All treatments aim to increase human body's resistance to diseases and prevention by improving the inter-connections among self-controlled systems (Lu et al., 2004).

CM Clinical Activities

CM, as a CAM in developed or western countries is typically practised in small clinic settings which are very identical to the Primary Care or General Practice (GP) (Ben-Arye et al., 2008; GP NSW, 2011; North, 2008). It follows the common GP clinical activities which include three major processes: reception; physician consultation and diagnosis; prescription and treatments (GP NSW, 2011; AHPRA, 2014).

Reception: appointments (booked and walk-in) scheduling is commonly the starting point of a medical care for both the patients and the clinics (GP NSW, 2011; AHPRA, 2014). It is one of the most resource demanding daily tasks (GP NSW, 2011; AHPRA, 2014). A first-time-visit patient is asked to fill in a form which provides the clinic with the patient's personal details and medical histories. This information is usually stored in the GP clinic file system electronically. However, most CM clinics are still recording these records on paper (Lin et al., 2013; 2014c). Our observation on ten CM clinics in Melbourne Australia indicates that men-made administration problems occur under this manual system. In summary they are: 1) file lost and misplace. Patient files can be misplaced at different categories, storage locations. This is because: a) clinics categorise and store patients file in a surname – given names sequential order. Some patients such as the Chinese usually read and write their surname first. This is the opposite of the Europeans who usually put their given names before their surname. b) different pronunciation and word. When Chinese names are recorded by PinYin (like English alphabets) without tones, it can be pronounced and referred to a range of different characters or words (Lin et al., 2014c). Hence, searching for the patient's file involves challenges, efforts and clarifications. 2) file management obstacles. Paper recording and storage make patient information update and management less efficient. 3) handwriting problems. Everyone writes differently, so it is sometimes difficult to read and understand the handwritten records.

In CM clinics, the receptionist also handles payments and insurance claims. As CM is not covered by Medicare Australia, patients must cover the cost privately. Some private insurance companies give certain percentage of rebate on acupuncture and remedial massage (Zheng, 2014).

Physician consultation and diagnosis: CM diagnosis methods are unique and different from WM, this is stated in details in the previous sections. To date, many CM diagnosis are recorded manually into the patients' files by physicians during the consultation. CMBA has launched policies, standards, and requirements on patient files. All CM clinics in Australia should record and report the mandatory elements of patient personal details in English (CMBA, 2014). Where records are maintained in a language other than English, should a copy of a patient's records be requested by the patient, or required by the CMBA or an authorised third party, it is the responsibility of the CM practitioner to provide at their own expense an English translation of the patient's records or cover the cost of this service according to CMBA (2014).

Prescription and treatments: after consultation and diagnosis, the physician may give the patient a treatment plan. The patient may be referred to a specialist for more specialised treatments or be transferred to hospital for an emergency care. It is very common that the patient is required to come back for a subsequent treatment. CM prescriptions and treatments cover wide ranges of products. The most common prescription is Chinese herbal medicine with acupuncture treatments (Kaptchuk, 2000; Liao, 2011; Liu & Liu, 2009). CMBA require CM practitioners provide information on treatments/therapies being used (including herbal, pharmaceutical, manipulative, dietary, and psychological); diagnosis, treatment principles, and recommended treatment plans; all procedures conducted including details of all acupuncture points and stimulation method; any medicine prescribed, administered or supplied for the patient or any other therapeutic agent used (including name, strength, quantity, dose, instructions for use, number of repeats and details of when started or stopped); discussion about possible side effects or alternative forms of treatment; details of how the patient was monitored and the outcome in progress notes (CMBA, 2014).

Herbal prescription is usually prepared by dispenser(s) after receiving the written prescription from the physician (Chi, 1994; Lu et al., 2004; Xue & O'Brien 2003). There are usually multiple packs of the same herbal combinations for each prescription. These packs are double checked by a second dispenser for accuracy (Chi, 1994; Lu et al., 2004; Xue & O'Brien 2003). Instructions of how to prepare and take the medicine are written and given to the patient. Any further questions can be answered before the patient exits the clinic.

CM Diagnosis and Treatment Processes

The above mentioned CM clinical activities and processes give us the understanding of CM clinic basic daily operations. The comparison of these operations to typical GP is important in analysing and developing a suitable IS/IT solution for the CM clinics. To achieve this, it is first necessary to map the processes. Figure 2 demonstrate this in details.

The CM processes in Figure 2 are a close match to WM clinics. Swisher et al (2001) analysed and modelled WM clinic processes which consist of: registration; check-in; examination (including pre-examination and post-examination); exit interview; and check-out (Swisher et al., 2001). In Swisher's model, a patient books a visit with a clinical staff prior to consultation in the registration process. In Check-in, patient's initial medical information is collected before examination. Next a physician collects more extensive medical information from the patient (pre-examination) if necessary; diagnoses the patient and prescribes treatments (examination); additional medical information is collected if any (post-examination). A physician performs the final consultation and diagnosis in exit interview process

Figure 2. CM Patient diagnosis and treatment processes
(Adopted from Lin et al., 2014c)

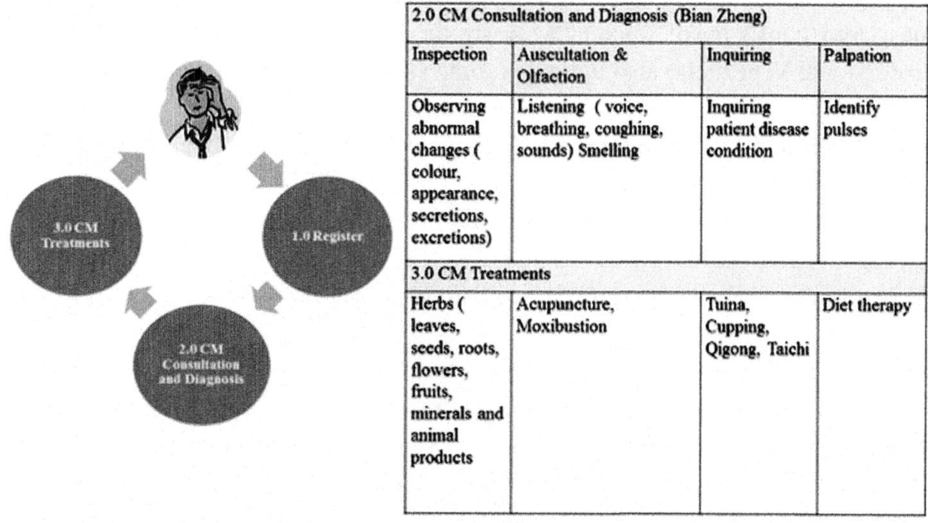

2.0 CM Consultation and Diagnosis (Bian Zheng)			
Inspection	Auscultation & Olfaction	Inquiring	Palpation
Observing abnormal changes (colour, appearance, secretions, excretions)	Listening (voice, breathing, coughing, sounds) Smelling	Inquiring patient disease condition	Identify pulses
3.0 CM Treatments			
Herbs (leaves, seeds, roots, flowers, fruits, minerals and animal products	Acupuncture, Moxibustion	Tuina, Cupping, Qigong, Taichi	Diet therapy

(Swisher et al., 2001). Comparing these WM processes with CM, we have found that Swisher's registration process matches the CM 1.0 process in Figure 2. The check-in and examination processes match CM process 2.0. The post-examination is really the 3.0 process in Figure 2. Instead of having exit interview and check-out, we realise that the processes can flow back and be repeated for some patients. This may suggest that CM clinics can expect as much benefit from a IS/IT solution as we are now witnessing in WM clinics.

Problems and Challenges of CM

Today CM clinics still operate its clinical activities manually; many CM practitioners use their first language to record patients' syndromes and treatments (Lin et al., 2013, 2014c). This creates language difficulties to others. It is also hard to implement standards, and to encourage an internationally recognised and registered practice. A patient's medical record can come in many forms including films, images, telegraphs, and electronic medical record (EMR). CM doctors found it difficult to store these crucial evidences in analysing and diagnosing the patient without the proper and adequate technology and equipment. As an ancient treatment to human diseases, CM today has a huge collection of herbs and medical equipment. Managing these medicines and equipment manually is a continuous resource and space-demanding task to the CM clinics.

Research has attempted to build and transfer the voluminous information and knowledge in Chinese herbs, acupuncture, syndromes, and treatments to a knowledge-based system which can be retrieved online or through Intranet. Some CM expert systems and applications are developed for certain diseases or particular treatment. For example, a Chinese acupuncture expert system can assist physician on acupuncture prescription, needle insertion position, and acupuncture points usage (Lam et al., 2012). The existing research and developments have some limitations: 1) only include or focus on limited or small amount of Chinese herbs with no or limited resources in Chinese acupuncture or vice versa (Yang et al. 2009), hence it is incomprehensive. 2) lack of evidence support on information production (Yang et al. 2009). 3) not an IS/IT system solution for CM clinics and practitioners to handle their daily key processes (Lin et al, 2013; 2014c). 4) no system functions and features on clinical medicine management (Lin et al.,2013, 2014c). 5) there is not a suitable synthesis to support or give a solid base or foundation for the IS/IT developments (Lin et al.,2013, 2014c; Yang et al. 2009). Further, a study of the current CM clinic management system (consisting of SmartTCM Australia, TCM Herbalist Israel, TCM Organiser Canada, and Shen Professional Venezuela) also indicates some significant concerns including:

- Incorrect use of the Chinese language as well as non-comprise to other languages except Chinese and English (Lin et al, 2014a).
- Not a secure multi-user and access which can accommodate administrator, physician, and dispenser (Lin et al, 2014a).
- Cannot be used on multi system and device (Lin et al, 2014a).

The most important limitation of the above all is that the synthesis of IS/IT developments so far has been mainly studied and applied to WM. It is our contention that blindly adopting these theories and technologies is not the best solution for CM. This view is supported in practice when we look at Enterprise Resource Planning (ERP) systems such as SAP and Oracle as they have tried to conquer the Chinese market by simply applying the same tools and techniques without first understanding and mapping the underlying circumstances and requirements. Xue et al. (2005) noted that "most ERP systems are designed by western IT professionals and the structures and processes embedded in these systems reflect western cultures. Implementation failures tend to occur when Chinese companies attempt to adopt foreign ERP systems." (Xue et al., 2005, p. 280). To avoid similar failures, it is therefore necessary to systematically examine the basis of the synthesis. Search and form a theoretical foundation that is suitable for CM practice. This is described in details in the next sections where we analyse the different inquiring and knowledge management systems.

SOLUTIONS AND RECOMMENDATIONS

The preceding section has indicated that CM practice is distinct and different from WM, simply adopting the existing IS/IT solutions which are designed and developed for WM, is fundamentally flawed and would thus not be the best approach for CM developments (Lin et al, 2013, 2014c). To form a foundation and synthesis for CM, this section reviews and analyses the basics of inquiring and knowledge management (KM) systems. In so doing, we propose a new theory that is more suitable for CM developments. Once this is done, then any CM system developments such as a CM Clinic Management System (CMCMS) can be built-on-top.

Inquiring Systems

Churchman defined the five inquiring systems: Leibnizian, Lockean, Hegelian, Kantian, and Singerian (Courtney et al, 2005; Churchman, 1971). Each of them represents a type of inquiring organisation from a system view of knowledge creation, examination, and management (Wickramasinghe, 2005).

Leibnizian, Lockean, and Singerian Inquiring System

Leibnizian inquiring system is a closed system with a set of built-in elementary axioms that are used along with formal logic and analysis to generate more fact nets (Churchman, 1971; Courtney et al., 2005; Hall & Croasdell, 2005;). Knowledge creation is limited as the Leibnizian system use only formal logic and mathematical analysis to make influences about cause and effect relationships (Courtney, 2001; Hall & Croasdell, 2005; Mason & Mitroff, 1973; Parrish & Courtney, 2012). They focus on reliability and replication. Organisational memory and knowledge expand within its internal boundary to achieve accuracy and repetition. Therefore they deal with problems that are highly structured with few unknown variables (Courtney, 2001; Hall & Croasdell, 2005; Mason & Mitroff, 1973; Parrish & Courtney, 2012). KM is concentrated on manipulating the organisation's explicit knowledge such as documents describing goals, plans, and standard operating procedures. Courtney (2001), Hall and Croasdell (2005), Mason and Mitroff (1973), Parrish and Courtney (2012) have all explained that tacit knowledge gets little emphasis in this organisation which leads to difficulties to adapt and maintain in a changing and non-consequential environment. IS/IT most suited to the Leibnizian inquiring systems are types of expert systems. Nonaka et al (1998) explained this form of KM in the combination mode of knowledge creation. He stated, "combination involves the conversion of explicit knowledge into more complex sets of explicit knowledge" (Nonaka et al., 1998, p. 674), and new knowledge is generated as an externalisation of editing and systemizing.

Lockean inquiring system is a close system in which community members sharing a common language and mindset supported by strong relationships and communication (Courtney, 2001; Hall & Croasdell, 2005; Mason & Mitroff, 1973; Parrish & Courtney, 2012). Lockean organisations develop organisational beliefs, practices, and rituals. These values are passed on, shared and perpetuated within the organisation through attention to symbolic references such as legends and/or well-respected authorities (Courtney, 2001; Hall & Croasdell, 2005; Mason & Mitroff, 1973; Parrish & Courtney, 2012). Knowledge is socially constructed through observation and discussion. Examples of IS/IT used in Lockean inquiring system are: repositories such as data warehouses (storing observations), data mining (analysing the observations), and groupware tools like emails (facilitating the communication and sharing) (Courtney, 2001). According to Courtney (2001) the Lockean organisations exemplifies Nonaka's socialisation mode of knowledge creation. Socialisation is about sharing individual's tacit knowledge to those "if the self becomes part of a larger self" (Nonaka et al., 1998, p. 674).

Singerian inquiring system is guided by two basic premises. The first is to establish a system of measures which specifies steps to be followed in resolving disagreements (Churchman, 1971; Courtney et al., 2005; Hall & Croasdell, 2005). The second is the strategy of agreement. When disagreements occur for various reasons, and when models fail to explain a phenomenon, new variables and laws are introduced to provide guidance and overcome inconsistencies (Courtney, 2001; Hall & Croasdell, 2005; Mason & Mitroff, 1973; Parrish & Courtney, 2012). Problem fragmentation or partitioning helps Singerian organisations make sense of the situation by sorting out the known and unknown, then it processes the unknown further, generating cycles of disagreement and agreement until the problem is fully investigated and understood from all sides (Courtney, 2001; Hall & Croasdell, 2005; Mason & Mitroff, 1973; Parrish & Courtney, 2012). The Singerian has the purpose of creating exoteric knowledge for choosing the right means for one's end. Knowledge must be connected to measurable improvements that are judged not only by organisational standards but also by what is good and ethical for all of society (Courtney, 2001; Hall & Croasdell, 2005; Mason & Mitroff, 1973; Parrish & Courtney, 2012). The Singerian inquirer believes that problems and knowledge domains are non-separable; everything is connected to everything else; from any source, discipline, and profession; and so they are analysed as wholes. Knowledge of all forms is considered which include: tacit and explicit, deep and shallow, declarative and procedural, exoteric and esoteric (Courtney, 2001; Hall & Croasdell, 2005; Mason & Mitroff, 1973; Parrish & Courtney, 2012). Nonaka's socialisation and externalisation modes are emphasised in the Singerian inquiring system style as a discourse may involve many perspectives. The Singerian approach is best supported by network based such as groupware and web-based to allow virtual information gathering and learning because of its need to include a wide range of individual stakeholders (Courtney, 2001; Hall & Croasdell, 2005; Mason & Mitroff, 1973; Parrish & Courtney, 2012). Repositories and document management systems are supportive tools for information gathering and dissemination process.

Hegelian Inquiring System

Hegelian inquiring system is based on the belief that the best way for knowledge creation is by observing a debate between two conflicting ideas (Courtney, 2001; Hall & Croasdell, 2005; Mason & Mitroff, 1973; Parrish & Courtney, 2012). There are three major players in the Hegelian system. The first player constructs a strong conviction of a fundamental thesis with great efforts of maximizing supporting materials. The second player does the same thing as the first only with an opposite worldview of the thesis - antithesis. The third player analyses the debate and constructs a new and larger worldview that is synthesis of the thesis and antithesis. In this style, knowledge is gained by reflecting and resolving diametrically opposed perspectives (Courtney, 2001; Hall & Croasdell, 2005; Mason & Mitroff, 1973; Parrish & Courtney, 2012). Hegelian organisations have little structure or formal mechanism for guidance; however it is assisted by group support systems that include negotiation and arbitration. Knowledge to be managed in such environments consists of information from the three players and the interaction dialogues (Courtney, 2001; Hall & Croasdell, 2005; Mason & Mitroff, 1973). IS/IT solutions that support Hegelian inquiring systems include: groupware that is designed to support and facilitate arguments among stakeholders in order to help them understand the specific elements of each other's proposals; repositories that hold the debate data; document management software and/or analysis tools for developing points to support either the thesis or the antithesis (Courtney, 2001; Hall & Croasdell, 2005; Mason & Mitroff, 1973).

In a Hegelian inquiring system, knowledge creation can be seen as consisting of Nonaka's socialisation and externalisation (Courtney, 2001). Socialisation as it involves three players' interaction and debating. It is through this social process, tacit and explicit knowledge of the thesis and antithesis are externalized (Courtney, 2001; Hall & Croasdell, 2005; Nonaka et al., 1998).

Kantian Inquiring System

The Kantian inquiring system is designed to incorporate both multiple perspectives and facts to determine models that are best-fit for the situation (Churchman, 1971; Courtney et al., 2005; Hall & Croasdell, 2005). Using Leibnizian fact nets to support its data analysis, Kantian inquiring systems perform various modelling techniques to interpret and explain the causal connections between perspectives and the observations (Courtney, 2001; Hall & Croasdell, 2005; Mason & Mitroff, 1973; Parrish & Courtney, 2012). Kantian organisation depends on communication, organisation memory, understanding of the modelling, stability of rules and regulations. In this style, knowledge is managed in both empirical and theoretical approach (Courtney, 2001; Hall & Croasdell, 2005; Mason & Mitroff, 1973; Parrish & Courtney, 2012). The perspectives can be heavily analytical as it uses multiple analytical methods for interpreting data. Learning is disseminated through the group members and KM may be enhanced by the use of a system design to discover and distribute information (Courtney, 2001; Hall & Croasdell, 2005; Mason & Mitroff, 1973; Parrish & Courtney, 2012). The Kantian inquiring system tends to be sensible to the environment. It is focused on flexibility, relationships, organisational development through contingency theory and the best-fit between itself and the environment; hence it can react quickly and effectively to problems and changes. This type of inquiring system is suitable for moderately uncertain situations, unstable environments and complex problems of high-to-moderate structure (Courtney, 2001; Hall & Croasdell, 2005; Mason & Mitroff, 1973; Parrish & Courtney, 2012).

The Kantian inquiring system can be seen in Nonaka's internalisation mode which includes both tacit and explicit knowledge (Courtney, 2001; Hall & Croasdell, 2005; Nonaka et al., 1998). The system uses machine-learning algorithm and models input by experts to analyse incoming information and add the processed information/models to the organisation's memory, according to Courtney (2001), Hall and Croasdell (2005), Nonaka et al. (1998). Examples of IS/IT in Kantian are: World Wide Web (www), databases, model management systems, decision support systems, and effective information systems.

Inquiring Systems for WM

Healthcare Information Systems (HIS) have been largely developed to produce expert systems, theorem-proving systems, problem-solving and decision-support systems, algorithm-generating systems, databases, and repositories in WM (Ferlie et al., 2012; Liao, 2003). Hence the existing HIS developments and solutions are mostly in the categories of Leibnizian and Lockean inquiring systems. As mentioned earlier, Leibnizian inquirer creates fact-net, expert systems perpetuating experiential knowledge. This can be seen in HIS, for example, electronic knowledge repositories, storing codified knowledge for future reuse; Clinical decision support systems (DSS), linking characteristics of patients with chest pain to software algorithms recommending specific action (Ferlie et al., 2012). This kind of DSS take information from various data sources and use these data to provide assistance with the structured portion of the semi-structured decision (Parrish & Courtney, 2012). This is an early form of a Kantian inquirer stated by Parrish and Courtney (2012), as the human decision maker must rely on intuition and experience to assist them with the unstructured portions. Singerian inquiring system's great emphasis on ethical behaviour can be seen in most HIS where medical ethics and professionalism are mandatory and expected to maintain strictly in practice. An example of this is a DSS which is developed and implemented with the guidance and principles of patient safety, quality performance, regulations, and policies (Parrish & Courtney, 2012).

Inquiring System for CM

The unique characters, diagnosis, and treatments of CM indicate that CM healthcare is a complex open environment. There are many variables, inputs, and perspectives to consider and communicate. This is a feature common to Kantian inquiring systems as it generates hypotheses on the basis of the inputs received from various knowledge sources (Churchman, 1971; Courtney et al., 2005). The Kantian inquiring system is also able to use explicit and tacit knowledge to consider the many interpretations of the inputs. Knowledge is compared allowing the inquirer to consider ways and/or different modelling to create and incorporate new knowledge (Churchman, 1971; Courtney et al., 2005).

We also see that CM exhibits features common to Hegelian inquiring systems since CM tries to resolve conflicts and proposes enlarged synthesis. As a result the problem is completely dissolved (Courtney et al., 2005; Hall & Croasdell, 2005; Morr & Subercaze, 2010). Hegelian's ability to understand all behaviours, forms, processes, arguments, and technologies support CM's comprehensive and systematic view of human diseases. CM philosophy emphasises inner self-controlled system connectivity and balance between Yin and Yang energy. Any disorder is a result of failure and/or imbalance of the system (Huang & Chen, 2007; Lu et al., 2004; Zhao et al., 1994). Hence resolving, strengthening, and rebalancing the system with duality wisdom (Wickramasinghe, 2005) is a key in CM practice.

Additionally, as Kantian and Hegelian rely on Leibnizian inquiring system's fact net to generate knowledge (Courtney, 2001; Hall & Croasdell, 2004; Moody & Shanks, 1999), then Leibnizian inquiring system is used as part of the knowledge base. This includes, for example: repositories, models, CMBA regulation and guidelines for CM practitioners in Australia, and the CM Portal. Furthermore, Singerian inquiring systems' strong emphasis on ethical conduct is extremely important to any HIS and is thus also relevant in the CM context. Patient autonomy, welfare and social justice must be considered and built-in as principles and guidelines in any CM IS/IT developments and solutions.

Table 2. Mapping inquiring systems to CM and WM

Inquiring Systems	Hegelian	Kantian	Singerian	Leibnizian	Lockean
Western Medicine					
Chinese Medicine					

(Adopted from Lin et al., 2014b) source: HICSS 2015

Table 2 illustrates the inquiring systems based on our discussion. From this table, we can see the different IS/IT design and development focus between the two types of medicine practices. WM IS/IT developments are mainly in the Leibnizian and Lockean inquiring systems with Singerian inquirer's ethical guidance (highlighted in a dark colour). Furthermore, research tends to indicate some early Kantian inquiring systems using DSS in WM (highlighted in a lighter colour). Our research suggest that CM IS/IT developments should be primarily in the category of Hegelian and Kantian inquiring systems (highlighted in a dark colour) with the support and principles from Singerian and Leibnizian inquiring systems (highlighted in a lighter colour). No colour, or white in Table 2 represents no IS/IT solution to date that fits this type of inquiring system respectively in WM or CM.

Knowledge Management (KM) Systems

KM systems are designed and developed to support and enhance knowledge intense tasks, processes, and projects for the purpose of knowledge creation, storage, retrieval, transfer, refinement, reuse, revision, and feedback (Maier & Hadrich, 2011). Typical KM systems contain data and knowledge sources; infrastructure services; integration services; knowledge services; personalisation services; and access services (Maier, 2007; Maier & Hadrich, 2011).

Data and knowledge sources include organisational internal and external information and knowledge, data warehouse, document management, personal information management, contents from Internet, WWW, and groupware (Maier, 2007; Maier & Hadrich, 2011). This research analyse the CM clinic's information and knowledge in these categories through the case study. For example, how does the clinic manage its medicine documentations? What are the key elements in managing this with IS/IT?

Infrastructure services provide basic functionality for synchronous and asynchronous communication, data and electronic assets management, extraction, transformation, and loading (Maier, 2007; Maier & Hadrich, 2011). For example, Intranet infrastructure services provide messaging, teleconferencing, and file transferring. In this case the research looks into the clinic's IT infrastructure services for messaging and files transferring.

Integration services help to meaningfully organise and link knowledge elements from a variety of sources. Integration is often used to analyse the organisation knowledge base and manage the multi-dimensional metadata (Maier, 2007; Maier & Hadrich, 2011). The research looks into how the clinic manages external information and knowledge such as films and laboratory test results in assisting diagnosis and treatments.

Knowledge services involve 1) discovery functions such as searching, mining, navigation, and visualisation (Maier, 2007; Maier & Hadrich, 2011). 2) publication functions like structuring, formats, and contextualisation (Maier, 2007; Maier & Hadrich, 2011). 3) collaboration functions include skill/expert management, knowledge sharing, awareness, and experience management (Maier, 2007; Maier

& Hadrich, 2011). 4) learning functions that use tools and techniques for authoring, managing courses, tutoring, learning paths, and examinations (Maier, 2007; Maier & Hadrich, 2011). In this category, the research analyses if any expert knowledge system is used in the clinic; if the physicians use any DSS in assisting diagnosis and treatments; how does the clinic manage its reporting and standards required by the CM authorities; how do the clinic practitioners search, order, and manage their medical/herb information; what are the major concerns and key elements in this area when using IS/IT?

Personalisation services can organise a portion of the KM system contents and services for specialists and/or specific roles (Maier, 2007; Maier & Hadrich, 2011). For example personalised or role-oriented knowledge portals; personal information management and digital assistant. The research looks into if there are any personal devices and applications that the practitioners are using or like to use; how the clinic manages these personalisation services. User access level of the clinic medicine practice is also studied.

KM architecture and characteristics are important elements which must be considered in CM developments. Table 3 summaries the systems that are suitable for CM information systems.

Table 3. Information systems for CM

| | | CM Inquiring Systems | | | | | |
	Lockean	**Singerian**	**Leibnizian**	**Kantian**	**Hegelian**	**KM Systems**
Inputs	Goals, decisions, standards, procedures	Units, standards	Fact net	Knowledge sources, organisation memory	Mission statements	Data and knowledge sources; infrastructure services; integration services; knowledge services; personalisation services; access services
Given	Organisation memory, structure, and culture	System of measures	Standards, operating procedures, rule base	Tacit and explicit knowledge, working theories	Opposing views	
Process	Negotiation, communication, consensus building	use variables to overcome inconsistency	Cause and effect analysis, inference	Knowledge scanning, association building	Arbitration	
Output	Ambiguous reduction	New measures, exoteric knowledge	Error detection and correction, suggested course of action	Integrated and timely knowledge	Conflict resolution, enlarged perspective, new strategic direction	
Knowledge perspective/mode	Socialisation	Socialisation, externalisation	Combination	Combination	Socialisation, externalisation	
IS/IT	Communication repositories, groupware, networks	Groupware, networks, repositories, document management	Models, Decision Support Systems (DSS), expert systems, document management	Database, knowledge and model bases, management systems, www	Repositories, groupware, negotiation systems	

(Adopted from Lin et al., 2014b) source: HICSS 2015

Figure 3. CMCMS design processes

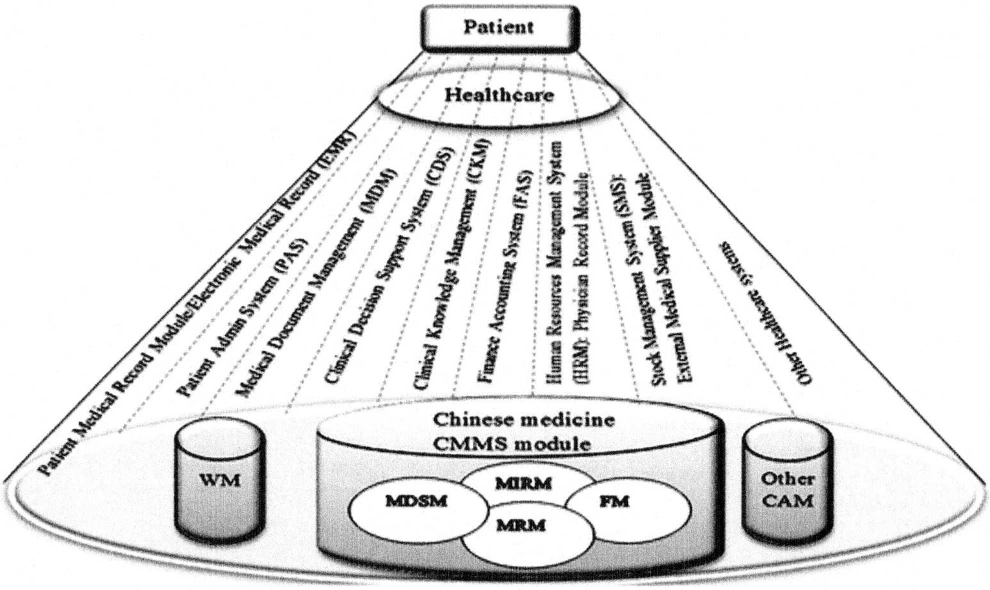

FUTURE RESEARCH DIRECTIONS

For CM to be integrated with WM in developed countries like Australia, there is more pressure for it to be more evidence based and have a more scientific and systematic structure in its delivery. We contend that IS/IT tools and techniques can play a key role in achieving this goal. As an extension of the proposed synthesis, this research looks into developing the CM clinic management system (CMCMS).

The CMCMS Study

The CMCMS development uses a mixed methodology of Case Study (CS) and Design Science (DS) to guide the various activities. CS is a commonly used and well-recognised research strategy in Healthcare Services and IS research (Yin, 1994, 1999). It attempts to examine a contemporary phenomenon in its real-life context, Yin (1994, 1999) stated. Through a typical CS, the research domain can be examined and a deeper understanding of the key and critical circumstances and conditions can be unearthed (Flick, 2014; Yin, 1994, 1999). Additionally, CS tools and techniques such as semi-structured interviews, thematic and artefact analysis provide valuable data and information for developing the CMCMS and thus are incorporated. DS methodology has its roots in the field of engineering and science (Hevner et al., 2004). It "seeks to create innovations that define the ideas, practices, technical capabilities, and products through which the analysis, design, implementation, management, and use of information systems can be effectively and efficiently accomplished" Hevner et al. (2004, p.76) said. DS is often used in developing executive information systems and system support emerging knowledge processes with effective development methods and system solutions for particular user group requirements (Hevner et al., 2004). This study goes through four DS processes: 1) analyse the existing situation: in this process the clinical data and research requirement are reviewed and analysed; semi-structured interviews are

Figure 4. CMCMS environment and modules
(Adopted from Lin et al., 2014c) Source: IJBET 2014

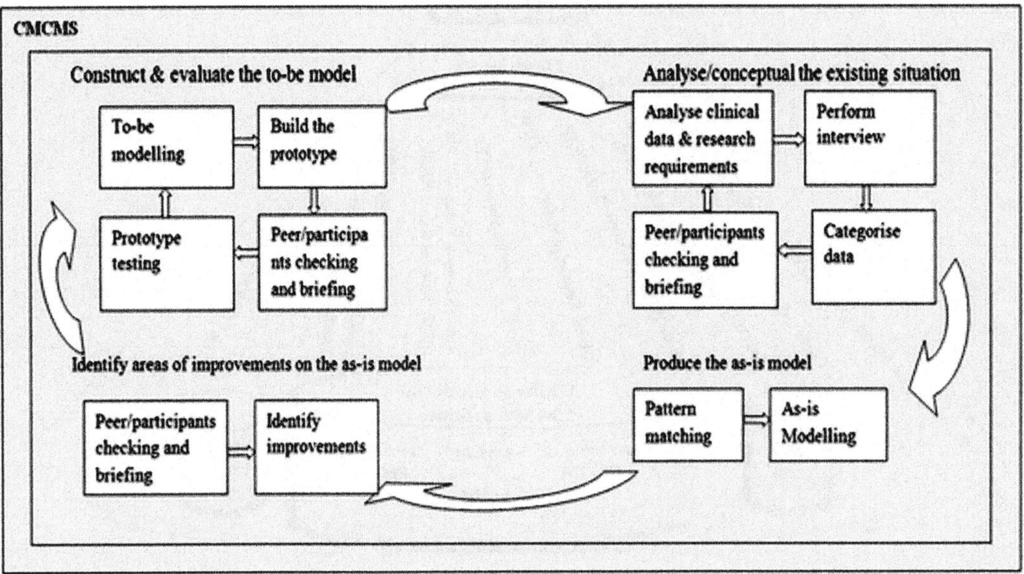

carried out in the case clinic guided by the interview questions; data is collected, categorised and peer reviewed. 2) situation design: the existing clinical (as-is) situation is modelled and analysed. Existing models and patterns from the literature are compared and mapped in this process. 3) improvements: areas of improvements, design, reengineering are identified with peer and domain experts contribution and advices. 4) evaluation: a range of IT tools and techniques are used in designing the system solution. These include: Business Process Modelling, Unified Modelling Language (UML) diagrams, and prototyping. The prototype and modules are then evaluated with specification, expectation, and precise scope. Figure 3 portrays these four processes.

The Conceptual Model

The CMCMS conceptual model identifies the environment, players, components, and integrations of CM system developments with other sectors and systems of healthcare. The primary driver/player in this diagram is the patient. That is because without the patient, none of the services are necessary. Therefore, all activities, systems, healthcare sectors are sharing a fundamental goal – a patient centred healthcare services (Epstein et al., 2010) with quality and efficiency.

At the need of care, a patient can trigger any of the components in Figure 4. The listed systems and modules under healthcare can be shared and information can be accessed and used across sectors. The broken line/link has the indication of communication and integration. The CMCMS has few internal modules which are: Medicine Item Record Module (MIRM), Medicine Decision Support Module (MDSM), Forecast Module (FM), and Medicine Reports Module (MRM). The MIRM contains detailed information about medicine items such as item name, category, item model, location at the clinic, vendor, manufacturer, reorder level, stock level, discontinued comments, transaction number, quantity, current on-hand quantity, transaction type, and payment information. The MDSM can support demand analysis, point-of-use, economic order quantity, reorder point system, can-order system, and safety stock. The FM can provide information for the clinic on what medicine should be ordered, in what amount, and in which season. MRM handles clinic medical reports including: medicine usage report, medicine order report, financial and payment report, patient medicine prescription report, and patient treatment report.

CONCLUSION

This chapter compares CM with WM in clinical activities and processes; diagnosis and treatments; IS/IT utilisations and clinical management systems. It advocates that IS/IT solutions and developments can support superior CM delivery. This in return can assist in achieving WHO's goal of having both types of medicines practiced alongside with complements to each other - a high level harmonisation and a more patient-centred approach. This chapter also discussed that CM IS/IT developments should follow a synthesis that is a combination of Churchman's Hegelian and Kantian inquiring systems with the support from Leiblizian and Singerian inquiring systems. This new synthesis extend Churchman's inquiring systems theory into a new domain within healthcare and combining the inquiring system with a design science approach for actually designing and developing a proposed solution. The proposed CMCMS provide an example and suggestion for CM clinics to migrate from manual system to a IS/IT solution which can be also used as assistance for both the CMBA and the individual CM practitioners in maintaining regulations and standards.

REFERENCES

AHPRA. (n.d.). *Australian Health Practitioner Regulation Agency*. Retrieved 14 October, 2014 from https://www.ahpra.gov.au/

Ben-Arye, E., Frenkel, M., Klein, A., & Scharf, M. (2008). Attitudes toward integration of complementary and alternative medicine in primary care: Perspectives of patients, physicians and complementary practitioners. *Patient Education and Counseling, 70*(3), 395–402. doi:10.1016/j.pec.2007.11.019 PMID:18201857

Bodeker, G., & Kronenberg, F. (2002). A public health agenda for traditional, complementary, and alternative medicine. *American Journal of Public Health, 92*(10), 1582–1591. doi:10.2105/AJPH.92.10.1582 PMID:12356597

Chi, C. (1994). Integrating Traditional Medicine into Modern Health Care Systems: Examining the role of Chinese Medicine in Taiwan. *Pergamon, 39*(3), 307-321.

Churchman, C. W. (1971). *The design of inquiring systems: basic concepts of systems and organisation*. New York: Basic Books.

CMBA. (n.d.). *Chinese Medicine Board of Australia*. Retrieved 14 October, 2014 from http://www.chinesemedicineboard.gov.au/

Courtney, J. F. (2001). Decision making and knowledge management in inquiring organisations: Toward a new decision-making paradigm for DSS. *Decision Support Systems, 31*(1), 17-38.

Courtney, J. F., Haynes, J. D., & Paradice, D. B. (2005). *Inquiring organisations: moving from knowledge management to wisdom.* IGI Global. doi:10.4018/978-1-59140-309-8

Epstein, R. M., Fiscella, K., Lesser, C. S., & Stange, K. C. (2010). Why the nation needs a policy push on patient-centered health care. *Health Affairs, 29*(8), 1489–1495. doi:10.1377/hlthaff.2009.0888 PMID:20679652

Feeley, T. W., Sledge, G. W., Levit, L., & Ganz, P. A. (2013). Improving the quality of cancer care in America through health information technology. *Journal of the American Medical Informatics Association.*

Ferlie, E., Crilly, T., Jashapara, A., & Peckham, A. (2012). Knowledge mobilisation in healthcare: a critical review of health sector and generic management literature. *Social Science & Medicine, 74*(8), 1297-1304.

Flick, U. (2014). An introduction to qualitative research. *Sage (Atlanta, Ga.).*

GP NSW. (2011). *A Guide to understanding and working with General Practice in New South Wales.* Retrieved 14 October, 2014 from http://www.gpnsw.com.au/__data/assets/pdf_file/0015/3444/AND145_GPNSW_Guide_WEB.pdf

Hall, D. J., & Croasdell, D. (2005). *Inquiring organisations: an organisational form perspective.* IGI Global. doi:10.4018/978-1-59140-309-8.ch001

Hesketh, T., & Zhu, W. X. (1997). Traditional Chinese Medicine: One country, two systems. *British Medical Journal, 315*(7100), 115–117. doi:10.1136/bmj.315.7100.115 PMID:9240055

Hevner, A. R., March, S.T., Park, J., & Ram, S. (2004). Design Science in Information Systems Research. *MIS Quarterly, 28*(1), 75 - 105.

Hojabri, R., & Manafi, M. (2012). Impact of using telemedicine on knowledge management in healthcare organisations: A case study. *African Journal of Business Management, 6*(4), 1604-1613.

Hsu, E. (Ed.). (2001). *Innovation in Chinese medicine* (Vol. 3). Cambridge University Press.

Huang, M. J. & Chen, M. Y. (2007). Integrated Design of the Intelligent Web-based Chinese Medical Diagnostic System (CMDS) - Systematic Development for Digestive Health. *Expert Systems with Applications, 32*(2), 658-673.

Kaptchuk, T. J. (2000). *Chinese Medicine - The Web That Has No Weaver.* An Imprint of Elbury Press, Random House, Rider.

Lam, C. F. D., Leung, K. S., Heng, P. A., Lim, C. E. D., & Wong, F. W. S. (2012). Chinese Acupuncture Expert System (CAES) - A useful tool to practice and Learn Medical Acupuncture. *Journal of Medical Systems, 36*(3), 1883-1890.

Liao, S. H. (2003). Knowledge management technologies and applications - literature review from 1995 to 2002. *Expert Systems with Applications, 25*(2), 155-164.

Liao, Y. Q. (2011). *Traditional Chinese Medicine.* Cambridge University Press.

Lin, C. H., Yang, A. W. H., Pittayachawan, S., Vogel, D., & Wickramasinghe, N. (2014a). Investigating the possibility for IS/IT to support the delivery of Chinese medicine. In *Proceedings of The First AIS-Journals Joint Author Workshop in ECIS*. Tel Aviv, Israel: ECIS.

Lin, C. H., Yang, A. W. H., Pittayachawan, S., Vogel, D., & Wickramasinghe, N. (2014b). Inquiring Knowledge Management Systems - A Chinese Medicine Perspective. In *Proceedings of the 2015 48th Hawaii International Conference on System Sciences (HICSS 2015)*. IEEE.

Lin, C. H., Yang, A. W. H., Pittayachawan, S., & Wickramasinghe, N. (2013). Using IS/IT to support the delivery of Chinese medicine: The design of a Chinese medicine clinic system. In *Proceedings of Australasian Conference on Information Systems*. Academic Press.

Lin, C. H., Yang, A. W. H., Pittayachawan, S., & Wickramasinghe, N. (2014c). *Using IS/IT to support the delivery of Chinese medicine: a Chinese medicine clinic management system. International Journal of Biomedical Engineering and Technology*.

Liu, Z. W., & Liu, L. (2009). *Essentials of Chinese Medicine*. Springer.

Lu, A. P., Jia, H. W., Xiao, C., & Lu, Q. P. (2004). Theory of Traditional Chinese Medicine and Therapeutic Method of Diseases. *World Journal of Gastroenterology, 10*(13), 1854-1856.

Lukman, S., He, Y., & Hui, S. C. (2007). *Computational methods for Traditional Chinese Medicine: A survey*. Elsevier.

Maier, R. (2007). *Knowledge management systems: Information and communication technologies for knowledge management*. Springer.

Maier, R., & Hädrich, T. (2011). *Knowledge Management Systems*. IGI.

Mason, R. O., & Mitroff, I. I. (1973). A program for research on management information systems. *Management Science, 19*(5), 475-487.

Moody, D. L., & Shanks, G. G. (1999). Using knowledge management and the internet to support evidence based practice: a medical case study. In *Proceedings of the 10th Australasian Conference on Information Systems* (pp. 660-676). Academic Press.

Morr, C. E., & Subercaze, J. (2010). *Handbook of Research on Developments in E-Health and Telemedicine: Technological and Social Perspectives*. IGI Global.

Nonaka, I., Reinmoeller, P., & Senoo, D. (1998). Management Focus The 'ART' of Knowledge: Systems to Capitalize on Market Knowledge. *European Management Journal, 16*(6), 673-684.

North, N. (2008). *Immigrant doctors practising non-Western medicine: a study of self-employed immigrant Chinese and Indian doctors practising non-biomedical traditions of medicine, New Settlers Programme*. Massey University.

O'Brien, E., Coats, A., Owens, P., Petrie, J., Padfield, P. L., Littler, W. A., & Mee, F. (2000). Use and interpretation of ambulatory blood pressure monitoring: Recommendations of the British Hypertension Society. *BMJ: British Medical Journal, 320*(7242), 1128–1134. doi:10.1136/bmj.320.7242.1128 PMID:10775227

Parrish, J. L. Jr, & Courtney, J. F. (2012). Inquiring Systems: Theoretical Foundations for Current and Future Information Systems, Information Systems Theory. *Springer New York, 2012*, 387–396.

Swisher, J. R., Jacobson, S. H., Jun, J. B., & Balci, O. (2001). Modeling and analyzing a physician clinic environment using discrete-event (visual) simulation. *Computers & Operations Research, 28*(2), 105-125.

Wang, Z. G., Chen, P., & Xie, P. P. (1999). *History and development of traditional Chinese medicine.* Science Press.

WHO. (2013). *WHO Traditional Medicine Strategy 2014 – 2023*. World Health Organisation. Retrieved 14 October, 2014 from: http://www.who.int/medicines/publications/traditional/trm_strategy14_23/en/

Wickramasinghe, N. (2005). The phenomenon of duality: A key to facilitate the transition from knowledge management to wisdom for inquiring organisations. In *Inquiring organisations: moving from knowledge management to wisdom* (pp. 272–315). IGI Global. doi:10.4018/978-1-59140-309-8.ch013

Wickramasinghe, N. (2013). Implicit and Explicit Knowledge Assets in Healthcare. In *Pervasive Health Knowledge Management* (pp. 15–26). Springer New York. doi:10.1007/978-1-4614-4514-2_3

Xue, C. C., & O'Brien, K. A. (2003). A Comprehensive Guide to Chinese Medicine Chapter 2: Modalities of Chinese Medicine. World Scientific Publishing.

Xue, C. C., Zhang, A. L., Lin, V., Myers, R., Polus, B., & Story, D. F. (2008). Acupuncture, chiropractic and osteopathy use in Australia: A national population survey. *BMC Public Health, 8*(1), 105. doi:10.1186/1471-2458-8-105 PMID:18377663

Xue, C.L, Zhang, A. L., Lin, V., Costa, C. D., & Story, D. F. (2007). Complementary and Alternative Medicine Use in Australia: A National Population-Based Survey. *The Journal of Alternative and Complementary Medicine, 13*(6), 643-650.

Xue, Y., Liang, H., Boulton, W. R., & Snyder, C. A. (2005). ERP implementation failures in China: case studies with implications for ERP vendors. *International Journal of Production Economics, 97*(3), 279-295.

Yang, A. W., Allan, G., Li, C. G., & Xue, C. C. (2009). Effective Application of Knowledge Management in Evidence-based Chinese Medicine: A Case Study. *eCam, 6*(3), 393-398.

Yin, R. K. (1994). *Case Study Research: Design and Methods* (2nd ed.). SAGE Publications.

Yin, R. K. (1999). Enhancing the quality of case studies in Health Services Research. *Health Services Research, 34*(5), 1209.

Zhao, Y. K., Tsursui, T. Endo, A. Minato, K., & Takahashi, T. (1994). Design and development of an expert system to assist diagnosis and treatment of chronic hepatitis using traditional Chinese medicine. *Informatics for Health and Social Care, 19*(1), 37-45.

Zheng, Z. (2014). *Acupuncture in Australia: regulation, education, practice, and research.* Integrative Medicine Research.

Zhu, B., & Wang, H. C. (2011). *Basic Theories of Traditional Chinese Medicine.* Jessica Kingsley Publishers.

Chapter 9
Strengthening Implementation of Guidelines at Primary Health Care

V. Horner
University of South Africa, South Africa

A. Coleman
University of South Africa, South Africa

ABSTRACT

Implementation of guidelines in the health system is a complex and considerable undertaking. After the health administration has developed guidelines, a dissemination strategy needs to be put in place. Dissemination involves distribution of printed guidelines booklets, training of health care providers, provision of the equipment needed for implementing the guidelines, improvements to facilities, and supervision and monitoring by managers. This chapter reports on the Basic Antenatal Care Information System (Bacis) study in South Africa which pertains to an e-health decision support systems that is intended as an aid for nurses and managers at primary health care. The Bacis program study is important because there are few published studies from developing countries on implementation of e-health decision support systems at primary health care and their effectiveness in improving care.

INTRODUCTION

In their classic reference, Field and Lohr (1990) define clinical practice guidelines as "…systematically developed statements to assist practitioners and consumers about appropriate health care actions for specific circumstances…" Clinical practice guidelines are meant to aid practitioners in delivering a high quality of care. In developing countries, primary health care is done by nurses and not doctors. This is due to the structure of the health system in developing countries, where doctors, being a scarce resource, are found higher up in the health system (Massyn, et al., 2004). However many cases presenting at primary health care in developing countries are often very challenging. Health administrators in developing countries now look to guidelines to assist these frontline care providers in carrying out their duties.

DOI: 10.4018/978-1-4666-9446-0.ch009

Implementation of guidelines in the health system is a major undertaking, which takes place over a number of years (Grimshaw, Thomas, et al., 2004). The first phase is guideline development. In this phase the best available evidence is reviewed in order that the guidelines are supported by this evidence. An important constraint in guideline development in developing countries is that the guidelines recommendations must suit local conditions and must make use of available resources. This is a challenge because the health system of a developing country has a high burden of disease and little resources. Therefore guidelines recommendations must rely on cost effective health care interventions. After guideline development a dissemination plan must be devised. The dissemination plan involves distribution of the printed guideline booklets, training of nurses, provision of the equipment that is needed for guidelines implementation, alteration in clinic processes, and supervision and monitoring of the implementation.

Dissemination often runs into problems. Horner, Rautenbach et al (2014) in South Africa found that the implementation and dissemination of the national guidelines on maternity care ran into the following problems, among others:

- Firstly the training program on the guidelines was not carried out effectively. For example the health administration was using the train the trainer approach, whereby clinic representatives were trained on the guidelines. After their training, the clinic representatives were expected to train their colleagues when they returned to the clinics. However this was not happening. As a result not all nurses were trained on the guidelines.
- Secondly there were problems with availability of the printed guidelines booklets. Therefore nurses had no reference at hand, and relied on colleagues who had gone for training.
- Finally tools to support monitoring and evaluation of guideline implementation were inadequate. Therefore managers do not have detailed data to assist them in their planning.

In the light of these challenges in guidelines implementation and dissemination this chapter explores the role that can be played by e-health decision support systems to strengthen implementation of guidelines at primary health care. The focus of the chapter is the case study on the Basic Antenatal Care Information Systems (Bacis), which is a case study on an e-health decision support system which was developed and piloted in South Africa (Horner, et al., 2013).

RATIONALE FOR E-HEALTH DECISION SUPPORT SYSTEMS

Computerised decision support systems were chosen in the Bacis program study because it has been shown by studies from developed countries that decision support systems can improve adherence of nurse and doctors with clinical practice guidelines (Grimshaw, et al., 2004; Balas, et al., 2000; Lobach & Hammond, 1997; Dowding, 2013; Zielstorff, 1998; Boxwala, et al., 2004). However developing and lower to middle income countries have only recently started using health information technology systems (Blaya, Hamish & Holt, 2010). For example South Africa has only recently developed an e-health strategy (Department of Health, 2012). Therefore the evidence base on implementation of e-health in developing countries is still accumulating.

Further the health system in South Africa is that of a developing country, with a high burden of disease and inadequate resources. Where information systems have been implemented in developing countries there are often challenges of data quality and lack of information management skills. This presents a challenge for implementation of the e-health strategy. Therefore there is interest to see how e-health systems can be implemented in a developing country such as South Africa, especially at primary health care level, as well as their effectiveness in improving the quality of care rendered to patients. At present there are few published studies on utilization of decision support systems in the context of primary health care and developing countries (Blaya, Hamish & Holt, 2010). The Bacis program study addresses this gap in studies on decision support systems from developing countries.

Blaya, Hamish and Holt (2010) report on a systematic review of e-health system implementations in developing countries. Their review included electronic health record systems, laboratory systems, pharmacy systems and decision support systems, among several categories. For the category decision support systems, some of the systems that were included in their review are an expert system for mechanically ventilated newborns in Thailand and a personal digital assistant (PDA) application for integrated management of childhood illnesses in Tanzania. In the first system the nurses felt that they had better judgment after implementation of the system, and in the second system, there was an improvement from the nurses in completion of the questionnaire when compared to the paper system.

The target audience of this chapter are managers in the health sector as well as e-health system designers. The chapter caters for the reader who is looking for an introduction to the field of e-health decision support systems in developing countries, as well as the advanced reader who is looking for data on implementation.

The main body of this chapter now follows. It begin with a description of the Bacis program, then the methodology used in piloting it, then the results of piloting, then the discussion, and chapter conclusion, and finally the future directions in the research area of decision support systems at primary health care.

OVERVIEW OF BACIS PROGRAM

Features of the Bacis Program

The Bacis program was developed at the South African Medical Research Council by the researcher (XXX), with the assistance of medical experts (Horner, et al., 2013). Its scope is identification of high risk pregnancies and management of low risk pregnancies at primary health care level. The acronym Bacis is in fact pronounced "basis" despite its spelling. In full it stands for Basic Antenatal Care Information System (Bacis). Its name combines the names: Basic Antenatal Care Checklist and information systems. This is to highlight the point that the Bacis program is an information system which implements the national guidelines on maternity care in South Africa and the Basic Antenatal Care (BANC) checklist.

Maternal health care was chosen as the focus of the Bacis program because it is one of the priority areas in the health services in South Africa (Department of Health, 2007; Pattinson, 2004; Department of Health, 2008; Pattinson, 2007). In fact improving maternal health care indicators is one of the eight Millennium Development Goals of the United Nations (Millenium Project, 2006).

Within maternal health care the focus of the Bacis program is on antenatal care. About twenty five percent of all maternal health complications happen during antenatal care, about forty percent happen during labour, and the remainder happen during postnatal care (Pattinson, 2007). These distributions show the importance of antenatal care. Further the confidential enquiry into maternal deaths in South Africa, states the following "…about 20-30% of all maternal deaths in South Africa occur from preventable factors, such as delays in referral and inadequate antenatal care response…" (Department of Health, 2008) Therefore antenatal care presents an important opportunity to improve the quality maternal health care.

Because of the importance of maternal health it was possible to bring together the various stakeholders in maternal, child and women's health in the health district where the Bacis program was piloted. These stakeholders provided stewardship for the project, and they assisted in obtaining permissions and aided the system's introduction at the clinics during piloting. Development of the Bacis program took six months, this was followed by six months of validation of its rule base, then a further nine month of piloting. Funding for the project was obtained from the National Research Foundation in South Africa and the national Department of Science and Technology.

The Bacis program uses patient specific information entered during an antenatal visit in order to perform:

- Risk classification;
- Identification of patients for referral; and
- Scheduling of maternity care interventions.

To perform these tasks the Bacis program uses its rule base and knowledge base that have been developed in collaboration with medical experts. However, the final decision is taken by the nursing sister. The Bacis program is only intended as an aid in the decision making process, i.e. it is a decision-support system.

The extended list of features of the Bacis program is the following:

- Referral criteria;
- A rule base of antenatal care protocols;
- A date function for calculation of expected date of delivery and visit schedule;
- Reminders and popup alerts for abnormal screening values;
- System created reminders;
- User defined reminders;
- Data entry and data validation prompts;
- Data completeness checks;
- Range checks and error checks for data input;
- Tick box fields and dropdown lists for ease of data entry;
- Comment fields for making unstructured notes; and
- An electronic antenatal care record consisting of all the data elements contained in the antenatal card of the Department of Health, implemented in Microsoft Access.

Menus of the Bacis Program

The Bacis program has six main menus: (1) history; (2) examination; (3) screenings; (4) pregnancy plan and reminders; (5) pregnancy outcomes; and (6) audit and quality assurance. Each menu is placed in a tab menu on the Bacis program interface. Figure 1, Figure 2 and Figure 3 show sample screenshots of the Bacis program interface. The first four tab menus cover the tasks and information of an antenatal care visit. These correspond to the headings of antenatal care described in the Basic Antenatal Care checklist

Figure 1. Pregnancy history, and an alert

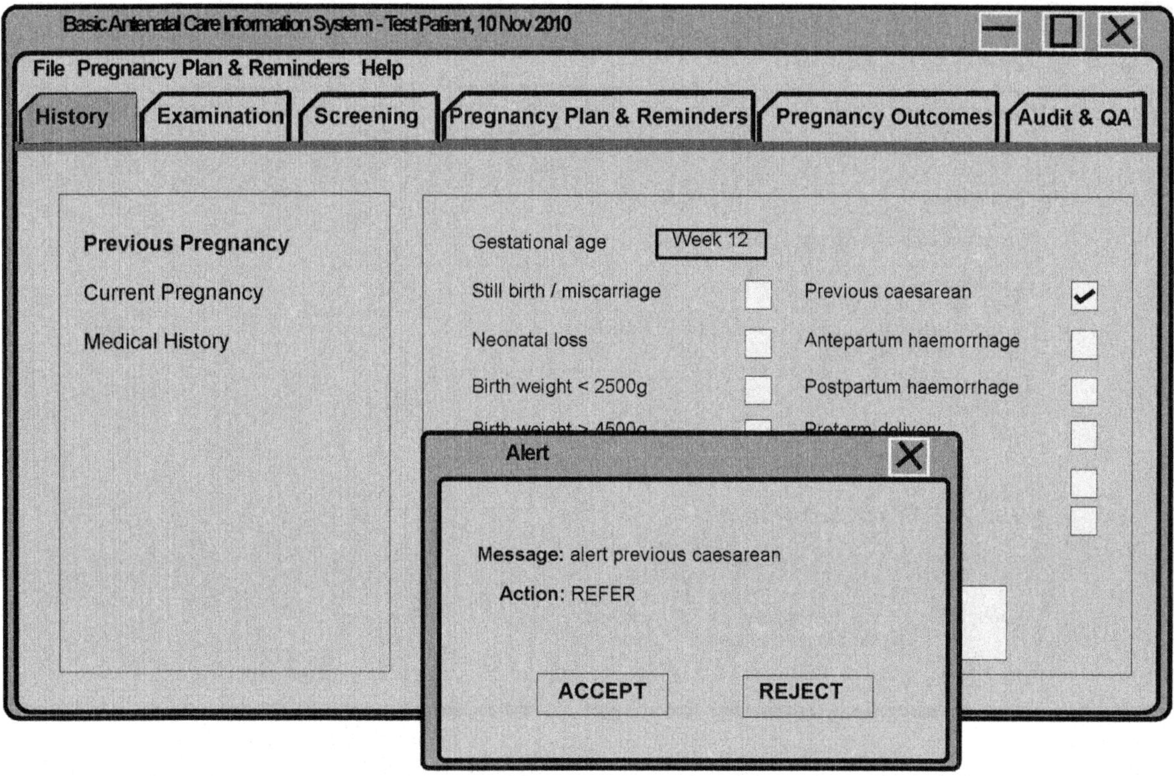

Figure 2. Screening

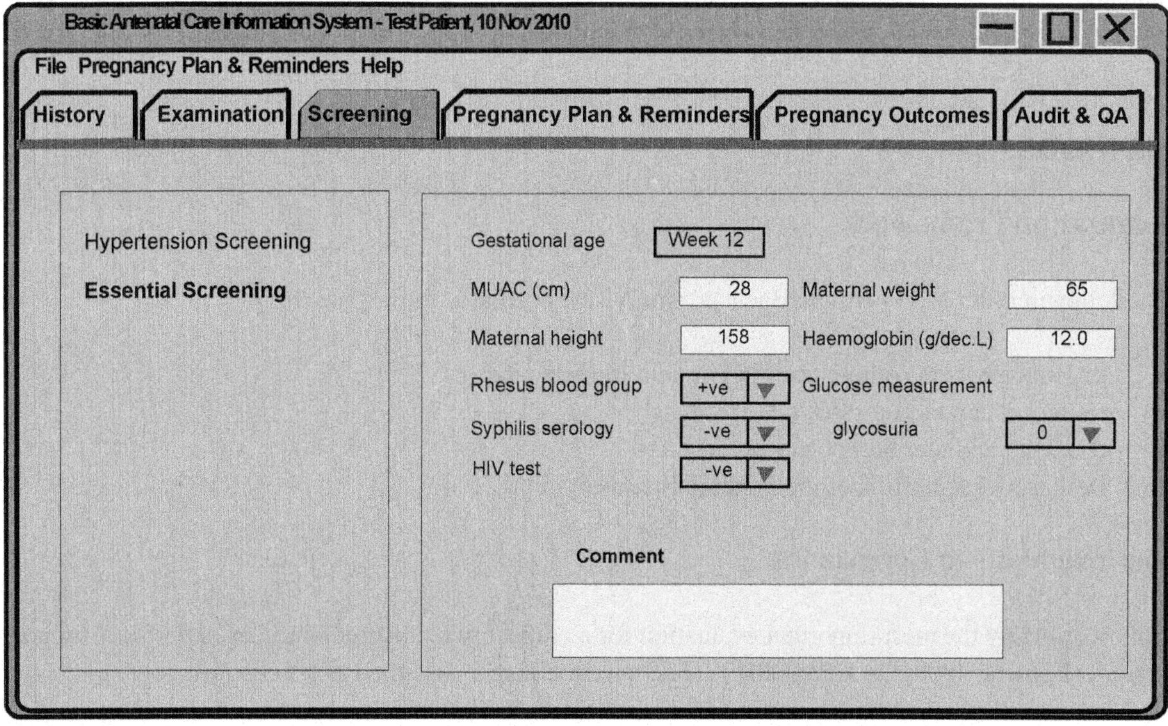

Figure 3. Pregnancy plan and reminders

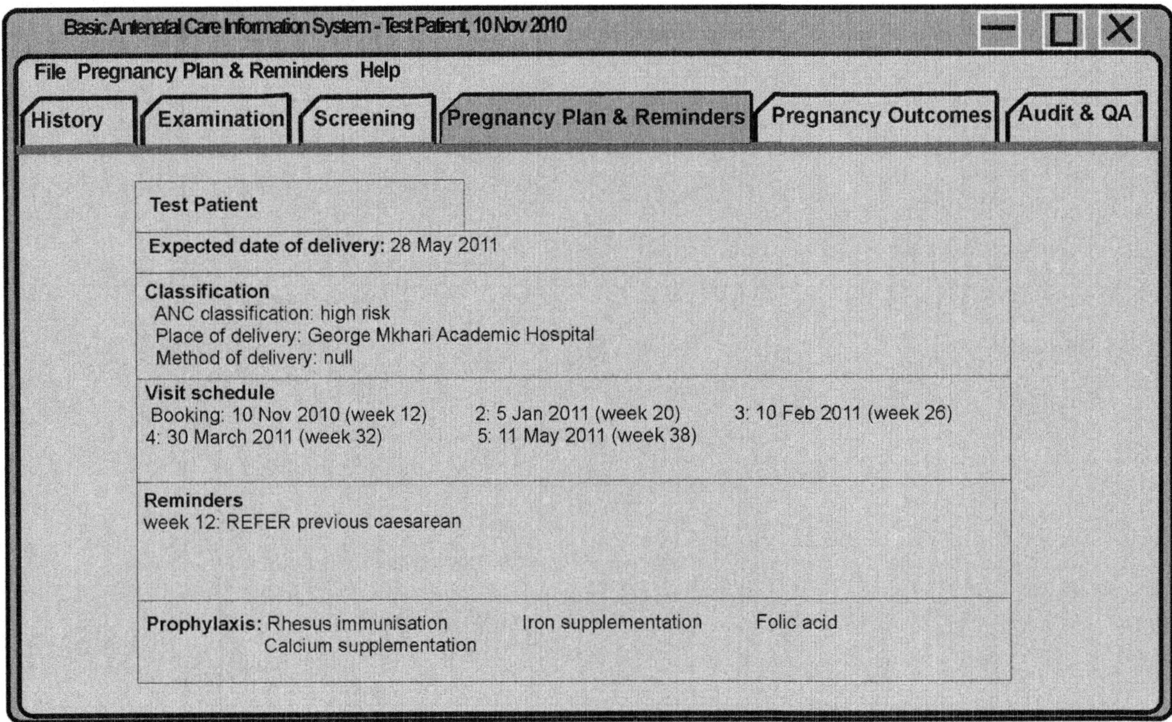

and in the national guidelines on maternity care (Pattinson, 2007; Department of Health, 2007). The fifth menu is for capturing some outcomes of the pregnancy, and the sixth menu is intended to assist clinic managers with performing audit of antenatal care at their facilities. Each tab menu has various fields and sub-fields associated with it. The full listing of the menus of the Bacis program is in Horner (2013).

METHODS

Evaluation Framework

The following four aspects of the Bacis program were evaluated during the study:

- Improvements in compliance after system implementation;
- System accuracy and safety;
- Usability and user acceptance review; and
- Resources implication of the system implementation.

Improvements to Compliance

This is arguably the most important evaluation for a clinical practice guideline-based decision support system (Berners, 1999; Dowding, 2013). The question here is whether the decision support system is able to improve compliance or not, and by how much. The results of this evaluation are the ones that will convince health sector managers on adoption of the system.

System Accuracy and Safety

Checking system accuracy is sometimes called system validation (Berners, 1999). The aim is to ascertain system safety as well as to measure system performance. Measures of performance and accuracy such as sensitivity and specificity in diagnosis are carried out under this heading (Webb & Bain, 2011). The accuracy of the system is often compared to a gold standard in diagnosis.

Usability Review and User Acceptance Testing

Usability checks whether the system is acceptable to the user community (ISO, 1998). Even if a system has passed system verification and validation it must still undergo usability and user acceptance testing. User acceptance testing can be done following models such as the technology assessment model, or other user acceptance models that are appropriate for the system under review (Davis, 1989).

Resources Implications of System Implementation

Introduction of an intervention has implications on the department of health's resources such as personnel, finances, and time. The resources needed for the system's implementation must therefore be assessed so that they are known. Consideration must be made of systems theory inputs such as: human resources, time, equipment, infrastructure, finances, and policies (Alliance for Health Policy and Systems Research, 2007).

Study Setting and Study Subjects

After its development of about a year, the Bacis program was field piloted for nine months at three primary health care clinics in Tshwane Health District. The three study clinics are located in three semi-rural townships: Winterveldt, Temba and Soshanguve. All three townships are located at some distance from the Pretoria central business district. The three townships are spread in a radius of about 45 kilometres from the Pretoria central business district. The population of Winterveldt is estimated at about 80 000, Temba at 50 000 and Soshanguve at more than 300 000. The townships consist of formal dwellings as well as shacks, with many backroom dwellings. They have high unemployment (40%) and high HIV prevalence (22%) (Jacobs, Punt & Bothloko, 2009). The profiles of these three townships fit those of typical underserved areas in South Africa, with a high burden of health issues. The three study clinics serve these three townships. The characteristics of the three study clinics are listed in Table 1.

The Bacis program was used by three study nurses for treating antenatal patients during the study, as well as a data entry clerk who was assisting the nurses at one of the study clinics. The data clerk was assisting the nurse with data capture of the patient information on the Bacis program. Two of the nurses used the system for three months and for all their patients at the first clinic. One nurse used it for nine months at the second clinic. And the data capturing clerk used it for nine months at the third clinic. In total the Bacis program was used by the study nurses to treat more than nine hundred (900) patients. The characteristics of the study nurses are shown in Table 2.

Table 1. Characteristics of the study clinics

Characteristic	Winterveldt	Temba	Soshanguve
1. General monthly patient load: (primary health care, chronic diseases, tuberculosis, HIV, and child health and maternity care)	13 000 patients per month	9 000 patients per month	19 000 patients per month
2. Antenatal care: average number of new bookings per month	210 patients	63 patients	166 patients
3. Average number of referrals in labour per month	78 patients	35 patients	181 patients
4. Average number of deliveries per month	104 patients	54 patients	200 patients
5. Staffing: professional nurses with midwifery	36 nurses	26 nurses	48 nurses
6. Staffing: advanced midwives at clinic	1 nurse	4 nurse	12 nurse
7. Estimated unemployment levels*	40%	40%	40%
8. Estimated household income per month *	R500	R500	R500

* Taken from: Profile of the North West Province: demographics, poverty, income, inequality and unemployment (Jacobs, Punt & Bothloko 2009).

Data Collection and Analysis

Piloting of the Bacis program was done between December 2010 and July 2011. Quantitative as well as qualitative methods of data collection and analysis were used in the study. The four aspects of the Bacis program that were chosen for this study were addressed as follows.

Improvements in Compliance

A comparative design was used to measure improvements in compliance, before introduction of the system, and after its introduction. The source of data was the patients' records. In this regard two patient record reviews were carried out on patients treated by the nurses, one before introduction of the system, and the second review after its introduction. The record review criteria consisted of eighteen standard antenatal care protocol items (18 antenatal care tasks) which were taken from the national guidelines

Table 2. Characteristics of the study nurses who used the Bacis program during piloting

Item	Value
1. Prior experience in using a health information for more than six months.	all 3 nurses
2. Prior experience in using an antenatal care or maternity care system.	2 nurses only
3. Prior experience in databases, such as Microsoft Access.	all 3 nurses
4. Participations in research or a survey before the Bacis program study.	all 3 nurses
5. Education: professional nurse.	all 3 nurses
6. Education: midwifery	all 3 nurses
7. Education: advanced midwifery	none
8. Knowledge of BANC (Bacis antenatal care checklist)	all 3 nurses
9. Training on the guidelines and the BANC (Bacis antenatal care checklist)	2 nurses only

Table 3. Quality criteria

Item	Item
1. previous pregnancy history	10. blood pressure
2. current pregnancy history	11. proteinuria
3. general medical history	12. maternal weight and height
4. general examination	13. Rh
5. severe symptoms	14. RPR
6. SFH	15. HIV
7. Foetal heart rate age>28 weeks	16. haemoglobin
8. Foetal lie and presentation	17. glycosuria
9. pregnancy infections	18. prophylaxis

*SFH: symphysis fundal height, Rh: rhesus factor, RPR: rapid plasma reagin.

on maternity care (Department of Health, 2007; Pattinson, 2007). Table 3 shows the criteria that were used in measuring compliance. Basic descriptive statistics were used for reporting the compliance data, and the t-test was used to test statistical significance at the 5% level of significance.

Compliance was measured as a combination of *completion* and *response*. Completion the first part of compliance checked whether the protocol item (i.e. antenatal care task) was carried out when due. If risk factors arose or abnormal values were observed, then a medical response was expected as the second part of compliance. The separation of compliance into completion and response was made because sometimes a task is performed by the nurse, and perhaps a risk factor correctly identified, however the medical response by the nurse may be incorrect or inadequate. In the record review missing information was scored as not completed.

The response adequacy is computed as the number of times that the response was adequate divided by the number of risk factors identified in the review. Similarly the percentage for completion is the number of times the item was actually carried out, divided by the number of times it was due.

System Accuracy and Safety

The sensitivity of the Bacis program was measured during the study. This measure compared the number of patients the system correctly classified as high risk against those it failed to correctly classify as high risk. Data for this was taken from the Bacis program as well as the referral registers at the study clinics and at the referral hospitals.

Usability and User Acceptance Testing

To assess user acceptance, semi-structured interviews were carried out with the three study nurses. The interviews had the following three themes. (1) Relevance of the content of the Bacis program. This theme compared the match between the content of the Bacis program with actual practice; (2) Usability and cognitive aspects of the Bacis program, such as the time needed by the users to learn the Bacis program and difficulties in completing its tasks; And, (3) usefulness of the reminders and alerts of the Bacis program as well as the method used for issuing them. These three themes match the two headings of the technology assessment model. The themes of the technology assessment model are perceived usefulness of the system, and perceived ease of use (Davis, 1989). The technology acceptance model was used in the study because it is a common model for user acceptance testing. It has been validated by many other studies, and it is therefore a good indicator of user acceptance of a system.

Resources Implications of System Implementation

Data on resources implications of the system is drawn from the experience of development and piloting of the Bacis program as well as analysis of documentation of the Department of Health on implementation plans for e-health in South Africa. The following systems theory inputs were considered: human resources, time, equipment, infrastructure, finances, and policies (Alliance for Health Policy and Systems Research, 2007).

Ethics Approval

Ethics approval for the study was obtained from the Medunsa Research Ethics Committee, which is in the Faculty of Health Sciences at the University of Limpopo, Medunsa Medical Campus. Consent was obtained from the nurses and patients to participate in the study and consent forms were also signed by them. The study was performed in compliance with the World Medical Association Declaration of Helsinki on Ethical Principles for Medical Research Involving Human Subjects (World Medical Association, 2001).

RESULTS

Improvements in Compliance

Compliance before Introduction of the Bacis Program

The following gaps in the quality of care were identified:

- **Previous Pregnancy History:** Completion is good at 100%, but the response is poor.
- **General Examination:** Completion is low at 67.4% and the response is not optimal at 85.4%.
- **Symphysis Fundal Measurements (SFH):** Completion is not optimal at 87%.
- **Foetal Lie and Presentation:** Completion is not optimal at 87.0%.
- **Severe Symptoms:** Response is low at 66.6%.
- **Pregnancy Infections:** Response is low at 66.6%.
- **Blood Pressure Screening:** Completion is optimal at 100%, but response poor.
- **Essential Screening (Rh Screening, RPR Screening and Hb Screening):** Completion is not optimal at 88.0%, 84.0% and 84.0% respectively.
- **HIV Screening:** Testing of pregnant women is optimal at 100%, but prevention of mother to child transmission of HIV (PMTCT) protocols are not followed correctly.
- **Folic Acid, and Iron Supplementation:** The supplementation is only being given to 30.4% of women.

Table 4. Compliance before introduction of the Bacis program versus after

Item	Completion (%)		Response Adequate (%)		Compliance (%)	
	Before	After	Before	After	Before	After
1. Previous pregnancy history	100.0	99.0	0.0	30.1	84.0	90.0
2. Current pregnancy history	96.0	100.0	100.0	0.0	96.0	95.0
3. General medical history	100.0	99.0	100.0	100.0	100.0	99.0
4. General examination	67.4	85.4	50.0	25.0	67.4	83.4
5. Symphysis fundal height (SFH)	87.0	93.4	*	*	87.0	93.4
6. Foetal heart rate, gestational age>28 weeks	100.0	92.1	*	*	100.0	92.1
7.Foetal lie and presentation, gestational age>34 weeks	87.0	86.1	*	*	87.0	86.1
8. Severe symptoms	*	*	66.6	100.0	97.8	100.0
9. Pregnancy infections	*	*	66.6	74.0	95.7	95.4
10. Blood pressure	100.0	100.0	0.0	25.0	95.7	98.0
11. Proteinuria	95.7	100.0	*	*	95.7	100.0
12. Maternal weight and height	58.7	94.0	*	*	58.7	94.0
13. Rhesus factor (Rh)	88.0	84.0	0.0	0.0	84.0	82.0
14. Rapid plasma reagin (RPR)	84.0	84.0	100.0	100.0	84.0	84.0
15. HIV	100.0	100.0	50.0	0.0	92.0	89.0
16. Haemoglobin (Hb)	84.0	84.0	100.0	50.0	84.0	83.0
17. Glycosuria	93.5	98.0	*	*	93.5	98.0
18. prophylaxis	30.4	45.0	*	*	30.4	45.0
Mean values	**85.7**	**90.3**	**57.6**	**45.8**	**85.1**	**89.3**

* Indicates that item was not applicable for measure, the reasons for this are explained.

Compliance after Introduction of the Bacis Program

Although 18 protocol items were considered in the review, severe symptoms and pregnancy infections were not included for 'completion' because there are no fields for them in the antenatal cards. This made it difficult to determine whether severe symptoms and pregnancy infections were completed or not completed based on the record review only.

Further, for 'response', only those items where serious issues arose in the study were included. Proteinuria, and maternal weight and height both had minor issues arising in the study and were therefore not included for 'response'. Foetal heart rate, foetal lie and presentation, and glycosuria had no issues arising in the study and were therefore not included for 'response'. Prophylaxis was only considered under completion because it is not a risk factor.

Though protocols exist for assessing the response to symphysis fundal measurements, they could not be consistently applied in the record review because of missing information and some inconsistencies that were identified. Hence, of the eighteen (18) protocol items, only eleven (11) were evaluated for response.

In view of the sample sizes for the two groups, the T-test statistical test was used to test for significant differences in compliance before and after introduction of the Bacis program at the 5% ($\alpha = 0.05$) level of significance.

In terms of overall compliance there was an improvement from 85.1% to 89.3% in compliance after introduction of the Bacis program. Although this improvement was not statistically significant, when results were stratified into specific categories, the Bacis program showed statistically significant improvement over the checklist system in the categories for compliance at booking, patients younger than 18 years and patients booking after week 20. Table 5 shows the results stratified according to antenatal category.

System Accuracy and Safety

Firstly, during system development the designer and the study obstetrician created tests cases to test each of the 49 rules of the Bacis program to determine whether they yielded a correct answer or not. Further a meeting, lasting for a full day, was held with maternity nurses and managers from the eight community health centres in Tshwane Health District and two district managers in order to review the Bacis program. During piloting the nurses were also asked to report errors. Corrections to the system were therefore made during the study to ensure its safety. Finally at the end of piloting the Bacis program correctly identified as high risk 35.5% of patients that were referred, it failed to correctly identify 17.4% as high risk, and 47.1% were referred in labour which is out scope for the Bacis program. The sensitivity of the Bacis program is therefore 67.2%.

Usability Review

Usability of the Bacis program was evaluated using the following three themes:

- Relevance of the content of the Bacis program;
- Learning and cognitive aspects of the system; and
- Usefulness of its reminders and alerts.

Table 5. Compliance by antenatal patient category

Item	Before Intervention (%)	After Intervention (%)	P-Values at 95% Confidence
1. Compliance overall	85.1	89.3	0.14
2. Compliance at booking (1ˢᵗ visit)	82.7	90.2	0.016 **
3. Compliance at follow up visits	87.4	86.6	0.87
4. Compliance for patients booking before week 20	89.9	89.7	0.96
5. Compliance for patients booking after week 20	82.8	89.2	0.040 **
6. Compliance for patients younger than 18 years	78.7	92.0	0.0023 **
7. Compliance for patient older than 18 years	85.6	89.0	0.27
8. Compliance for primigravida patients	87.3	91.9	0.18
9. Compliance for multi-gravida patients	83.7	88.1	0.16

** The double star indicates that result is statistically significant.

Relevance of the Content of the Bacis Program

In all the interviews the nurses generally felt that the clinical content of the Bacis program matched their understanding of antenatal care, though they raised a number of points on some of the steps that it followed. For example, in the beginning of the study, in the meeting held to review the Bacis program, the nurses asked why hypertension screening was not part of the examination menu in the high level menus of the Bacis program and why proteinuria was not next to glycosuria. The reason for this was explained by the study obstetrician, and thereafter the nurses accepted the explanation saying that "… it was a minor adjustment to the steps they normally followed…"

Learning and Cognitive Aspects

On the question of whether it was easy or difficult to learn to use the Bacis program, the nurses said that "…it was a simple program which guided one along the process of antenatal care…" The younger nurses, who are more computer literate, said it was simple in their perception, while the older nurses said that they felt too old for computers. Generally, the impression gained was that many nurses are computer literate and that implementation of the Bacis program would be welcome to them given its benefits.

Usefulness of System Reminders and Alerts

The nurses reported that they found its reminders useful on the whole. They were happy with both the data input alerts as well as the clinical reminders. They said that "... the program guided one along the steps of the Basic Antenatal Care (BANC) checklist. What to do and when to refer ..." They further said that "... if they did not agree with a reminder, the system offered them an option to ignore or to override it ..." which they said offered them flexibility.

The conclusion was that the nurses on the whole found the Bacis program to be an acceptable tool for them as a decision aid. One of the strengths of the Bacis program is that its data is intended for use by the nurses rather than for reporting to higher levels in the health system hierarchy. It is hoped that this will motivate the nurses to use it.

Resources Implication of System Introduction

Human Resources, Time, and Policies

Firstly, training of nurses in utilisation of the Bacis program will be a challenge, as this will involve many nurses, and the training requires a substantial commitment in time from the participating nurses. Time is a big problem at the clinics in South Africa.

Secondly integration of the Bacis program with the clinics' workflow also needs further attention. Currently patient held paper records have to be completed, which are used for the duration of a woman's pregnancy. The patient-held paper records are important because there is no electronic patient record in

South Africa. In this scenario the Bacis program becomes an extra item in the duties of the nurses. This may explain the difficulty in finding a nurse at Temba clinic where a data capturing clerk was used instead.

On policies, the Department of Health has put in place a number of important policies for enabling implementation of e-health systems, such as the e-health strategy (Department of Health, 2012). These policies are welcoming and supportive of implementations of e-health systems in South Africa.

Equipment, Infrastructure, and Finances

Implementation of the Bacis program depends on availability of computers at the clinics. Currently this is not the case in South Africa. However the e-health strategy of the Department of Health makes provisions for computers and software such as Microsoft Access.

DISCUSSION

Four aspects of the Bacis program were evaluated: improvements in compliance, system accuracy, user acceptance, and resources utilisation. On the whole for these four aspects the results were successful.

The Bacis program had a statistically significant improvement in compliance for three out of nine important antenatal patient categories. These nine categories were either demographic information items or clinical information items. The three categories which had statistical significance in the results includes the most important category of booking. Booking is the first visit of a pregnant mother. Most pregnancy screenings are carried out during this first visit, as well as risk classification. Therefore this study on the Bacis program was considered successful. However a follow up study needs to be done, which will have a larger sample, and therefore yield a significant result for most of the categories.

The Bacis program is safe because it uses the process of the national guidelines on maternity care. And secondly the Bacis program is meant to be used by a professional nurse, who makes the final decision. In other words it is a decision support system. In terms of usability, the nurses on the whole were satisfied with the Bacis program according to the usability review. On resources utilization, the Bacis program implementation was judged to be feasible. There was however the issue pertaining to the time needed for entering information in both the Bacis program as well as the patient held cards. The nurses however said that the extra time needed for entering information in the Bacis program in addition to the patient cards can be offset by the benefits of using the system. Its benefits include increased compliance with the guidelines, as well as its role as an aid for facility managers in performing quality assurance.

Another important outcome from the Bacis program study is validation of its rule base. The rule base of the Bacis program was formulated as production rules. Production rules can be understood by domain experts as well as engineers. Unlike database schemas and many other formalisms which are understandable to engineers only, production rules can be understood by people who are not engineers. Production rules therefore facilitate communication between medical experts and engineers. Communication between the medical experts and engineers is often a big challenge when developing knowledge based systems in health care (Patel, et al., 1998). Though the formalism of rules was not previously known to the medical experts in the study, after learning it in the study, the medical experts made use of it even in tasks not related to the Bacis program. For example the medical experts used the 49 rules from the Bacis program study in an audit of antenatal care at one of the study clinics (Horner, et al., 2014). The rules enabled reviewer objectivity. This was possible because production rules have a format for describing strict criteria, and the format of production rules has an unambiguous formal meaning. Therefore validation of the rule base of the Bacis program was one of the important results from the study.

Finally the Bacis program study provided data on the detailed care activities that are carried out during antenatal patient visits at the study clinics. This is important because most studies on antenatal care in South Africa provide data on antenatal attendance and other aggregate indices, but few provide the detailed data on care activities that are received by the patients. From this detailed data gathered in the study it was possible to clearly identify gaps in the quality of antenatal care at the clinics as well as the opportunities for improvements.

CONCLUSION

The focus of this chapter was on the Bacis program study. The Bacis program is an e-health decision support system for strengthening implementation of the national guidelines on maternity care in South Africa. In the chapter implementation of the Bacis program was elaborated-on as well as the system's effectiveness in improving the quality of care rendered to patients. This work is of value to managers in the health sector as well as designers of e-health systems.

FUTURE RESEARCH DIRECTIONS

The area of research of guidelines-based decision support systems in developing countries is one that has great potential for future research. For example guidelines based decision support systems can be extended to other domains of care in South Africa such as lung disease or chronic care. Another area of potential future research is in the area of decision support for community health workers. In many developing countries there is currently a drive to introduce community health workers. Community health workers extend the reach of the health services into the community. These community health workers can play an important role in preventative care, chronic care, improving compliance of patients with treatments, as well as the early detection of health problems. There is therefore an opportunity in providing decision support for the community health workers in developing countries.

REFERENCES

Alliance for Health Policy and Systems Research. (2007). *Briefing Note 1*. Geneva: Alliance for Health Policy and Systems Research. Retrieved in January 2013, from http://www.who.int/alliance-hpsr/resources/alliancehpsr_briefingnote1.pdf

Balas, A. E., Weingarten, S., Garb, C. T., Blumenthal, D., Boren, S., & Brown, G. D. (2000). Improving preventative care by prompting physicians. *Archives of Internal Medicine, 160*(3), 301–308. doi:10.1001/archinte.160.3.301 PMID:10668831

Berners, E. S. (Ed.). (1999). *Clinical decision supports systems.* New York: Springer-Verlag. doi:10.1007/978-1-4757-3903-9

Blaya, J. A., Hamish, S. F., & Holt, B. (2010). e-Health technologies show promise in developing countries. *Health Affairs, 29*(2), 244–251. doi:10.1377/hlthaff.2009.0894 PMID:20348068

Boxwala, A. A., Peleg, M., Tu, S., Ogunyemi, O., Zeng, Q. T., Wang, D., & Shortliffe, E. H. et al. (2004). GLIF3: A representation format for sharable computer-interpretable clinical practice guidelines. *Journal of Biomedical Informatics, 37*(3), 147–161. doi:10.1016/j.jbi.2004.04.002 PMID:15196480

Davis, F. (1989). Perceived usefulness, perceived ease of use, and user acceptance of information technology. *Management Information Systems Quarterly, 13*(3), 319–240. doi:10.2307/249008

Department of Health. (2007). *Guidelines for Maternity Care in South Africa* [national guidelines on maternity care]. Pretoria, South Africa: Department of Health, South Africa.

Department of Health. (2008). *Confidential Enquiry into Maternal Deaths 2007* [report on enquiry into maternal deaths]. Pretoria, South Africa: Department of Health, South Africa.

Department of Health. (2012). e-Health Strategy, 2012 – 2016. Pretoria, South Africa: Department of Health, South Africa.

Dowding, D. (2013). Using computerized decision support systems. *Nursing Times, 109*(36), 23–25. PMID:24245371

Field, M. J., & Lohr, K. N. (1990). *Clinical practice guidelines: directions of a new paradigm.* Washington, DC: National Academy Press.

Grimshaw, J. M., Thomas, R. E., MacLennan, G., Fraser, C., Ramsay, C. R., Vale, L., & Donaldson, C. et al. (2004). Effectiveness and effeciency of guideline dissemination and implementation strategies [technical report, health systems research agency]. *Health Technology Assessment, 8*(6). doi:10.3310/hta8060 PMID:14960256

Horner, V. (2013). *Development and piloting of an e-health decision support system for improving compliance of primary health care staff to the maternity care guidelines and protocols.* (PhD thesis). University of Limpopo, Medunsa Medical Campus, Garankua, South Africa.

Horner, V., Rautenbach, P., Mbananga, N., Mashamba, T., & Kwinda, H. (2013). An e-health decision support system for improving compliance of health workers to the maternity care protocols in South Africa. *Appl.Clin.Inf., 4*(1), 25–36. doi:10.4338/ACI-2012-10-RA-0044 PMID:23650485

Horner, V., Rautenbach, P., Mbananga, N., Mashamba, T., Olurunju, S., Kwinda, H., & Ramahlo, T. (2014). Audit of antenatal care at a community health centre in Tshwane North sub-district, Gauteng Province. *South African Family Practice Journal, 56*(2), 153–158. doi:10.1080/20786204.2014.10855354

ISO9241-11. (1998). *Ergonomic requirements for office work with visual display terminals (VDT) – Part II: Guidance on usability.* International Organisation for Standardisation.

Jacobs, E., Punt, C., & Bothloko, C. (2009). *A profile of the North West Province: demographics, poverty, income, inequality and unemployment* [technical report; Internet]. PROVIDE Project. North West Provincial Government, South Africa. Retrieved in 2012, from: http://ideas.repec.org/p/ags/provbp/58055.html

Lobach, D. F., & Hammond, W. E. (1997). Computerized decision support based on a clinical practice guideline improves compliance with care standards. *The American Journal of Medicine, 102*(1), 89–98. doi:10.1016/S0002-9343(96)00382-8 PMID:9209205

Massyn, N., Day, C., & Dombo, M et al. (Eds.). (2004). *District health barometer*. Durban, South Africa: Health Systems Trust.

Millennium Project. (2006). *Goals*. United Nations. Retrieved in Jan 2013 December, from: http://www.milleniumproject.org/goals

Patel, V. L., Allen, V. G., Arocha, J. F., Jose, B. A., & Shortliffe, E. H. (1998). Representing clinical guidelines in GLIF: Individual and collaborative expertise. *Journal of the American Medical Informatics Association, 5*(5), 467–483. doi:10.1136/jamia.1998.0050467 PMID:9760394

Pattinson, R. C. (2004). Maternal health. [report by health systems research agency] In *South African Health Review 2003/2004* (pp. 89–99). Durban, South Africa: Health Systems Trust, South Africa.

Pattinson, R. C. (2007). *Basic Antenatal Care (BANC) Handbook* [training manual for nurses]. Pretoria, South Africa: University of Pretoria, South Africa.

Webb, P., & Bain, C. (2011). *Essential epidemiology*. Cambridge: Cambridge University Press.

World Medical Association. (2001). World Medical Association Declaration of Helsinki: Ethical principles for medical research involving human subject. *Bulletin of the World Health Organization, 79*(4), 373–374. PMID:11357217

Zielstorff, R. D. (1998). Online practice guidelines: Issues, obstacles, and future prospects. *Journal of the American Medical Informatics Association, 5*(3), 227–236. doi:10.1136/jamia.1998.0050227 PMID:9609492

KEY TERMS AND DEFINITIONS

Antenatal: This is the extended period, which covers the gestation period, but before labour and delivery. About half of all maternity referrals are supposed to happen during the antenatal period according to the national guidelines on maternity care in South Africa. Therefore this is an important part of maternal health care.

Confidential Enquiry into Maternal Deaths: Following the experiences of developed countries, the confidential enquiry into maternal deaths (CEMD) was set up in South Africa in the late 1990s. Maternal mortality was made a notifiable event by law. Maternal mortality is defined as the death of a pregnant woman irrespective of gestational age, or the death of a woman within forty two (42) days after the end of her pregnancy. A panel of experts sits to review each maternal death. The aim of the panel is to describe the trend of diseases causing maternal death as well as as the avoidable factors, missed opportunities and substandard care related to the deaths. The first report on the confidential enquiry into maternal deaths in South Africa was published in 1999, and it covered the years 1998 and 1999. The second report covered the period 1999 to 2001, and was published in 2002. The third report was published in 2005, and covers the period 2002 to 2004, the fourth report covers 2005 to 2007, and the most recent is the period 2008 to 2010.

Decision Support System: A decision-support system is a system which uses a vast store of high quality knowledge derived from evidence. It is used to assist practitioners in their duties. It is developed using the methodology of knowledge engineering.

Field Prototype: A prototype evolves through a number of stages. The first prototype is normally used by the development team only, and is usually very primitive. The first prototype may not be safe or appropriate for the users. As the development process advances more sophisticated and better prototypes are built until there is one which can be tested with the users. A field prototype is intended for use by the users in the actual deployment environment, outside of a lab or other such tightly controlled environment.

Labour: Labour in maternity care is a synonym for childbirth, which is the culmination of a pregnancy. A full term pregnancy happens between gestational age of thirty eight up to week forty two. Before gestation week thirty six it is classified as preterm labour and after week forty two as post term labour. The duration of labour and delivery varies from eight hours to twenty hours. About half of all referrals are supposed to happen during labour according to the Guidelines for Maternity Care in South Africa.

Perinatal Mortality: This index combines stillbirths and neonatal deaths, and is also used as a measure of the quality of maternity services. The sources of perinatal deaths may be antenatal care, postnatal care or management during labour.

Primary Health Care: In the health system primary health care refers to the lowest level facilities in the health systems, which are the clinics. These are the first points of contact between the community and the health system. Patient may be referred to higher level facilities from primary health care if their problem is beyond their capacity. The principle of primary health care originated in the 1970s, in a movement which sought to improve health care in the developing countries, which then were called the third world, where the situation in health care was desperate with high infant mortality rates and many diseases in the population. The idea was to have outreach centres to the community and even into households, generally away from the hospitals in order to improve access to health care services. The training of primary health care nurses in South Africa began in the 1970s. This was a new responsibility for nurses as they could now assume some of the responsibilities and duties of doctors in these outreach centres such as diagnosis and writing prescriptions. To help in the penetration as far as households, auxiliary health workers were also trained. There are three levels above primary health care in South Africa. These are level one hospitals, level two hospitals, and right on top are the tertiary hospitals. Each level has its prescribed capacity. Using maternity as an example the capacity of each level is as follows. Primary health care may have midwives and advanced midwives, but no resident doctors normally. There may be a visiting doctor on some days. Clinics may deliver low risk pregnancies, but high risk pregnancies must be referred. Level one hospitals have advanced midwives and resident doctors.

In terms of equipment they have blood transfusion services, x-rays and other services. They may have a visiting obstetrician. Level two hospitals in addition to all the above, have a resident obstetrician, and can manage severe cases. In the hierarchy, tertiary hospitals are at the top, and they have all the medical specialties, such as cardiology, neurology, etc.

Rule Base/Knowledge Base: A knowledge base is the module of a decision-support system which stores the knowledge of the system. The knowledge base is used during decision-support. The knowledge is stored in an encoded form. The encoding format may be rules or frames or any other knowledge representation format.

Chapter 10
General Practitioners' Adoption and Use of ICT

Quazi Omar Faruq
Victoria University, Australia

ABSTRACT

The influence of ICT in General Practice varied from a solo practice to a GP specialist of a primary healthcare team. Different factors influence the GP to use ICT. After 2nd World War the national legislative requirement influenced more to adopt ICT, of which most important is the Medicare or Medicaid payment and also the richness of the environment (measured by network readiness index). Shift to group practice or corporate level practice requires ICT support to handle automated actions (i.e. completing repetitive jobs, answering frequently asked questions by webpage). Role of telecommunication and IT service providers, and that of entrepreneurs for information management are also discussed. While discussing the challenges in implementing ICT in future model of GP service it focuses on the slow usage of computer and other IT products by doctors, as noted in the past decades.

INTRODUCTION

This chapter will explore the use of ICT in General Practice of Doctors in healthcare system. In doing so, it will first identify the role of general practitioners in the modern healthcare system, particularly in primary healthcare (PHC), and then demonstrate the role of ICT to improve the quality of those roles and the adoption of ICT by the practitioners in the present time. The issue will be discussed in the context of changing role of general practitioners, from a solo private practitioner to a team member of a broader primary healthcare system.

When we talk about General Practice (GP) in developed capitalist or socialist countries it refers mostly to medical graduates from colleges teaching allopathic regime but what about traditional medical healers, ayurvedic and homeopathic practitioners. As it is hard to collect accurate data on this issue this chapter will focus on modern allopathic practitioners only, even though there is evidence that other groups are also utilising some of the benefits of ICT.

DOI: 10.4018/978-1-4666-9446-0.ch010

General practice has a familiar concept in developed countries but how far it applies to other countries where it might also be known as family physician or private physician. Today in many countries, like US, UK, European Union, Australia & also some Asian & African countries, GP is a speciality. Medical graduates now have to complete fellowship programmes before being considered as general practitioner (Simon 2009). As a practitioner they are no more the sole decision maker about a client as they are a team of primary health care service. GPs are now gatekeeper of the health service.

Information technology is becoming an integral part of many services including health service. Different factors influence the general practitioner to use ICT in practice. After the Second World War most important factor is the national legislative requirement to adopt certain electronic media to gain funding or to participate in incentive programme. In developed countries adoption of ICT is more influenced by richness of the environment which could be measured by different indicators like network readiness index (NRI) and priorities of national policy. Increasing influence of ICT also increasing the cost of running business which is driving GPs to group practices instead of solo practice, some are even moving to corporate level functioning.

In underdeveloped countries among several factors adoption of technology depends on the proven advantage of the technology along with its cost-effective accessibility in the service. So, this chapter also looks into the factors influencing the acceptance and deterrence of ICT in practice in reference to developed and underdeveloped countries perspective. This growth also allures other entrepreneurs to form partnership for information management. Telecommunication and IT service providers like Telstra or others have come forward to introduce products for tele-health.

It will also focus on challenges in implementing future development of ICT in general practice. One important challenge is the slow usage of computer and other IT products by doctors.

Hope this chapter would be of interest to IT Specialists, healthcare professionals, and Business Managers in Healthcare Organisations, academics: undergraduates, postgraduates, and researchers involved in healthcare sector.

INTRODUCTION

Until the mid-1900 medical graduates had the option to join an institution or to work on their own at their preferred area, with very little or no obligation to any legislation but the ethics. Even if physicians were working at institutions they were private practitioners at some time of their life. Almost all doctors were in general practice (GP) with duties in medicine, surgery or other specialities with a sign of "Physician and Surgeon" at their door and as a solo practitioner (Bryan, 1971: Plianbangchang, 2011). Earlier GP service was not totally regulated by any national programme, even though there might have weak professional bodies like general practitioner's forum. As there was no legislative control so in some instances complexities arouse among practices resulting from professional jealousy e.g. criticising publicly about one's ability to diagnose measles (Bryan 1971). Doctors were more interested to treat a person rather than maintaining records. Doctors' prescription was in many cases nothing but a scribble on a paper, only deciphered by pharmacists. Over time there were questions about the legibility and completeness of the handwritten prescriptions (Albarrak AI et.al, 2014). Even though the practice changed in developed socialist countries in most underdeveloped countries GP service is still direct fee for service, where client pay upfront. Initially GP service was driven by business interest and clinical skill with little interest in management quality (Jowett & Danielyan, 2010).

Today General Practice in a developed country setting is a medical speciality to provide person centred, continuing, comprehensive and coordinated whole-person health care to individuals and families in their communities (RACGP, 2014). In most countries GP system is guided by professional body like College of General Practitioners to set boundaries on different activities of a practitioner e.g. recommending working hours to avoid stress. So, today business interest is not totally waived but quality prevails over other interest. Increased emphasis on primary health care is considered by some as the death of general practice (Martin and Sturmberg, 2005) in developed countries.

Previously community members had the option to receive health service either from hospitals or from private practitioners where fees depended on the popularity of the practitioner or on their acquaintance to elite members of the society. Overtime this attracted the politicians and social reformers to criticise the major expense of personal income (more than 40%) to maintain health and well-being of the society (Bryan 1971, Jowett & Danielyan, 2010)). This initiated the search for cost effective and efficient health care funding system.

Since the adoption of Alma Ata Declaration in United Nations, in 1978, many countries took initiative to strengthen primary healthcare to ensure quality health to its citizens, but the adoption of the system was different. Some countries integrated GPs as the first line of contact in health care. In some primary healthcare delivery model GPs are in central role of the team (Atun, 2004; Macinko, et al, 2003), while in other model GPs run isolated solo practice. The key role of General Practice in UK and that of Family practice in USA in the primary care led National Health Service was initiated around 1995 (Onion & Berrington, 1999). The benefit of that initiative is reflected in the better health and fewer health inequalities of its citizens (Starfield, Shi, Macinko, 2005). The individual country efforts are enhanced by international body like World Organization of National Colleges, Academies and Academic Associations of General Practitioners/Family Physicians (WONCA). WONCA now has 126 Member Organizations in 102 countries with membership of about 300,000 family doctors (WONCA 2014). It organises meeting with General Practice Society of member countries along with health ministry officials and community leaders to strengthen the key role of GP/ FP in primary health care of a country.

In countries with regulated primary healthcare general practitioners became the gate keeper of public health system. Entry to the secondary or tertiary level hospitals is regulated by referral from GP or through emergency. A primary care provider may be called a general practitioner or, family doctor to guide individual and also their family on a variety of health care and wellness issues. In developed countries the integrated Primary health care (PHC) service has transformed the focus of general practice towards multidisciplinary team (Nurses, allied health workers and other groups who has increasingly expanded role in primary care) and a wider system (Martin & Sturmberg, 2005). This takes away some of the decision making role of GPs, as in PHC decision making is the role of specialists or the team.

Increased focus on primary health care, particularly in developed socialist countries, helped formalising or regulating the role of GP and also upgrading the profession in a specialist category. To be a GP a medical graduate now needs to complete the fellowship and or other specialist courses. Today the role of GP can vary between (or even within) countries. In urban areas of some countries their roles tend to be narrower and focused on the care of chronic health problems; the treatment of acute non-life-threatening diseases; the early detection and referral to specialized care of patients with serious diseases; and preventative care including health education and immunization. In rural areas of those countries and in most developing countries a GP may be routinely involved in pre-hospital emergency care, the delivery of babies, community hospital care and performing low-complexity surgical procedures.

SCOPE OF ICT IN GENERAL PRACTICE

To understand the scope of ICT it is important to dissect the general practice into its roles. The definition of GP is changing with the influence of national and international policy of healthcare in a country.

Before 19th century general practice meant a physician (qualified from a college) doing a solo practice to provide medical consultation to any person. Besides a receptionist inclusion of a nurse was the beginning of organised GP chamber, which is recorded between sixties and seventies in US, Canada, NZ and a bit later in Australia (Dunt et.al. 1991, DiCenso et al. 2010,). Healthcare is always information intensive starting from history taking to prescribing medication and follow-up. Good GP practice meant well organised record keeping or filing up individual information. After Second World War the concept changed from a self-regulated physician to a programme integrated professional, by being involved in the national primary healthcare programme. At this point many considered the death of the general practice, as it is regulated by primary health care system (Martin and Sturmberg, 2005).

Today as a member of the primary health care team GP need to participate in the prevention and health promotion programmes to provide early intervention for those at risk. They have to provide the services of a counsellor and act as changing agent for the individual and community. They need to provide first hand service to manage acute, chronic and complex conditions within the practice population, taking into account the uniqueness of each individual for health and illness. To ensure quality of care GP need to understand individual client, share knowledge and gain their trust to apply best available care. At some situations GP also need to coordinate clinical team, resources and services. All these require effective and up-to-date communication system.

Up to the early part of 19th century doctor's reputation were more dependent on their bedside manner or personal communication besides their professional skills, as not all doctors had the skill or knowledge to cure most diseases (Thomas, 2006). Today ensuring updated quality service GP needs more scientific knowledge about disease and its management process by continuous upskilling in all aspects of the service encompassing all age group, gender, body system and disease process but doctor-patient interaction or patient education should be maintained. In doing that it is important to gain information on updates related to diagnostic and therapeutic skills with an understanding to manage new challenges (e.g. SARS or Ebola virus prevention) either through participation in centre based learning or distant learning. They should be acquainted with service provision and service providers for referral. In a busy life availability of customised learning materials to be used at own environment is most effective. Besides the formal institutional learning peer group discussion is very effective to overcome day to day challenges, for which networking is important which could be solved by broadband internet, Facebook, blogging etc.

In providing person centred care GP needs to collect lot of information to ensure quality service for all and also share with other specialist but also need to ensure privacy and security of the information. Security could be ensured by data encryption and decryption, which needs the assistance of ICT. In order to maintain balance between ethics, profession and legislation information update is crucial.

For effective management of the client's condition it is also important to prescribe a solution in client's socio-economic perspective, which needs to analyse cost effectiveness of the service besides the quality, that is better managed by good software. Also accurate record keeping, good planning, acceptable monitoring system and progress evaluation is the key for chronic illness management. All these needs ICT support.

Today a GP has to manage following activities to effectively fulfil his or her role in the health care team (RACGP, 2014):

- Client management through history taking, examining, investigate, provide treatment
- Using appropriate equipment by understanding the availability of state of the art item in the profession, procuring and maintaining it,
- Ensuring physical and mental fitness
- Record keeping with efficient and quick retrieval system, maintaining privacy & confidentiality
- Time management by visiting clients in allocated time,
- Referring clients to other services with updated knowledge about services and adopting easy and quick referring procedures,
- **Knowledge Gathering and Updating:** By attending training, seminar, reading literature
- **Empowering Clients:** By disseminating knowledge (e.g. handbill, video),
- **Conflict Management:** To avoid conflict between ethics, profession and business interest.

Management of a disease process requires effective coordination in the chain of services that includes doctor's initial assessment, investigation by a facility to establish diagnosis, selecting proper mode of treatment, arranging right medication or intervention and follow up. If doctor's prescription is not legible to the pharmacist or spelling of the client's name is different along the chain then the risk of treatment error would outweigh the benefit. Studies show that the rate of completeness in patient identification would increase in electronic prescription compared to hand written ones and such errors could be reduced significantly (Albarrak et.al. 2014). In Australia, a survey in 2006 suggested as many as 10% clients in GP care experienced an adverse drug event (Miller, Britt & Valenti, 2006).

Also, ICT would improve the speed of communication between GP and pharmacist as well as reduce the error of medication delivery to clients i.e. correct medication to right person could be ensured. In electronic prescription system it is possible to avoid drug interaction by utilise decision support tools e.g. drug-drug, drug –dose & drug-allergy interaction.

Treating a client could be in a fixed place or at remote area and it could vary from simple advice, regular visit or urgent procedure like surgery. Remoteness of the clients position from the GP is always a challenge in healthcare. ICT could be of immense help in urgency, remoteness and convenience. Today availability of mobile devices and that of social media like Facebook can enable a client to discuss with GPs (via a tele-health communication platform) without even a journey to the GP clinic.

Advances in technology have made it possible to get digital images of an X-ray or ultrasound, and also wider access to broadband internet enables a doctor to contact a lab requesting the digital image of the ultrasound or x-ray immediately after the procedure for instant review, if it is an emergency. Any change in a person's prescription could be quickly done by sending an email to the pharmacist, who can prepare new Webster pack in few minutes and can send it to patient by express mail.

All those discussion suggests there is wide scope for ICT in the general practice and may include, but not be limited to, followings:

- Patient Administration systems
- Tracking and Reporting systems for patient-centric healthcare data or other clinical data
- Analytical programs or frameworks, related to diagnostics or research

- Clinical Decision Support Systems
- Financial transactions for private payment or public funding
- Population statistics and forecasting systems
- Legal and ethical framework
- Upskilling framework to update clinical or other skills
- **Communication:** Either for Face to face or Distant communication
- **Assisting Time Management:** Through real time 'appointment diary' i.e. automatically changing the information to avoid conflict of time, schedule reminder e.g. pop-up windows to remind client's for "Follow-up" or next activity

The future of GP is again in verge of changing status as some countries are moving towards total digital service with minimum doctor patient physical contact. In the proposed system clients will be able to communicate with the physician without even leaving their own place (i.e. home or office or other places) as tele-health will eventuate that dream. All that suggests in future GP would have limited choice to escape ICT use.

ADOPTION OF ICT IN TODAYS PRACTICE

Before the twentieth century humanity experienced two major paradigm shifts directly related to the world of work: the agricultural revolution and the industrial revolution. The present paradigm shift is Information Revolution, that is not restricted to computers but to information and communication technology (ICT) encompassing and affecting all products, services, processes and systems relating to the generation, transmission and storage of information (Pelgrum, W.J., Law, N., 2003).

Like all new technologies adoption is mostly dependent on two important factors – one is user's own benefit analysis i.e. how the user perceives the technology and how much value to put on it, the other important factor is the seriousness of the national programme or on the national legislation e.g. incentive to adopt it or punitive actions to ignore it (Hall and Khan, 2003). Besides that user's perspective, of gaining competitive advantage and compliance to regulation, availability of enriched environment is a compelling force to adopt technology. For example, if there is high speed broadband internet and plenty of devices to satisfy individual needs then adoption is very rapid? In the following paragraph some of the important factors influencing the ICT use in general practice will be discussed.

User Initiatives

Use of ICT in general practice in early 19th century could be traced by the existence of mobile radio-controlled services for emergency or after hour calls and also tape recording education materials distributed among selected groups (Bryan, 1971). Today due to intense competition and soaring cost of resources solo practices are declining in recent years with rise in group practices to participate in the national primary care (Britt et.al 2013). Large group practice or corporate practice like super clinic adopts ICT for resource management including human resource and for scheduling services.

Consumer pressure is also a factor for GPs to adopt ICT (MacGregor et.al 2006), as today many people access the internet and google the problem or the available solutions to problem and at a GP visit they expect their concerns be valued by GP. This requires GP to search the media by themselves to network with peers and to explain issues either in their own computer monitor or in other media to satisfy clients concern.

GP Locum service is always an important aspect of the community healthcare. Today almost all GP use iPhone or other smartphone to receive calls from agencies allocating them jobs and use mobile EFPOTS or other transaction equipment for billing. To share knowledge they use Facebook or other social media from mobile devices.

Survey of rural GP in Australia suggests Diffusion theory's "relative advantage" and the "usefulness" factor of "Technology Acceptance Model (TAM)" plays a role in using ICT in practice (Deering, Tatnall, and Burgess, 2010).

Legislation and National Initiatives

After the World War II the issue of "personal health" become an important public issue demanding more to be done which drove the governments to adopt a formal healthcare system in the second half of the 20th century (Thomas, 2006). That in turn influenced the formulation of national health policy with emphasis on primary healthcare and GP's becoming the first contact point of the service. Most developed countries are now focusing on eHealth that is defined broadly as "the use of Information and Communication Technologies (ICT) across the whole range of healthcare functions" to cope with the challenges currently faced by healthcare systems (Codagnone & Lupiañez-Villanueva, 2013). Unfortunately, many underdeveloped countries are still lacking that vision and even though they might have a national health policy there is lack of effort to implement it.

In Australia, "Medicare Benefits Schedule" has influenced a lot for ICT usage among GPs. The schedule encourages recording each consultation, develop care plan for patients with chronic illness to ensure providing organised, systematic and practical care (Zwar & Davis, 2012). Use of ICT saves GP time to ensure the eligibility of a client for particular funded plan of treatment. The Practice Incentives Program (PIP) managed by Medicare on behalf of the Department of Health and Ageing is very important (PIP 2014). The PIP encourages GP to be accredited or registered by fulfilling the Royal Australian College of GP (RACGP) Standards for general practices. Payments are made through the PIP for improved use of information management and technology (IM/IT) and other conditions. It helped raise the use of computers among GP from 15% in 1997 to 70% in 2000 (McInnes, Saltman and Kidd, 2006).

Some countries are pushing the healthcare practitioners including GP for optimum use of ICT e.g. starting in 2015, US hospitals and doctors face cuts to their Medicare and Medicaid reimbursements if they haven't adopted meaningful health information technology (HIT) that includes electronic prescribing systems and other elements of Health Information Technology for Economic and Clinical Health (HITECH) Act (Toland, 2011). Moving to a fully electronic system, US expect substantial savings in their health budget.

In UK electronic notes transfer program enables patients' electronic health records to be transferred directly and securely between GP practices (GP2GP, 2014). It improves patient care as GPs will usually have full and detailed medical records, electronic health record (HER), available to them for a new patient's first consultation. It will avoid transcribing errors and omissions, also provide important information about allergies, vaccination, referrals etc. This is an initiative of the Health and Social Care Information Centre (HSCIC), set up as an Executive Non Departmental Public Body (ENDPB) in April 2013 under the Health and Social Care Act 2012. At present even though majority of practices in UK use computerised systems, not all information could be transferred electronically from one practice to other, when a client moves. So, paper-based transfer is the option (printing-off from electronic health records) which the new practice needs to re-enter in their own systems. The new practice often does not have the benefit of the medical history at first consultation as the paper-based transfer system can take weeks to months to complete.

Professional Initiative

Overtime doctors' themselves took several initiatives to educate peers and bring professionalism either through colleges or through publications like journals, to improve quality. In Australia Royal Australian College of General Practitioners (RACGP), Australian College of Rural & Remote Medicine (ACRRM) contributed a lot to standardise the practice along with promoting the use of ICT among GPs through online registration, journals, webinar, WebTV. GPs are not able to get PIP payment without RACGP registration.

Entrepreneur Initiative

Volume of information increases with the growth of general practice, requiring its skilful handling not only for organising but also to ensure client privacy and safety. So, opportunity arouse for entrepreneur to develop new ventures to serve the GP, particularly for data management. Selecting right item from wide options like media selection (out of Windows, Linux, Android) and 3G or 4G platform is not easy for GPs. So many data management businesses have come into play.

Virtual doctor consultation is going to be a reality in Australia as Telstra launched its e-Health division in collaboration with Swiss company Medgate (Telstra 2014a, Ramli 2014; Swan, 2014). This is promised to connect client to doctors, doctors to different providers of healthcare service and to provide access to healthcare information as and when desired within five years i.e. by 2020. Already two providers signed with Telstra one is Northern Territory government to improve remote healthcare and "Silver Chain Group" a large not for profit health and community care organisation signed for the low risk age-care client's post-surgery issues. In this venture other partners of Telstra are – Fred IT group (related to pharmacy), HealthConnex (related to data security), Entra Health Systems (for integrated communication), Verdi, Medinexus, ReadyCare and HealthEngine (Telstra 2014a). This would surely impact the GP service in its future modus operandi. ReadyCare a new service that connects people to GPs over the phone for consultations and HealthEngine helps patients find and book health appointments anywhere, any time (Telstra 2014b). This will enforce GPs to learn more about ICT use to be in business.

Use of tele-health proposed by Telstra could be an advantage if GP can easily and safely share their experience, related to the client's condition and procedures, with others (specialists, or primary healthcare team). This would also help them to compare the management of other doctors, locally, nationally or internationally, and guide to improve.

HealthLink, established in 1993, in NZ provides nearly all of the clinical communications used in New Zealand and is the largest provider of clinical messaging services in Australia, also operates in the Pacific Island nations and Canada It is developing systems and services to facilitate exchange of clinical information through data-centres across a country. It helps reduce the health professionals time in data management and communication with different service providers e.g. pathology, radiology, referring patients etc. It enables the electronic delivery of pathology and radiology results and discharge summaries. It also provides a large managed security infrastructure and is a pioneer in the development of 'cloud-based' online forms technology. (Health Link 2014)

Patients First is a joint initiative of General Practice New Zealand and The Royal New Zealand College of General Practitioners, started in April 2010, to integrate and transfer patient information in primary healthcare from one health care provider to another (e.g. hospital to community settings). It involves the Health IT Board, Ministry of Health and the Health Quality and Safety Commission. Its services include but not limited to improving the availability of health-related statistical data and facilitating the sharing of resources, knowledge and information among health care providers, in New Zealand. Patients First's initiative of New Zealand ePrescription Service (NZePS) delivers electronic prescriptions directly to pharmacies, resulting in a reduction of transcription effort and improved accuracy of content. GPs don't need to handover a prescription to a client (Patients First, 2014).

GP Partners Australia, an initiative of South Australia, was established in 2011 to support GPs for managed service (e.g. security, backup and efficient network), managed infrastructure (e.g. clinical application & workstation problem solution), and other ad-hoc support.

Global Initiatives

Some international forums are pushing the ICT usage across the globe so that GP in all countries can get the benefit of it. To ensure the existence of positive environment for ICT use in a country, different indicators are formulated by global organisations. Network Readiness Index (NRI) calculated by the "World Economic Forum" considers different indicators like Internet access, adult literacy, mobile phone subscription, the availability of venture capital, patent applications and e-government services to gauge the social and economic impact of digitization (World Economic Forum 2013). In 2013 top ten countries with high NRI are – Finland, Singapore, Sweden, Netherlands, Norway, Switzerland, UK, Denmark, USA, Taiwan (China). Latin America, the Caribbean and sub-Saharan Africa countries are lagging behind.

United Nations Conference on Trade and Development (UNCTAD) has established an ICT diffusion index, which is based on connectivity, access and policy. Also the ICT Development Index (IDI) is a composite index combining 11 indicators into one benchmark measure to monitor and compare developments in ICT across countries (ITU, 2012).

It is expected that countries with high NRI would influence more ICT usage among GP's, even though national policy and the existence of other initiatives would have impact.

Today physical structure of communication system has improved a lot (e.g. data transfer through non-linear fibre optics has a capacity of 1 Tb / second). This makes real time image and video transmission easier and faster (Agrawal, 2012). Countries like Australia are taking advantage of that, as expressed by Telstra Health Division to boost the telemedicine and eHealth programme (Telstra, 2014a).

EU has set "Digital Agenda for Europe" and has formulated "eHealth Action Plan" in 2012 to reach a target for eHealth in the region. EU is trying to improve its ICT use in health sector along with better performance in Electronic Health Records (EHR), Health Information Exchange (HIE), Telehealth, and Personal Health Records (PHR) (Codagnone & Lupiañez-Villanueva, 2013). The 2013 survey in EU countries suggest that levels of adoption are influenced by GPs individual characteristics and attitudes as well as by country level effects, and by the perception of impacts and barriers. The majority of GPs place more emphasis on barriers than on benefits, and identify lack of financial incentives and resources, lack of inter-operability, and lack of a regulatory framework on issues of confidentiality and privacy as the main barriers.

USAGE OF ICT IN PRACTICE

The use and the influence of ICT in general practice gained momentum since late 19th century even though main focus was the use of computer rather than ICT as a whole (Bolton '97; Marcus ' 89; Murray '91; Ryan '89; Warshawsky'93).

Each year Australian Divisions of GP report the number of practices known to be using IM/IT. These data provide a national indication of the extent of IM/IT uptake in general practice, and for what purposes IM/IT is being used. It shows ICT usage for "Electronic diagnosis & treatment (EDT)" is relatively more common among GP and other uses include "Patient information database', "Practice administration", "Electronic Data Availability and exchange" (PHCRIS, 2006-07).

Use of computer and software at clinical consultation has become almost universal (96%) among GPs in Australia and OECD countries (Codagnone & Lupiañez-Villanueva, 2013; Britt et.al, 2013). More than 90% GPs are now producing prescriptions electronically, preparing electronic medical records. Around 70% are checking for drug–drug interactions, ordering laboratory tests, run recall systems, and record progress notes (McInnes, Saltman and Kidd, 2006). Few (40%) are using ICT to generate lists of patients requiring long term follow up e.g. clients on an immunisation schedule needing vaccines and those taking the same medication needing follow up. Some researchers found around 80% GPs use computer for ordering laboratory tests, updating patient allergy information, generating patient health summaries, billing and appointment scheduling, while few GP does other functions like creating and updating disease management plans, recording progress notes, accessing educational material for patients, and conducting clinical audits (Deering, Tatnall, and Burgess, 2010).

The 2013 survey in EU countries shows that use of basic ICT (a computer connected to Internet) in the GP consultation room has become almost universal. Situation is not so rosy while discussing the use of ICT in Electronic Health Records (EHR), Health Information Exchange (HIE), Telehealth, and Personal Health Records (PHR). There is a concern that the transition from paper-based record to electronic record is slow. (Codagnone & Lupiañez-Villanueva, 2013). According to this EU survey

- **HER Means:** Systems that are used by healthcare professionals (doctors and nurses) to enter, store, view, and manage patient health and administrative information and data.
- **HIE:** Is the process of electronically transferring / sharing / enabling access to patient health information and data.
- **Telehealth:** Is the use of broadband-based technological platforms for the purpose of providing health services, medical training and health education over a distance.
- **PHR:** Are electronic systems allowing patients to have secure access to, and manage, their health information.

GP's are happy to use an ICT as long as it is simple and quick, which is reflected by the finding that near universal use of electronic prescribing is related to relative easiness of completing the job by mouse clicks and PIP payment incentive (Deering, Tatnall, Burgess, 2010). Same study finds that relatively poor typing skills hinder the completion of electronic progress notes.

Survey shows that 87% of doctors use personal mobile devices for clinical use, of those 62% have medical apps on their smartphones (Avant 2014). Smartphones also helps them to get reference materials handy and do calculations quickly.

ICT is helping GP in document management, indexing, storage either onsite or in a third party server. It is allowing staff to concentrate more on customer service.

ICT is playing an important role in disseminating primary healthcare knowledge at practices. Many GP chambers are fitted with big screen TV to disseminate knowledge to clients while they are waiting for consultation. Live internet TV continuously displaying eye catching video on health issues not only breaks the boredom of waiting but also helps educating clients on health issues. Digital boards displaying multiple health related messages at random order after varied interval with impressive design at the same point, draws attention of clients as it breaks the monotonicity of traditional fixed board display. Automated services are answering simple queries of clients. Webpages created for practices are informing clients about the available facility and are loaded with answers for frequently asked questions. This helps GP to focus more on specific issues related to client health.

Digital imaging system has reduced hazards related to x-ray plates or ultrasound plates. GPs can now communicate with peers or specialists with better quality images, with remote chance of being discoloured or faded. This also gives opportunity to review the images again and again to enhance their knowledge.

Scanning images of document and attaching to email is a very common approach to refer a client.

So, ICT has improved the images and functionality of the practices in the last few decades.

CHALLENGES IN IMPLEMENTING ICT

Push for technology is always a hot topic in all centuries but getting the best result out of it is a time factor along with educating and motivating human factor, for desired level of success.

ICT is expected to improve health-care quality, safety, and efficiency in general practice. In the 20th century one important drive to implement "Health information technology (HIT)" was to combat patient management errors and quality-of-care deficits (Miller, Britt & Valenti, 2006). Patient management errors, including diagnostic error and prescription error, were meant to be reduced but evidence suggests that even after decades of computer use diagnostic error is still a concern. (Avant, 2014; AHIT blog, 2014). In reviewing the issue it is revealed that some factors contributing to diagnostic error - insufficient time with patients, unreliable tools, knowledge limitations, limited access to test results, fragmentation of care etc. needs more attention (Avant 2014). It is a concern then that while using the proposed tele-health in future two factors might still contribute to errors those are knowledge limitation and unreliable tools. Doctors are familiar with direct examination of a client at their chamber, how much accuracy they could achieve by examining a digital appearance of a person i.e. on TV screen. Also when the GP will require certain investigation where from client will get that and how reliable that test would be.

GP are using different devices (smartphones, tablets etc) and apps for communication but there is still no clear guideline to use those devices for data safety. Besides communication (including personal or corporate emails), present day smart devices, used by doctors, also store personal information and business related information. It is a mini version of a briefcase carried by doctors in early 19th century, but much more resourceful than the old briefcase. Loss of a smart device can compromise client privacy and damage to GP's business, as shown by "Project Honey Stick" of Symantec in 2012 (Avant 2014).

So it is important to educate GPs with different security options to evade opportunist data thieves by – locking devices with password, remote locking or content wiping, data encryption requiring a PIN to access. GP also need knowledge in selecting the device and security plan of the service provider, they should research about it before procuring one not just going to a shop and buying it.

Implementing the quality assurance guideline in the virtual consultation could be another challenge to face indemnity issues, as client may call at any time from any place using different devices faking personal ID or generating conflicting information. GP need more guideline to ensure the best outcome of each case.

It would be a challenge to measure the outcome and select a procedure to improve it. The cost of making a virtual GP consultation for a client needs consideration. Would Medicare or other social services cover the cost of such consultation or the system will leave poor clients out of standard quality service.

General Practice or Family Practice has definitely changed its form in the past decade and is forced to have further changes in future due to the ICT impact. Solo practice is at extinction due to the emergence of corporate style health facility to accommodate investment in equipment to which ICT would add extra, would that compromise client service due to the commercialisation of care? In the old style general practice a doctor was able to spend more time at consultation but in the new system a tendency to provide mechanised instant service might compromise doctor-patient relationship.

With the rollover of the tele-health would the term general practice (or GP) be relevant as the first contact doctor can instantly communicate with other PHC team members and specialists of choice from anywhere of a country or globe making care plan or treatment plan quickly. Future GP role, if it persists, would definitely include tele-diagnosis with more digital knowledge e.g. to diagnose by facial image, to arrange webinar fashion board-meeting with client and other professionals across the world (rather than today's single one on one client consultation), to perform tele-procedure guided by other professionals etc. This might need extra time for a junior doctor to become a GP, would that contribute to more doctor shortage or automation of minor jobs would free doctors time to provide care to more clients per hour than the present situation.

In late nineteen century researchers expressed concern about the slow progress in transition from paper-based to electronic based record management (Hersh, WR '95), after several decades of national effort to influence ICT usage not enough GP even in developed countries are using it, as is evident by lack of interest to update "electronic progress notes" or access client information for vaccination update or continuation of long term medication. So, to ensure maximum use of ICT at all aspects of GP role how much effort would require in education (e.g. medical education curriculum) or professional development (through RACGP or ACRRM) or other legislative and incentive programmes.

Low- and middle-income countries face the most severe challenges in ensuring a sufficient, fit-for-purpose healthcare delivery system. The Ebola epidemic in West & Central Africa demonstrates the weak health systems with insufficient workforce & related resources to be able to respond to emerging needs (WHO, 2014). Would GP in those situations be able to use ICT based service, as their NRI rating is low? Would the cost of ICT be at affordable range to provide better healthcare to the vast population of those countries?

REFERENCES

Agrawal, G. P. (2012). *Nonlinear Fiber Optics*. Retrieved from http://www.amazon.com/Nonlinear-Fiber-Optics-Edition-Photonics/dp/0123970237

AHIT blog. (2014). *U.S. Food and Drug Administration has begun collecting reports involving electronic health and IT errors, some of which have resulted in death.* Australian Health Information Technology Blog. Retrieved from http://aushealthit.blogspot.com.au/2011/08/what-is-problem-with-e-health-could-it.html

Albarrak, A. I., Al Rashidi, E. A., & Fatani, R. K. (2014, March). Assessment of legibility and completeness of handwritten and electronic prescriptions. *Saudi Pharmaceutical Journal, 13.* doi:10.1016/j.jsps.2014.02.013

Atun, R. (2004). What are the advantages and disadvantages of restructuring a health care system to be more focused on primary care services? Geneva: WHO Regional Office for Europe's Health Evidence Network (HEN).

Avant. (2014). *Doctor's guide to smarter phone use.* Retrieved from http://connect.avant.org.au/i/320049

Boerma, W.G.W., & Mulder, P. H. (2008). *Health care and general practice across Europe.* The University of Michigan.

Bolton, P. (1997, October). Through the looking glass. Computers & general practice. *Australian Family Physician, 26*(10), 1167–1169. PMID:9339591

Britt, H., Miller, G. C., Charles, J., Henderson, J., Bayram, C., & Pan, Y. et al.. (2010). *General practice activity in Australia 2009-10.* Canberra: Australian Institute of Health and Welfare.

Britt H, Miller GC,, Henderson J, Bayram C, Valenti L, Harrison C, Charles J, Pan Y et al. (2013). *General practice activity in Australia 2012- 13.* The Family Medicine Research Centre, General Practice Series Number 33, November 2013. Sydney University Press.

Codagnone, C., & Lupiañez-Villanueva, F. (2013). Benchmarking Deployment of eHealth among General Practitioners, 2013 Final report. European Commission. Doi:10.2759/24556

Deering, P., Tatnall, A., & Burgess, S. (2010). Adoption of ICT in Rural Medical General Practices in Australia: an Actor-Network Study. *International Journal of Actor-Network Theory and Technological Innovation, 2* (1), 54-69.

DHS (Department of Health and Ageing). (2004). *Medicare definition of a GP.* Retrieved from http://www.health.gov.au/internet/wcms/publishing.nsf/Content/pcd-publications-gpinoz2004

DiCenso, A., Martin-Misener, R., Bryant-Lukosius, D., Bourgeault, I., Kilpatrick, K., Donald, F., & Charbonneau-Smith, R. et al. (2010, December). Advanced Practice Nursing in Canada: Overview of a decision support synthesis. *Canadian Journal of Nursing Leadership, 23*(special issue), 15–34. doi:10.12927/cjnl.2010.22267 PMID:21478685

Dunt, D., Temple-Smith, M., & Johnson, K. A. (1991). Nursing outside hospitals: the working experience of community nurses: job characteristics. *International Journal of Nursing Studies, 28*(1), 27–37. doi:10.1016/0020-7489(91)90047-7 PMID:1856030

First, P. (2014). Retrieved from http://www.patientsfirst.org.nz/about

Gp2Gp. (2014). Retrieved from http://systems.hscic.gov.uk/gp2gp/implementation/gp2gpfactsheet.pdf–

Gandevia, B. (1971). A History of General Practice in Australia. *Canadian Family Physician Medecin de Famille Canadien*, (October), 51–59. PMID:20468689

Hall, B. H., & Khan, B. (2003). Adoption of new technology. In D. C. Jones (Ed.), *The New Economy Handbook*. San Diego, CA: Elsevier/ Academic Press.

Hersh, W. R. (1995, December). The electronic medical record: Promises and problems. *Journal of the American Society for Information Science*, *46*(10), 772–776. doi:10.1002/(SICI)1097-4571(199512)46:10<772::AID-ASI9>3.0.CO;2-0

ITU. (2012). *International Telecommunication Union, CH-1211*. Retrieved from http://www.itu.int/en/ITU-D/Statistics/Documents/publications/mis2012/MIS2012_without_Annex_4.pdf

Jowett, M., & Danielyan, E. (2010). Is there a role for user charges? Thoughts on health system reform in Armenia. *Bulletin of the World Health Organization*, *88*(6), 472–473. doi:10.2471/BLT.09.074765 PMID:20539867

Link, H. (2014). Retrieved from https://www.healthlink.net/en_AU/about-us/company-profile/-

MacGregor, R. C., Hyland, P. N., Harvie, C., & Lee, B. C. (2006). An Examination of the Driving Forces Behind ICT Adoption in Australian Rural and Regional Medical Practices. In Proceedings of IIT06 Conference. Dubai, UAE: IEEE.

Macinko, J., Starfield, B., & Shi, L. (2003). The contribution of Primary Care Systems to health outcomes within Organisation for Economic Cooperation & Development (OECD) countries, 1970 – 1998. *Health Services Research, 38*(3), 831 – 865. DOI: 10.1111/1475-6773.00149

Marcus, A. (1989, February 4). Computers and general practice. *Lancet*, *1*(8632), 278. doi:10.1016/S0140-6736(89)91288-9 PMID:2563438

Martin, C.M., & Sturmberg, J.P. (2005). General practice — chaos, complexity and innovation. *MJA, 183*(2), 106-109.

McInnes, D. (2006). General practitioners' use of computers for prescribing and electronic health records: Results from a national survey. *The Medical Journal of Australia*, *185*(2), 88–91. PMID:16842064

Miller, G. C., Britt, H. C., & Valenti, L. (2006). Adverse drug events in general practice patients in Australia. *The Medical Journal of Australia*, *184*, 321–324. PMID:16584364

Murray, T. S. (1991, August). Computer assisted learning for general practice. *The British Journal of General Practice*, *41*(349), 344–345. PMID:1777283

Onion, D. K., & Berrington, R. M. (1999, March-April). Comparioson of UK General Practice and US Family Practice. *ABFP*, *12*(2), 164–172.

PHCRIS. (2006-07). *PHCRIS Fast Fact - IM/IT use in Australian general practices, 2003-04 to 2006-07; Annual Survey of Divisions (ASD) Report series, 2003-04 to 2006-07*. Retrieved from http://www.phcris.org.au/fastfacts/fact.php?id=5029

PIP. (2014). *Practice Incentive Programme*. Retrieved from http://www.medicareaustralia.gov.au/provider/incentives/pip/-

Plianbangchang, S. (2011). *Regional Consultation on Strengthening Role of Family/Community Physicians in Primary Health Care*. Jakarta, Indonesia: Academic Press.

Quinn, G. P., & Keough, M. J. (2002). *Experimental Design and Data Analysis for Biologists*. Cambridge University Press. Retrieved from http://books.google.com.au/books?hl=en&lr=&id=VtU3-y7LaLYC&oi=fnd&pg=PP17&dq=GP+and+IT&ots=czom2Bqkiy&sig=iVsd0AsJx11cM5WmUIwSU8nh21I#v=onepage&q=GP%20and%20IT&f=false

RACGP. (2014). Retrieved from http://www.racgp.org.au/becomingagp/what-is-a-gp/what-is-general-practice/

Ramli, D. (2014). Telstra inks eHealth deal with Medgate. *The Australian Financial Review*. Retrieved from http://www.afr.com/p/technology/telstra_inks_ehealth_deal_with_medgate_dfUoP2yhYylu0uxVskoPDI

Ryan, M. P. (1989, May). A system for general practice computing in Scotland. *Health Bulletin, 47*(3), 110–119. PMID:2807896

Simon, C. (2009). From Generalism to Specialty—A Short History of General Practice. InnovAiT.

Starfield, B., Shi, L., & Macinko, J. (2005, September). Contribution of Primary Care to Health Systems and Health. *The Milbank Quarterly, 83*(3), 457–502. doi:10.1111/j.1468-0009.2005.00409.x PMID:16202000

Swan, D. (2014). *Telstra targets healthcare with new deals*. Business Spectator. Retrieved from http://www.businessspectator.com.au/news/2014/10/22/technology/telstra-targets-healthcare-new-deals

Telstra. (2014a). *Our partners in health*. Retrieved from http://www.telstra.com.au/personal/telstra-health/about/our-partners/-

Telstra. (2014b). *Readycare and Healthengine will transform how Australians connect with healthcare*. Retrieved from http://www.telstra.com.au/personal/telstra-health/products/telehealth/clinical-consultation/

Thomas, R. K. (2006). The History of Health Communication. In Health Communication. Springer US. Doi:10.1007/0-387-26116-8_4

Toland, B. (2011, August 7). Electronic records no panacea for health care industry. *Pittsburgh Post-Gazette*. Retrieved from http://old.post-gazette.com/pg/11219/1165767-114-0.stm?cmpid=nationworld.xml

Walley, T., & Mantgani, A. (1997, October 11). The UK General Practice Research Database. *Lancet, 350*(9084), 1097–1099. doi:10.1016/S0140-6736(97)04248-7 PMID:10213569

Warshawsky, S. (1993, December). General practitioner records on computer. *Family Practice, 10*(4), 474. doi:10.1093/fampra/10.4.474 PMID:8031369

WHO. (2014). *Brochure*. Retrieved from http://www.who.int/hrh/documents/strategy_brochure9-20-14.pdf

Wikipedia. (2014). *General Practitioner*. Retrieved from http://en.wikipedia.org/wiki/General_practitioner

WONCA. (2014). *WONCA in brief*. Retrieved from http://www.globalfamilydoctor.com/AboutWonca/brief.aspx

World Economic Forum. (2013). *Global Information Technology Report 2013.* Retrieved from http://www.weforum.org/reports/global-information-technology-report-2013

Zwar, N., & Davis, G. P. (2012). General Practice. In Understanding the Australian Health Care System (2nd ed.). Elsevier Health Sciences.

APPENDIX: ABBREVIATIONS

HER: Electronic Health Record.
FP: Family Practice.
GP: General Practice.
HIE: Health Information Exchange.
PHC: Primary health care.
PHR: Personal Health Record.
SARS: Severe Acute Respiratory Syndrome caused by SARS coronavirus.

Chapter 11
Utilisation of Health Information Systems for Service Delivery in the Namibian Environment

Ronald Karon
Namibia University of Science and Technology, Namibia

ABSTRACT

The use of Health Information Systems (HIS) is considered to be a major contributing factor to health-care service delivery. However, the utilisation of HIS which includes use and management is critically challenging in the public health sector in many developing countries. The manifestation of the challenges results in poor service delivery, which includes patient deaths. This is the main motivation for this study, to investigate how HIS can be used to improve service delivering in the hospitals from developing countries perspective. The study was carried out in Namibia, using two hospitals in the public healthcare. The study adopted the qualitative case study. The study revealed that the use of parallel systems, lack of systems integration, lack of portable devices and users' incompetency are some of the factors which impact the use and management of HIS in hospitals.

INTRODUCTION

Maximizing Healthcare delivery through technology integration is such an important topic worldwide as Healthcare is critically important to everyone's life. Healthcare concerns itself with the wellbeing or health of individuals within a community. As such ways in how healthcare service delivery can be improved has been trending globally. Today the incorporation and use of Health Information Systems (HIS) can aid in enhanced healthcare service delivery. Given this importance of healthcare quality, this chapter aimed to investigate the use of HIS in the Namibian public health sector. The objectives of the chapter in attaining the aim was to understand how HIS is utilised by medical practitioner' and administrator', the factors encountered in using the HIS and the impact that the use of HIS has on service delivery within the public health sector.

DOI: 10.4018/978-1-4666-9446-0.ch011

BACKGROUND

The essentiality of maximizing Healthcare quality cannot be over emphasized in our world at present. Kulkarni (2006, p. 8) defined Healthcare as "the prevention, treatment, and management of illness and the preservation of mental and physical well-being through the services offered by the medical and allied health profession". The importance of healthcare continues to receive increasing attention particularly on the aspect of service delivery to the needy. Cline and Luiz (2013) argued that Healthcare service delivery could be improved by incorporating HIS into hospital processes and activities. Dalziel (2008) defines HIS as "a computer program that organizes clinical data through acquisition, storage and distribution of information" (p. 3). HIS functions involves the use of information technology (IT) which basically are the use of computers, telecommunications and other information processing technologies within healthcare organizations to automate the work processes (Kulkarni, 2006).

The need to improve and maintain healthcare service delivery is a global concern. The areas of improvement include hygiene and the production of health environments (Yen-Han, 2013). Healthcare is critical to every nation in that the economic growth and productivity can be negatively hampered should health conditions of communities deteriorate due to poor healthcare services (Vichianin, 2007). According to Xiao (2012), the U.S. government embarked on an effort to increase healthcare quality and minimize healthcare costs by incorporating technology, such as the use of HIS, into the existing healthcare system. Barrette (2011) argued that technology investment in healthcare is escalating, greatly believed to yield enhanced healthcare quality. The Institute of Medicine (IOM) defines healthcare quality as "the degree to which health services for individuals and populations increase the likelihood of desired health outcomes and are consistent with current professional knowledge" (Vichianin, 2007, p. 18).

However in developing countries there are many factors that could have an impact on the utilisation of HIS, more specifically in the public health sector. In Ghana for example there is minimal government contribution and support toward healthcare service delivery efforts (Melesse, 2010). Some other factors include under-resourced facilities or resistance by healthcare professionals to adopt the use of HIS which could be contributed by a lack of understanding about the positive outcomes attributed to the use of HIS within healthcare (Cline & Luiz, 2013). In Namibia, the national health information system (NHIS) was implemented in 1990, soon after the country had its independence. The primary purpose of the NHIS was to provide ample information on a large number of health indicators and to optimize healthcare service delivery (Haoses-Gorases, 2005). The NHIS had since undergone several improvements, in an effort to address the gaps and challenges it is confronted with, such as integration issues.

HIS enables and supports the automation of work processes and activities in hospitals and clinics which adopts practices, such as capturing of patient data electronically instead of the use of a paper-based system. According to Lorenzi and Riley (2004), HIS will allow for easier and faster retrieval and management of patient information when required. The authors further argued that prompt diagnosis will be possible as medical practitioners would have faster access to a patient' medical history which is a support base in determining diagnosis (Lorenzi & Riley, 2004).

The optimisation of functionalities such as the work flow processes using HIS within healthcare would ultimately improve the overall healthcare service delivery (Hersh, 2009). An example is the use of electronic health records (EHRs) in countries, such as the United States of America. Liong (2008) defines an EHR as "…a computerized clinical information system that stores and displays patient information in legible and organized ways, and facilitates the recording and retrieval of clinical information about patients" (p. 1).

It is argued in some quarters that HIS has proven to provide optimal access to healthcare patient records and lowered overall costs within healthcare. An example is the electronic storage of patient data instead of physical files which consume space, facilities and incur administrative costs such as purchasing of files and filing cabinets (Lorenzi & Riley, 2004). However there are certain areas that continue to be challenging the use of HIS in healthcare. This includes privacy and security of patient information on the network. According to Sondheimer et al, (2009) there is a public awareness of the risks or possible loop holes that may lead to the unauthorized access of private information.

Another factor that could influence the use of HIS is nurse's attitude toward the HIS possibly contributed by the generation age gap (Fasolino, 2009). Dalziel (2008) posits that older nurses are prone to have a less positive attitude toward the use of HIS. Furthermore, Jackson (2013) states that there are some challenges attributed to the use of an EHR such as "decreased communication between other disciplines, the quality of care being delivered, and in some cases hindered their work by impairing critical thinking" (p. 4).

The demand for healthcare services will continue to increase as long as there are lives. As such, there is inevitable need for continuous improvement for efficiency and effectiveness of healthcare service to the society at large. The use of HIS is generally accepted as the way through which healthcare operations can be improved (Hersh, 2009). Thus, various stakeholders, namely healthcare experts, policy makers, investors and consumers points to the important role that HIS plays in the healthcare industry (Wu, et al., 2006). Hence the hope that HIS will continue to yield a positive impact if used and managed appropriately (Pisk, 2010).

MAIN FOCUS OF THE CHAPTER

Improper healthcare systems or infrastructures are some possible factors contributing to poor healthcare service delivery, which is especially challenging in the public health sector of developing countries. The manifestation of such challenges results in poor service delivery, which includes patient deaths.

Research Methodology

Based on the aim and objectives of the study the qualitative research method was employed. According to Bricki and Green (2007) a qualitative research focuses on behavioural aspects of specific settings, rather than numeric values. It was thus befitting to adopt the qualitative approach as the research questions sought to understand how and why HIS was used in the delivering of healthcare service. For the study to be specific and in-depth a case study approach was applied. Al-Mutairi and Mohammed (2011) defines a case study as "an empirical inquiry that investigates a contemporary phenomenon within its real-life context, especially when the boundaries between phenomenon and context are not clearly defined" (p. 2). The authors further explained how the case study approach "allows an investigation to retain the holistic and meaningful characteristics of real-life events such as individual life cycles, organization and managerial processes..." (p. 2).

Two public hospitals were selected as cases in the study. Both hospitals are situated in Windhoek, Namibia. The primary rational for had selected the two hospitals include accessibility and functionality. The two hospitals granted access to be used as cases in the study. The core functions of the hospitals

Figure 1.

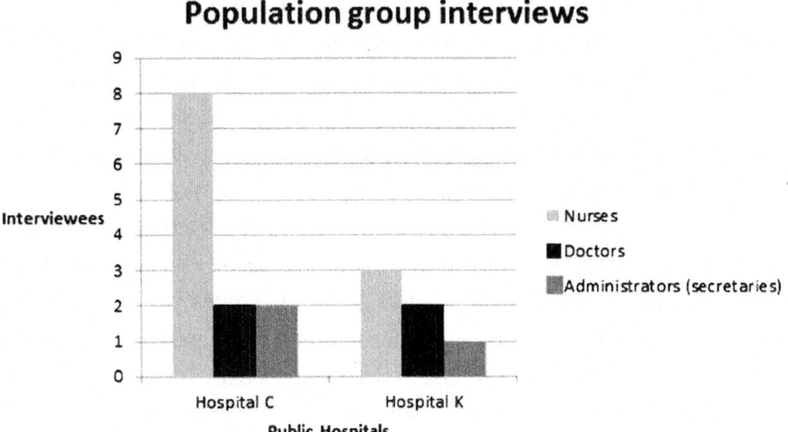

are very distinct from each other. Hospital K is a referral, meaning that it is more of a first aid point, where diagnosis is carried out. Thereafter, the patient is referred to another hospital, such as Hospital C. Hospital C is more of a specialist hospital.

The semi-structured interview technique was used for data collection, as interaction was required to obtain individual and group's opinion and perspectives on the use and management of the HIS. The participants were medical practitioners and administrators in the two cases. The interviews were conducted, using the English language and two local Namibian languages, namely Khoekhoe (also known as Nama/Damara) and Afrikaans. This was according to the interviewee's preference. The interviewees from both hospitals were labelled CH001, CH002, etc. and KH001, KH002, etc. respectively. Quotes from the interviewees were referenced in accordance to page and line numbers, E.g. "CH001, 4:88".

As illustrated in Figure 1, at the point of saturation, a total of eleven (11) nurses, four (4) doctors and three (3) administrators (secretaries) were interviewed at the two hospitals. Saturation is at the point where the researcher noticed that there was no new information forth coming from the interviews. Eight (8) nurses were interviewed at Hospital C and three (3) nurses at Hospital K. Doctor's interviewed were two (2) from both hospitals. There were two (2) group interviews conducted with nurses, which ranged from two to three nurses at a time. Both group interviews were conducted at Hospital C. Additionally, two (2) administrative staff members were interviewed at Hospital C and one (1) at Hospital K.

Nurses were interviewed first, followed by the doctors. This order was followed simply to determine or separate the nurses' views and perceptions from that of doctors. This is primarily because nurses are the first contact point for patients. Additionally, the researcher conducted group interviews with nurses mainly because it was impossible to get one-on-one interviews with some of them due to the demanding working environment.

Data Analysis

The data was analysed, using the interpretive technique. Interpretivism relates to understanding and obtaining meaning about objects and subjects of the phenomenon being studied (Noble, 2012). The analysis was carried out to examine and understand how HIS was used in the Namibian public health sector. Analysis was performed separately on the two cases using the three research questions below that were designed to attain the objectives and aim of the study.

1. How do the medical practitioners make use of the current HIS for service delivery?

The medical practitioners, which include Nurses and Doctors made use of the HIS in different ways, and for various purposes, more particularly at Hospital C. This was attributed to their different functions and tasks. In order to clearly define how the practitioners used the HIS, the researcher followed and tried to make sense of the process involved in a patient's visit to the hospital.

The nurses are the first contact point with regards to patient care at both hospitals. Patient's first visit to Hospital C begins with registration at reception (CH001, 1:4). Patients are required to provide their demographic details, such as identification number, medical aid number (if available), name, surname, date of birth, residential address and contact number (CH010, 2:64-65). However patients at Hospital C can bypass the registration point and be directly admitted to a ward if it was an emergency. According to one of the nurses, patients can only be referred to Hospital C from two health facilities, "Hospital K and other regions" (CH004-Group, 1:3). A patient is referred from other regions only if the patient cannot be helped at the initial region (CH02, 1:8-9). In cases where a patient is directly taken into a ward the nurses would check for the patient's vital signs, such as blood pressure and thereafter the secretary registers the patient using the HIS. However the HIS neither automatically allocates a doctor nor sends alert messages to specialists on duty. This makes the manual system valid and important. A nurse posited that the "manual file system is used for storing and managing hardcopies of files" (CH001, 2:36). As a result Hospital C operates parallel systems simultaneously, the HIS and the paper based system.

Based patient information obtained, including bio-data, a first time patient is provided with a Medical Registration (MR) number which is automatically generated by the HIS. In addition to the MR number the patient's face is captured using a webcam (CH010, 1:14). The patient's facial image is captured and stored on the system along with the MR number. A card is than produced electronically for the patient, similar to that of a driver's license or identification card. According to a nurse "the MR number also appears on the patient's hospital passport which is in a paper form" (CH010, 2:65-67). Furthermore another nurse stated the importance of a patient's MR number particularly for tracing purposes. The medical staff, more specifically, nurses or secretaries should be able to trace relatives for notification purposes (KH0001, 70:73).

The MR number is a number unique to a patient and when this number is punched into to the electronic system, it displays all medical information of the patient. Medical information such as doctor's appointments or "previous bills and outstanding accounts" can be viewed (CH001, 1:31-32). The MR number is also handwritten on the physical file of a patient by staff on duty at the time. Sometimes, human error occurs as a result, making the process inaccurate. Such human errors can be detrimental as one patient could be mistaken for another.

The MR number does not have authentication, meaning the number can be changed by any individual intentionally or unintentionally (CH003, 1:14). This can have fatal implications as a patient could be mistaken for another. Additionally wrong bills could be sent to patients, as they are generated based on the produced MR number without a validation mechanism. Billing is said to be generated by the accounts office (CH010, 3:79-80).

Doctors at Hospital C can also access patient medical records on the HIS. One of the nurses explained that the doctor uses the MR number to access patients' details (CH010, 2:36-37). For example doctors in the department that deals with HIV make use of the HIS to record patient medical information, for treatment eligibility and their current state of health (CH01, 1:27-30). Every user is assigned login details with little differentiation in accessibility privileges. The doctors attained more access rights and hence could access all patient information, nurses on the other hand could do the same but only to close proximity (CH01, 2:34-36).

When a patient needs to see a doctor, the patient's information is entered by the secretaries and the secretary books the patient for an appointment using the HIS. The doctors can use the HIS system to place medication orders on behalf of patients or instruct a pharmacy at the hospital to prepare medication for a specified patient (CH01, 2:52-54). Laboratory test results could also be retrieved via the HIS but this was not done yet at the time of the study. One doctor explained "It's supposed to be that way but it haven't started working that way, so we are still waiting" (CH01, 2:56-57).

Hospital K on the other hand only utilised a paper-based system. Nurses and doctors including administrators carried out their tasks manually. Upon visiting Hospital K, a patient presents a hospital passport and moves on to pay a service fee at reception. From reception the patient is moved to the casualty area where they wait to be screened by a nurse (KH003, 1:2-3). This is to determine the patients' medical urgency. One of the interviewees explained "the nurse conduct the process of observations, and ask the patient about his or her medical history. Thereafter the nurse recommend whether the patient require the attention of a doctor or not" (KH003, 2:43-45). In case of an emergency, such as vehicle accidents involving several people, the nurse on duty make use of the triage method to determine which of the patients need urgent medical attention. A nurse explained that "the triage method is when you are treating patients according to their situations. For example, a patient with severe bleeding is placed ahead of those without physical injuries" (KH003, 1:15-19).

Patient demographics at Hospital K are recorded in files by nurses or doctors (KH001, 2:46-53). These physical files are stored in a designated storage room at the basement of the hospital (KH0001, 1:23-24). Basically all recording, retrieval, access and storage processes are manual.

2. What are the factors which influence HIS usage for service delivery within the Namibian environment?

There were various factors identified which influenced the use of HIS for service delivery in the two hospitals. The factors ranged from inadequate staff training to not enough computers in the hospital wards.

It was empirically revealed that the use of HIS in Hospital C had some benefits, but at the same time there were concerns on the effective use of the system. According to an interviewed nurse there was a time factor. This includes the time it takes to type patient data on a computer, while dealing with a lot of patients requiring attention in a ward simultaneously (CH008, 2:36-38). It is because the nurses are under staffed and there is a lack of sufficient computers in a ward. Each ward at the Central Hospital only has one computer (CH008, 2:36).

Another factor which influences the use of HIS for healthcare service delivery is the advanced age of some nurses. They are considered to be very slow in typing and affect service when many patients needs to be treated, hence electronic data capturing becomes a hindrance (CH001, 2:73-75). According to one of the nurses HIS training at Central Hospital took only about three to five days, which was considered insufficient by the nurses (CH004-Group, 1:20). Additionally the availability of the HIS was a major concern at the hospital, as a doctors stated that "the system (HIS) is always offline and on (mostly offline) and this type of situation goes for days before it can be fully restored" (CH01, 2:64). The doctor further stated that the template used in the HIS system is inadequate for their department and does not meet the departmental requirements (CH01, 2:65-66).

HIS was not in use at the time of this study at Hospital K but that the medical practitioners were nonetheless being prepared to use HIS to carry out their duties. A secretary that was interviewed at Hospital K stated that "we received two days of training which was very short" (KH0001, 2:46-48).

FINDINGS AND DISCUSSIONS

Based on the analysis of the data presented above, four critical factors were found to influence the use of HIS in the two Namibian public hospitals. The factors are parallel systems, lack of integration, lack of portable devices and human incompetence. The factors are discussed as follows.

Parallel Systems

The HIS and manual system were used in parallel in carrying out the hospital's processes and activities, sometimes, simultaneously at the time of the study. The utilisation of parallel systems at Hospital C was attributed to the fact that the HIS was needed to be fully stable before the manual process could be phased out. As such, the manual system was still considered vital should the use of HIS fail to be efficient in its operation. The plan was to systematically phase out the manual system once the data have been completely captured, processes migrated, and the functions well understood by the users.

Similar to many hospitals, at Hospital C the first point for a patient is at the reception. Patients are required to provide their personal and medical details to the administrator at reception. The patient data is captured on the system and the patient receive a Medical Registration number which is generated by the HIS. The Medical Registration number is a unique medical identifier for the patient which is also recorded on the patient's traditional passport. The Medical Registration number when entered would display all the patient's medical demographics on the HIS. Furthermore, the face of the patient is captured, using a web camera. A hospital card which is similar to a driving license or identification card is issued to the patient to complete the process of registration. This is in an effort to eventually do away with the traditional patient hospital passports that is a shape of a medium sized rectangular booklet, which is prone to wear and tear.

However, patients can bypass the reception point when in critical condition, such as a life threatening situation or unconsciousness. In such cases the patient is sent directly to a ward for first aid attendance by nurses. Depending on the situation and condition of the patient, doctors are assigned. Every ward has one computer and there are administrators assigned to these wards. The administrators are responsible for registering the patient on the HIS, answering telephone calls, filing, etc. this means that a patient can be registered at both the reception point or at the ward.

The nurses are responsible for recording the recovery progress of the patient, using the HIS. The nurses are also responsible for discharging a patient on the system, where in such a case the availability of that particular patient bed will be visible on the system. However, not all the nurses could make use of the system appropriately. Hence majority still relied on the manual process to carry out their tasks. As a result the manual system could be seen as a duplicative effort, causing slower responses to activities.

As empirically revealed, retrieval and access to patients' medical records are faster, when using the HIS. Since patient medical information is contained in the HIS, the billing and payment processes are faster consolidated. Re-registering of patients every time a patient returns to the hospital will not be necessary as patient information that was provided upon first registration is kept on the HIS. Both hospitals have a centralised storage room where all paper files for many years are stored.

Lack of Integration

The HIS was not fully utilised at the time of this research at Hospital C. This was due to integration challenges. The department of HIV for example was one of the affected departments at the Hospital requesting that some of their departmental requirements be met in order to efficiently use the system. This was because of their unique tasks within the health environment, such as counselling of patients before HIV tests. As a result the use of the manual file system continued to be prevalent in the hospital's operations. Some of the doctors indicated that the lack of integration of the systems caused duplication of work load, as the recording of information needed to be done in two different systems. During such a process, accuracy and consistency are not guaranteed because of the double workload.

Lack of Portable Devices

Another challenging factor that the doctors were confronted with is accessibility to the system from anywhere and at any given time. This was primarily to enable the doctors to record patient medical information as they move through the different wards, as well as to access the information outside the hospital for their private scrutiny. This could have been achieved with the use of portable devices. However, the HIS did not accommodate the integration of portable devices such as laptops and smart phones. Additionally the network connection was unstable. The inability to use portable devices once again contributed to a double workload as upon return of the doctors to their offices they had to re-capture the manually recorded patient data on the HIS.

User Incompetency

The competency of the users, which included doctors and nurses, were vital in the effective use and management of the HIS. Nurses at Hospital C were confronted with competency challenges such as lack of familiarity with the computer keyboard causing an inability to type patient medical information accurately and at a faster pace. However this challenge was more prevalent with the older generation of nurses. The implication was that it takes longer to complete registration of patients due to slow typing, thereby causing a delay in responding to urgently needed medical attention by other patients.

The incompetency of users in the use and management of the HIS was also attributed to a lack of proper training. According to some nurses training was offered but for only three to five days. Thus it was considered insufficient to get a grip of the system's functionalities.

With regards to Hospital K, it was established that the patient registration, admission and communication processes were manually done and were not computerized at the time of the study. For example, when a patient gets registered, a file is opened and patient information is recorded therein. The same process applied to patient admissions. Every patient has a hospital passport where medical history is recorded by a nurse or the doctor. Within this operandi, if a nurse intended to communicate a certain diagnose to a doctor, he/she did so by writing on the patient's hospital passport. This system has been there for a very long time and the medical personnel have become very comfortable with it. This has also contributed to the lack of interest in emerging technologies such as the HIS. The four factors are further outlined below with recommendations on how these challenges could be addressed.

Research shows that the above identified factors are commonly faced by most healthcare organisations, especially in developing countries. The use of parallel systems at the one hospital was attributed to the HIS not fully functional and stable at the time of the study and was rather considered to be a pilot run until such a time all major challenges are resolved and full functionality and stability of the system is proven.

The lack of sufficient training contributed to user incompetency which was a major factor that negatively impacted the use of HIS at the Hospital. Nurses and doctors for one had little confidence in using the HIS. It was found that the use of HIS was especially challenging to older Nurses, hence they opted to rather continue using the traditional paper based system. The administrators on the other hand were more optimistic in using the HIS as they claimed would enhance patient information retrieval and billing processes. Training thus was a factor that was necessary in boosting the confidence of the HIS users.

In addition to parallel systems and user incompetency', a lack of portable devices was another factor. Doctors especially indicated that the lack of portable devices caused a double workload since data capturing had to be done manually and needed to be re-captured on the computerised system. Not only was the lack thereof a challenge but that if there were portable devices the integration of these devices to the HIS for remote access would be a challenge.

As such a lack of integration was the final factor. The lack of integration results in ineffective operation of the HIS, causing poor information flow between sectors and units in the healthcare. Unmet user requirements were indicated to be attributing to a lack of integration as different departments have different functions. For example the department of HIV required doctors to take tests and provide counselling and these requirements were different from the doctors doing rounds in the wards.

Based on the outcome of this study, it is evident that to effectively use and manage the HIS for enhanced service delivery the aforementioned challenges need to be addressed. It is recommended that an awareness campaign about the HIS be conducted at the healthcare, as awareness about the system, its functionalities and benefits were lacking. Proper communication about the system functionalities and benefits were necessary. It is suggested that communication about the system be channelled through all levels. More emphasis must be placed on the benefits the use and management of the HIS would bring to healthcare service delivery. In that way all stakeholders, especially the end users of the system would be motivated and buy into the idea of using the system.

Additionally it is suggested that user requirements studies be carried out by the respective IT personnel in the healthcare to ensure that the system meets all departmental user requirements, which would allow for integration of departments and portable devices with the HIS. Training is the underlying success of the effective use of the system. Research showed that older medical practitioners were found to be less enthusiastic about the use of technology in carry out their duties, as such good training would motivate the use of the HIS and dissolve possible barriers in using the system.

CONCLUSION

The wellbeing of a collective of individuals in a nation in terms of health reflects in productivity and economic growth. Therefore healthcare service delivery is vital and can be optimized by introducing HIS in healthcare facilities. HIS allows for manual operational processes in healthcare to be computerised, such as the use of electronic health records (EHR) whereby patient records are electronically produced, stored and retrieved, enabling faster access, bulk storage and accuracy. Readability of electronically recorded patient data as supposed to bad handwriting from some doctors is another advantage.

Many developing countries are challenged with both technical and non-technical challenges as revealed in the analysis of the data for Hospital K and Hospital C in this chapter. The main challenges that were found in the study were the use of parallel systems, lack of integration, lack of portable devices and user incompetency. It was thus recommended that efforts be directed to sufficient training of the HIS users to encourage competency and confidence in using the system. Additionally addressing integration issues was necessary, as the HIS require optimised utilisation to explore its potentials to the fullest in order to improve the service of healthcare to the communities in Namibia. Optimal human interaction with the HIS is vital to avoid redundant Healthcare service delivery. The interaction seemingly had a significant influence on the integration of HIS, which could foster collaboration and consolidation of processes and activities.

It is eminent that research efforts and the practical application thereof be directed toward how Healthcare delivery can be maximised and managed by adopting the use of IT, as sustained community health care development can positively impact the economic growth and productivity of a nation. Thus this chapter aimed to investigate the utilisation of HIS for service delivery in the public health sector from a developing country's perspective.

REFERENCES

Adler-Milstein, J. R. (2011). The use of information technology in US health care delivery. *Proquest Dissertations and Theses*, 1.

Aftahi, S. R. (2013). Spirituality in a heealthcare organization: An exploratory qualitative inquiry. *Proquest Dissertations and Theses*, 52-53.

Akerman, E. A. (2006). Attitudes toward computers and computerization in Canadian critical care nurses. *Proquest Dissertations and Theses*, 1.

Al-Mutairi, M. S., & Mohammed, L. A. (2011). *Cases on ICT Utilization, Practice and Solutions. Tools for managing day-to-day issues.* New York: Information Science Reference. doi:10.4018/978-1-60960-015-0

Al-Mutairi, S. M., & Mohammed, L. A. (2011). *Cases on ICT Utilization, Practice and Solutions. Tools for managing Day-to-Day issues.* New York: Information Science Reference. doi:10.4018/978-1-60960-015-0

Alexander, R. C. (2009). Fostering student engagement in the history through student-created digital media: A qualitative and quantitative study of student engagement and learning outcomes in 6th-grade history instruction. *Proquest Dissertations and Theses*, 62.

Amendola, M. L. (2008). An examination of the leadership competency requirements of nurse leaders in healthcare information technology. *Proquest*, 14.

Amershi, H. (2006). Leading information technology (IT) integration within vancouver coastal health. *Proquest Dissertations and Theses*, 2.

Barrette, E. G. (2011). The impact of health information technology on demand for hospital inpatient services. *ProQuest*, 93-94.

Baumbach, J. (2006). Nurse practitioner utilization of information technology. *Proquest Dissertations and Theses*, 7.

Bogdan, R., Biklen, C., & Knopp, S. (1998). Qualitative research in education. An introduction to theory and methods. Boston: Allyn and Bacon.

Brikci, N., & Green, J. (2007). *A guide to using qualitative research methodology*. Academic Press.

Brown-Davis, C. B. (2009). Managed care and minority healthcare access in Georgia: A qualitative study of the quality and accessibility of care provided to the minority elderly population of Dekalb county. *Proquest Dissertations and Theses*, 12-13.

Chang, J. (2007). Nursing informatics competencies required of nurses in Taiwan: A Delphi method. *Proquest Dissertations and Theses*, 1-2.

Cline, G., & Luiz, J. (2013). Information technology systems in public sector health facilities in developing countries: the case of South Africa. *BMC Medicial informatics and decision making*, 13.

Craig, H. D. (2013). Using Diffusion of Innovation theory to determine Missouri providers' perception of telemedicine. *Proquest Dissertations and Theses*, 10.

Czanderna, K. H. (2013). A qualitative study on the impact of a short term global healthcare immersion experience in bachelor of science nursing students. *Proquest Dissertations and Theses*, 68-69.

Daly, G. (2012). Nursing perceptions of electronic documentation. *Proquest*, 3.

Dalziel, C. A. (2007). Factors that enhance nurses' use of health information systems to support clinical decision-making. *Proquest*, 1.

Dalziel, C. A. (2008). Factors that enhance nurses use of health information systems to support clinical decision making. *Proquest dissertations and theses*.

Dalziel, C. A. (2008). *Factors that enhances nurses use of health information systems to support clinical decision making*. ProQuest Dissertations and Theses.

Dienemann, J., & Castle, B. V. (2003). The impact of healthcare informatics on the organisation. *Jona*, 557-558.

Edwards, D. (2011). Analyzing decision-Making styles and strategic planning techniques for information technology in non-profit organisations. *Proquest Dissertations and Theses*, 24.

Farquharson, P. H. (2009). The perception of information technology investment and its impact on productivity at small private colleges. *Proquest*, 6.

Fasolino, T. (2009). *Nursing related factors influencing medication error incidence on medical surgical units*. Proquest.

Goodwin, C. S. (2013). Healthcare organizational metaphors and implications for leadership. *Proquest Dissertations and Theses*, 1.

Grgurović, M. (2010). Technology-enhanced blended language learning in an ESL class: A description of a model and an application of the diffusion of innovations theory. *Proquest Dissertations and Theses,* 21-25.

Grossman, C. S. (2014). Succession planning and knowledge transfer in higher education. *Proquest Dissertations and Theses,* 70.

Haoses-Gorases, L. (2005). *Utilisation of health information system (HIS) in Namibia: focus on challenges and opportunities faced by health care delivery system.* Academic Press.

Hersh, W. (2009). A stimulus to define informatics and health information technology. *BMC Medical Informatics and Decision Making, 9*(1), 24. doi:10.1186/1472-6947-9-24 PMID:19445665

Hobbs, S. D. (2007). Clinical nurses' perception of nursing informatics competencies. *Proquest Dissertations and Theses,* 1.

Hofler, L. D. (2007). A case study of the relationship between the North Carolina center for nursing and nursing workforce issues in the state of North Carolina through the lens of planned change. *Proquest Dissertations and Theses,* 33.

Iacono, J., Brown, A., & Holtham, C. (2009). Research methods: A case example of participant observation. *Electronic Journal of Business Research Methods,* 40.

Jackson, A. C. (2014). The effect of suspension as a deterrent to student misconduct. *Proquest Dissertations and Theses,* 110.

Jackson, A. S. (2013). Impact of electronic health records on nurses' information seeking and discriminating skills for critical thinking. *ProQuest,* 4-5.

Jensen, T. A. (2013). Nurses' perceptions of nursing care documentation in the electronic health record. *Proquest Dissertations and Theses,* 1.

Jones, S. M. (2012). The development of trust in the nurse-patient relationship with hospitalized Mexican American patients. *Proquest Dissertations and Theses,* 179.

Jones-Zeigler, C. M. (2011). Computerization in practice: The lived experience of experienced nurses. *Proquest,* 1-2.

Kelley, T. F. (2012). Information use with paper and electronic nursing documentation by nurses caring for pediatric patients. *Proquest Dissertations and Theses,* 15.

Kulkarni, V. A. (2006). *Implementation of electronic health records: Modeling and evaluating healthcare information systems for quality improvements in the U.S. healthcare industry.* Academic Press.

Liong, A. S. (2008, March). *Descriptions of nurses experiences with electronic health records (EHR): A phenomenological study.* Academic Press.

Liong, A. S. (2008). Descriptions of nurses experiences with electronic health records (EHR): A phenomenological study. *Proquest Dissertations and Theses,* 1-2.

Lorenzi, N., & Riley, R. (2004). *Managing technological change: organizational aspects*. New York: Springer. doi:10.1007/978-1-4757-4116-2

Maerten, E. (2009). Study of the first woman president hired by a board of regents in Oklahoma president Emerita of Southwestern Oklahoma state university Dr. Joe Anna Hibler. *ProQuest Dissertations and Theses*, 65-66.

Mallet, R. K. (2014). The influence of organizational subculture on information technology project success in the healthcare sector: A qualitative, multi-case study. *Proquest Dissertations and Theses*, 57.

Mann, C. (2013). Experience of adjunct novice clinical nursing faculty: An interpretive case study. *Proquest Dissertations and Theses*, 88-89.

Melesse, M. (2010). Gender, equity and access to health care: The Case of Ghana's Health Financing Reform. *ProQuest*, 11.

Miller, B. A. (2008). Exploring the use of information technology for enhancing interagency coordination. *Proguest*, 10.

Minor, M. O. (2009). What is the efficacy of using an integrated model in measuring sense of community (SOC) in accelerated degree completion programs? *Proquest Dissertations and Theses*, 8.

Monier, J. P. (2011). Community development in rural America: The power to exchange capital resources in Norton county, Kansas. *Proquest Dissertations and Theses*, 11.

Ngafeeson, M. N. (2013). Understanding user resistance to information technology: Toward a comprehensive model in health information technology. *Proquest Dissertations and Theses*, 113.

Noble, E. (2012). The role mentoring plays in a white female novice teacher's perceptions of her enculturation into a culturally diverse campus. *ProQuest Dissertations and Theses*, 11-12.

Noseworthy, J. (2012). A solitary journey: Interpretive description of women's experiences of perinatal loss in labour. *Proquest Dissertations and Theses*, 40.

Pack, J. (2011). Multiple intelligences and experiential learning styles: A mixed method study of registered nurses' attitudes toward computers and web-based learning. *Proquest*, 1.

Pagano, M. W. (2013). Toward improved security and privacy in modern healthcare. *Proquest Dissertations and Theses*, 10.

Perron, M. D. (2014). Residential substance abuse treatment experiences of baby boomers: A qualitative study. *Proquest Dissertations and Theses*, 6-51.

Perron, M. D. (2014). Residential substance abuse treatment experiences of baby boomers: A qualitative study. *Proquest Dissertations and Theses*, 6-39.

Peterson, L. A. (2006). Information technology use in nursing and nursing education as reported by beginning nurses. *Proquest Dissertations and Theses*, 2.

Peterson, L. A. (2006). Information technology use in nursing and nursing education as reported by beginning nurses. *Proquest*, 2.

Pisk, R. M. (2010). *Physician satisfaction and workflow intergration factors associated with electronic medical record implementation in a pediatric hospital.* Proquest.

Roberts, S. A. (2007). The impact of Information Technology on small, medium, and large hospitals: quality, safety and financial metrics. *Proquest Dissertations and Theses,* 14.

Roberts, S. A. (2007). The impact of Information Technology on small, medium, and large hospitals: quality, safety and financial metrics. *Proquest,* 14.

Rogers, E. M. (1983). *Diffusion of innovations.* New York: Free Press.

Royce, M. (2008). A step beyond inclusion: A case study of what one principle did to improve achievement for students with disabilities. *Proquest Dissertations and Theses,* 63-69.

Sondheimer, N., Katsh, E., Clarke, L., Osterweil, L., & Rainey, D. (2009). *Dispute prevention and dispute resolution in networked.* Academic Press.

Spoelstra, S. (2006). Asking the question: What is organization? *Proquest Dissertations and Theses,* 18.

Thompson, C. D. (2014). Benefits and risks of electronic medical record (EMR): An interpretive analysis of Healthcare consumers' perceptions of an evolving health information systems technology. *Proquest Dissertations and Theses,* 43.

Tian, R. (2013). Effect of work complexity and individual differences on nursing IT utilization. *Proquest Dissertations and Theses,* 19.

Tonge, S. I. (2014). Exploring juvenile delinquency and the justice system: Social workers' perspective. *Proquest Dissertations and Theses,* 55-57.

Tucker, M. T. (2009). Application of the Diffusion of Innovations theory and the health believe model to describe the EMR use among Alabama family medicine physicians: A rural and urban analysis. *Proquest Dissertations and Theses,* 29-34.

Vichianin, Y. (2007). *How to healthcare information and communication technology (HICT) interventions affect access to public sector healthcare delivery in a developing country? A case study of professionals' perception in saraburi province.* Thailand: ProQuest.

Weng, S.-J. (2008). A framework for efficient resource allocation in healthcare. *Proquest Dissertations and Theses,* 1.

Winzenreid, J. E. (2009). Exploring cultural norms and behaviors that define an ethical environment in charitable nonprofit organizations. *Proquest Dissertations and Theses,* 21.

Wu, S., Chaudhry, B., Wang, J., Maglione, M., Mojica, W., Roth, E., et al. (2006). *Systematic review: impact of health information technology on quality, efficiency, and costs of medical care.* Academic Press.

Xiao, N. (2012). Essay on the impact of health information technology on healthcare providers and patients. *ProQuest,* 1-2.

Yen-Han, L. (2013). Healthcare reform in mainland China: The relationship of healthcare reform and economic development in Chinese rural and urban areas. *ProQuest Dissertations and Theses,* 1.

KEY TERMS AND DEFINITIONS

Administrator: A secretary at the reception area of a hospital.

Healthcare Service Delivery: A duty carried out by health professionals at a hospital in meeting medical or health related needs of a patient or community.

Healthcare: A hospital that provides health related services to a community.

Hospital C: A pseudonym for a public hospital in Windhoek, Namibia. It is mainly a specialist hospital.

Hospital K: A pseudonym for a public hospital in Windhoek, Namibia. It is mainly a referral hospital.

Medical Practitioners: Qualified Nurses and Doctors.

MR-Number: Medical Registration number that a patient receives upon first time visit or admission to a hospital.

Chapter 12
RFID Applications in Healthcare–State–of–the–Art and Future Trends

Amir Manzoor
Bahria University, Pakistan

ABSTRACT

Implementation of RFID technology-based healthcare services is on the rise. The purpose of this chapter is a thorough, systematic review of the existing literature to provide a discussion of current trends and future directions in this domain. Findings indicate that tracking is the key RFID enabling function. Automatic data collection and transfer is an RFID function also frequently used in relation to assets, staff, and patients. Finally, RFID is employed for sensing, most often in relation to patients, but also to assets. The chapter concludes by highlighting future research directions where the deployment of RFID technology is likely to transform the healthcare sector.

INTRODUCTION

The healthcare industry is one of the largest sectors in many economies (Payton et al., 2011). Healthcare sector in USA created approximately 14.3 million jobs in 2008. This sector was expected to provide an additional 3.2 million jobs by 2018 (United-States-Department-of-Labor, 2010). At present, global healthcare sector is facing many challenges such as increasing operating costs, increasing number of medication errors, and ageing patient population. US healthcare expenses were expected to reach almost 20% of the GNP by 2017. That amounted to an increase of 15% in healthcare expenditure since 1963 (Middleton, 2009; Wurster et al., 2009). In Canada, healthcare expenses were expected to be almost 7.1% of the GNP by 2020, an increase of 1.1% since 2000 (Brimacombe et al., 2001). In Australia, healthcare expenses were estimated at 10% of the GNP (GS1-Australia, 2010). Each year, approximately 1.5 million Americans suffered from medication errors and these errors resulted in significant additional healthcare costs (National-Academy-of-Sciences, 2007). A study done in 2002 estimated that the population of people aged 85 and above in western countries would increase by 350% in 2020 (Wiener & Tilly, 2002). Another

DOI: 10.4018/978-1-4666-9446-0.ch012

study estimated that by 2050 the population of older Americans would increase by 135% (Newell, 2011). It is evident that there would be an increased pressure on healthcare expenditure, which will become more complicated given that, due to the economic crisis, several countries are facing critical challenges in providing healthcare services. Healthcare is a very different business due to various reasons. Patients are not typical consumers, they do not always make the decision as to when, and where they will seek which type of care and at what cost. Healthcare providers are not as autonomous as any other typical business could be. Various stakeholders, such as legislators, regulators, and payers often affect both clinical and business decisions of caregivers. For healthcare providers, efficiency is not merely good fiscal practice. It must be a critical component of their mission (Fosso Wamba, Anand, & Carter, 2013; Lefebvre, Castro, & Lefebvre, 2011). Healthcare sector today provides strong institutional powers and policies for an effective use of information technology (IT). Healthcare sector considers adoption and effective use of IT a critical goal of modern healthcare system to enable better support service delivery (Menachemi & Brooks, 2006; Payton et al., 2011). IT offer many opportunities for healthcare transformation through business process reengineering. Effective use of IT could provide minimized data-entry errors, real-time access to patient data, improved clinical trials, streamlined processes, increased transparency, reduced administrative overhead, creation of new high-tech healthcare markets and jobs and improved overall healthcare management of individuals (PCAST, 2010; Burkhard et al., 2010). The estimated potential safety savings from adoption and use of interoperable electronic medical records systems in USA was approximately US$142–371 billion (Sherer, 2010). RFID technology is considered the next IT innovation expected to expand healthcare transformation (Fosso Wamba et al., 2008; Ngai et al., 2009a,b; Oztekin et al., 2010a,b; Fosso Wamba, 2011). In order maximize efficiency and reduce waste, healthcare providers need to answer some tough questions such as what they have, where they have it, and where it needs to go. In order successfully track equipment and people, healthcare providers need a flexible and scalable system that provides automatic tracking with no dependency on clinical staff. One such system is RFID-bases system. All the capabilities enabled by RFID technology have the potential to facilitate new value creation in healthcare service innovation (Dominguez-Péry et al., 2011).

In short, RFID-enabled healthcare transformation projects could lead to tremendous benefits. These benefits include improved patient care, improved patient security, and safety, and improved organizational performance (Reyes et al., 2011). Use of RFID in healthcare can enable "new work practices to develop higher order capabilities for improving cost management, enhancing patient safety, and enabling regulatory compliance in hospital settings" (Lewis et al., 2009, p-8). The high operational and strategic potential of the RFID technology is effective in the healthcare market. The value of the RFID market rose from about $ 5.63 billion in 2010 to almost $ 5.84 billion in 2011(Das & Harrop, 2011). The global market turnover for RFID readers and RFID tags alone was expected to reach $8.9 billion by 2015 (MarketResearch.com, 2011). In 2011, almost 150 million RFID tags were in use in the healthcare supply chain (Pleshek, 2011). The sale of RFID tags and systems was expected to reach almost $ 1.43 billion in 2019, an increase of 51% from 2009. Such an increase is due to the widespread of RFID-enabled healthcare applications, including the item-level tagging of drugs and various medical disposables, real-time locating systems for healthcare staff, patients and assets for improved efficiency and reduced losses, the compliance with safety requirements, and the availability of assets (Harrop et al., 2009).

The objective of this chapter is to provide an overview of RFID applications in healthcare. This overview would serve as a foundation for healthcare professionals with limited knowledge of information and communication technologies (ICT) to determine further directions of how RFID can be employed to solve their problems.

STAKEHOLDERS, THEIR ISSUES, AND RFID SOLUTIONS

Key stakeholders of healthcare sector can fall into following some major categories. The first category includes those involved in healthcare program operations e.g. Management, program staff, partners, and funding agencies. The second category includes those served or affected by the healthcare programs e.g. patients or clients, advocacy groups, community members, and elected officials. Third category includes those who are intended users of the evaluation findings e.g. persons in a position to make decisions about the program, such as partners, funding agencies, and the general public or taxpayers.

Stakeholders of healthcare industry face many issues today. In USA alone, more than 500 patients per day are killed sue to errors, accidents and infections in hospitals. This number does not include the mortality and suffering from millions of procedures that never needed to be done in the first place. At the same time, the employers and other purchasers paying for this care are losing "patience" with the slow pace of change in cleaning up the mess (Binder, 2013).

Role of RFID in Healthcare

RFID uses radio waves to communicate between an RFID reader (also called RFID interrogator) and an electronic tag affixed to an object. RFID tags (active, passive, or semi-passive) are also called RFID chips or transponders. RFID tags can serve as a digital data store and each tag is encoded with a unique identifier that is tied to a database. Tags can be read using handheld or mobile readers, shelf or tabletop readers, or readers that can be installed at doorways. RFID readers communicate with the tags and retrieve the information to be sent to a host computer. This host computer acts as a RFID middleware and ensures communication between the RFID infrastructure and the different organizational systems (Asif & Mandviwalla, 2005). RFID operates without line-of-sight, provide dynamic item tracking to ensure patient safety, improved supply chain efficiency, improved overall safety, and operational efficiency. RFID systems greatly streamline inventory and asset tracking, virtually eliminating human error. Use of RFID systems provide detailed records of the movement of assets.

Issues and RFID Solutions

Following are some of the major issues faced by healthcare industry today and examples of various RFID solutions implemented by healthcare providers.

Asset Tracking and Management

Every hospital has high-value assets (such as wheel chairs, IV pumps, instruments, beds, etc.). If these devices move untraceable and we have no clear mechanism to determine their location, hospital staff can be unable to provide timely patient care. The turnover of these assets is essential for efficient operations of healthcare facility. While constant reporting on exact asset location is not required in all cases, but healthcare provider must be able to know the movement and have the ability to track where the asset goes. A wheel chair may cost around $150. However, it could cost $7,000 worth of clinical time per weak and up to 75% of maintenance time to search a wheel chair. To ensure effective performance of medical equipment regular, scheduled maintenance according to manufacturers' specifications is required. A typical hospital bed costs around $1200. Hospitals incur costs when no bed is available and patients spend extra time in an area that required heavy resources (such as ICU) (Motorola, 2013). Most healthcare providers could make their operations better by increasing efficiency, especially in managing vast supplies of medical equipment. It is estimated that on average 15% of a typical hospital's mobile assets are lost or stolen during their useful life. That translates to an average cost of approximately $3,000 per item (Motorola, 2013). RFID is a highly adaptable technology that can be used to track and better manage critical healthcare assets and patients by enabling real-time identification, tracking, and tracing (Symonds et al., 2007; Bendavid et al., 2010; Fisher & Monahan, 2008). Based on particular needs, RFID-based solutions can include any mix of handheld, mobile, or fixed position readers and RFID tags can be used for virtually any type of item or for people. RFID-based systems can be implemented and be incrementally expanded. RFID tags are widely available, affordable, and inexpensive compared with Real Time Location System (RTLS) tags. RFID technology is a viable mean of checking, tracking, and tracing pharmaceutical products. RFID allows proper management of incident audit trails between the medical equipment and the healthcare staff (Booth et al., 2006). RFID readers doesn't require a line of sight to capture data and their range can be adjusted and modified to meet specific environmental needs and RFID tag types. Since RFID readers are capable of simultaneously capturing the data of multiple assets, the time required to take inventory can be reduced drastically. The RFID readers can be installed at strategic location where there is extensive movement of critical assets to detect and record inventory of such assets. This enables the healthcare provider quickly locate the assets based on their last known location. This quick asset location provides many benefits. These benefits include improved patient care and staff productivity, faster patient and room turnover, improved incremental revenue, tighter asset control, lower replacement costs, reduced patient care delays, reduced capital expenditure, speedy equipment requests, faster equipment delivery, enhanced equipment flow processes, and resource planning. Using data collected using RFID, healthcare providers can easily comply with requirements of the regulatory bodies.

Purdue Pharma L.P., a US-based pharmaceutical company, implemented individual item RFID tagging on its prescription pain relief medicine bottles to follow the products' movements throughout the supply chain (Burt 2005 and Havenstein 2005). Siemens and Isar River University Hospital, Munich, Germany ran a project with RFID tagging of materials to test the use of active and passive RFID tags to track items used during surgery, and to track the surgical process itself to make sure item utilized during surgery are not inadvertently left behind inside a patient's body (Bacheldor, 2007o). The Royal Alexandra Hospital used a hospital-wide RFID asset tracking virtual asset library. The purpose of this library was to improve the use of assets, ensure the medical devices are available when needed, streamline routine scheduled maintenance, and reduce health and safety risks that could result if scheduled inspection plans are not met (Vilamovska et al., 2008; Britton, 2007). Southern Ohio Medical Center deployed a RFID-based asset tracking system to increase its efficiency of asset and equipment tracking. Medline Industries, a US distributor of medical supplies, marketed a RFID-based asset tracking system to detect any surgical asset left behind in patients after an operation. All surgical assets had RFID tags embedded. Hospital personnel passed a handheld wand containing an antenna connected to the RFID interrogator over the patient to pick up the RF signals of any tagged items left in the patient's body. (Sullivan, 2006). US-based Wayne Memorial Hospital deployed RFID technology for real-time asset location tracking and management. Hospital staff was able to keep track of the location and status of tagged assets (such as infusion pumps and wheel chairs) (Bacheldor 2007; RAND Corporation 2009). The UMass Memorial Medical Center (UMMC) in Massachusetts implemented RFID cabinets. These cabinets stored, tracked, and managed the utilization of high cost cardiac rhythm devices and supplies. UMMC was able to achieve approximately 38% reduction in inventory of selected high volume, high cost items (Collette and Johnson 2008). Ter Gooi Hospital employed Wi-Fi-based active RFID tags to track the location of infusion pumps and EKG machines (Wessel, 2007c). Benefits from the application included better use of staff time, improved efficiency, and more timely care (Bacheldor, 2007s). Trondheim Hospital deployed an RFID-based uniform-tracking system. The system provided real-time inventory visibility of uniforms. With this system, Trondheim Hospital was able to reduce the space and labor costs with increased inventory accuracy. Texi, a Norway-based solution provider, developed an RFID system for the hospital inventory management where the RFID tags sewn into the garments were read by RFID readers. These RFID readers were installed in inventory closets and bins for soiled garments. The system provided 90% savings in space costs and resulted in an estimated (US$ 6 million) in space saving (O'Connor, 2007d). Bon Secours Richmond Health System deployed a RFID enabled mobile asset management system to track and manage critical mobile medical equipment. This system was one of the largest RFID-based asset management system in USA (Vilamovska et al., 2008; Swedberg, 2008b; Harrop et al,2007).

Inventory Management

Healthcare providers need to know when various consumables are nearing re-order status, with minimal staff monitoring. Inefficiency also affects inventory management and hospitals often face issues of misplaced, out of stock or expired medical supplies. This happens because no definitive system exists to monitor inventory changes. When there exist high usage levels and access by multiple users, monitoring stock level is often ignored. This absence of monitoring results in inaccurate inventories and unnecessary rush orders to meet patient needs. Many hospitals typically overstock IV because it is a commonly used medical supply often lost or misplaced. This overstocking typically costs hospitals $150,000 per year (Motorola, 2013). Hospitals may overstock other consumables as well such as dressings and instruments. This overstocking could result in tying up an average of 30% of hospital's capital (Motorola, 2013). Multiple RFID tags can be read at once to provide constant monitoring of inventory in a drug or supply cabinet. This way healthcare provider can better manage purchasing, reduce excessive inventories, and reduce delays in patient care. Fixed RFID readers, installed at supply room doors, are able to automatically and continuously record the asset location as it moves from one place to another. Handheld RFID readers provide on-the-spot reading of RFID tags and can be used to count inventory or locate a specific asset that could be misplaced in the supply room. RFID readers are capable of simulataneously capturing data of hundreds of assets. These readers can issue alerts when preset critical levels of inventory are reached. As such, use of RFID tags significantly reduces the time required for taking inventory of all assets in areas such as patient rooms, labs, procedure areas and stockrooms. Another benefit of the real-time, updated, and accurate inventory is to avoid out-of-stock situations for critical supplies needed for patients that would otherwise require rush orders at premium prices. With RFID reader and tagged supplies, items can be automatically dispensed and charged to the patients for proper billing, reduced lost and stolen supplies, reduced replacement costs, and increased revenue by eliminating non-charged consumables. Alerts can be issued to purchasers for expiring products to get timely re-orders.

DePuy Orthopedics, Inc., is a designer, manufacturer, and distributor of orthopedic devices and supplies. DePuy implemented RFID to track kits of critical operating room products shipped to sales agents and hospitals. Each kit and each part had an RFID tag attached. The system provided improved operational efficiency and labor productivity, time reduction in per-kit processing time and 99.99% read accuracy (ODIN 2008).

Time Management

Clinical time with patients is a critical resource for hospitals and many a times clinical staff spends too much time on non-patient care activities. Hospital nurses could spend an average of 20% of their time simply searching for portable medical equipment (Motorola, 2013).

Patient Tracking

Even with carefully designed plans of patient tracking, mistakes can happen. About 100 babies are switched at birth in U.S. hospitals every year (Motorola, 2013). Many patients need to walk around the facility as part of the recovery process. Many patients are vulnerable (such as people with mental disorders) and such hospitals need to restrict their movement. Practical solutions are required to balance patient freedom with patient safety. Errors in patient identification can lead to medication errors, delay in patient care, and lost valuable clinical time. One solution is RFID tagged wristbands. Patients wear these wristbands to enable positive patient identification (PPID). With positive patient identification, medication and treatment errors are reduced and patient movement can be recorded unobtrusively as they move around the facility. RFID readers are installed at key places to automatically record movement of patients and alerts can be issues to hospital staff in case vulnerable patients leave the designated areas.

Ospedale Treviglio-Caravaggio, an Italy-based hospital, implemented RFID to track admitted patients as they are admitted. Typically, when new patients arrived and admitted, the hospital followed a series of procedures for diagnosis or therapy. The patients were moved from one medical service area to another. This movement was difficult due to the dynamic nature of the system. For example, if x-ray procedure took long time, patients were taken for another procedure. Use of RFID allowed hospital administration to track the location of those patients or the procedures they had undergone (Swedberg, 2008a). Birmingham Heartlands Hospital used RFID-enabled wristbands to track patients and procedures, identify patients, and decrease incidents harmful to patients. (Bacheldor, 2007r). Xtag developed a RFID- based baby tagging system for safety and security. The system could also be used to track wandering patients in elder care facilities. The babies and elder patients wore an RFID bracelet with an embedded battery-powered RFID tag. The Xtag system offered one of the most secure protection system for the prevention of abduction attempts on the market in the world. The RFID tag was tamper proof and generated an alarm if the strap is cut, the tag is slipped of the ankle, the tag is removed underwater while bathing, or if the tag is disguised or damaged. RFID readers were designed to work with existing access control systems and picked up the signal and transmitted location data to the system (Maselli, 2003). ProSolutions, a Canadian firm specializing in RFID systems and integration, developed a RFID-based system (called BlueTag system) that protected newborn babies, Alzheimer's patients, and other individuals staying in hospital. The BlueTag system leveraged active ultrahigh-frequency (UHF) RFID tags embedded in bracelets and is used in 50 maternity wards in 10 countries around the world. (Bacheldor, 2008a).

Healthcare IT Asset Management

Since typical IT equipment in healthcare environments is mobile, the inventory management can be time-consuming and misplaced or stolen equipment can increase costs because hospitals incur costs of hardware and staff costs of searching and re-deploying. There exist very stringent regulatory requirements related to security and control of financial and clinical records. The loss of medical equipment can also result in loss of data and consequently provide severe regulatory implications. Handheld RFID readers can provide a quick and efficient mean for hospital staff to track and manage inventory of equipment. Fixed RFID readers, installed at strategic and high-traffic locations can help keep track of important equipment (such as laptops and workstations on wheels (WOWs)) containing sensitive information.

RFID enable IT asset management provides faster service, improved security, accounting, and helps ensure and demonstrate compliance with HIPAA regulations regarding data security. With an up-to-date and accurate database of assets, hospitals can easily deploy the required upgrades and security updates on the assets. Any interruption in work (due to missing items or data) and time required to take inventory of assets can be effectively optimized.

File and Data Tracking

Healthcare regulatory requirements to safeguard patient records against loss or unauthorized access (e.g. by visitors, patients and other non-hospital personnel) are stringent and apply to both paper and digital records. There exist a variety of documents and data files that constitute patient records. These documents and data files may include charts, physician and pharmacy orders, and laboratory reports and imaging files. The dilemma here is that these documents must be circulated to be useful. RFID-based security solutions can be deployed to provide limited but secure clinical access on an as-needed basis to patient records while racking access. Handheld RFID readers can be used to locate a misfiled RFID-enabled files and folders minimizing the staff time needed to search for documents. Fixed RFID readers can track the movement of these files and folders around the facility. This feature could also help in forensic investigation. RFID technology is hard to counterfeit and provides greater security for sensitive financial and clinical patient-related information.

Huntsville Hospital used a RFID solution to verify a patient's identity and document the surgical process, from admission to discharge. Passive RFID tags were attached with patients. The objective of the system was to improve efficiency and communication that would directly improve surgical start times (Bacheldor, 2007k). The Emergency Health Centre (EHC) in Houston, Texas deployed a real-time RFID-based location tracking system to improve its patient care. On admission, patients wore RFID-enabled wristbands. These wristbands were tracked by RFID readers to record how much time patients spent to receive the needed medical care. Hospital staff received alerts from the system when beds and rooms were clean and ready for occupation. Emergency medical information service provider MedicAlert Foundation and California State University-Stanislaus (CSU) tested RFID-enabled medical cards to provide a more efficient method of collecting and forwarding patients' health-related data at the point of medical service (Swedberg 2007c).

A number of RFID-related software applications were developed in Taiwan. Some of these applications focused on the use of radio frequency identification (RFID) technology to prevent spread of the severe acute respiratory syndrome (SARS) disease. These applications include computerized systems for monitoring the body temperature of healthcare personnel and patients in the hospital, track potential virus carriers and, when necessary, map their movements throughout hospitals and keeping track of people under quarantine in facilities separate from hospitals (Ioan, Turcu, Turcu, & Cerlinc, 2010).

Anti-Counterfeiting

Drug counterfeiting is an increasing global problem that results in patient's loss of money. Patients not only get inferior, non-economical products but also face significant health threats because these drugs contain dangerous substances. Pharmaceutical companies lose financially due to counterfeit drug trade and governments lose in terms of lost taxes and resources spent to combat counterfeiting. Worldwide counterfeit sales are increasing at about 13 percent annually, which is twice the rate of legitimate pharmaceuticals sales. Counterfeit sales were expected to reach $75 billion mark by 2010 (National Association of Boards of Pharmacy, 2009). RFID technology can help pharmaceutical companies, distributors, and hospitals to combat and deter drug counterfeiting. Counterfeit pharmaceutical products are a major threat to patient safety today. This is because these products may contain hazardous ingredients (Fuhrer &Guinard, 2006) and they may cause important financial losses to pharmaceutical firms (Dahiya, 2008). According to some estimates, almost 10% of pharmaceutical products marketed worldwide in 2010 were counterfeit (Lefebvre et al., 2011) and resulted in about US$ 75 billion in financial losses by the pharmaceutical industry (Dahiya, 2008). In this context, major US regulatory bodies (e.g., Food and Drug Administration) have issued adoption mandates. These mandates require pharmaceutical firms to adopt a unique identifier (or e-Pedigree) for the tracking and tracing of pharmaceutical products throughout the supply chain. These actions have caused a renewed interest in the adoption and use of RFID technology in healthcare sector. Some studies have even suggested that "RFID is an enabling technology that saves lives, prevents errors, saves costs and increases security. It removes tedious procedures and provides patients with more freedom and dignity" (IDTechEx, 2006, p-1).

Patient Care

RFID technology offers an improved means of reducing errors in patient care, including adverse drug effects, allergies, patient–medication mismatches and medication dosage errors (Thuemmler et al., 2007; Tu et al., 2009; Aspden, Wolcott, Bootman, & Cronenwett, 2007). RFID technology can enable healthcare stakeholders to monitor all steps related to the patient blood collection and transfusion process, including the identification of blood bags at the collection point, the tracking and tracing of products from the collection point to the healthcare facility, and blood transfusion to a dedicated patient (Najera et al.,2011). Also, this technology makes it easier to manage patients with chronic conditions (Cresswell & Sheikh, 2008; Michael et al., 2008).

A hospital in Saarbrücken, Germany, used radio frequency technology to track bags of blood to record transfusions and ensure that patients get blood intended specifically for them. This RFID solution added significant security so the hospital can make sure the correct blood product is given to each patient (Wessel, 2006b). Italy's National Cancer Institute in Milan and Ospedale Maggiore hospital in Bologna used RFID technology to increase efficiency and safety in the management of the transfusion process. RFID tags were placed on blood bags and patient wristbands and staffs used handheld computers to register patients upon arrival, verify patient-blood group, and recognize patients and transfusion units at any time (Sini et al, 2008; Wessel, 2006h). Amsterdam Medical Centre used RFID to track and trace medical equipment, monitor the movements of patients and staff, and track and trace blood products. The goal of using RFID was to optimize schedules so more patients could be treated. A RFID-based system was deployed by St Vincent's Hospital, Alabama to provide patient-tracking and real-time clinical information. The system resulted in improved quality of patient care and increased revenues (Bacheldor, 2007e; Gambon, 2006). A concept developed by New Jersey orthopaedic surgeon Lee Berger, the noninvasive Ortho-Tag uses radio-frequency identification (RFID) technology designed at University of Pittsburgh to give physicians easy access to information about implants and patients often at the end of a long paper trail (Swedberg, 2008c). Arthur Koblasz developed a body-worn RFID tag. The body-worn RFID tags may include an upper body RFID tag located in a wrist band and a lower body RFID tag located in a sock worn by the monitored person. The RFID instrumentation located in the premises may include one or more antennas located in the floor, door, bed frame, and mattress. The systems may also activate response actions upon detecting specified movements, such as sending an alert message to a patient monitoring system, activating an alarm, activating a camera, and/or playing a recorded message to the person. The purpose was to prevent or detect specific types of movements of the person, such as falls from which the person has not recovered (Koblasz, 2007). The International Medical Centre of Japan implemented a Point of Act System (POAS) to provide real-time input at the point of action. POAS. POAS collected, managed and used consumption data at the point of care (e.g. hospital bed). POAS (Akyama, 2007).

Medication Error Reduction/Medication Compliance

According to National Coordinating Council for Medication Error Reporting and Prevention, a medication error is any preventable event that may cause or lead to inappropriate medication use or patient harm while the medication is in the control of the health care professional, patient, or consumer. Such events may be related to professional practice, health care products, procedures, and systems, including prescribing, order communication, product labeling, packaging, and nomenclature, compounding, dispensing, distribution, administration, education, monitoring, and use. RFID can play an important role in reducing these errors.

Germany's Jena University Hospital, the largest hospital in the German Federal State of Thuringia, used passive RFID tags to track medication in real-time from the hospital's pharmacy to intensive care and individual patients. Patients wore an RFID bracelet used for digital matching of medication to the individual patient. Handheld scanners read these bracelets and nurses gained instant access to detailed patient information displayed on a screen. The aim of using RFID was to reduce medication errors and improve workflow (Wessel, 2006c, 2007a). Jacobi Medical Center in New York used handheld computers match the RFID tags on patients' wrists with bar-coded information on packets of medication to minimize medication errors and provide patients only the medication that has been prescribed to him or her. This system saved nurses time and allowed the nurse more time for direct patient care (Crounse, 2005). Medixine is a Finnish company that specializes in disease management. Medixine developed a system using RFID and mobile phones to make sure Alzheimer's patients take their medication (Collins, 2004). A European trial, sponsored by Novartis and conducted by ECCT, an Eindhoven-based provider of medical consumer electronic devices, used battery-powered RFID tags embedded within medication blister packs. The trail showed that monitoring patients' compliance with medication prescriptions can help them comply with their medication schedule—thereby improving the benefits of taking the drug (Collins, 2006d). A groups of pharmaceutical companies including Merck and Novartis used RFID tags, along with a range of bar code technologies, on individual items to detect dispensing errors and counterfeit drugs before they reached patients (Collins, 2004b). St. Clair Hospital, Pittsburgh, implemented a bar code software system to eliminate medication-dispensing errors (Swedberg, 2005).

Workflow Improvement

Memorial Medical Center in Long Beach, California implemented a RFID-based people/asset tracking system to improve the operations of its emergency department (Cross, 2006). The new system provided extensive data about emergency department use and patients trends and played key role in the quality improvement initiatives led by the hospital to reduce patients waiting time. This system also provided increased patient safety, better use of staff time, and increased facility capacity (Vilamovska et al., 2008).

US-based Providence Health Center implemented a RFID-based real-time locating system to track patients, staff, and equipment. The objective of the system was to improve its patient and operational processes and tracking of medical devices. RF signals emitted from active RF tags attached with patients/staff/equipment were received by RFID readers. These readers were typically mounted on the walls (Bacheldor, 2007j). Using a grant from Robert Wood Johnson Foundation, Shelby County Regional Medical Center in Memphis, Tennessee deployed a RFID-based patient tracking system to better manage its overcrowded emergency department. As a result, the typical patient stay time in trauma unit increased from 25% to 80% (Gearon, 2005b).

COSTS OF HEALTHCARE RFID IMPLEMENTATION

The cost of the RFID technology (tags, readers, middleware, consulting, process design, troubleshooting, training, etc.) will impact return on investment (ROI) and value of RFID implementation. Direct RFID costs include the costs of RFID tags, RFID infrastructure, and RFID middleware. These direct costs are one key barrier to widespread adoption of healthcare RFID. According to Page (2007), the cost of RFID infrastructure can run from $200,000 to $600,000 or more for a facility-wide RFID tracking system in a medium-sized hospital. Davis (2004) reports that the costs for an RFID system can run from $20,000 to over $1 million depending on the size of the area where the technology is deployed and the application. According to Harrop et al., (2008), the prices of RFID tags will fall substantially in the near future. We can also make similar assumptions about prices of RFID infrastructure and middleware. One way to reduced RFID costs is by substituting RFID-designated reader networks with an existing Wi-Fi network (at the cost of worse granularity and network overload), or by using handheld devices at all times (leading to loss of user-friendliness).

ISSUES OF HEALTHCARE RFID IMPLEMENTATION

There exist many important barriers to wider-scale RFID implementation in healthcare (Ting, Kwok, Tsang, & Lee, 2011; Lefebvre, Castro, & Lefebvre, 2011; Fosso Wamba, Anand, & Carter, 2013; Middleton, 2009; Buyurgan, Landry, & Philippe, 2013; Garfinkel & Rosenberg, 2006; Wamba, 2012; Ting, Kwok, Tsang, & Lee, 2011; Cheng & Chai, 2012; Yao, Chu, & Li, 2010).

Privacy, Security, Data Integrity, and Legal Issues

Healthcare RFID implementation raise many issues pertaining to the protection of the privacy, security, integrity, legal issues, and ownership of the data collected through RFID applications. Within and across healthcare sectors, these issues are not addressed either fully or consistently. Benefits of using RFID in healthcare can be achieved when patients feel confident about security and privacy of the data being transmitted, security of technology, and the related policies (Sotto, 2008). According to Sotto (2008), there can be four categories of privacy concerns with respect to the use healthcare RFID. These concerns include the inappropriate collection of health information through RFID technology, the intentional misuse, or unauthorized disclosure of the data by an authorized data holder, the intentional interception of the transmitted/stored in RFID applications information and its subsequent misuse by unauthorized parties, and the unauthorized alteration of the data kept by an RFID application. To resolve the first issue, patients can be allowed to opt out of RFID systems, and by not using RFID chip to store any medical data on the RFID chip. Such data should instead be stored in a secure server in compliance with the Health Insurance Portability and Accountability Act (HIPAA) (Hagland, 2005). Encryption and authentication techniques can be used to address third issue. Halamka et al. (2006) suggests that RFID chips should serve exclusively for identification, and not authentication or access control.

RFID tags are susceptible to many of the same data security concerns associated with any wireless device. Passive tags in particular are considered to be *promiscuous* (automatically yielding their data to any device that queries the tag. This characteristic of tags raise concerns about skimming, interception, interference, hacking, cloning, and fraud, with potentially profound implications for privacy. While a variety of security defenses exist, such as shielding, tag encryption, reader authentication, role-based access control, and the addition of passwords, these solutions can raise complexity and costs. If RFID tags contain personal information, which could include health information, or data linked to personally identifiable individuals, without the proper security or integrity mechanisms in place, privacy interests become engaged. Personal health information is among the most sensitive types of information. As such, it requires stronger justifications for its collection, use and disclosure, rigorous protections against theft, loss and unauthorized use and disclosure, strong security around retention, transfer, and disposal, and stronger, more accountable governance mechanisms (Cavoukian, 2008).

Technical Issues

There exist many technical issues related to RFID implementation. Some of these issues include the reliability and interoperability of RFID technologies, non-interference of RFID technology with other clinical information systems, and lack of RFID industry standards and best practices. This lack of standardization can also cause interoperability issues for RFID solutions offered by various providers. Practice of non-complying their RFID solutions with current medical regulations (HIPAA) is another barrier to RFID implementation (Fisher & Monahan, 2008). Vendors also do not normally tailor systems to specific healthcare provider needs and that could lead to maladaptation of technology. According to Fisher and Monahan (2008), limited standards also limit interoperability between RFID and existing systems in hospital. To solve these issues, European Union (EU) in 2007 adopted formally an ultra-wideband (UWB) frequency range for RFID healthcare application use in EU member countries. A significant implication of this decision was that RFID solution providers using UWB will need to alter their solutions to meet several new frequency limitations.

Operational/Managerial Issues

There exist a large number of operational/managerial issues related to healthcare RFID implementation. These issues include lack of guaranteed return on investment (ROI), lack of standardization in the risk calculations for identical RFID applications, difficulties in choosing the optimal mix of RFID technologies, lack of RFID best practices, implementation costs, implementation uncertainties, integration of the RFID systems into the existing IT systems, uncertain maintenance costs, and the limited availability of integrated RFID solutions. ROI of RFID implementation may not be guaranteed due to wide variability of RFID technologies and of settings within which they are deployed. Implementation costs and uncertainties are also due to the relatively little experience with healthcare RFID implementation (Anand & Wamba, 2013; Buyurgan, Landry, & Philippe, 2013). Lack of RFID best practices is because RFID technology is still relatively a young technology. Some other challenges to RFID implementation include building RFID infrastructure and bundling applications within hospital (Hagland, 2005). According to Dempsey (2005), hospitals also need to understand that there exist different types of RFID and each type has a different place in healthcare. Dempsey (2005) further suggests that RFID implementation can result in various organizational challenges and change in organizational processes.

Cultural and Ethical Issues

These issues include concerns about the surveillance potential of RFID, lack of understanding of the privacy and security threats associated with healthcare RFID, ethical, cultural, and social perceptions about RFID and its functions, and lack of potential patient acceptance due to the factors listed above (Wurster, Lichtenstein, & Hogeboom, 2008). According to Fisher and Monahan (2008), a closer examination is required of the social and organizational factors that contribute to the success or failure of RFID systems. The results of this examination should be intertwined in the preparatory work for RFID deployment. Expanding capability of interoperable RFID technology is increasing fear of potential privacy threats (Fisher and Monahan 2008). RFID implementation in healthcare has received much attention from those in healthcare community concerned about patient privacy. Boulard (2005) and O'Connor (2005c) argues that true threats of RFID implementation related to personal data security and privacy have largely been misunderstood. These misunderstandings have resulted in many anti-RFID movements (Albrecht, 2007) and lobbying initiatives concerned with fear of surveillance threats (Boulard, 2005).

This lack of understanding of the real threats and benefits of healthcare RFID implementation can have sever implications for realization of true potential of RFID in improving the safety and quality of healthcare. This issue could become more serious if widespread awareness of RFID among consumers is not developed in near future. By 2009, only 18% Europeans were aware of RFID (Slettemeås, 2009). This implies that these issues can be harder to overcome among older populations. The acceptance of RFID by these older populations is key for the success of any healthcare RFID solution. National and global legislation, that addresses the privacy and legal issues, can help achieve this acceptance.

PRACTICAL/MANAGERIAL IMPLICATIONS AND RECOMMENDATIONS

Knowing the current state of operation is half the battle in improving it. Real-time information, collected, stored, and analyzed, provides the foundation from which healthcare professionals can glean the sort of business intelligence that can optimize workflow, improve utilization of valuable resources, and improve patient care and their outcomes. Data from RFID sensors provides capabilities to trigger event notifications, provide situational awareness regarding participant status in a workflow, track and manage assets, and even track and contain disease outbreaks. RFID data from multiple systems can be integrated and streamed in real-time into multiple clinical and administrative databases, and Big Data analysis tools can then be applied to dig deeper meaning from the relationships between seemingly disparate data types.

Healthcare providers can benefit from every extra minute saved. RFID tags worn on healthcare professionals ID badges and RFID tags on various assets create a perspective of action and location over time. This gives healthcare providers an objective look at how they're moving their assets/personnel through the hospital and how much time healthcare personals are actually spending with patients versus walking around trying to find needed information and equipment. Adjustments to design or process as a result of this knowledge may help staff feel less pressured as they move through their day, leaving them more capacity to focus on care and minimizing mistakes.

When compared to similar Automatic Identification and Data Capture (AIDC) technologies (e.g., bar-coding),RFID technology presents a vast range of advantages including: a unique item/product level identification, no need for line of sight, multiple tags reading, more data storage capability and data read/write capabilities (Asif & Mandviwalla, 2005). However, the high implementation costs of the technology remains a major inhibitor for its widespread adoption and use, as well as the substantial gap between the technology implementation costs and the RFID-enabled benefits (Bensel et al., 2008). Furthermore, the lack of common standard and the low operational performance level of RFID in a harsh environment continue to hamper its adoption.

There are many ways in which RFID solutions provide a justifiable return on investment, including productivity gains from automated workflow, better staffing-to-demand ratio, lower instances of HAIs, reduced staffing turnover and better protection against damages due to improved risk management. One of the most impactful areas may be increasing Medicare reimbursements for care based on patient survey results. This serves as a major incentive for hospitals to do all they can to ensure patients are not only objectively well cared for, but that they are aware of the quality of their care, feel positively about their experience and report as such. RFID tracking and monitoring provides an unbiased baseline by which providers can measure their performance and make timely improvements, and also serves as evidence of the quality of care provided. It is a transparent model that proves to patients that providers take their perceptions seriously, and aim to excel. It is also a reminder that they must be authentic in their reporting of the care they received. The practical balance of providing quality care efficiently has real impacts on the success of a healthcare organization, but so too does the patient perception of the quality of care.

Legacy information systems may need to be modified to accommodate the RFID system, technology, and information. Depending on the operating environment, the intended purposes, the technology contemplated, and the deployment method being considered, RFID technologies may not deliver sufficient accuracy or performance results to be suitable for mission-critical applications and uses. RFID systems are information systems that automatically capture, transmit and process identifiable information. Informational privacy involves the right of individuals to exercise control over the collection, use, retention and disclosure of personally identifiable information by others. RFID systems inherently poses privacy issues (Garfinkel & Rosenberg, 2006) and warrant a holistic systems approach to privacy. RFID tags contain unique identifiers. RFID tag data can be read at a distance, without line-of-sight even without consent of the individual who may be carrying the tag. This has compelling implications for informed consent. RFID information systems can also capture time and location data, upon which item histories and profiles can be constructed, making accountability for data use critical. Healthcare providers need to know what data is collected, how and for what purposes, where it is stored, how it is used, with whom it is shared or potentially disclosed, under what conditions, and so forth. There are inherent tensions between the, at times, competing interests of organizations and individuals over the disposition of the personal health information, especially over the undisclosed or unauthorized revelation of facts about individuals and the negative effects they may experience as a consequence. RFID information technologies can exacerbate a power imbalance between the individual and the collecting organization (Cavoukian, 2008).

Literature identifies many enablers for healthcare RFID implementation (Payton, Pare, Le Rouge, & Reddy, 2011; Cao, Baker, Wetherbe, & Gu, 2012; Wamba, 2012; Mehrjerdi, 2010; Wilkerson & McDonald Jr, 2007; Motorola, 2013; Newell, 2011; Ajami & Carter, 2013; Yao, Chu, & Li, 2010).

The primary enabler for the use of RFID in healthcare delivery is the improvement in the quality of care. This quality of care is associated with implementation and capabilities of RFID. The improvement in the quality of care can be in terms of process control and capacity to support modern medicine practices, reduction of harmful incidents, improved resource use, delivery of safe, fast and unambiguous identification, and the creation of an operationally integrated hospital information system. Some short-term advantages of healthcare RFID include distant patient management (at home), biometric data collection, and telemetry and intelligent outpatient care. Given the increasing number of older people in many parts of the world including Europe, these benefits can be promising. RFID is also more efficient as compared to alternative solutions.

Use of RFID allows healthcare providers, analysts and researchers to identify a clear business case for specific RFID solutions that meet their needs best. For example, documentary evidence exists that shows good ROI of RFID inventory and asset management applications. Similarly, evidence shows clear benefit of installing real-time location systems for staff, patients and assets within healthcare facilities (Brimacombe, Antunes, & McIntyre, 2001). According to Murphy (2006), real-time RFID systems can provide clinical timesaving of up to two days a week. There are other uses of RFID (such as RFID-supported haemovigilance systems) that help provide positive, correct, patient-procedure and patient medication. All of these lead to improved patient care and bring direct (monetary) and indirect (e.g. reduced liability and additional treatment costs) benefits for healthcare providers. The falling RFID tag prices and vendor initiative for creating interoperable, cost-effective solutions are some other reasons that provide strong case for RFID adoption.

Healthcare is a complex system and as such the key to success of RFID implementation is the process of implementation. One reason for this is that the healthcare RFID is a relatively young and still developing technology. In its current state, RFID lacks established best practices and involve multiple technology that differ significantly in their functionality and purpose. Staged implementation is often recommended in case of RFID implementation. A staged implementation involves a well-planned and successful pilot, understanding of various RFID implementation-related issues (such as costs, types of tags, system operation, mix of technologies to be used, understanding of business processes, stakeholders analysis, support from top management, vendor selection, and staff training) (Murphy, 2006).

RFID is technically superior to alternative technologies and provide many significant benefits such as real-time data availability, ability to store more data, security of data using encryption, and user-friendliness.

Governments are involved at both national and international level to support healthcare RFID implementation. Governments provide various incentives (such as promulgation of explicit patient safety standards for healthcare RFID applications, the adoption of quality standards in national healthcare systems, and financial incentives for healthcare RFID adoption by healthcare providers (Motorola, 2013).

In the world of healthcare, "the more you know, the better." RFID applications, partnered with data evaluation technology, are a powerful tool in establishing a standard of applied awareness. Hospitals can derive a competitive advantage from this awareness that can dramatically change the way healthcare is deployed and managed to optimize hospital operations and patient outcomes.

FUTURE RESEARCH DIRECTIONS

There is plethora of opportunities for future research in this area. Prior research on IT-enabled firm performance suggests that the role and articulation of 'the underlying mechanisms' through which IT capabilities improve firm performance remain unclear" (Mithas et al., 2011, p-238). How the management of these new RFID-enabled healthcare capabilities should be realized to enhance healthcare performance? This area needs further research.

Fosso Wamba and Chatfield (2009) found that business value creation and realization from RFID projects was dependent on many contingency factors such as strong leadership, second-order organizational learning, resources commitment, and organizational transformation. Whether these factors are still relevant and the degree to which they still exist in healthcare sector today is a question that needs further research. This question is important given the fact that the context of the healthcare sector today provides high level of complexity (LeRouge et al., 2007). Another area that needs further investigation is technological, organizational and environmental factors that may have an impact on the adoption and use of RFID-enabled healthcare applications by applying current dominant IS adoption theories (Fichman, 2000).

One of the key challenges of the healthcare sector is the difficulty of measuring the exact healthcare delivery costs to each patient, which allows a comparison of the costs with the outcomes (Kaplan & Porter, 2011). In this context, an area that needs future investigation is the assessment the business value of RFID-enabled item level tagging to evaluate its impact on the healthcare outcome and costs. Furthermore, to understand the influence of different healthcare stakeholders on their peers, it would be interesting to examine the business value from the co-adoption of RFID technology and other healthcare ISs (e.g., ERP, electronic medical records (EMR) systems etc.). Prior studies on IT adoption (Riggins & Mukhopadhyay, 1994) show a positive correlation between the level of business process reengineering and the use of and value gained from Its (Fosso Wamba & Chatfield, 2009). Therefore, additional research is needed to empirically investigate how to reengineer healthcare-related processes (patient, asset and staff) to achieve higher levels of business value from RFID-enabled healthcare projects.

Future research should also look at better strategies to incorporate RFID into healthcare processes and operations. Future studies need for example to identify the scope of the RFID-enabled healthcare project, then assess the potential impact of the technology in terms of incremental and/or process transformation. This assessment should also include the cascade effect that can be created by applying RFID at certain parts of the organization and/or operations. Developing a holistic performance measurement and management system to assess the value generated by RFID-enabled healthcare operations should be also included into future research.

CONCLUSION

This chapter presented a comprehensive overview of RFID technology adoption in the healthcare Industry including RFID applications and issues in the healthcare. More specifically, the chapter provided several examples of real-world RFID applications in the healthcare sector to illustrate emerging trends, and how various factors are influencing benefits creation from RFID technology in the healthcare sector.

This chapter also posits that the realization of the full business benefits from RFID-enabled healthcare applications will depend on many enablers namely better healthcare delivery, clear business case for certain RFID applications, smart implementation, technological superiority of RFID applications, and government incentives/support. The chapter also highlighted several avenues for future research on healthcare RFID. It can be said that there is a need for more healthcare RFID research. Also, given the sensitive nature of medical information, there is a need for more research on data management, security and privacy issues.

This chapter contributes to our understanding of RFID implementation in healthcare sector and its contribution to the efficiency of healthcare sector. The chapter also indicates that the policy makers should be aware of the opportunity to use RFID in healthcare and their policies and strategies should be formulated accordingly. Furthermore, effective use of RFID require various enablers, most important of which is the government support to use of RFID in healthcare. Furthermore, the ethical/cultural issues related to RFID implementation require close collaboration among RFID products manufactures and healthcare providers.

REFERENCES

Ajami, S., & Carter, M. W. (2013). *The advantages and disadvantages of Radio Frequency Identification (RFID) in Health-care Centers; approach in Emergency Room (ER)*. Academic Press.

Anand, A., & Wamba, S. F. (2013). Business value of RFID-enabled healthcare transformation projects. *Business Process Management Journal, 19*(1), 111–145. doi:10.1108/14637151311294895

Asif, Z., & Mandviwalla, M. (2005). Integrating the supply chain with RFID: A tech-nical and business analysis. *Communications of the Association for Information Systems, 15*, 393–427.

Aspden, P., Wolcott, J., Bootman, J. L., & Cronenwett, L. R. (2007). *Preventing medication errors*. National Academies Press.

Bacheldor, B. (2006, May 8). Report Sees Sharp Rise in Pharma RFID. *RFID Journal.*

Bacheldor, B. (2007a, October 29). Denver Health Adopting a Hospital-Wide RTLS System. *RFID Journal.*

Bacheldor, B. (2007b, October 9). Health Facility Uses RTLS to Provide 'Concierge' Care. *RFID Journal.*

Bacheldor, B. (2007c, April 23). Pharma RFID Adoption Still Slow. *RFID Journal.*

Bacheldor, B. (2007d, April 24). Siemens Launches RFID Pilot to Track Surgical Sponges, Procedures. *RFID Journal.*

Bacheldor, B. (2007e, April 10). Tags Track Surgical Patients at Birmingham Heartlands Hospital. *RFID Journal.*

Bacheldor, B. (2007f, December 12). Tergooi Hospital Uses RFID to Boost Efficiency. *RFID Journal.*

Bacheldor, B. (2008, February 13). BlueTag Patient-Tracking Comes to North America. *RFID Journal.*

Bendavid, Y., Boeck, H., & Philippe, R. (2010). Redesigning the replenishment process of medical supplies in hospitals with RFID. *Business Process Management Journal, 16*(6), 991–1013. doi:10.1108/14637151011093035

Bensel, P., & Gunther, O. et al.. (2008). Cost–benefit sharing in cross-company RFID applications: A case study approach. In *29th International Conference on Information Systems (ICIS)* (pp. 1–17). Paris, France.

Booth, P., Frisch, P. H., ... (2006). Application of RFID in an integrated healthcare environment. In *Conference proceedings: Annual international conference of the IEEE Engineering in Medicine and Biology Society.* IEEE Engineering in Medicine and Biology Society. doi:10.1109/IEMBS.2006.259389

Boulard, G. (2005). RFID: Promise or Peril? It may be easier than ever to track information, but it is causing concerns over privacy and civil liberties. *State Legislatures Magazine., 31*(10), 22–24. PMID:16397978

Brimacombe, G. G., Antunes, P., & McIntyre, J. (2001). *The future cost of health care in Canada, 2000 to 2020: balancing affordability and sustainability.* Conference Board of Canada.

Britton, J. (2007). An investigation into the feasibility of locating portable medical devices using radio frequency identification devices and technology. *Journal of Medical Engineering & Technology, 31*(6), 450–458. doi:10.1080/03091900701292141 PMID:17994419

Burkhard, R. J., & Schooley, B. et al.. (2010). Information systems and healthcareXXXVII: When your employer provides your personal health record—Exploring employee perceptions of an employer-sponsored PHR system. *Communications of the Association for Information Systems, 27*, 323–338.

Buyurgan, N., Landry, S., & Philippe, R. (2013). RFID Adoption in Healthcare and ROI Analysis. In *The Value of RFID* (pp. 81–96). Springer. doi:10.1007/978-1-4471-4345-1_7

Cao, Q., Baker, J., Wetherbe, J., & Gu, V. (2012). *Organizational adoption of innovation: Identifying factors that influence RFID adoption in the healthcare industry.* Academic Press.

Cavoukian, A. (2008, January). *RFID and Privacy-Guidance for Health-Care Providers.* Information and Privacy Commissioner of Ontario. Retrieved from http://www.longwoods.com/articles/images/rfid-healthcare.pdf

Cheng, C.-Y., & Chai, J.-W. (2012). Deployment of RFID in healthcare facilities—experimental design in MRI department. *Journal of Medical Systems, 36*(6), 3423–3433. doi:10.1007/s10916-011-9796-9 PMID:22072278

Collins, J. (2004a, November 16). Purdue Pharma Tags OxyContin. *RFID Journal.*

Collins, J. (2004b, November 19). Six U.K. Drug makers Pilot RFID. *RFID Journal.*

Collins, J. (2006d, June 20). Novartis Trial Shows RFID Can Boost Patient Compliance. *RFID Journal*.

Cresswell, K. M., & Sheikh, A. (2008). Information technology—Based approaches toreducing repeat drug exposure in patients with known drug allergies. *Journal of Allergy and Clinical Immunology, 121*(5), 1112-1117.

Cross, M. (2006). Keeping the ER on track. *Health Data Management, 14* (9), 68–69.

Crounse, B. (2005). *RFID: Increasing patient safety, reducing healthcare costs, 2005*. Available at http://www.microsoft.com/industry/healthcare/providers/businessvalue/housecalls/rfid.mspx

Dahiya, S. (2008). Counterfeit medicines: The global hazard. *Latest Reviews, 6*(4), 1–4.

Das, R., & Harrop, P. (2011). *RFID Forecasts, Players and Opportunities 2011–2021*. IDTechEx.

Davis, S. (2004). Tagging along. RFID helps hospitals track assets and people. *Health Facilities Management, 17*(12), 20–24. PMID:15637841

Dempsey, M. (2005). Weaving through the hopes and hype surrounding RFID. *Biomedical Instrumentation and Technology Supplement*, 19–22.

Dominguez-Péry, C., & Ageron, B. et al.. (2011). A service science framework to enhancevalue creation in service innovation projects: An RFID case study. *International Journal of Production Economics*.

Fichman, R. G. (2000). The diffusion and assimilation of information technology innovations. In R. Zmud (Ed.), *Framing the domains of IT management: projec-ting the future through the past*. Cincinnati, OH: Pinnaflex Educational Resources, Incorporated.

Fisher, J. A., & Monahan, T. (2008). Tracking the social dimensions of RFID systems in hospitals. *International Journal of Medical Informatics, 77*(3), 176–183. doi:10.1016/j.ijmedinf.2007.04.010 PMID:17544841

Fosso Wamba, S., Anand, A., & Carter, L. (2013). A literature review of RFID-enabled healthcare applications and issues. *International Journal of Information Management, 33*(5), 875–891. doi:10.1016/j.ijinfomgt.2013.07.005

Fosso Wamba, S., & Chatfield, A. T. (2009). A contingency model for creating value from RFID supply chain network projects in logistics and manufacturing environments. *European Journal of Information Systems, 18*(6), 615–636. doi:10.1057/ejis.2009.44

Fosso Wamba, S., Lefebvre, L. A., Bendavid, Y., & Lefebvre, É. (2008). Exploring the impact of RFID technology and the EPC network on mobile B 2B ecommerce: A case study in the retail industry. *International Journal of Production Economics, 112*(2), 614–629. doi:10.1016/j.ijpe.2007.05.010

Fosso Wamba, S., & Ngai, E. W. T. (2011). Unveiling the potential of RFID-enabled intelligent patient management: Results of a Delphi study. In *44th Hawaii international conference on systems science*. Koloa, HI: IEEE.

Fuhrer, P., & Guinard, D. (2006). Building a smart hospital using RFID technologies. In *European conference on eHealth* (pp. 131–142). Fribourg, Switzerland: Academic Press.

GS1-Australia (2010). *Healthcare industry*. Author.

Gambon, J. (2006, August 28). RFID Frees Up Patient Beds. *RFID Journal*.

Garfinkel, S., & Rosenberg, B. (2006). *RFID: Applications, security, and privacy*. Pearson Education India.

Gearon, C. (2005). Technology. Behind the hype. *Hospitals & Health Networks, 79*(6), 22, 24.

Hagland, M. (2005). Nine tech trends: Bar coding and RFID. *Healthcare Informatics*.

Halamka, J., Juels, J., Stubblefield, A., & Westhues, J. (2006). *The security implications of RFID for Healthcare and Pharmaceuticals 2008-2018*. IDTechEx. Retrieved from http://www.idtechex.com/research/reports/rfid_for_healthcare_and_ pharmaceuticals_2008_2018_000146.asp

Harrop, P., Das R., et al. (2009). *RFID for Healthcare and Pharmaceuticals 2009–2019*. IDTechEx.

IDTechEx (2006). *Rapid adoption of RFID in healthcare*. Author.

Ioan, T., Turcu, C., Turcu, C., & Cerlinc, M. (2010). RFID-based Information System for Patients and Medical Staff Identification and Tracking. In C. Turcu (Ed.), *Sustainable Radio Frequency Identification Solutions*. InTech. Retrieved from http://www.intechopen.com/books/sustainable-radio-frequency-identification-solutions/rfid-based-information-system-for-patients-and-medical-staff-identification-and-tracking

Kaplan, R. S., & Porter, M. E. (2011). How to solve the cost crisis in health care. *Harvard Business Review, 89*(9), 46–64. PMID:21939127

Lefebvre, É., Castro, L., & Lefebvre, L. A. (2011). Assessing the prevailing implementation issues of RFID in healthcare: A five-phase implementation model. *Int. J. Electron. Comput. Comm. Tech, 5*(2), 110–117.

Lefebvre, E., & Romero, A. et al.. (2011). Technological strategies to deal with counter-feit medicines: The European and North-American perspectives. *International Journal of Education and Information Technologies, 5*(3), 275–284.

LeRouge, C., Mantzana, V., & Wilson, E. V. (2007). Healthcare information systems research, revelations and visions. *European Journal of Information Systems, 16*(6), 669–671. doi:10.1057/palgrave.ejis.3000712

Lewis, M. O., Sankaranarayanan, B., ... (2009). RFID-enabled process capabilities and its impacts on healthcare process performance: A multi-level analysis. In ECIS 2009 proceedings. Verona, Italy: ECIS.

MarketResearch.com. (2011). *RFID readers and tags? A global market overview*. Author.

Maselli, J. (2003, May 27). Xtag Unveils Infant Security System. *RFID Journal*.

Means, C. (2008). *Mobile technology gets boost with vendor collaboration*. Retrieved from http://healthcareitnews.eu/content/view/765/45

Mehrjerdi, Y. Z. (2010). RFID-enabled healthcare systems: Risk-benefit analysis. *International Journal of Pharmaceutical and Healthcare Marketing, 4*(3), 282–300. doi:10.1108/17506121011076192

Menachemi, N., & Brooks, R. G. (2006). EHR and other IT adoption among physicians: Results of a large-scale state wide analysis. *Journal of Healthcare Information Management, 20*(3), 79–87. PMID:16903665

Michael, M. G., Fusco, S. J., & Michael, K. (2008). A research note on ethics in the emerging age of überveillance. *Computer Communications, 31*(6), 1192–1199. doi:10.1016/j.comcom.2008.01.023

Middleton, B. (2009). *Re-engineering U. S. health care with healthcare information technology- promises and peril.* Academic Press.

Mithas, S., & Ramasubbu, N. et al.. (2011). How information management capability influences firm performance. *Management Information Systems Quarterly, 35*(1), 237–256.

Motorola. (2013). *RFID solutions for healthcare reducing costs and improving operational efficiency.* Retrieved from http://www.motorolasolutions.com/web/Business/Solutions/Industry%20Solutions/RFID%20 Solutions/RFID_in_Healthcare/_documents/_staticfiles/Application_Brief_RFID_in_Healthcare.pdf

Murphy, D. (2006). Is RFID right for your organization? Understand your process before implementing a solution. *Materials Management in Health Care, 15*(6), 28–33. PMID:16859241

Najera, P., Lopez, J., & Roman, R. (2011). Real-time location and inpatient care systems based on passive RFID. *Journal of Network and Computer Applications, 34*(3), 980–989. doi:10.1016/j.jnca.2010.04.011

National-Academy-of-Sciences (2007). *Preventing medication errors: Quality chasm series.* Author.

National Association of Boards of Pharmacy. (2009). *National Association of Boards of Pharmacy (NABP), About the issue.* Available at http://www.dangerouspill.com/about_the_issue.html

Newell, S. (2011). Special section on healthcare information systems. *The Journal of Strategic Information Systems, 20*(2), 158–160. doi:10.1016/j.jsis.2011.05.002

Ngai, E. W., Poon, J. K., Suk, F. F. C., & Ng, C. C. (2009a). Design of an RFID-based healthcare management system using an information system design theory. *Information Systems Frontiers, 11*(4), 405–417. doi:10.1007/s10796-009-9154-3

Ngai, E. W. T., Moon, K. K. L., Riggins, F. J., & Yi, C. Y. (2008). RFID research: An academic literature review(1995–2005) and future research directions. *International Journal of Production Economics, 112*(2), 510–520. doi:10.1016/j.ijpe.2007.05.004

Ngai, E. W. T., Xiu, L., & Chau, D. C. K. (2009b). Application of data mining techniques in customer relationship management: A literature review and classification. *Expert Systems with Applications, 36*(2, Part 2), 2592–2602. doi:10.1016/j.eswa.2008.02.021

O'Connor, M. C. (2005, February 17). Surveys Reveal Dubious Consumers. *RFID Journal.*

O'Connor, M. C. (2007, February 6). RFID Tidies Up Distribution of Hospital Scrubs. *RFID Journal.*

Oztekin, A., Mahdavi, F., Erande, K., Kong, Z. J., Swim, L. K., & Bukkapatnam, S. T. S. (2010a). Criticality index analysis based optimal RFID reader placement models for asset tracking. *International Journal of Production Research, 48*(9), 2679–2698. doi:10.1080/00207540903565006

Oztekin, A., Pajouh, F. M., Delen, D., & Swim, L. K. (2010b). An RFID network design methodology for asset tracking in healthcare. *Decision Support Systems, 49*(1), 100–109. doi:10.1016/j.dss.2010.01.007

Page, L. (2007). Testing gives way to implementation. Hospitals tune in to RFID. *Materials Management in Health Care, 16*(5), 18–20. PMID:17552344

Payton, F. C., & Pare, G. et al.. (2011). Health care IT: Process, people, patients and inter-disciplinary considerations. *Journal of the Association for Information Systems, 12*(2/3), i–xiii.

Payton, F. C., Pare, G., Le Rouge, C. M., & Reddy, M. (2011). Health care IT: Process, people, patients and interdisciplinary considerations. *Journal of the Association for Information Systems, 12*(2), 3.

PCAST. (2010). *Report to the President realizing the full potential of the health information technology to improve healthcare for Americans: The path forward. President's Council of Advisors on Science and Technology (PCAST)*. Executive Office of the President.

Pleshek, J. (2011). *RFID will see double-digit growth in the healthcare market*. Retrieved 21 December, 2011, from http://wtnnews.com/articles/8824/

Reyes, P. M., Li, S., et al. (2011). Accessing antecedents and outcomes of RFID implementation in health care. *International Journal of Production Economics*.

Riggins, F. J., & Mukhopadhyay, T. (1994). Interdependent benefits from interorganizational systems: Opportunities for business partner reengineering. *Journal of Management Information Systems, 11*(2), 37–57.

Sherer, S. (2010). Information systems and healthcare: An institutional theory per-spective on physician adoption of electronic health records. *Communications of the Association for Information Systems, 27*(7), 127–140.

Sini, E., Locatelli, P., & Restifo, N. (2008). Making the clinical process safe and efficient using RFID in healthcare. *European Journal of ePractice, 2*. Available at http://www.epractice.eu/en/document/287903

Slettemeås, D. (2009). RFID—the "Next Step" in Consumer–Product Relations or Orwellian Nightmare? *Challenges for Research and Policy, 32*(3), 219–244. doi:10.1007/s10603-009-9103-z

Southard, P. B., Chandra, C., & Kumar, S. (2012). RFID in healthcare: A Six Sigma DMAIC and simulation case study. *International Journal of Health Care Quality Assurance, 25*(4), 291–321. doi:10.1108/09526861211221491 PMID:22755482

Sullivan, L. (2006). *Medline Markets RFID System for Surgical Sponges*. RFID Journal.

Swartz, N. (2005). FDA Okays Implanted Chip for Health Care. Information Management Journal. *Lenexa, 39*(1), 16.

Swedberg, C. (2005, September 12). Pittsburgh Hospital Pilots Hybrid System. *RFID Journal*.

Swedberg, C. (2007, February 16). MedicAlert Aims to RFID-Enable Medical Records. *RFID Journal*.

Swedberg, C. (2008a, January 3). Medical Center Set to Grow With RFID. *RFID Journal*.

Swedberg, C. (2008b, March 18). Surgeon Designs System to Monitor Orthopedic Implants and Promote Healing. *RFID Journal*.

Symonds, J., & Parry, D. et al.. (2007). An RFID-based system for assisted living:Challenges and solutions. *The Journal on Information Technology in Healthcare*, 5(6), 387–398. PMID:17901606

Thuemmler, C., Buchanan, W., & Kumar, V. (2007). Setting safety standards by designing a low budget and compatible patient identification system based on passive RFID technology. *International Journal of Healthcare Technology and Management*, 8(5), 571–583. doi:10.1504/IJHTM.2007.013524

Ting, S. L., Kwok, S. K., Tsang, A. H., & Lee, W. B. (2011). Critical elements and lessons learnt from the implementation of an RFID-enabled healthcare management system in a medical organization. *Journal of Medical Systems*, 35(4), 657–669. doi:10.1007/s10916-009-9403-5 PMID:20703523

Tu, Y.-J., Zhou, W., & Piramuthu, S. (2009). Identifying RFID-embedded objects in pervasive healthcare applications. *Decision Support Systems*, 46(2), 586–593. doi:10.1016/j.dss.2008.10.001

United-States-Department-of-Labor. (2010). Healthcare: Career guide to industries U.S.D. o. labor. VeriChip cloning. *Journal of the American Medical Informatics Association*, 13(6), 601–607.

Vilamovska, A. M., Hatziandreu, E., Schindler, R., Oranje, C., Vries, H., & Krapels, J. (2008). *Study on the requirements and options for RFID application in healthcare, July 2008*. Retrieved from http://ec.europa.eu/information_society/activities/health/docs/studies/200807-rfid-ehealth.pdf

Vilamovska, A. M., Hatziandreu, E., Schindler, R., Oranje, C., Vries, H., & Krapels, J. (2008). *Study on the requirements and options for RFID application in healthcare, July 2008*. Retrieved from http://ec.europa.eu/information_society/activities/health/docs/studies/200807-rfid-ehealth.pdf

Wamba, S. F. (2012). RFID-enabled healthcare applications, issues and benefits: An archival analysis (1997–2011). *Journal of Medical Systems*, 36(6), 3393–3398. doi:10.1007/s10916-011-9807-x PMID:22109670

Wessel, R. (2006a, February 27). German Clinic Uses RFID to Track Blood. *RFID Journal*.

Wessel, R. (2006b, June 9). German Hospital Expects RFID to Eradicate Drug Errors. *RFID Journal*.

Wessel, R. (2006c, September 26). RFID-enabled Locks Secure Bags of Blood. *RFID Journal*.

Wessel, R. (2007, June 1). Jena University Hospital Prescribes RFID to Reduce Medication Errors. *RFID Journal*.

Wiener, J. M., & Tilly, J. (2002). Population ageing in the United States of America: Implications for public programmes. *International Journal of Epidemiology*, 31(4), 776–781. doi:10.1093/ije/31.4.776 PMID:12177018

Wilkerson, J. L., & McDonald Jr, C. L. (2007). RFID in Healthcare. *The Journal of Organizational Leadership & Business*, 1–8.

Wurster, C., & Lichtenstein, B. P. et al.. (2009). Strategic, political, and cultural aspectsof IT implementation: Improving the efficacy of an IT system in a large hospital. *Journal of Healthcare Management*, *54*(3), 191. PMID:19554799

Wurster, C. J., Lichtenstein, B. B., & Hogeboom, T. (2008). Strategic, political, and cultural aspects of IT implementation: improving the efficacy of an IT system in a large hospital. *Journal of Healthcare Management, 54*(3), 191–206, discussion 206–7.

Yao, W., Chu, C.-H., & Li, Z. (2010). The use of RFID in healthcare: Benefits and barriers. In *RFID-Technology and Applications (RFID-TA), 2010 IEEE International Conference on* (pp. 128–134). IEEE.

KEY TERMS AND DEFINITIONS

Active RFID: Active RFID is a method of automatic identification that uses ID tags which are self-powered.

AIDC: Automatic identification and data capture (AIDC) are methods of automatically identifying objects, collecting data about them, and entering that data directly into computer systems. AIDC require no human intervention.

Battery-Assisted Passive RFID: Battery-assisted Passive RFID is a method of automatic identification that uses ID tags that has a small battery on board and is activated when in the presence of an RFID reader.

Counterfeit Medicine: A medicine which is illegal and may be harmful for human health because it may be contaminated, contain the wrong or no active ingredient, or have the right active ingredient but at the wrong dose.

Haemovigilance: "Haemovigilance is a system of monitoring, identification, reporting, investigation and analysis of adverse events near-misses and reactions related to transfusion and manufacturing.

Passive RFID: Passive RFID is a method of automatic identification that uses ID tags that uses the radio energy transmitted by the reader.

RFID: RFID (radio frequency identification) is a technology that uses radio frequency signals to uniquely identify an object, animal, or person.

Chapter 13
Integrated Hospital Information System Architecture Design in Indonesia

Putu Wuri Handayani
Universitas Indonesia, Indonesia

Puspa Indahati Sandhyaduhita
Universitas Indonesia, Indonesia

Achmad Nizar Hidayanto
Universitas Indonesia, Indonesia

Ave Adriana Pinem
Universitas Indonesia, Indonesia

Haya Rizqi Fajrina
Universitas Indonesia, Indonesia

Kasiyah M. Junus
Universitas Indonesia, Indonesia

Indra Budi
Universitas Indonesia, Indonesia

Dumilah Ayuningtyas
Universitas Indonesia, Indonesia

ABSTRACT

Implementing Hospital Information System is an ultimately important practice that should be performed by hospitals in order to deliver accurate, timely, complete, and easily accessible data/information in an integrated manner. Given the specific characteristics of Indonesia, the objective of this research is to design an Information System Architecture as part of the Enterprise Architecture based on The Open Group Architecture Framework in order to support the Hospital Information System implementation in Indonesia. This research focuses on the hospitals basic processes, viz. the emergency processes, the inpatient processes and the outpatient processes. The integration aspect of the architecture should connect the hospitals with other related stakeholders. This research is a qualitative study by conducting interviews and observations in three government public hospitals, several directorate generals of the Indonesian Ministry of Health and a representative from the WHO. The result of this research is an integrated Information System Architecture model.

DOI: 10.4018/978-1-4666-9446-0.ch013

INTRODUCTION

Hospitals as one of the public entities are expected to provide optimal services to the public and other stakeholders. To provide optimal services, information technology can be used, which has been acknowledged by the Directorate General of Health Development (*Direktorat Jenderal Bina Upaya Kesehatan*) of the Indonesian Ministry of Health by endorsing the use of information technology (IT), such as information systems, in the healthcare sector. The use of information technology in the healthcare sector is commonly known as e-health (Rawabdeh, 2007). The information system that is specifically designed for hospitals is widely known either as the Hospital Information System (HIS) or the Clinical Information System (CIS) (Petroudi & Giannakakis, 2011). According to Petroudi and Giannakakis' study, the Hospital Information System can provide solutions in producing effective and efficient operational processes in a hospital by integrating the entire process from the registration process to the payment process in conjunction with all of the required information.

The Hospital Information System is not only important for supporting operational processes in the hospitals but also important for the government, which is a stakeholder, because it can effectively and efficiently provide data of citizens' health information to enable the government to make decisions regarding healthcare facilities and healthcare programs to manage and finance healthcare facilities and medical research (World Health Organization, 2001). In addition, Law Number 14/2008 on the Public Information Disclosure, the President Regulation Number 12/2013 regarding Health Insurance, and the Minister of Health Regulation Number 1691/Menkes/Per/VIII/2011 regarding Hospital Patient Safety agree that hospitals should be able to provide accurate, timely, and complete health data/information that is easily accessible for the public and other relevant stakeholders. Thus, implementing the Hospital Information System is an important practice that should be performed by hospitals to not only produce effective and efficient operational processes but also to provide and deliver accurate, timely, complete, and easily accessible data/information in an integrated manner.

Pursuant to the Regulation of the Minister of Health Number 1144/Menkes/Per/VIII/2010 regarding the Organization and Working Procedure of the Ministry of Health, Article 106 states that the Directorate General of Health Development shall: (1) formulate and implement policies in the area of health development; (2) formulate norms, standards, procedures, and criteria in the area of health development; (3) provide technical guidance and evaluations in the area of health development; and (4) implement the administration of the Directorate General of Health Development. To date, although the Directorate General of Health Development acknowledges the importance of e-health, which includes the Hospital Information System, the Directorate General of Health Development has only issued one regulation (Kementrian Kesehatan RI, 2011), the Regulation of the Minister of Health Number 1171/MENKES/PER/VI/2011 on the Hospital Reporting System (HRS), which manages the reporting mechanisms and defines the types of reports that are required by the Ministry of Health from each hospital as the basis to determine health policies in Indonesia. In addition to the Directorate General of Health Development, the Indonesian Government has enacted Government Regulation Number 46/2014 concerning the Health Information System that defines the scope of health information as encompassing the health effort, health research and development, health funding, health workers, medical tools and equipment, health management and regulations, and community empowerment. Likewise, this regulation also lacks the standard procedures and guidelines in determining the business processes and data that are required to be exchanged between the hospitals and other relevant stakeholders. Therefore, despite the urgency to implement the Hospital Information System, the lack of regulations and the absence of standard procedures and guidelines contribute to the small number of public hospitals implementing the Hospital Information System. In addition, the lack of financial support also decreases the number (Health Metrics Network, 2008).

It can be inferred that the development of the procedures and guidelines for implementing the Hospital Information System in an integrated manner is very important to ensure the effective, efficient, and secure delivery of quality healthcare; however, the implementation of an integrated Hospital Information System in Indonesia poses a big challenge because Indonesia is a large archipelago in which the network and internet infrastructures are still not equally distributed throughout the country. These constraints limit hospitals to having loosely coupled integration architecture between hospitals and other related stakeholders, and a higher quality system is necessary to improve the quality and speed of healthcare work processes as well as to improve the availability and quality of data and information. Thus, it is expected that the rapid development of IT-related method/methodology can offer alternatives to these challenges. One of the best practices that is widely used in the industry is an approach called Enterprise Architecture, which can provide guidance for developing an integrated information system architecture (Niemi, 2006).

Enterprise Architecture (EA) can be defined as (1) a conceptual framework that depicts the primary components of an enterprise/organization and the relationship among these components and the environment and (2) the principles governing its design and evolution (Rood, 1994; IEEE, 2000). Enterprise Architecture Framework (EAF), such as TOGAF (The Open Group Architecture Framework), serves as an instrument that can be used as a guideline to design IT architecture and logic structure, to organize complex information, and to address IT/IS and business needs (Sajid & Ahsan, 2014). TOGAF defines the scope of applications of products and services that are in the domain of business and industry, technical infrastructure based on open system building blocks, including the definition of business process architecture, information system architecture, data architecture, and technology architecture. The phases of the enterprise architecture development method using TOGAF consist of a preliminary definition of frameworks and principles, architecture vision, business architecture, and information system architecture (McSweeney, 2000). A study conducted by Costetchi et al. (2014) shows that e-health enterprise system architecture provides a framework to support e-health in delivering coherent and interoperable e-health solutions that can form a true integrated e-health system aiming to deliver shared data and applications to healthcare participants. Therefore, it can be inferred that an enterprise architecture approach can be used as a frame of reference for designing information architecture in a planned, purposeful, and efficient manner.

Unfortunately, there are only a few studies related to enterprise architecture in the healthcare domain. Costetchi et al. (2014) designed an e-health framework that can be applied to meet both general and specific objectives called the Romania Healthcare Framework for Rare Diseases. The dimensions that are highlighted in the framework are the contextual level (strategy, objective, and goal), business architecture modeling, healthcare network, healthcare information system, technical/infrastructure architecture, data architecture, application architecture, technology/equipment architecture, and knowledge and educational/research/training. Thus, enriching the previous studies and considering the characteristics of Indonesia to develop an integrated Hospital Information System is needed to ensure an efficient integration of various systems from central to regional healthcare units. Furthermore, this architecture could also be implemented in other hospitals, especially in the developing countries that have similar characteristics to Indonesia.

Since an Enterprise Architecture Framework is deemed able to guide the development of an integrated architecture, the objective of this research is to design an Information System Architecture as part of the Enterprise Architecture based on TOGAF in order to support the Hospital Information System implementation in Indonesia. In the long term, it is expected that this Enterprise Architecture approach can improve the quality of hospital services and the provision of data to the Ministry of Health. Therefore, the scope of this research is defined as follows:

1. The focus is on basic hospital processes, such as emergency processes, inpatient processes, and outpatient processes, each of which include the registration, medical treatment, medical record management, billing, and payment process steps.
2. The integration aspect should connect the hospitals with the Ministry of Health, the provincial or the district/city Health Office, the National Population and Family Planning Board (*Badan Kependudukan dan Keluarga Berencana Nasional*/BKKBN), the Health Social Security Agency (*Badan Penyelenggara Jaminan Sosial/BPJS - Kesehatan*), international organizations, such as the World Health Organization (WHO), the manufacturers and suppliers of medical devices, and the public.
3. Designing the information system architecture in government public hospitals.

BACKGROUND

Hospital Information System (HIS)

The Hospital Information System (HIS), also often called the Clinical Information System (CIS), is a comprehensive, integrated information system designed to manage the administrative, financial, and clinical aspects of a hospital (Petroudi & Giannakakis, 2011). The aim of the Hospital Information System is to achieve the best possible process for patient care and administration by electronic data processing (Petroudi & Giannakakis, 2011). The Hospital Information System is an instance of the Health Information System (Haux, 2006). The Health Information System includes all health care systems involving patient care that must be integrated to generate consistent, valid, and correct data. To accommodate that objective, the Hospital Information System needs to provide services that can be used to exchange data with other health care systems.

It is common in a hospital environment that a number of systems are developed separately. To integrate entire business process in a hospital, Lu et al. (2005) designed the Enterprise Hospital Information System. The architecture was supposed to integrate three aspects in implementing the enterprise system: data integration, workflow integration and function integration. This enterprise system covered the Clinical Terminal, PACS (Picture Archiving and Communication System), Hospital Information System, and LIS (Laboratory Information System).

Indonesia has considered the Hospital Information System to be an important aspect in the health system. This is supported by Regulation Number 36/2009 issued by the Indonesian Minister of Health regarding Health. This regulation concerns health information system utilization and the integration across multiple sectors in healthcare. The Indonesian Health Information System Roadmap for the period from 2011-2014 (Pusat Data dan Informasi, 2012) states that one of the Ministry of Health's strategic plans is to effectuate the collection, the storage and the data dissemination system automatically through the utilization of information technology.

Though the benefits of a Hospital Information System have been emphasized, there is only a limited number of hospitals that have implemented the Hospital Information System (Bina Upaya Kesehatan, 2013). Although the Directorate of the Referral Health Effort (*Direktorat Bina Upaya Kesehatan Rujukan*) has launched a very basic package of the Hospital Information System, which is an open source Hospital Information System called SIMRS GOS (*Sistem Informasi Manajemen Rumah Sakit Generic Open Source*), hospitals still encounter obstacles in implementing the Hospital Information System. In addition, SIMRS GOS only implements very basic functions and does not have a clear and detailed architecture. The lack of funds, (IT) human resources, and an IT infrastructure are some elements that negatively influence hospital management decisions in implementing the Hospital Information System. Another issue that should be considered is the compatibility issue between the Hospital Information System and other existing systems and how these systems can be well-integrated.

The Open Group Architecture Framework (TOGAF)

According to Rood (1994), architecture is defined as a representation or model of components that build the system and the relationship of these components (Rood, 1994). Another definition of architecture is defined by ANSI/IEEE Std 1471-2000, as the "fundamental organization of a system, embodied in its components, their relationships to each other and the environment, and the principles governing its design and evolution" (IEEE, 2000, p.3). Based on these definitions, Enterprise Architecture (EA) can be defined as: (1) a conceptual framework that depicts the primary components of an enterprise/organization and the relationship among these components and the environment and (2) the principles governing its design and evolution (Rood, 1994; Winter & Fischer, 2007).

Enterprise Architecture is an architectural discipline that merges strategic business and IT objectives with opportunities for change and governs the resulting change initiatives (Jensen, Cline, & Owen, 2011). Enterprise Architecture is also a strategic planning tool and can be used as a reference architecture for modeling to develop a master plan that acts as an integrating force between aspects of (Dennis, 2010):

1. **Business Planning:** Including goals, visions, strategies and governance principles
2. **Business Operations:** Including clinical and business terms, organization structures, processes and data
3. **Automation:** Including application systems and databases
4. **The Business's Enabling Technological Infrastructure:** Including computers, operating systems and networks.

Enterprise Architecture goals can be divided into two categories: external and internal (Lange & Mendling, 2011). The external goal is related to fulfilling the regulatory requirements (Lange & Mendling, 2011). The internal goal is related to organizational goals, such as a business-IT alignment with the objective to align business with IT implementation, a cost reduction objective to reduce IT and business processes related to costs, standardization/consolidation that aims to simplify the architecture, management/governance with the objective to improve the decision making process, and agility with the objective to improve processes and IT flexibility. These goals would help organizations quickly respond to the change of environment and improve interoperability and integration (Lange & Mendling, 2011; National Institute of Health, 2011).

Enterprise Architecture Framework (EAF) is an instrument that can be used as a guideline to design IT architecture and logic structures, to organize complex information, and to address IT/IS and business needs, such as The Open Group Architecture Framework (TOGAF) (Sajid & Ahsan, 2014). TOGAF was introduced in 1995; it is based on the United States Department of Defense Technical Architecture Framework for Information Management (Sajid & Ahsan, 2014). TOGAF is an architectural framework that provides guidelines to design, evaluate, and build suitable architectures for enterprises/organizations. TOGAF includes the application of products and services that are in the domain of business and industry and the technical infrastructure based on open system building blocks, including the definition of business process architecture, application architecture, data architecture, and technology architecture. The phases of the Enterprise Architecture development method using the TOGAF framework consists of the preliminary definition of the framework and the principles, the architecture vision, the business architecture, and the information system architecture (McSweeney, 2000).

The preliminary definition of the framework and principles is a phase in which several aspects, such as the enterprise, the requirement for the architecture work, the architectural principles, the framework to be used, and the relationship between management frameworks are defined. The architecture vision phase is a phase in which a vision of capability and business value that will be delivered as a result of the proposed enterprise architecture is developed. It also defines the scope of the architecture, the key stakeholders, the business principles, the objectives, and the key business requirements. In the business architecture phase, the business architecture that represents the fundamentals of the organization based on the business strategy is built. The business architecture also defines the governance and the business processes of the organization. Two modeling methods that can be used to design business architecture are Unified Modeling Language (UML) and IDEF-0. During the information system architecture phase, the application and the data architecture are formed. The application architecture phase depicts the blueprint of each individual system needed by the organization based on their interactions and their relationships in the core business processes of the organization. The data architecture phase describes the logical and the physical data set structure and the data management resources (TOGAF 9.1, 2013).

Figure 1 describes a TOGAF content meta-model that could be used as a stand-alone framework for architecture within an enterprise. This content meta-model provides definitions of all types of building blocks that may exist within an architecture, showing how these building blocks can be described and related to one another (i.e., data entities held within applications and technologies implement those application) (TOGAF 9.1, 2013).

Indonesian Healthcare System

Access to health information will be effective and efficient if each stakeholder has implemented a Health Information System (Health IS), which has been considered by WHO to be one of the six major components of a health care system in a country (World Health Organization, 2011). Due to the development of the silo (computer-based) systems both within the Ministry of Health and almost in every health care facility (i.e., hospitals and clinics), the implementation of the Indonesian Health Information System still faces several obstacles, such as data redundancy and the inefficient use of resources in central and regional units (Pusat Data dan Informasi, 2012). Thus, a major challenge for the Ministry of Health, as explicitly stated in the Indonesia Health Information System Roadmap 2011-2014, is to integrate different application components where integrity and different types of integration need to be achieved (Winter, et al., 2011). In order to solve these problems, the Ministry of Health has formulated

Figure 1. TOGAF Content Meta-model
(TOGAF 9.1, 2013)

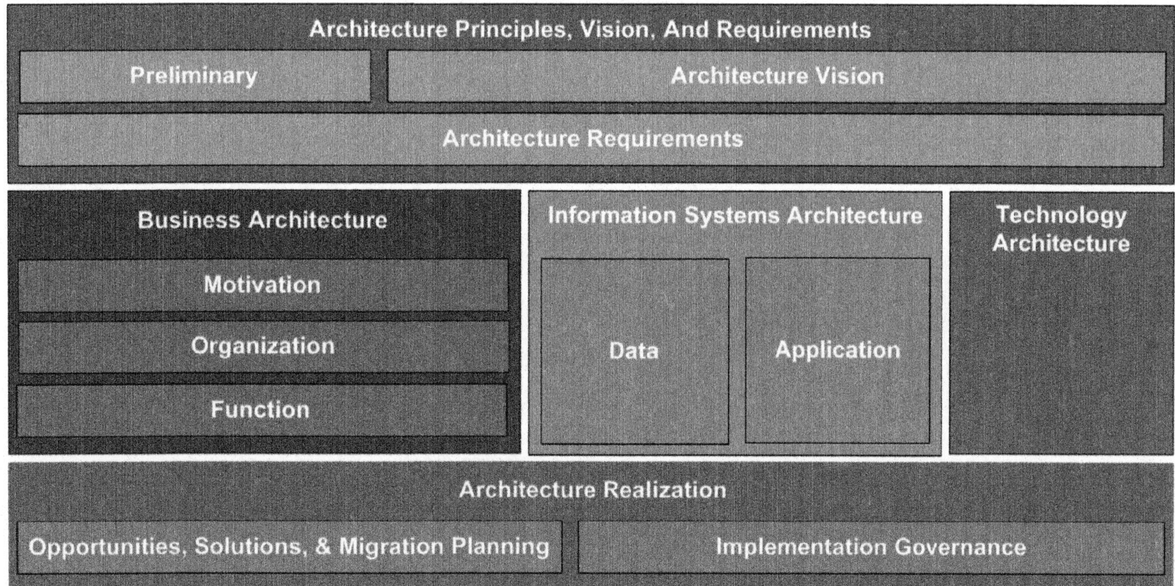

a plan in the Indonesia Health Information System Roadmap 2011-2014 to build a National Health Data Repository that can accommodate all health data from all sources (i.e., the hospitals and the HSSA). In the future, this data repository is expected to be implemented in hospitals, province and city/district Health Offices, and other related stakeholders. In order to support that policy, which is also pursuant to the Regulation of the Minister of Health Number 82 Year 2013 regarding the Hospital Information System, every hospital in Indonesia must implement a Hospital Information System; however, most of the hospitals to date still do not have an appropriate plan to implement a Hospital Information System due to the lack of IT knowledge and awareness as well as funding issues. Therefore, the design of the Enterprise Architecture for a Hospital Information System is deemed to be urgently required.

The Indonesian Healthcare System involves several stakeholders who manage the flow of health information, health services, products, and funding. The key players in the Indonesian Healthcare System are the hospitals. Hospitals, as depicted in the Hospital Supply Chain (Figure 2), should be able to provide the Ministry of Health, the provincial or the district/city Health Office, the National Population and Family Planning Board (*Badan Kependudukan dan Keluarga Berencana Nasional*/BKKBN), the Health Social Security Agency (*Badan Penyelenggara Jaminan Sosial/BPJS - Kesehatan*), international organizations, such as the WHO, the manufacturers and suppliers of medical devices, and the public with health care information..

As shown in Figure 2, the flow of products, information, and funding from each party in the supply chain is affected by specified policies or regulations by the external parties. Related data/information about products and funding can be exchanged between the parties in the supply chain with external parties and vice versa. In the internal and upstream supply chain, the medical device procurement process is conducted by the integration between the suppliers and the manufacturers of the medical devices and the hospital. The downstream supply chain focuses on the basic process steps, such as the registration, medical treatment, medical record management, and billing. The payment will be made by the social

Figure 2. The Hospitals Supply Chain

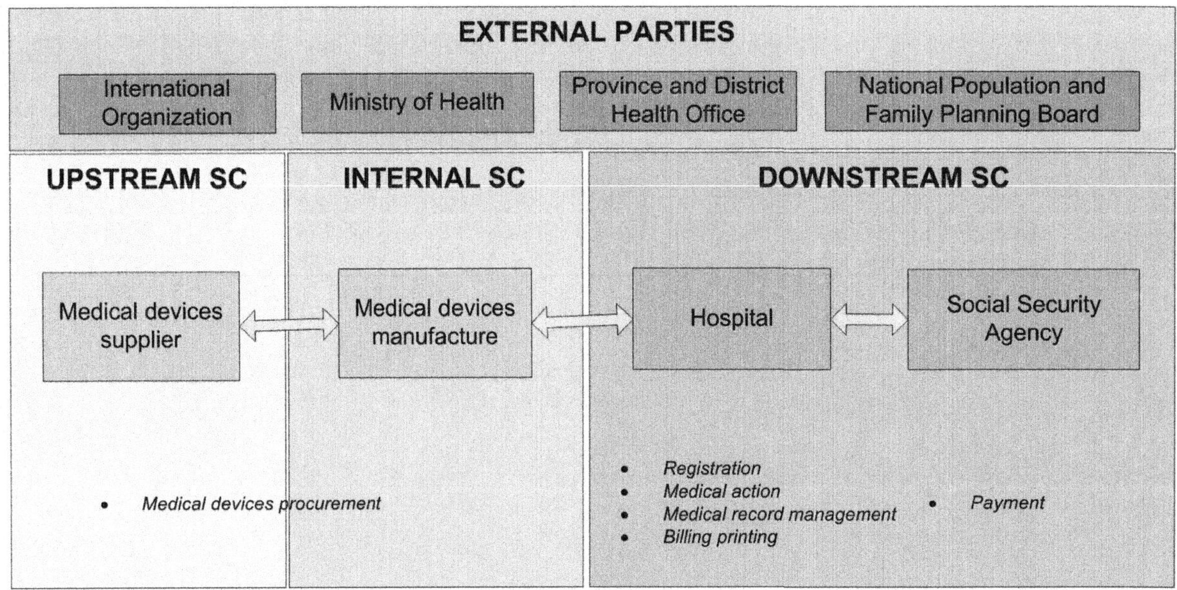

security agency. Figure 3 explains the detailed flow of information among the health care stakeholders mentioned in Figure 2.

The highest level of data exchange occurs between the WHO and the Ministry of Health and between the Ministry of Health and the BKKBN. The data exchange between the Ministry of Health and the WHO is conducted manually (requires paperwork). It involves the exchange of the groups of data

Figure 3. The Health Services Integration

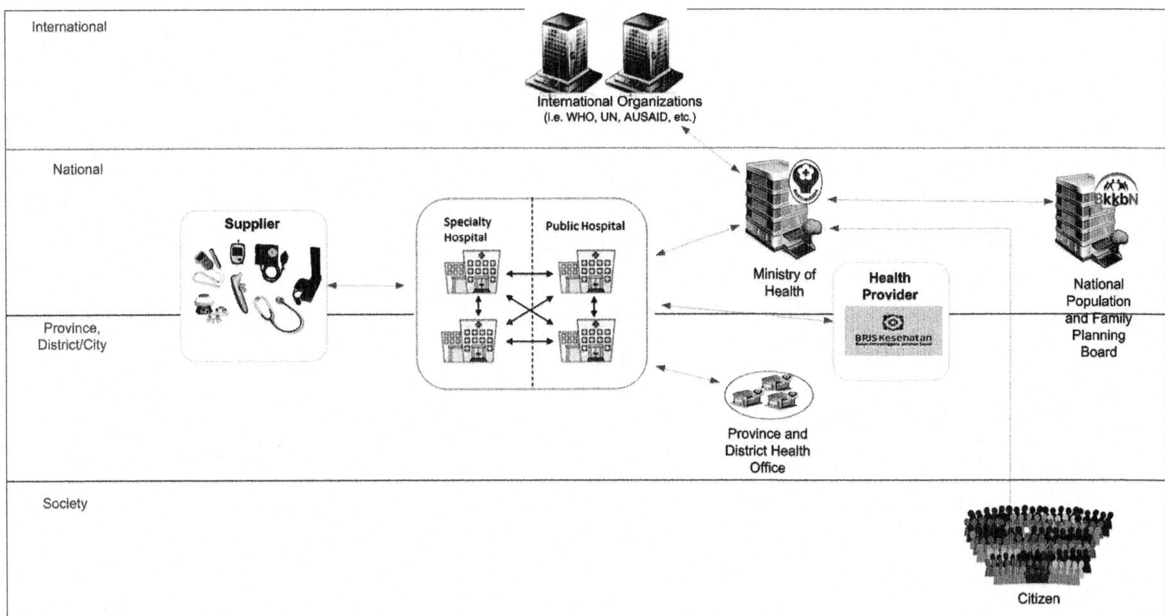

which consists of diseases, environmental health, maternal and child health, health care facilities, health care, and the budget. The data exchange between the Ministry of Health and the BKKBN is specific to maternal and child health data.

The primary data exchange occurs between the hospitals and the Ministry of Health. The data is obtained by the Ministry of Health from all hospitals in Indonesia through the hospital reports submitted periodically by the hospitals. The hospitals' annual report submission is regulated by the Regulation of the Indonesian Ministry of Health Number 1171/MENKES/PER/VI/2011 regarding the Hospital Reporting System (HRS) (*Sistem Informasi Rumah Sakit* or *SIRS*), which requires hospitals to submit their annual reports to the Ministry of Health. The hospitals' annual reports are sent directly by the hospitals to the Ministry of Health via the Hospital Reporting System (HRS), a web-based application developed and managed by the Directorate of the Referral Health Effort (DRHE) of the Ministry of Health. The submission is performed by uploading the report file to the Hospital Reporting System website. The hospitals' annual reports include the profile data and the hospitals' performance. In addition to the Hospital Reporting System, the Directorate of the Referral Health Effort also develops and manages the Medical Equipment Procurement Application (MEPA) (*Aplikasi Pengadaan Alat Kesehatan*/ASPAK), a web-based application for submitting hospital data regarding the facilities, the infrastructures, and the medical equipment that are owned and managed by the hospitals. The submission is performed by uploading the data to the MEPA. For hospitals with IT infrastructure constraints, they can send the hardcopy of the data manually to the nearest district/city Health Office, and the district/city Health Office will forward the data to the Ministry of Health through the Hospital Reporting System or the Medical Equipment Procurement Application website.

In addition to the highest level data exchange and the primary data exchange, community groups require access to health information that is managed by the Ministry of Health, which includes data of the health facilities, diseases, maternal and child health, health insurance, budgeting, nutrition, medicine, and research and development. Thus, the Ministry of Health should provide information services for the community groups to provide the corresponding data.

Moreover, to achieve internal and upstream supply chain performance excellence, the hospitals must collaborate with the manufacturers (and if possible also with the suppliers) of the medical devices to perform the procurement process of the medical equipment. The associated data include the device name, the brand, the type, the serial number, the price, the manufacturers, and the distributors. On the other hand, to manage the patients' claims, the hospitals must collaborate with the healthcare providers, namely the Health Social Security Agency (HSSA). The data exchanged in this process include the patients' names and the diagnosis of the patients' illnesses.

Pursuant to the Regulation of the Indonesian Minister of Health Number 001/2012 regarding the Individual Health Care Referral System, the health facilities in Indonesia are divided into three categories:

1. **First Health Facilities:** Primary healthcare provided by doctors and dentists in a health center, health center care (*puskesmas/pusat kesehatan masyarakat*), integrated health service posts (*posyandu/ pos pelayanan terpadu*), private hospitals with general medical services (*rumah sakit pratama*), health center clinics, government and private clinics that provide general medical services, private practice doctors or dentists, and physician practices or family dentists located within the region or city

2. **Second Health Facilities:** Specialized health services performed by a specialist physician or dentist who uses knowledge and medical technology in a public or special district hospital

3.   **Third Health Facilities:** A sub-specialized health service performed by a physician or dentist sub-specialists who use their knowledge of health and technology in a public hospital, specialized center, or national referral hospital

Pursuant to the Ministry of Health Regulation Number 340/Menkes/Per/III/2010 regarding Hospital Classification, the classification of hospitals is generally divided into public and specialized hospitals. Public hospitals are hospitals that are owned by the government as well as by private parties that provide health care services to all areas and for all types of diseases. Specialty hospitals are hospitals that are owned by the government as well as by private parties that provide health care in one specific area or for one particular type of disease based on disciplines, age groups, organs, or types of diseases. Public and specialty hospitals are spread throughout the province and districts/cities. According to the range of facilities and service capabilities, the public hospitals are classified into the A class, the B class, the C class, and the D class. Specialized hospitals are similarly ranked. The A class hospitals have a larger number of facilities and wider service capabilities than the B class hospitals, and so forth.

Based on the Regulation of the Minister of Health of the Republic of Indonesia Number 001 of 2012 and the regionalization of the area, the distribution of health care facilities is divided into:

1.   **The District Level:** Inpatient health centers, community health centers, mobile clinics
2.   **The City Level:** Class C hospitals, class D hospitals, private hospitals with general medical services
3.   **The Provincial Level:** Class A hospitals, class B hospitals, specialized Hospitals, national referral hospitals

The health care referral system is the provision of services that defines the delegation of tasks and responsibilities of health care services on a reciprocal basis. The referral system is required for patients covered by the National Health Insurance (NHI) (*Jaminan Kesehatan Nasional – JKN*) and registered for the Health Social Security Agency (HSSA) (*BPJS-Kesehatan*). The coverage includes the medical referral (based on the Regulation of the Indonesian Minister of Health Number 001/2012) defined as follows:

1.   Consult patients for diagnostic purposes, treatment, operative measures, etc.
2.   Deliver the materials (specimens) for a more complete laboratory examination
3.   Bring more competent or specialized medical staff to improve the quality of medical care

The vertical referral is a referral between different health care levels from a lower level to the higher level or vice versa, while the horizontal referral is a referral for health services on the same level. The vertical referral and the horizontal referral is performed whenever the referrer cannot provide health care services according to the patients' needs because of the limited facilities, equipment, and/or medical staff. A vertical referral from a lower level to a higher one is normally done when patients require a specialist or sub-specialist for medical treatments. The refer-back process from a higher level health facility to a lower one can be performed when the following occurs (Regulation of the Indonesian Minister of Health Number 001/2012):

1.   The patients' health problems can be treated by a lower level healthcare facility and its corresponding competency and authority

2. The competency and authority of the first or the second level of the healthcare facility can better handle the patients' needs than the higher ones
3. The patients' follow-up treatments can be handled by the lower level of the health facility as well as for reasons of convenience, efficiency, and long-term care
4. The higher level healthcare facility cannot provide health services that correspond to the patients' needs due to the limited facilities, infrastructure, equipment, and/or medical staff

Figure 4 describes the flow of the inter-hospital referral in accordance with the scope of this study. The referral process must obtain prior approval from patients and/or their families after the patients and/or families receive an appropriate explanation from the hospital authority and health personnel, which includes the following information (Regulation of the Indonesian Minister of Health Number 001/2012):

1. Diagnosis and treatment and/or medical treatment necessary
2. Reason for referral and destination
3. Risks that can arise if a referral is not done

Figure 4. The Referral Flow Process among Hospitals

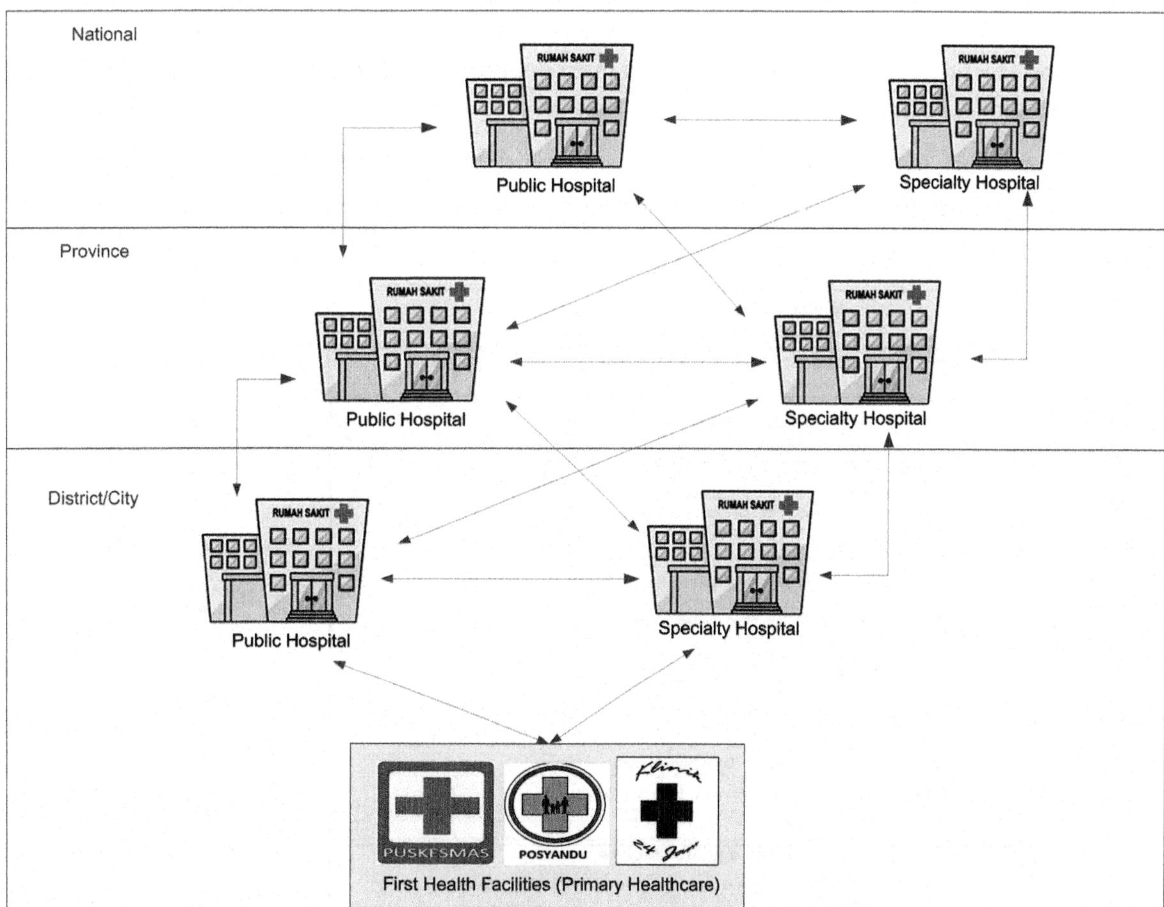

4.   Referral transport
5.   Risks or complications that may arise during the trip.

All of the information above is also included in the cover letter that contains the identity of the patient, the results of the examination (history, physical examination, and investigation), the working diagnosis, the therapy and/or the measures that have been provided, the purpose of the referral, and the name and signature of the medical staff who provided the services.

By having an integrated health data repository, as shown in Figure 5, the Ministry of Health can manage effective governance to make an efficient use of IT resources and budgets. This will help in achieving the Millennium Development Goals (MDGs) of the national health development: eliminating health services disparities and the barriers in accessing health services. In order to provide fast and mobile access to all related stakeholders, the Health Information System could be accessed through a smart phone, tablet, and the internet.

METHODOLOGY

We conducted the TOGAF phases to develop this research beginning with defining the architecture's needs and principles, the business process architecture, the application architecture, and the data architecture. During the preliminary phase, we interviewed hospital management of the inpatient, the outpatient, and the emergency services departments in three public hospitals to obtain information regarding their architecture needs, required principles, business processes, and information systems. The business

Figure 5. The Future Plan of the Enterprise Architecture Model of the Indonesian Health Information System

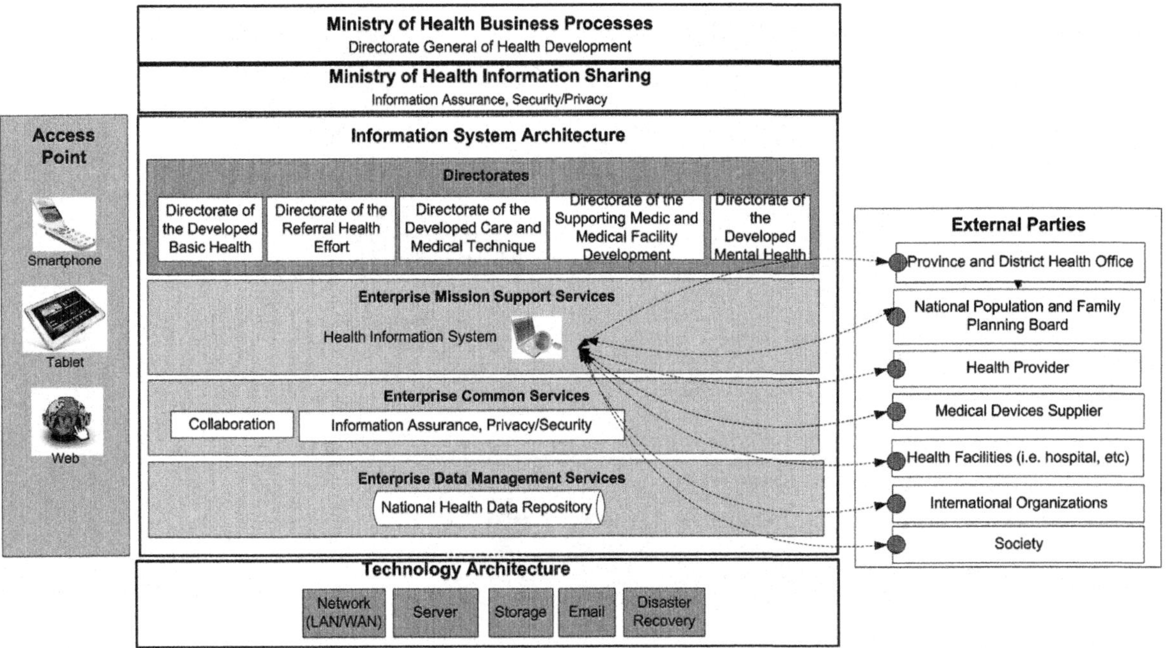

processes mapping for the inpatient, outpatient, and emergency services was completed by reviewing the current operations performed by the hospitals' administration and then confirmed by the guidelines issued by the Directorate of the Referral Health Effort of the Ministry of Health. The interview results and our document analysis were then formulated in swim-lane flowcharts in order to depict the hospitals' basic business processes. Then, the data catalog and the main service class diagram were formulated based on those basic processes.

Regarding to the Indonesian Healthcare System, the artifacts yielded from this research are as follows:

1. **Architecture Principles, Vision, and Requirements Phase:** Hospitals' value chain, architecture principles, list of actors, business needs, problems and solutions
2. **Business Architecture Phase:** Hospitals basic business processes, use of case diagrams of the hospitals' basic services
3. **Information System Phase:** Data catalog, class diagrams for the hospitals' basic services

Data Collection Procedure

This research was a qualitative research study using in-depth interviews and case studies. The interviews were conducted from January to August of 2014 with eleven people from the management department of three public hospitals. The three public hospitals were chosen as case studies in this research because: (1) they had high scores for the national accreditation assessment, (2) they had partially implemented the Hospital Information System, and (3) they were public hospitals with several facilities and services. In addition, to understand the national and international health regulations and procedures, additional interviews were conducted with experts from the Directorate of the Referral Health Effort, the Directorate of the Supporting Medic and the Medical Facility Development (*Direktorat Bina Pelayanan Penunjang Medik dan Sarana Kesehatan*), the Center for Data and Information (*Pusat Data dan Informasi*) and a representative from the World Health Organization (WHO) in Indonesia.

Instruments

Interviews with all respondents included open-ended questions. The questions were related to the hospitals' business processes and organizational structures, current IT-related problems, existing information system, and their expectations for the Hospital Information System development.

RESULTS

Respondent Demographics

The respondents consisted of the management personnel from one government public hospital, i.e., the Head of the Health Information Management Installation, the Deputy Chief of Emergency Nursing, the Head of the Hospital Management Information System, and the Deputy Chief of the General Inpatient section A, and two government district public hospitals, i.e., the Deputy Director of Services, the Head of the Hospital Management Information System, two Heads of the Medical Record Sub Division, the Head of the Emergency Unit, and two Heads of the Inpatient Rooms. The respondents were selected due to their expertise and experience in hospital management and the hospital information system. In addition, to understand the national and international health regulations and procedures, the interview processes involved four experts from the Ministry of Health, i.e., one expert from the Directorate of the Referral Health Effort, two experts from the Directorate of Supporting Medic and Medical Facility Development, one expert from the Center for Data and Information, and one representative from the World Health Organization (WHO) in Indonesia.

Information System Architecture Design

Defining Architecture's Vision, Principles, and Needs

The business value chain analysis introduced by Michael Porter in 1985 is used to describe activities that an organization performs and links them to the organization's competitive position. According to Porter, activity is divided into primary and support activities (Porter, 1985). Primary activities are directly concerned the creation or delivery of a product or service. Each of these activities is linked and supported by support activities to improve an organization's effectiveness or efficiency. Primary activities can be grouped into the areas of logistics, operations, service, marketing, and sales. The main areas of support activities are related to procurement, technology development, human resource management, and infrastructure.

According to Porter's value chain, organization activity is divided into primary and support activities. The primary activities include the activities undertaken to provide high quality health care to the patients, which includes patient registration, medical care, medical care support (i.e., laboratory and radiology), medical records management, inventory management, payment, and customer service. These primary activities are supported by marketing, nutrition, finance, human resource management, waste management, pharmacy, information technology, and research and education. Moreover, to achieve excellent health services, the primary activities should be supported by the Hospital Information System. Figure 6 describes the hospital value chain.

Based on the interviews and observations conducted in one government public hospital and two government district public hospitals, it can be observed that the government public hospital and one of

Figure 6. Hospital Value Chain

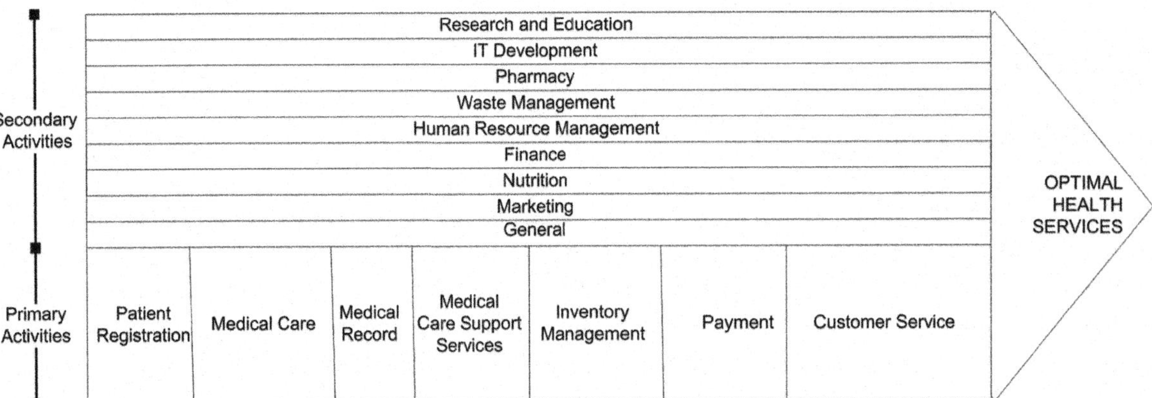

the government district public hospitals did not yet have an integrated Hospital Information System, but they did already have an IT unit and an IT manager as well as an adequate IT infrastructure and IT human resources. The other government district public hospital had implemented the Hospital Information System partially in the registration and billing modules but still did not have an IT unit, an IT manager, a sufficient IT infrastructure, or adequate IT human resources.

Based on the results of the interviews conducted in the hospitals regarding implementing the Hospital Information System, the business principles, the data principles, the application principles, and the technology principles required by the hospitals can be seen in Table 1.

Based on the identification of the hospitals' business activities from the interviews, the architecture principles and needs can be identified as the human actors and the basic business requirements required to implement the Hospital Information System. The basic business needs should be aligned primarily with the needs of the Ministry of Health as the national health policy maker. After mapping each actor to its business need, each problem is identified for each actor, and then each of the corresponding solutions is proposed to achieve the improvement target. Table 2 describes the mapping between the actors, the identification of business needs, the problems, and the proposed solutions.

Table 1. Defining Architecture Principles

Principle	Statement	Rationale	Implication
Business	5. Sustainability of excellent health care	Management can create policies for all major services to make the flow of information run smoothly, accurately, and in an integrated manner	If these policies have been formalized, the functions of each unit will work effectively and efficiently and will not interfere with the health services provided
	6. Service-oriented	The development of information technology-oriented architecture services can further facilitate the exchange of information between relevant stakeholders	Application developed and adapted to the business processes associated with it
	7. Comply with applicable laws	Organizational policies and business processes are executed following the rules and policies applicable	The management policy of the organization, data, and information technology must follow the rules of applicable law
	8. IT responsibility	The existence of IT managers in the organizational structure that is responsible for IT implementation activities	IT Unit is responsible for managing applications that support hospital business processes
Data	3. Data is an asset	The design of the data architecture must be able to see the data needs from the operator level to the management level	The existence of a data manager responsible for the availability of data
	4. Ease of data access	Authorization of data access rights for each user to respond quickly and maintain the data security	Information widely accessible, accurate and integrated
Application	3. Technology independence	Architecture development involving multiple platforms can prevent hospitals from depending on one particular party	Choosing a platform that can support interoperability
	4. Ease of use	Applications should be used easily by the user and involve users in the development of such applications	The design of user interface and displayed information provided by the application is easy to use and the information provided by the application is easily understood
Technology	2. Changes based on needs	Changes in IT should be done in response to hospital business needs	The need for IT planning that is aligned with future business planning

Table 2. Catalog of Actors, Business Needs, Problems, and Solutions

Actor	Basic Business Needs	Problem	Solution
Patient	Viewing patient medical record summary	Patient access to medical records is limited	Providing a Hospital Information System to facilitate patient access to medical records
Admission	Manage patients' data profile	Patient profile data scattered in several units often resulting in duplicate patient data	Providing a unified registration process along with an integrated Hospital Information System
Health workers	• Manage data relating to the clinical aspects of the order on each unit of measure (e.g. able to place an order for a package of measures or laboratory) • Can be integrated with other modules that are interconnected such as medical records, billing, support (lab, radiology)	Order clinical measures cannot be done in an integrated way	Providing an integrated Hospital Information System
Cashier	Manage patient billing data	Patient billing data is scattered in related medical units	Providing an integrated Hospital Information System
Hospital management and external parties (e.g. Ministry of Health, Province and District Health Offices, Health Providers, Medical Device Suppliers, hospitals)	Viewing hospital performance report	Hospital performance data is scattered in related medical units	Implement best practice processes and a Hospital Information System

Business Architecture

The government public hospital business processes begin when the patients complete registration in each unit of the targeted service. The patients who experience an emergency based on the results of the medical examination and need further treatment must register in advance at emergency registration; however, if it is not an emergency, the patient can be admitted in the outpatient registration section for further examination. If the patient is determined by medical personnel to require intensive care hospitalization, the patient must register with inpatient admissions subject to settling the payment process on an outpatient basis. Once the registration process is completed, the medical staff will perform the necessary medical treatment for patients throughout the subsequent medical action that will be recorded in the patients' medical records. If a patient is declared cured by medical personnel, then the patient will be provided with a bill according to the type of services provided. Billing is merged in one application for emergency room and inpatient services. In other cases, billing is printed separately. The payment process will be conducted in accordance with the billing documents received by the patient. If the patient is covered by both private and government insurers, then billing will be done by the hospital and vice versa. A patient who pays in person is required to pay in full either in cash or using a debit/credit card.

Figure 7. Government Public Hospitals Basic Business Processes Flowchart

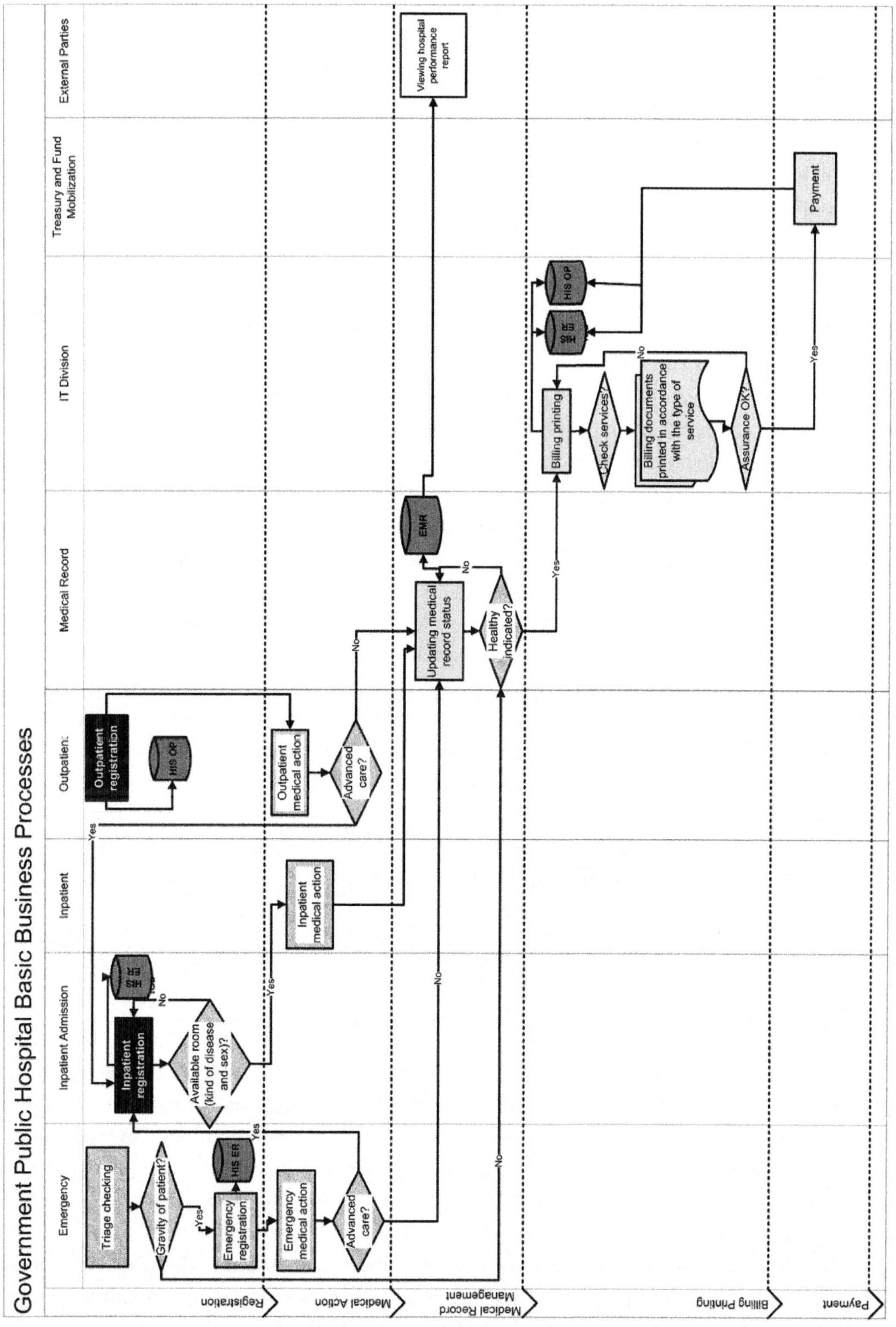

Currently, to support the business processes in government public hospitals (Figure **7**), there are three different applications where each application has functions to:

- Assist in the registration and management of billing for the inpatient and emergency department (Hospital Information System ER application)
- Assist in the registration and management of billing for the outpatient department (Hospital Information System ER application)
- Manage patient medical records (Hospital Information System OP application)

Based on Figure **7**, it can be seen that there are redundant processes carried out by more than one party and more applications involved in the current business processes in the department of central general state hospital. In addition, billing documents for all departments are still managed by IT unit.

On the other hand, one of the district general state hospitals had not implemented an integrated Hospital Information System and did not have an IT unit and adequate number of IT human resources as well as an adequate infrastructure. IT managers were in a sub-section of the Medical Records Department. The other district general state hospital had implemented an integrated Hospital Information System and had an IT unit in the finance department. In addition, these hospitals were supported by employees categorized as civil servants, regional honors (contract employee with a salary paid by the local government), and honor employees of the public service board (contract employee with a salary paid by the hospital).

According to the Head of Medical Records, there are still barriers in Hospital Information System implementation, such as lack of human resources in terms of both number and capacity (related workload) of the human resources for the use of a Hospital Information System. With the change of status as the Public Service Board in 2010 (PPID, 2013), according to the Deputy Speaker Services Director, the hospital must be able to independently obtain financing to support its operations, including paying salaries of honor employees of public service boards. Financial support from the local government is limited to the construction of facilities, such as buildings. In addition, as a referral hospital, the hospital may not refuse warranty patients, so the possibility of 'buddy' for inpatient cases to a higher class of service often cannot be avoided. Most patients who come to the government public hospitals are assurance patients. According to the way the payments are made by the patients, the patients served by this hospital are divided into cash and insurance patients (i.e., public and private social security, *Jaminan Kesehatan Masyarakat* [*Jamkesmas*] and *Jampersal* [extension of Jamkesmas], cooperation association with the company or factory and *Jamkesda*). Figure 8 shows the details of the basic business process services provided by government district public hospitals.

Government district public hospitals' basic services include emergency, outpatient, and inpatient services. As shown in Figure 8, the patients who come to the hospitals can receive these services. Patients who require emergency room services must first perform a triage examination to determine the severity of the patients' conditions. After that, the patients will receive medical treatment, and the patients must register as an emergency patient and are required to pay for administrative costs, physician services, and treatment. If the patients require medical personnel to undergo intensive treatment, the patients will complete inpatient registration.

Inpatient services require the patients to receive a room in accordance with the disease, gender, and economic circumstances of the patients. If a room is available, the patients are required to register for hospitalization. Medical treatment received by the patients will be recorded in the patients' medical record documents. If the patients are allowed to go home, they will then complete the payment, and the

Figure 8. Government District Public Hospitals' Basic Business Processes Flowchart

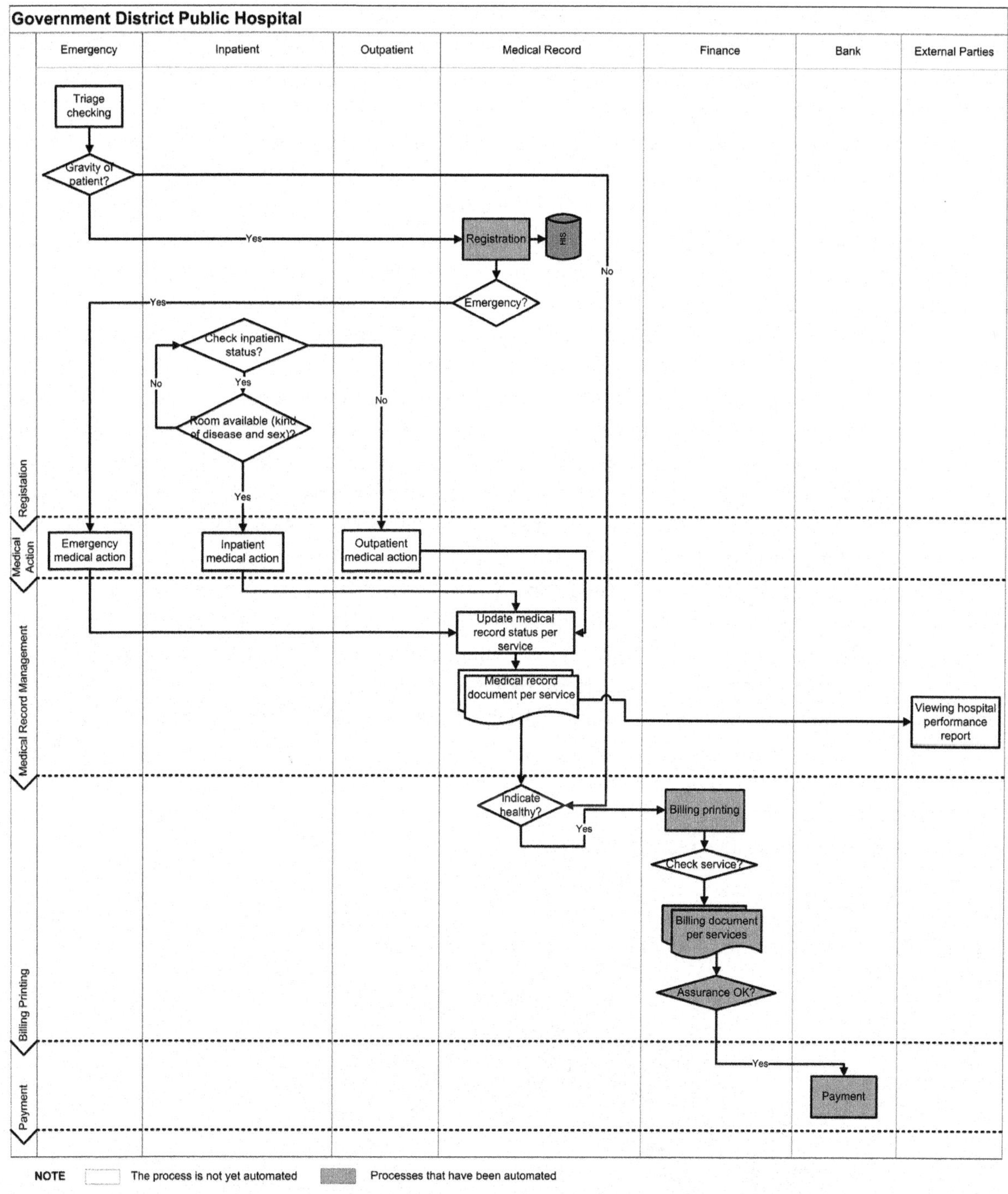

bill is printed. Outpatient services begin with patient registration. At the time of registration, the patients are required to pay for administrative costs, physician services, and medical treatment. After registering, the patients will receive medical treatment, and all medical treatments will be recorded in the patients' medical record documents. The information contained in the medical records is very important for hospital management to plan their healthcare facilities and services, conduct medical research, and to provide healthcare statistics to all required stakeholders. This designates medical record management as the center of integration between related units in the hospital. If the hospital is able to take care of a patient, the hospital should accept this patient for treatment; otherwise, this hospital should refer the patient to other hospitals, as stated in Figure 8.

Figure 7 and Figure 8 show that the hospitals' generic processes begin with the registration process performed in an integrated manner for the inpatient, the outpatient, and the emergency unit (Figure 9). There is only one registration process for the three basic services. Once the registration process is completed, the medical personnel will conduct the medical action/treatment according to the type and level of severity of the patient's condition. Then, all flow of activities performed by the medical personnel will be recorded automatically in the medical records of the patients. After the patient is declared healthy and discharged by the medical personnel, the billing process (printing) can be performed, and, subsequently, the payment process can be completed by the patient.

From a business standpoint, the registration process should be able to accommodate the three basic services. The same should hold for the billing process. Therefore, at the implementation level, it is possible that a bill for more than one service can be printed on one single billing document. In addition, the roles and responsibilities to manage the billing document should not be managed by the IT unit but should be managed by the finance unit performed by cashier and supported by the application. Therefore, this study proposes a generic business process flow as an end-to-end service to patients, as described in Figure 10.

A future business architecture formulated using a use case diagram can show the relationships between actors and the associated modules in the Hospital Information System (Figure 11). The data in the Hospital Information System can be processed, preferably automatically, to produce periodic reports for the Ministry of Health via the Hospital Reporting System. Reports that are required to be submitted through the reporting application are as follows (Bina Upaya Kesehatan, 2011):

1. Hospital profile data
2. Hospital health workers
3. Hospital service activities recapitulation data

Figure 9. Government Public Hospital Basic Services' Business Processes

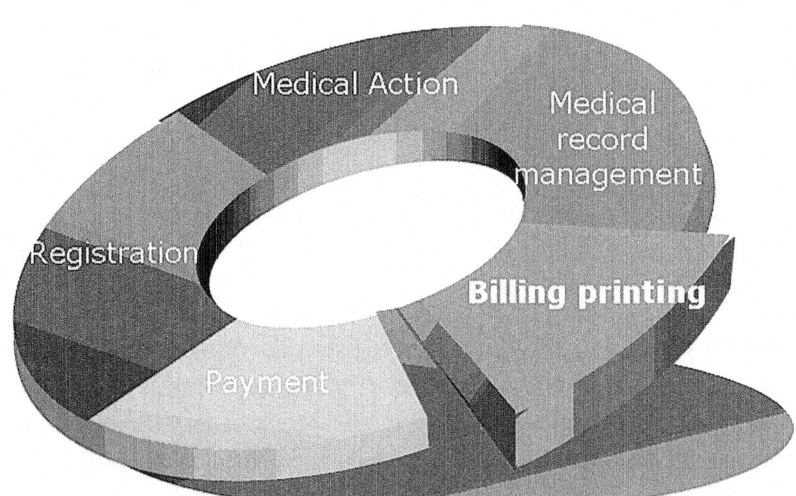

Figure 10. Proposed Government Public Hospitals' Basic Business Processes Flowchart

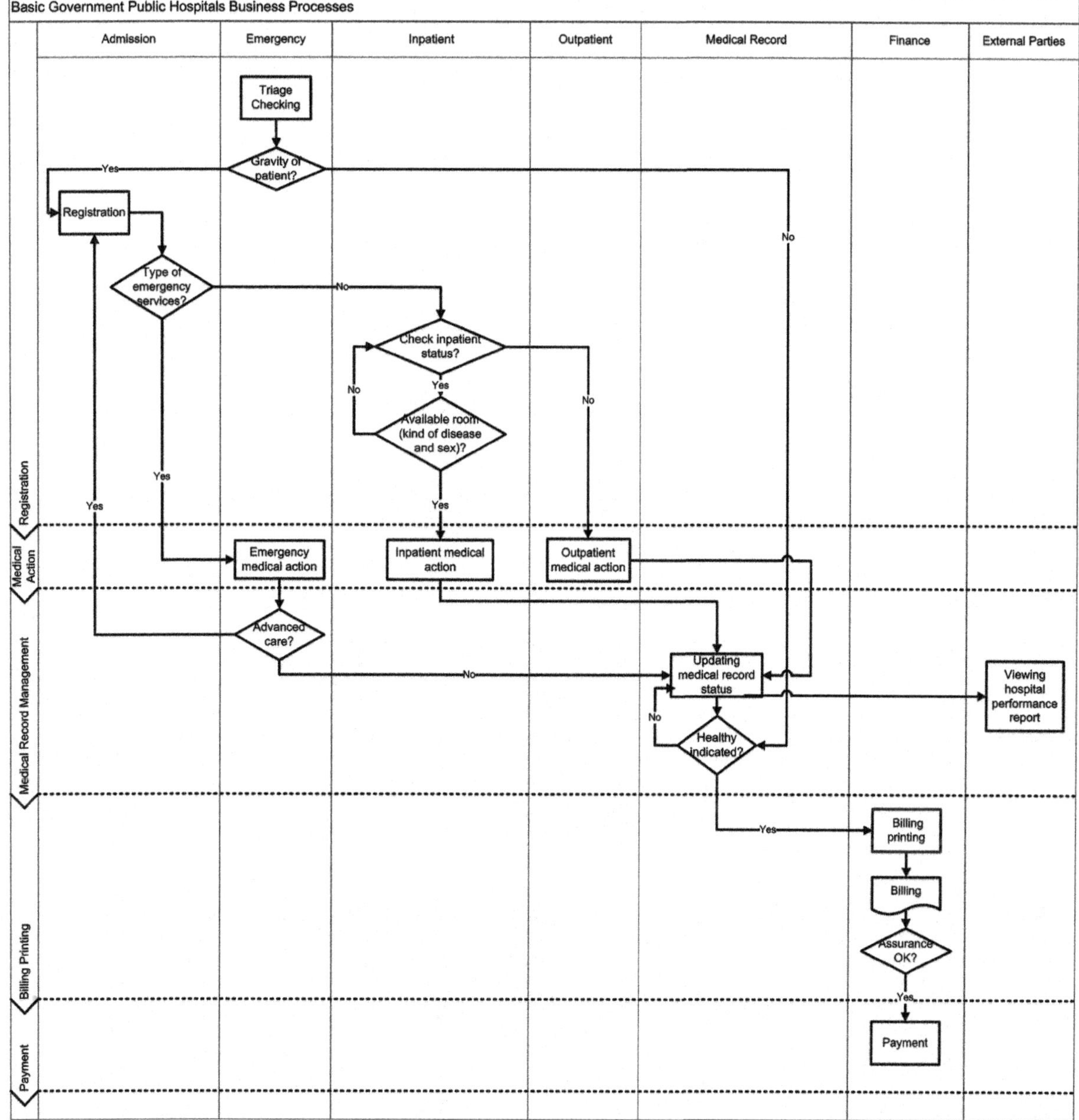

4. Disease/morbidity inpatients compilation data
5. Disease/morbidity outpatients compilation data.

Both the Ministry of Health and hospitals require the same data that can be provided by processes run by the hospitals. The medical record function may issue a summary of data related to the hospitals service activities and a compilation of diseases/morbidity for inpatients and outpatients. Details of data that should be prepared and automated by the hospitals can be seen in Table 3. Then, by analyzing and summarizing the medical record data, the external parties can access the hospitals' performance reports.

Figure 11. Government Public Hospital Basic Services' Use Case Diagram

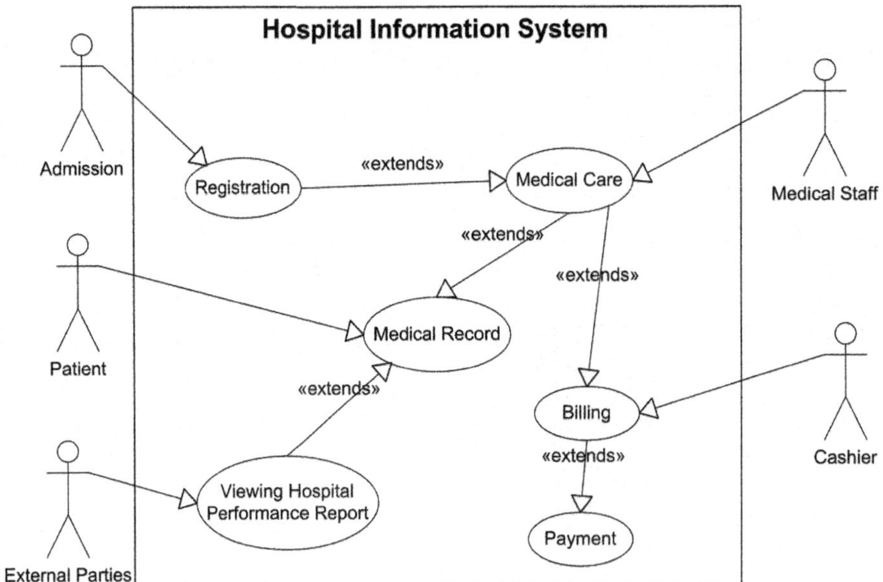

Table 3. Government Public Hospital Basic Services' Data Catalog

Process	Required Data Entity	By the Use of		
		Hospital	**Patient**	**Ministry of Health**
Registration	• Type of hospital • Emergency department facility • Facility per polyclinic • Facility per room • Disease type • Patient • Health workers	View the number of patient visits for each unit of service as well as a comparison of new and old patients	Managing the patient profile data	View the number of patient visits for each unit of service as well as a comparison of new and old patients
Medical Records	• Patient • Medical Records • Medical actions per emergency rooms • Medical action per inpatient rooms	Overall summary of patient medical record data can be processed to see indicators of hospital services, the activities of each unit of service, state of inpatient morbidity / road	Viewing medical record summary	Overall summary of patient medical record data can be processed to see indicators of hospital services, the activities of each unit of service, state of inpatient morbidity / road
Billing	• Patient • Billing	Overall summary of data can be processed to see billing statistics and payment methods of patients	Looking at the data transactions made while undergoing treatment	Overall summary of data can be processed to see billing statistics and payment methods of patients

Information System Architecture

Information system architecture can be designed by defining the data architecture and the application architecture with the required modules of the Hospital Information System to support the hospitals' operations services. Data architecture defines various types and sources of data needed to support the business process needs of the hospitals, the Ministry of Health, and the patients. As shown in Figure 9, each process requires several data in order to complete the hospital business processes (Table 3). The data are maintained by the corresponding business functions, such as admissions or registration staff, medical staff, and billing staff. The registration staff require data such as type of hospital, emergency department facility, facility per polyclinic, facility per room, disease type, patient profile, and health workers in order to generate reports of the number of patient visits for the hospital and to view the patient profile data and the summary of patient visits for certain hospitals in several periods, which is needed by the Ministry of Health. Next, the medical staff (in this case the steward of health data is the medical record staff) needs personal patient data, medical records, medical actions per emergency room, and medical actions per inpatient rooms in order to provide reports of the overall summary of patient medical records to identify the indicators of the hospitals' services, the activities of each unit of services, and the state of the inpatient morbidity/road, which is required by the hospitals and the Ministry of Health. The finance (billing) staff manages patient and billing data in order to view the summary of the billing statistics (including the payment methods) required by the hospitals and the Ministry of Health.

The health master data (e.g., patient, health workers, and disease types) as well as transaction data (e.g., billing and medical record) should be easily accessible by the emergency, the inpatient and the outpatient medical staff. The emergency, inpatient, and outpatient staff operate their facilities and administer medical actions that are conducted in their units. The data required by each major service units can be seen in Figure 12. The data sharing mechanism is conducted by defining the scope of common or shared data/information in the enterprise level and in the unit level. Sharing data can be easily done when there is a single repository accessible, e.g., through web services.

Finally, in order to describe the connectivity between data entities, a class diagram will be used (Figure 13). Figure 13 shows that patient data should be linked with medical activity data along with the facilities and the related health personnel. The data will be aggregated into a patient medical record entity. Some hospitals still separate the patients' medical records for emergency, inpatient, and outpatient activities. The billing entity will take the information from patients' medical records.

In accordance with the hospital's basic business processes that require a particular end-to-end process, the registration, the medical action, the medical record management, the billing, and the payment process, hospitals are required to implement Hospital Information System modules that at least consist of:

- **Registration Module:** Supports the integrated registration, scheduling, and queuing process for inpatient, outpatient, and emergency room departments
- **Order Communication System (OCS) Module:** Assists medical staff in performing medical procedures that need to be performed according to the disease suffered by the patient. This module involves the medical record module and other supporting modules, such as laboratory and radiology.
- **Medical Records Module:** Manages patient medical records (patient identification and numbering, patient's diagnose and procedure)
- **Billing Module:** Supports the process of calculating and printing the bill (billing) and payments (payment) made by the patient
- **Emergency, Inpatient and Outpatient Unit Module:** Support the activities in the emergency, inpatient, and outpatient medical departments

Figure 12. Primary Data for Government Public Hospitals' Basic Services

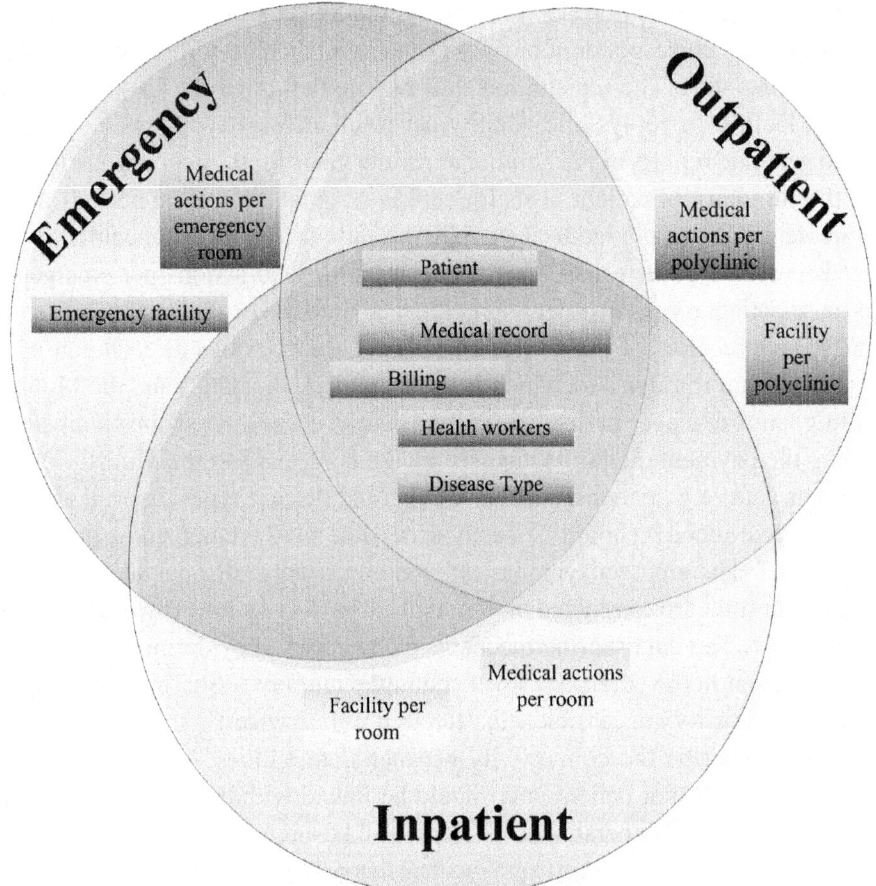

These modules are the core modules to support other hospital activities, making it easier for hospital management and staff to obtain and provide integrated and accurate data/information. Moreover, the best results could be achieved if the modules could also be integrated with other hospital modules and/or applications and health devices. Figure 14 depicts the integrated hospital information system architecture.

As shown in Figure 14, the integration point between hospitals and the external parties is located in the central integration modules, which are the billing, medical records, order communication system, referrals, and research and development modules. The integration between hospitals and the external parties can be performed using technologies such as service-oriented architecture, enterprise application integration technologies, and electronic data interchange. The information system architecture should also be supported by a technology architecture, such as the health communication standard (i.e. HL7, DICOM, CCOW), that is commonly used in the health care domain, network, server, storage, email, and disaster recovery. HL7 (Health Level Seven) and DICOM (Digital Imaging and Communications in Medicine) mainly support data integration, while CCOW (Clinical Context Object Workgroup) enables contextual integration (Winter, et al., 2011). Finally, in order to provide broad and fast access to all related stakeholders, the Hospital Information System could be accessed through smart phones, tablets, and the internet.

Figure 13. Government Public Hospital Basic Services' Class Diagram

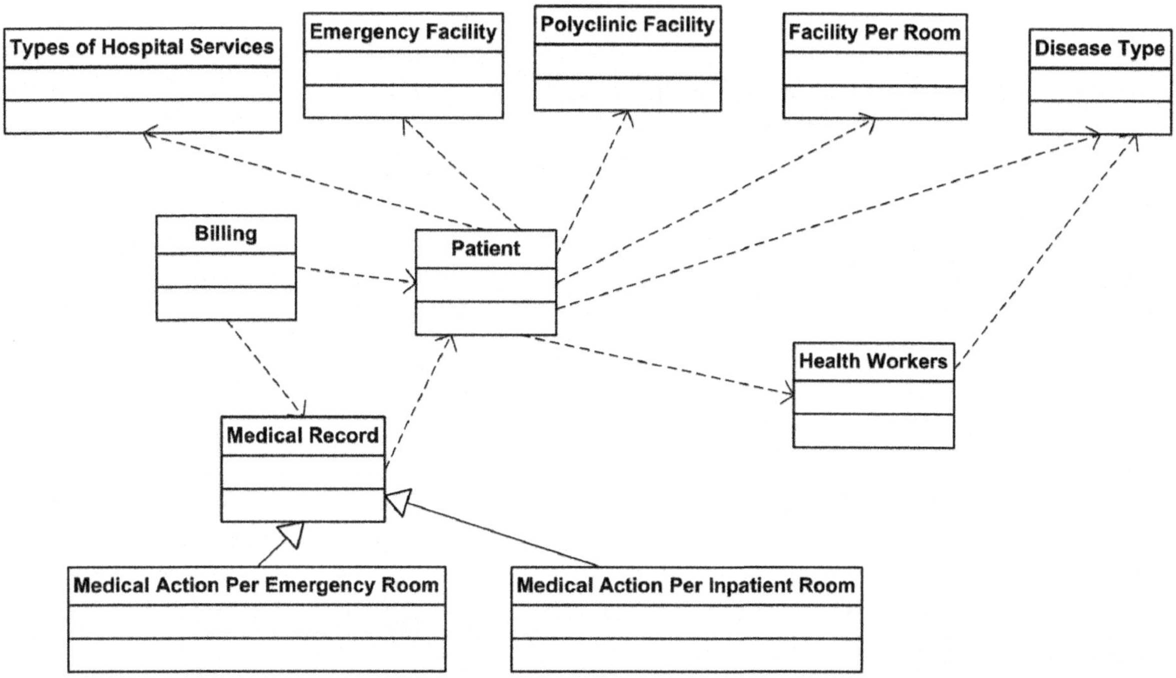

Figure 14. Government Public Hospital Information System Architecture

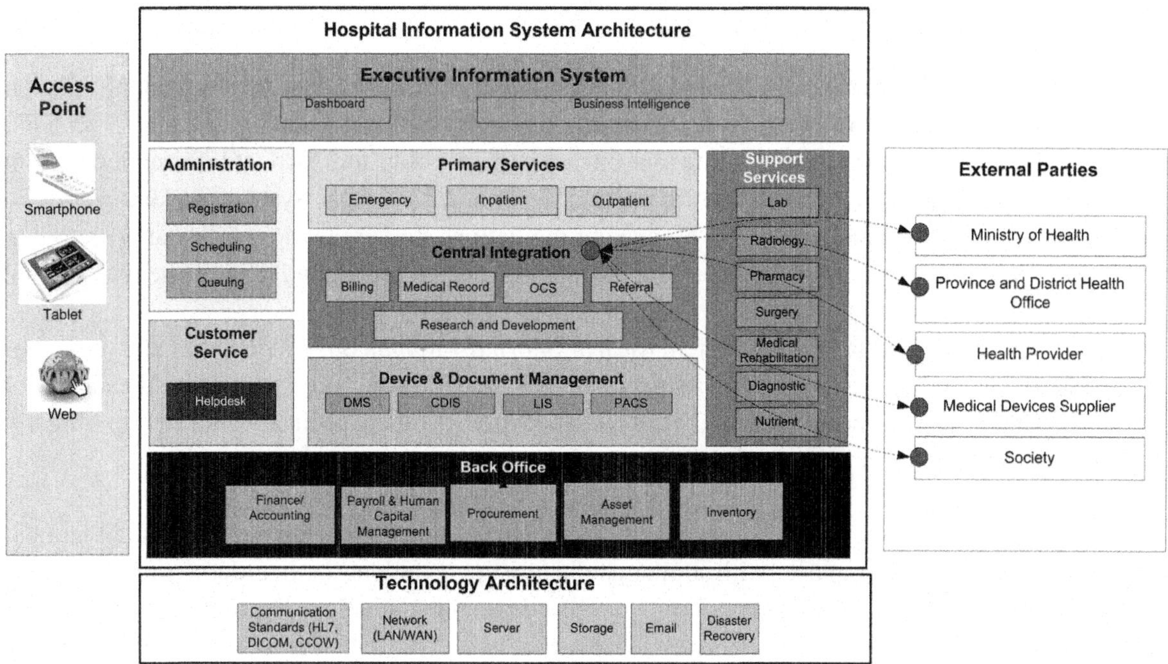

IMPLICATIONS

In order to implement an integrated hospital information system architecture, hospitals should assess their current business processes and applications. Based on existing processes and application assessments, hospitals could map their existing processes and applications using Figure 14. This research shows that hospitals have basic processes from the administration to the payment process in the emergency, inpatient, and outpatient units, so hospitals could adopt the information system architecture in Figure 14 for administration, primary services, and central integration modules. Other modules could be implemented according to the needs and characteristics of the hospital. Finally, in order to successfully implement this architecture, hospitals should be able to integrate the Hospital Information System with other related stakeholders (e.g., health care providers, medical device suppliers, and Ministry of Health).

In addition, based on the study by Handayani et al. (2014) and our analysis, the recommendations for the Ministry of Health are as follows:

1. The Ministry of Health needs to formulate IT governance policies for the hospitals so that the hospitals can define the position of the IT unit as well as the position of IT management and IT staff, including their career paths. This policy is required so that the hospital IT management can be well-integrated as part of the complete hospital management and can provide accountable support for the hospital operations.
2. The Ministry of Health needs to create a data dictionary (adjusted to the needs of health indicators and data/information for each unit in the Ministry of Health) and a standardized data exchange format that can support all platforms/technology to process the necessary data exchange between hospitals and the Ministry of Health. This is essential in order to support the integration of national e-health.
3. The Ministry of Health needs to compose an enterprise architecture guideline for Hospital Information System implementation, especially to help hospitals with limited IT budgets.
4. The Ministry of Health needs to create relevant assessment points for Hospital Information System implementations. This can be done by adding Hospital Information System implementation to the hospital accreditation criteria or by making regulations stating that hospitals that wish to join *BPJS - Kesehatan* programs (Health Social Security Agency) are required to implement a Hospital Information System.
5. The current Hospital Reporting System (*Sistem Informasi Rumah Sakit- SIRS*) has not yet implemented the validation and verification function. This function is required to improve the quality of data. The standard validation and verification procedure should be set in advance by the Ministry of Health to guide the process of validation and verification.

In principle, this hospital information system architecture could also be implemented in other hospitals in other developing countries with similar characteristics as Indonesia. In order to implement this architecture, there are several points that should be considered for adaptation. The architecture principle (Table 1) and the catalog of actors, business needs, problems, and solutions (Table 2) are relatively general, so it can be directly reused. If there is an additional constraint specific to the local context, e.g., in some countries, patient privacy is explicitly and strictly regulated, the principles and catalog can be easily extended to accommodate the issue. Second, since the business processes in this architecture are based on the referral system in Indonesia, specific referral systems should be examined and adjustments should be made regarding the health process (in the business architecture), the information flows, and the health data catalog (in the information system architecture, e.g., Table 3) within the architecture to formulize the appropriate business and information system architecture.

FUTURE RESEARCH DIRECTIONS

In order to design a complete enterprise architecture, future research should be conducted to define the information technology layers and to develop a hospital data dictionary. Other research that should be conducted in the future should focus on identifying the non-technical issues to increase awareness of their biggest impacts on the success of IT projects.

Theoretical Significance

Enterprise Architecture is one of the best practices that is currently widely used by the organization as a guideline to design IT architecture and logic structure, to organize complex information, and to address IT/IS and business needs (Sajid & Ahsan, 2014). TOGAF could be utilized to describe the organizational enterprise architecture because it provides guidelines to design, evaluate, and build the suitable architecture for an enterprise/organization. Until now, most healthcare organizations have not been aware and thus have not utilized enterprise architecture for their IT planning purposes.

This study shows that enterprise architecture, especially TOGAF, which provides quite extensive references, can be partially adopted to provide guidance for developing integrated information technology architecture to support hospitals' basic activities, namely the emergency unit, the inpatient unit, and the outpatient unit activities. The following steps and its corresponding artifacts of TOGAF utilized in this study are as follows: (1) Defining Architecture Principles, Vision, and Requirements (artifacts: architecture principle and value chain); (2) Defining Business Architecture (artifacts: catalog of actors, business needs, problems, and solutions); and (3) Defining Information Systems Architecture (artifacts: flowcharts, use case diagrams, data catalogs, information system architecture).

CONCLUSION

Hospitals are a public entity and therefore should provide optimal services to patients and other related stakeholders. Thus, hospitals should be encouraged to define their Information Technology (IT) standards and policies and subsequently implement health applications (e.g., Hospital Information System). One of the best practices that is widely used in the industry is Enterprise Architecture. Enterprise Architecture can provide guidance for developing integrated information system architecture, especially to support hospitals' basic activities from patient registration to the payment process. In order to develop a suitable enterprise architecture, hospitals should follow several required architecture principles related to business (i.e., sustainability of excellent health care, service-oriented environment, compliance with applicable laws, and IT responsibility), data (i.e., data as an asset and ease of data access), application (i.e., technology independence and ease of use), and technology (i.e., changes based on needs). The responding actors involved in the Hospital Information System are (1) the admission staff, which is responsible for the registration process; (2) the patients who wish to view a summary of their medical records; (3) the medical staff, which manages the patients' records; (4) the cashiers, who manage billing transactions; and (5) hospital management and external parties (i.e., health providers and the public) who wish to view hospital performance reports. Finally, to make hospital operations run efficiently and effectively, hospitals should at least implement the following IT application modules: registration, an order communication system, medical records, and payment.

ACKNOWLEDGMENT

We express our gratitude to the Directorate General of Higher Education for the *Program Penelitian Unggulan Perguruan Tinggi* (PUPT) Grant No. 1025/H2.R12/HKP.05.00/2014 and Universitas Indonesia for the continuous support particularly for the Directorate of Research and Community Engagement. Moreover, we would like to gratefully acknowledge the insightful contribution from Dr. R. Noviane Chasny, a Health Management Information Officer of the World Health Organization (WHO) Country Office for Indonesia.

REFERENCES

Bina Upaya Kesehatan Kementerian Kesehatan, R. I. (2011, November 8). *Juknis Sistem Informasi Rumah Sakit (SIRS) 2011*. Retrieved from www.buk.depkes.go.id

Bina Upaya Kesehatan Kementerian Kesehatan, R. I. (2013). *Ditjen BUK Sosialisasikan SIMRS Generik Open Source*. Retrieved from http://buk.depkes.go.id/index.php?option=com_content&view=article&id=376:ditjen-buk-sosialisasikan-simrs-generik-open-source&catid=1:latest-news

Costetchi, N., Danila, C., & Stanescu, A. M. (2014). Enterprise System Architecture to Sustain Cross-Domain e-Healthcare Applications. In Enterprise Interoperability VI (pp. 271-281). Springer International Publishing. doi:10.1007/978-3-319-04948-9_23

Dennis, S. (2010). IS World, 2003. *Journal of International Technology*.

Handayani, P. W., Hidayanto, A. N., Sandhyaduhita, P. I., Pinem, A. A., Fajrina, H. R., & Trisnanty, I. A. K. (2014). Critical Success Factors in Implementing Hospital Information System in Indonesia: Case Study Public Hospitals. In *Proceedings of the International Conference for Diversity, Technology and Innovation for Operational Competitiveness* (TIIM). Academic Press.

Haux, R. (2006). Health information systems- past, present, future. *International Journal of Medical Informatics*, 75(3-4), 268–281. doi:10.1016/j.ijmedinf.2005.08.002 PMID:16169771

Health Metrics Network. (2008). Retrieved from http://www.who.int/healthmetrics/library/countries/HMN_KEN_Assess_Final_2008_06_en.pdf

IEEE. (2000). *IEEE Recommended Practice for Architectural Description of Software Intensive Systems*. IEEE Std 1471- 2000.

Jensen, C. T., Cline, O., & Owen, M. (2011, March). *Combining Business Process Management and Enterprise Architecture for Better Business Outcomes*. IBM Redbook.

Kabupaten Bogor, P. P. I. D. (2013). *Profil RSUD Cibinong*. Retrieved from Pejabat Pengelola Informasi dan Dokumentasi (PPID) Kabupaten Bogor: http://ppid.bogorkab.go.id/?site=27

Kementrian Kesehatan, R. I. (2011, November 10). *Pertemuan Koordinasi Teknis IT Dalam Rangka E-Health*. Retrieved from http://buk.depkes.go.id/index.php?option=com_content&view=article&id= 224:pertemuan-koordinasi-teknis-it-dalam-rangka-e-health

Lange, M., & Mendling, J. (2011). An Experts' Perspective on Enterprise Architecture Goals, Framework Adoption and Benefit Assessment. *15th IEEE International Enterprise Distributed Object Computing Conference Workshops (EDOCW)*. Helsinki: IEEE.

Lu, X., Duan, H., Li, H., Zhao, C., & An, J. (2005). The Architecture of Enterprise Hospital Information. *Proceeding of the 2005 IEEE Engineering in Medicine and Biology 27th Annual Conference*, (pp. 6957-6960). IEEE.

McSweeney, A. (2000). *Enterprise Architecture and TOGAF*. The Open Group Architecture Framework.

National Institutes of Health. (2011, November 8). *Benefits of Enterprise Architecture*. Retrieved from https://enterprisearchitecture.nih.gov/Pages/BenefitsEnterpriseArchitecture.aspx

Niemi, E. (2006). Enterprise Architecture Benefits: Perceptions from Literature and Practice. *Proceedings of the 7th IBIMA Conference Internet & Information Systems in the Digital Age*. IBIMA.

Petroudi, D., & Giannakakis, N. (2011). New Technologies in Hospital Information System. In Clinical Technologies: Concepts, Methodologies, Tools and Applications, (pp. 2029-2034). IGI Global. doi:10.4018/978-1-60960-561-2.ch801

Porter, M. E. (1985). *Competitive advantage: creating and sustaining competitive performance*. New York: The Free Press.

Pusat Data dan Informasi Kementerian Kesehatan RI. (2012). *Roadmap Sistem Informasi Kesehatan tahun 2011-2014*. Jakarta: Kemenkes RI.

Rawabdeh, A. A. A. (2007). An E-health Trend Plan for the Jordanian Health Care System. *International Journal of Health Care Quality Assurance*, *20*(6), 516–531. doi:10.1108/09526860710819459 PMID:18030969

Rood, M. A. (1994). Enterprise Architecture: Definition, Content, and Utility. *Proceedings of the IEEE Third Workshop on Enabling Technologies: Infrastructure for Collaborative Enterprises*, (pp. 106-111). IEEE.

Sajid, M., & Ahsan, K. (2014). Enterprise Architecture for Healthcare Organizations. *World Applied Sciences Journal*, *30*(10), 1330–1333.

TOGAF 9.1. (2013). Retrieved from http://pubs.opengroup.org/architecture/togaf9-doc/arch/index.html

Winter, A., Haux, R., Ammenwerth, E., Brigl, B., Hellrung, N., & Jahn, F. (2011). *Health Information System Architectures and Strategies*. London: Springer-Verlag London Limited. doi:10.1007/978-1-84996-441-8

Winter, R., & Fischer, R. (2007). Essential Layers, Artifacts, and Dependencies of Enterprise Architecture. *Journal of Enterprise Architecture*, 1-12.

World Health Organization. (2001). *Medical Records Manual A Guide for Developing Countries*. World Health Organization.

World Health Organization. (2011, November 8). *Key Components of a Well-Functioning Health System*. Retrieved from http://www.who.int/healthsystems/EN_HSSkeycomponents.pdf

Chapter 14

Lessons Learned from the Implementation of an Emergency Department Information System

Paraskevas Vezyridis
University of Nottingham, UK

Stephen Timmons
University of Nottingham, UK

Heather Wharrad
University of Nottingham, UK

ABSTRACT

Clinical information systems are increasingly used in emergency departments across the English National Health Service. The implementation outcome is unpredictable and success is not guaranteed. This study identifies facilitating social and technical factors for implementing an Emergency Department Information System. This is a qualitative study, using interviews with 28 emergency department clinicians, administrators and managers. Project management documents, user guides, design blueprints and internal reports were also analysed. Lessons learned include the importance of acquiring an established, customised and user-friendly system, attracting funding, establishing communication channels between stakeholders, developing detailed implementation plans and tailored training programmes, investing in peer-support, and analysing the workflow impact of the system. Socio-technical factors, both in and out of the hospital, influenced the success of the implementation. By being systematic in addressing these socio-technical factors certain implementation barriers can be overcome.

INTRODUCTION

Emergency departments (EDs) require sophisticated information technology (IT) for managing their complex operations. Despite a rather low adoption rate (Landman, Bernstein, Hsiao, & Desai, 2010),

DOI: 10.4018/978-1-4666-9446-0.ch014

introducing such clinical information systems can assist EDs in the provision of quality care (Aronsky, Jones, Lanaghan, & Slovis, 2008). EDs are thus well equipped to improve their efficiency (Baumlin & Richardson, 2006) through more accurate forecasting of demand and better resource allocation (Stuart, 2004). This is particularly true as patient volume, crowding and acuity continue to rise (Shapiro et al., 2010), whilst the number of inpatient beds decreases (Baumlin et al., 2010).

However, the outcome of the implementation of a clinical information system in practice is often unpredictable and success is not always guaranteed. Even in cases where failure in the process of deploying a system is attributed to specific technical inconsistencies or deficiencies, there are always issues and parameters outside the sphere of influence of IT staff that need to be considered; issues that are rooted in the organisation or in the surrounding social environment in which the system is designed to operate (Berg, 1998). There is also the issue of time. Hillestad et al. (2005) assert, for example, that for a system to prove its efficiency a widespread adoption is required. Only after a certain period of time, process changes, and resource reduction will the potential cost effectiveness or quality improvements become clear. Thus, it is necessary to consider both technology and the organisation as concepts that intertwine with one another to produce something new. Despite technology's capacity to act as an agent for change, organisational change is often a prerequisite for the deployment of new technologies (Grimson & Grimson, 2002). This is because it is the established organisational norms and values that provide the context of this interaction and, often, determine the outcome of the implementation (Berg, 2001).

In this chapter, the authors attempt to contribute to an increasing body of knowledge around the lessons that can be learned from these types of programmes. They studied an Emergency Department Information System (EDIS) for patient registration and tracking in an ED of a large University NHS hospital in England: the first clinical information system that was successfully implemented under the National Programme for Information Technology (NPfIT). They have previously identified clinical users' initial reactions and interacting concerns with EDIS (Vezyridis, Timmons, & Wharrad, 2012). Here, by adopting a qualitative approach, based on interviews and document analysis, the study evolved around the identification and analysis of the *wider* social, technical, economic and policy factors, conditions and processes that have impacted upon its initial diffusion. The particular research questions were:

- Why was this particular system selected for deployment? Was the selection of this system internal or external to the organisation process?
- How was this project initiated and how did this implementation proceed?
- What are the practical lessons that can be learned from this implementation?

BACKGROUND

Emergency Department Information Systems

First pioneered in Australia in 1994 (New South Wales Department of Health [NSW DH], 1998), Emergency Department Information Systems can provide EDs with computing capabilities for electronic *registration* and *triage*, real-time patient flow and care *tracking*, *charting* (time-stamped patient care documentation and continuity, remuneration, benchmarking and critical pathways), *referencing* (information about medications, interactions, diagnoses, treatments and best practices), *prescribing, order entry* and finally *discharging* (clinical and non-clinical information for discharge, follow-up instructions and recommendations) (DeWoody & Loadman, 1999; Righini, 2002; Rowe et al., 2006; Shapiro et al., 2010). A fully functional EDIS may also provide access to past medical history, follow-up notes and electronic imaging, transmission of prescriptions to pharmacies and decision support (Landman et al., 2010). Therefore, it can be used as an effective set of tools for managing workload, forecasting demand and allocating resources (Stuart, 2004); improving all aspects of care, from throughput and turnaround times (Weiner, Baumlin, & Shapiro, 2007) to satisfaction for patients and staff alike (Wiler et al., 2010).

In the US, the implementation and use of EDIS is thought to improve workflows with quick (3-6 months) return on investment (ROI) (Rogoski, 2002), particularly for cost savings (coding, dictation, transcription, paper use, medication errors) and revenue captures (charges, reimbursement, increased patient visits) (Fisher & Tibbs, 2003; Anderson, 2005). Other cost, time, performance and satisfaction benefits claimed (due to automation) include (Neal, 2003; Fisher & Tibbs, 2003; Garvie, 2004; Anderson, 2005; Bouchard, 2005; Berghoef, 2006):

- Elimination of illegible prescriptions, lost patient records, duplications and *bottlenecks*.
- Improved clinical documentation for patient registration and tracking.
- Increased time for direct patient care.
- Increased clinical accountability and improved evaluation of clinical performance.
- Improved patient data protection.
- Reduced average length of stay for patients and, increased patient satisfaction and staff morale.

Challenges and Barriers of EDIS Implementation

However, although these systems claim to reduce expenditures, by replacing the costly paper record with technology, few cost-benefit analyses are available in the market for purchasers to make evidence-based decisions (Milbank Memorial Fund, 2000). Their methods and outcome measures, and also the accuracy and completeness of the information they collect (Coonan, 2004), are often questionable (Wiler et al., 2010). Numerous studies have highlighted reasons why these and other clinical information systems, despite their supposed potential, have not been widely accepted or fully integrated into health systems around the world.

For example, there can be certain features of the system or certain characteristics of the hospital that may have a negative impact on the implementation, such as multiple departments within the hospital with different cultures and work practices, adequacy of communication between vendors and hospital managers, the financial circumstances of the hospital, performance ratings, existing information technology infrastructure and timetables for replacement of existing systems (Hendy, Reeves, Fulop, Hutchings, & Masseria, 2005). There are also issues of high cost, a lack of mature products, the complexity of the clinical setting, users' computer competence and data input that challenge their deployment (Burton, Anderson, & Kues, 2004; Hier, Rothschild, Lemaistre, & Keeler, 2005). Other studies have found perceived implementation costs for training, change management, loss of revenue, operational control, disruption to practice, negative impact on clinician-patient relationship and work pressure as substantial barriers to the computerisation of clinical tasks (for more see Johnston, Leung, Wong, Ho, & Fielding, 2002). Importantly, clinicians' data privacy concerns around security breaches and tampering of patients' records are thought to negatively impact adoption (Yoon, Chang, Kang, Bae, & Park, 2012; Inokuchi et al., 2014). Since most of these systems have been developed for the Anglophone healthcare IT market, the system's language has also been identified as a significant barrier (Inokuchi et al., 2013).

Especially in the user context, factors include age, gender and personality characteristics, specialty and experience, expectations and interests, computer literacy, emotions and attitudes towards health informatics and, commitment of clinical leadership (Young, 1984; Anderson, Jay, Schweer, & Anderson, 1986; Cork, Detner, & Friedman, 1998; O'Connell, Cho, Shah, Brown, & Shiffman, 2004). A lack of clarity amongst the users about the advantages of such systems has also been identified (Sujansky, 1998). These user aspects have been identified in several theories, such as the technology acceptance model (TAM), the unified theory of acceptance and use of technology (UTAUT), the innovation diffusion theory (IDT), the theory of planned behaviour (TPB) and the theory of reasoned action (TRA). However, as Najaftorkaman, Ghapanchi, Talaei-Khoei, & Ray (2014) note in their systematic literature review these theories, while they identify most of the *individual, psychological* and *behavioural* factors in healthcare IT adoption, they tend to ignore other, sometimes equally important, *financial* (start-up and on-going costs, ROI), *legal* (security, privacy, liability, policies and standards), *environmental* (job security, vendor efforts, prior experience), *organisational* (age, size and type of practice, experience, ownership, workflows) and *technical* (system customisability, reliability and usability) factors.

Other experts such as Eason (2005) assert that clinical information systems will be abandoned if a user-centred, local design approach is not rolled out. He goes on to suggest that only by understanding local ambitions, studying sociotechnical design, establishing local planning teams and constantly reviewing systems' implications and users' experiences can the system be saved from failure. The selection of an appropriate system relies heavily upon issues of intuitiveness, user-friendliness and comprehensiveness, in order to persuade users to input the data (Rogoski, 2002) as well as on the system's ability to be integrated to existing IT infrastructures (Neal, 2003). The majority of successful stories of implementing an EDIS refer to the need of establishing a strategic interdisciplinary committee, consisting of nurses, physicians, clerical staff, information technologists, finance officers and departmental administrators, for selecting the system and leading the change management (Bouchard, 2005; Anderson, 2005; Taylor, 2006; Berghoef, 2006; Wickramasinghe, Tumu, Bali, & Tatnall, 2007). From there, the transition to computing usually begins by marketing the system internally and preparing for big learning curves. This is achieved by a *phased implementation* (Wickramasinghe, et al. 2007), where modules and core components are gradually installed and integrated to the main system, providing staff with time to get accustomed to new workflows and developing competent *super users* for training, demonstrating and assisting the other users around the system (Garvie, 2004; Taylor, 2006).

METHODS

Case Study Profile

The study was conducted in the ED of a large university NHS hospital in England. It serves a local population of 650,000 and treats approximately 400 attendees per day (60% discharged, 25% admitted and 15% referred as outpatients). With around 14-18 nurses, 6-7 doctors and 6 emergency department assistants (EDAs), all of various grades and experience, on duty at any given time and across its six sections (Areas 1, 2 & 3, paediatric, X-ray and Emergency Nurse Practitioners' offices), it is now one of the busiest in the UK.

The EDIS studied was implemented in October 2004 through a *phased implementation* (Wickrama-singhe et al., 2007) and under the Projects in Controlled Environments (PRINCE2) integrated project management framework (Office of Government Commerce [OGG], 2012). Previously, patient registration was completed by clerical staff at the reception desk using the hospital's main Patient Administration System (PAS), while nurses and physicians were using a single, three-page, paper form to record and store observations, investigations, clinical notes and drug prescriptions. Now, after (the electronic) registration at the reception desk by EDAs, clinicians can use EDIS to enter triage details, observations, clinical notes, consultations, prescribed medicines and investigations, view alerts and track patients around the ED. This *first phase* of the implementation also involved the interfacing to the trolley wait system and to PAS as well as the rollout of the module for the production of General Practitioners (GPs) letters. For accessing EDIS, there are password-protected desktop terminals in each staff station, the reception desk, the Sisters' office and the doctors' writing room, while 13 wall-mounted workstations were installed inside the cubicles. The system's hardware requirements were scoped at 100-150 concurrent users.

Data Collection

Data were collected through semi-structured interviews (approximately 4.5 years after implementation), while potential participants were recruited via purposive, snowball sampling. The only selection criterion was that participants had started working in the ED for at least a year before the implementation of EDIS. Each interview was 30 minutes long on average (15 hours in total) and all but two of them were digitally audio-recorded. Participants were asked to recall and describe their experience with EDIS implementation. Written materials about the implementation were also examined, including; project management documents (implementation planning study, project initiation, site specific tasks, project review), user guides, reference manuals, business cases, paper forms, contingency plans, minutes, policy documents, and financial reports. In this way, views and assumptions from people closer to the implementation and from the organisational viewpoint were collected, while the project management documents contributed to an understanding of the organisational and professional context of the implementation process.

Data Analysis

These documents and the interview transcripts were then organised and analysed with the use of Computer Assisted Qualitative Data Analysis Software (QSR NVivo 8). Through a thematic analysis (Dixon-Woods, Agarwal, Jones, Young, & Sutton, 2005), prominent, recurrent and inclusive thematic categories were identified. Then, these thematic headings and coding categories were cross-referenced for relevance, consistency and relationships. Careful consideration was given so as not to exclude activities, processes or accounts that offer limited explanatory value, however semi-statistical constructions like *most of the users* were used as to highlight stronger and prevalent themes.

The study was approved by the local Research Ethics Committee. Participants were given an information sheet and individual written consent was obtained. Data were stored securely, and all findings reported anonymously.

FINDINGS

Participants

Twenty-eight participants (23 female and 5 male), mainly ED clinicians, were interviewed for this study: 1 system administrator, 1 change manager, 2 EDAs, 1 operational services coordinator, 4 ENPs, 4 charge nurses (NICs), 15 nurses of various grades and experience.

Lesson 1: Timing

This study highlights the importance of choosing the right moment when implementing EDIS. By this, we mean building and maintaining a positive momentum by converging the interests and commitment of relevant stakeholders (ED, ICT teams and vendor).

This includes being alert for IT procurement funding and waiting until the system of choice is available. Here, the hospital's clinical, operational and strategic management had been investigating systems for 4 years and had identified this EDIS as their system of choice. However, cost was prohibiting its acquisition. With the advent of the NPfIT, the ED was finally able to acquire the system free of charge and with adequate technical and legal support under the Local Service Providers (LSP) scheme (Brennan, 2005). Yet, contracts with the LSP were still under central negotiation and the rollout was not planned until the next year (2005). To overcome this obstacle, the hospital's Director of ICT had the NPfIT and the LSP to agree to a tactical early adoption of the system. Sometimes, however, this momentum can be strengthened further by new requirements imposed on the ED from outside the hospital. In this particular case, there were several additional requirements that acted as an impetus for this implementation, since:

- From January 2005, it had to formally report to the DH on waiting times and achieve the 4hr wait target (DH, 2004).
- At the same time, investigations, consultations, special treatments, diagnostics and admissions had to be accurately recorded for correct payments, under the Payments by Results (PbR) financial scheme.
- From 2005, the Commissioning Data Set (CDS) was being mandated.
- Each December-March, it always faces *winter pressures*.
- At the end of 2004, the vendor's time slot to fully concentrate on this implementation was expiring and no onsite support would have been available afterwards.

In addition, following specific recommendations by NHS Estates (2003; 2004), a major refurbishment of the ED had been completed one year before implementation. The department now featured 9 resuscitation bays, compared to the previous 4, and 26 adult treatment cubicles for minor and major illnesses/injuries, compared to the previous 12.

The department layout changed radically...it's compartmentalised so without EDIS I don't think the new actual department layout and accommodation would have been as practical and as useful as it is now.

Therefore, as the working environmental, clinical, service and informational needs of the department changed drastically, the use of a clinical information system became a necessity. In fact, a key factor in the acceptability of EDIS was that it challenged the efficacy of existing, hand-written, systems for time-sensitive information management. For example, the traditional whiteboard and the paper records have limited calculative and sharing capabilities, making it difficult to handle patient tracking with pen and paper or magnetic strips in an ED which had recently doubled its capacity to treat patients.

We'd always been keen to have a new system for the new department because we knew by expanding it physically it was going to become more difficult to manage it practically…we needed a new way of managing the information that we had about patients with all the targets that have come in since…

I suspect that if we had to go back to the whiteboard and relying on a nurse's memory as to where a patient was at any given time, I think we would soon start to see a lot more four hour breaches…actually being able to track times of patients to see how we are doing and where the weak points are, that's a big advantage.

By securing additional funding for hardware upgrades to support the new software, and by making this project a high priority for the hospital, in March 2004 a tight (6-month) timescale for the implementation of EDIS was set.

Lesson 2: Project Management

The EDIS was, at the time, quite popular within the NHS, with several hospitals having implemented it already[1]. This was important, as it had already been modified, to a certain extent, to NHS practice. Therefore, the hospital project team had the opportunity to visit other sites and learn from their experience. It also meant that the hospital did not have to spend additional resources on in-house development of EDIS.

However, the hospital did not have a desired plan of action for this implementation. The Implementation Planning Study (IPS), devised by the vendor in collaboration with the hospital's project team, provided this detailed plan of how the implementation should be organised, what each member of the team had to do and what tasks and actions had to be carried out. In particular, it defined objectives, scopes and benefits, personnel and resources, hardware and software requirements, training, delineation of roles and responsibilities as well as risks and contingencies. It was, therefore, well received by the hospital implementation team.

… the idea of an implementation planning study was absolutely spot on, it was brilliant, it's the sort of thing that I wish we adopted more in that for three days we lived and breathed how we were going to do EDIS.

From there, four implementation teams, each with a project manager, were established. One team from the vendor and one from the hospital were responsible for the implementation until the go-live date, with the other two (again, one from the vendor and one from the hospital) assuming their responsibilities after that day. The vendor and ED project managers were responsible for developing the project management documents so that a plan was agreed and followed by both teams. The ED project manager was responsible for measuring whether the project was managed successfully and that an acceptable product was delivered.

While the whole of implementation on the *shop floor* was organised by the project managers and the above two teams, a hospital project board dealt with the overall management of the project at a higher level. This board had the overall responsibility, accountability and authority to provide direction and management for the success of the project. It consisted of a *Senior User* (an ED Consultant), the *Senior Supplier* (the hospital's Director of ICT) and a *Project Sponsor* (Executive member of the hospital). This structure, by taking advantage of the rapid deployment of EDIS, was found to be beneficial in the development of direct communication channels and, therefore, of a better working relationship with the vendor.

Importantly, *Clinical Leads* had a fundamental role in the implementation of EDIS and in change management. The authors have previously reported that clinical users' initial reactions to EDIS implementation evolved around issues of technology integration and transition to paperless practices, computer-based information provision as well as issues of computer literacy and system availability (Vezyridis et al., 2012). The Clinical Leads, as experienced clinicians, constituted the link between the shop floor, the vendor of the system and the project board, representing users' views during project team meetings, communicating to the users the organisational and technical processes to be followed, while actively advocating and promoting the system's benefits among their more apprehensive colleagues. They were also involved in user training and support. Lastly, they provided the vendor with detailed departmental workflows so as to analyse the system's organisational impact and make it compatible with the department's work practices.

One of the key things that I did was almost like a patient process looking at where each of the patients would go through, which gave the software team an understanding of how our Department worked... Once the software had been installed ..we were then involved in setting up all the various EDIS pages and settings and entering various diagnostic codes and things like that, in conjunction with the ICT teams as well..

However, the more configurations the systems had to undergo the more likely it was for the project to hit difficulties with severe deployment delays. A balance had to be reached. In the end, it was decided that the two subsequent phases, with more advanced and site-specific modifications, (e.g. interfaces to other hospital main systems and departments) could be completed later (under a maintenance and support services agreement) as the users and the department acquired greater working knowledge of the system. The first crucial phase concentrated on EDIS basic capabilities for patient registration and tracking, and tracking of tariff-based investigations, such as configuring modules (clinical workflow, task management, clinical documentation, orders, prescribing, alerts, allergies), interfacing to PAS and the trolley wait system, producing GP letters, web linking to Pathology and Radiology and, regional and site-specific code setting (diagnosis, minimum data set). Despite this, EDIS was unable to meet the hospital's reporting requirements and the department had to make its own arrangements for ad hoc reporting via a third party application.

Lesson 3: Training

Particularly in big departments, training all potential users is not an easy task. In this ED, approximately 275 members of staff, with a further 100 non-ED staff, were identified for training. After the vendor's recommendations, a *Train the Trainer* methodology was adopted. The vendor trained 8 core trainers who then trained 30 *super users*. Training sessions and documentation were organised by the vendor who also assisted in the delivery of training by the core trainers to the front users. Three two-hour training slots for each clinician-user were arranged 3-4 months before the go-live day, in a dedicated (close to the ED) computer room with around 15 workstations in place. Users were also encouraged to spend any available time playing with the system at their own pace.

The training programme included development of both basic Microsoft Windows and EDIS functionality skills. This was important as users were expected to navigate themselves between the various computer screens with two new devices (keyboard and a mouse) so as to locate, from an array, several *text boxes*, to *move* patients on the *map* area of the system, to *save* the cubicles for a patient that had gone for an x-ray or electronically discharge a particular patient and to *save* data input once they completed typing. At the same time, this increased attention to the development of keyboard and navigation skills was adding to the users' fear of mishandling the system and making mistakes that could not be rectified later on, affecting the quality of the information electronic patient records hold. In fact, one thing that users immediately realised, to their great disappointment, was that what gets *saved* it stays for good. While on paper they could write something down and later rub it or cross it out, in EDIS nothing could be deleted or even spell-checked. Therefore, all data entry and reporting had to be completed accurately, affecting speed of use.

In the end, the tight timescale for the implementation and the lack of adequate funding to buy out work time resulted in only a handful of super users being trained and ready for the go live day. Also, while pocket-sized user guides and manuals were developed to guide users through the system, their uptake was limited as their linear structure and technical language were abhorred by most clinicians without previous exposure to computer use.

Lesson 4: Support

During the crucial first weeks after go-live, support involved overstaffing the ED and placing computer competent clinical users, hospital IT staff and the clinical leads within the department to help those less competent. Initially they focused on the reception desk to support clerical staff in registering new patients via EDIS. *Handhold* sessions were also in place particularly for the clinical areas and for certain periods, talking staff though the use of the system.

Just being there really, I spent a lot of hours that week we went live here in the department, about 80, 85 hours actually physically present in the department, hand holding, showing them how to do things, making sure things were running smoothly.

Importantly, users who managed to grasp the system quickly were sharing information and knowledge with their colleagues about filling in text boxes, navigating through screens and menus, moving patients through the system, 'saving' clinical notes and rectifying data entry mistakes (Vezyridis et al., 2012). This additional support was very helpful particularly during those difficult hours when the department was experiencing immense pressures while opportunities to bleep the IT Helpdesk or the software trainers were not available (out-of-hours).

Lots of people were finding little ways around things, by working it out on the computer and then telling you, you know, I've found this, this is how you do it and you make it quicker. So you know, as we found little things we all just told each other.

… so you did have support if you were unsure about something and people were quite patient, you know, with people that are a bit stupid!

Implementation teams should also consider the issue of seniority and how it correlates with age and computer competence. This is important because these users not only had to familiarise themselves with a new, technologically mediated practice, but were also expected to provide technical support to other, junior members of staff. As professional seniority may be related to a bigger EDIS learning curve, this new role may not be embraced as expected, as the system disturbs their relationships with junior staff and displaces them from the centre of clinical network within the ED:

You've perhaps got a charge nurse or a sister…very experienced…can lead the whole department and has been the nurse in charge for years… and then suddenly they are put in EDIS and they were put way out of their comfort zones and people were looking to them to help them and they were frightened of it…

The role of the *system administrator* was also developed for departmental autonomy regarding training of new users, basic support, maintenance, user account management and reporting. From there, the system administrator (an EDA) could also liaise further with the hospital ICT team and the vendor for issues such as downtime resolution, scheduled upgrading and software modification.

Lastly, while wall-mounted EDIS terminals were also installed inside the cubicles for users to directly input clinical notes during patient assessment, these were not widely used. For most of the times, clinicians expressed their preference for paper note-taking at the bedside, particularly those who were feeling embarrassed by their lack of computing typing skills and speed. Also, there were times when these terminals were obstructed by medical equipment. Other reasons for not using these terminals included their fixed position on the wall which was not always ergonomically convenient for users of different heights, occasions when clinicians had to turn their back to a patient who seemed to be agitated or when it was preferable to keep certain information more confidential (e.g. domestic violence, mental health issues) and not having patients looking over their shoulders as they typed in their notes. This, however, resulted in congestion at the main staff desk as clinicians were trying to find an available desktop to work on.

DISCUSSION

The implementation of EDIS was completed successfully within a tight, but realistic, timescale. The 4hr wait time target acted as an impetus for several changes to take place. Before the system was introduced, the built environment and the reconfiguration of patient flows were drastically reconfigured, challenging traditional information management artefacts (dry-erase whiteboard, paper records), but causing overcrowding around computer terminals by clinicians waiting to get access to them for data input. A multidisciplinary hospital project team of enthusiastic and motivated members attracted adequate funding and, with the vendor's help, set out a detailed plan of action to carry out the implementation, including working out EDIS's impact on current workflows. Early adoption allowed for some customisation of the system to meet local requirements. Despite the preparation of a good number of super users and user manuals, adoption by users was facilitated by an inspiring and consistent clinical leadership as well as by intensive peer support post go-live. A summary of key recommendations for implementing EDIS is included in Table 1.

Some of these results have also been found by other researchers who examined barriers to successful IT implementations in similar settings (see Khalifa, 2013). For example, Avgar, Litwin, & Pronovost, (2012) believe an organisation is more likely to adopt health IT if the specific solution serves its strategic (performance) objectives and reinforces its organisational practices, the department has the operational capacity to innovate and the frontline staff has the necessary set of skills and involvement in the implementation process. Handel, Wears, Nathanson, & Pines, (2011), in their consensus paper, identified the analysis of "patient flow and integration into clinical work" (p. e47) and usability testing as crucial steps to determine the impact of the system on the delivery of care and to increase system's user-friendliness. Clayton et al. (2005) suggest that extended testing/piloting can determine user acceptance and number of concurrent users the system can sustain, while Ash, Stavri, Dykstra, & Fournier, (2003b) add high-level integration with legacy systems for speed and continuity of care. For all this, Dinh and Chu (2006), and Inokuchi et al., (2014) emphasise the importance of adequate funding, not only for software and hardware but also for on-going maintenance. It is also important to set realistic timescales (Handel & Hackman, 2010) to avoid disappointment and loss of enthusiasm by people on the *shop floor*.

In any case, contracting a suitable vendor, specialised in EDIS development and with a system open to modifications, is essential to a successful outcome. Da've (2004) considers an experienced, resourceful and financially healthy vendor to be better in guiding the implementation with minimum delays, adequate communication and support in the long run (Inokuchi et al., 2014). Also, the American College of Emergency Physicians [ACEP] (2009) seems to be more favourable of vendors knowledgeable of the ED clinical reality as they are more likely to have a system that meets the specific ED requirements. The vendor's role in EDIS implementation may extend further into the training of users and ACEP notes that this important and often neglected process has financial implications that should be equally addressed. They also suggest identifying competent core trainers for delivering repeated, short and flexible training sessions (ACEP 2009), while Clayton et al. (2005) emphasise the buy-out of as much staff time as possible to encourage participation.

For wider support, Ash et al. (2003a; 2003b) emphasise the importance of identifying active multidisciplinary project teams (clinicians, technologists and leaders) and, generally, having *special people* in all levels of leadership and support (administrative, clinical and technological). Handel and Hackman (2010) highlighted the need for recruiting experienced and enthusiastic Clinical Leads, characterised, as Ash et al. (2003b) have found, by advanced social (positive, persistent, influential and understanding) skills. In fact, a systematic review by Ingebrigtsen et al. (2014) found that skilled and experienced, with IT project management, clinical leaders are more visionary and motivated to commit long-term to successful organisational and clinical outcomes from the implementation. Serving as liaisons between clinical, technical and hospital staff, these champions can "ensure safe and efficient EDIS operations" (Farley et al., 2013, p. 403).

Table 1. Summary of Recommendations

Healthcare Organisation
• Ensure an active project board • Accurately identify all stakeholders and involved personnel (ICT, ED, vendor), and assign specific roles • Assemble two project teams, one from the hospital and one from the vendor • Assemble an experienced and mixed hospital project team (clinical and ICT) • Perform work and information flows analyses to determine organisational impact and resolve issues • Train project teams on hospital's procurement procedures • Develop and practice downtime contingency plans before going live • Develop adequate interfaces with any legacy hospital systems (e.g. trolley wait, PAS) • Perform extended testing/piloting (including usability testing) for user acceptance • Attract additional financial resources for supportive software and hardware (e.g. printers and printing material, spare equipment for breakdowns) • Expect delays in cabling the ED, ordering workstations and printers, development of local specifics and interfaces • Maintain open communication channels between ED and hospital ICT • Continuously monitor and evaluate data quality (from day one)
System Vendor
• Experienced in ED implementations in the context of NHS • Provides an Implementation Planning Study • Agree on regular ED visits, meetings and (de)briefings with hospital project team for onsite feedback and progress • Agree on specific communication channels between project teams • Provides advice and support on hardware acquisition (e.g. servers, cabling, terminals, network) and training programme • Clarify level of involvement and relationships between vendor, LSP and hospital • Clarify framework and level of technical support • Open and flexible to customise EDIS and develop interfaces to existing systems according to requirements • Clarify timescale for full concentration on implementation • Clarify framework and level of support after go-live, particularly on working hours
User Training
• Clarify training requirements with vendor and tailor programme to audience • Work on getting majority of staff trained and buy-out ED staff time • Locate a computer room, with demo software installed on terminals, close to (or within) the ED • Widely advertise training sessions across staff and provide flexible training hours • Develop repeated short sessions for each user rather than few long ones • Follow a *Train the Trainer* approach within the ED for autonomy • Identify computer proficient core trainers • Assign core training in software and in hardware use to EDIS vendor • Balance Microsoft Windows and mouse skills set across user base • Include training on workarounds and shortcuts (with caution) • Invest in super-user training • Be prepared to extend training as technical delays unfold
User Support
• Identify experienced and enthusiastic Clinical Leads and provide them with time and resources to be present in the ED, but be prepared for their burn out • Prepare hospital ICT team to step in when vendor becomes slow to respond • Rely more on face-to-face (e.g. meetings) and less on read communication • Engage middle management and staff • Make provisions for on call and out-of-hours ICT helpdesk • Invest in *handholding* and peer support for longer than expected • Raise awareness across the whole hospital of what is happening in the ED and why • Identify decision makers and problem solvers and place them on the *shop floor* • Identify skilled super-users and arrange a good number of them in each shift, but expect their limited, incremental contribution during first weeks after go-live • Develop user guides to fit staff's pockets, but expect an incremental reliance on them • Expect reduced departmental performance during the first weeks after going live

During go-live, Ash et al. (2003a) suggest an extensive period of *handholding* and peer support on the *shop floor* for several weeks when reduced performance is expected (Meadors, Benda, Hettinger, & Ratwani, 2014; Handel & Hackman, 2010), while Fenton, Giannangelo, & Stanfill, (2006) suggest providing users with on call and out-of-hours ICT helpdesk access. Since unscheduled system downtimes (network infrastructure and servers failures, power outages) (Hoot, Wright, & Aronsky, 2003) is the harsh reality in a computerised practice, Handel and Hackman (2010) note that contingency plans need to be developed and practiced well in advance. Lastly, we too, in accordance with Svenson, Pollack, Fallat, & Drapeau, (2003) and Gordon, Flottemesch, & Asplin, (2008), emphasise continuous monitoring and validation of EDIS data from day one for avoiding misclassifications (e.g. discharge, admission) or incorrect timestamps of ED events. Without adequate training and supervision, the department might end up having its staff misinterpreting these reporting terms, which could result in the production of inaccurate information for process evaluation and performance improvement (Avgar et al., 2012).

Study Limitations

As the study was limited to a single clinical setting, implementing one commercial system, generalisations should be made with caution. Other EDs may benefit from alternative approaches due to differences in size, resources, procurement and contractual arrangements, workflows, infrastructure, built environment, leadership, staffing levels and workload. In addition, the sample, although small, was of the appropriate size for the nature of the topic, objectives, design, quality of data and, importantly, ED-specific conditions (high levels of workload and staff turnover) which made difficult the recruitment of participants who met selection criteria. While poor recall of prior experiences in participants is always an issue in individual interviews, we were able to collect more crystallised accounts about the implementation processes that have persisted over time. We also complemented these qualitative findings with information from several project documents. Lastly, although this study examined an implementation that occurred 8 years ago, its findings are still relevant today. While adoption rates of fully functional EDIS remain low (Landman et al., 2010), the market is steadily growing. Particularly in England, more hospitals acquire Emergency Department Information Systems than ever before (e.g. Mid Staffordshire, Blackpool, Morecambe Bay) as the NPfIT (now under the responsibility of the Health and Social Care Information Centre) is far from complete.

FUTURE RESEARCH DIRECTIONS

The literature on case studies from EDs that have implemented EDIS is very limited, as any lessons learned usually stay with the respective organisation. Given the facts that this EDIS was one of the first to go live under the NPfIT and NHS hospitals today still have to use the same project management framework (PRINCE2), the findings of this study are particularly illuminating. The authors hope that through this paper, they promote inter-organisational knowledge sharing. However, more similar studies are required to conduct cross-case comparisons (Sheikh et al., 2011) so as to facilitate the safe adoption of best practices. These can be enriched by observations during implementation to explicate the subtle details and fine nuances of the complex interactions not included in interviews and written materials. Lastly, they, too, suggest that a more sociotechnical approach to the examination of processes, concerning both the people and the technologies involved (Greenhalgh et al., 2010), will better incorporate the local circumstances of individual settings into project management planning.

CONCLUSION

The authors have presented some valuable lessons from one implementation of EDIS at a large university hospital that other EDs might find useful when deploying similar systems. EDIS is a technology that can improve documentation, clinical flows and, consequently, patient care. However, it takes time and effort before such systems can find their place in the ED. While performance indicators might create the necessary impetus, these kinds of projects are complex in nature and should not be treated as straightforward deployments. From the design and installation of the system to user training and support, relationships between staff and with the vendor, careful planning and motivated stakeholder involvement are required for a successful outcome.

REFERENCES

American College of Emergency Physicians. (2009). *EDIS: primer for emergency physicians, nurses, and IT professionals*. Irving, TX: ACEP SEMI.

Anderson, J. G., Jay, S. J., Schweer, H. M., & Anderson, M. M. (1986). Why doctors don't use computers: Some empirical findings. *Journal of the Royal Society of Medicine, 79*, 142–144. PMID:3701749

Anderson, P. (2005). Building on Success. *Health Management Technology, 26*(5), 32–34. PMID:15932071

Aronsky, D., Jones, I., Lanaghan, K., & Slovis, C. M. (2008). Supporting Patient Care in the Emergency Department with a Computerized Whiteboard System. *Journal of the American Medical Informatics Association, 15*(2), 184–194. doi:10.1197/jamia.M2489 PMID:18096913

Ash, J. S., Fournier, L., Stavri, P. Z., & Dykstra, R. (2003a). Principles for a Successful Computerized Physician Order Entry Implementation. In *AMIA Symposium Proceedings*. Washington, DC: American Medical Informatics Association.

Ash, J. S., Stavri, P. Z., Dykstra, R., & Fournier, L. (2003b). Implementing computerized physician order entry: The importance of special people. *International Journal of Medical Informatics, 69*(2-3), 235–250. doi:10.1016/S1386-5056(02)00107-7 PMID:12810127

Avgar, A. C., Litwin, A. S., & Pronovost, P. J. (2012). Drivers and barriers in health IT adoption: A proposed framework. *Applied Clinical Informatics, 3*(4), 488–500. doi:10.4338/ACI-2012-07-R-0029 PMID:23646093

Baumlin, K. M., & Richardson, L. D. (2006). Emergency Department Information System (EDIS) Success: EDIS Implementation Improves Documentation and Increases Charges and Revenue. *Academic Emergency Medicine, 13*(5Supplement 1), s61. doi:10.1197/j.aem.2006.03.138

Baumlin, K. M., Shapiro, J. S., Weiner, C. Gottlieb, B., Chawla, N., & Richardson, L. D. (2010). Clinical Information System and Process Redesign Improves Emergency Department Efficiency. *Joint Commission Journal on Quality and Patient Safety, 36*, 179-1AP.

Berg, M. (1998). Medical work and the computer-based patient record: A sociological perspective. *Methods of Information in Medicine, 37*, 294–301. PMID:9787631

Berg, M. (2001). Implementing information systems in health care organizations: Myths and challenges. *International Journal of Medical Informatics, 64*(2-3), 143–156. doi:10.1016/S1386-5056(01)00200-3 PMID:11734382

Berghoef, H. (2006). (Good) growing pains. Michigan ED automates patient tracking, nurse documentation and charge capture to maintain excellent customer service, increase efficiencies and boost revenue. *Health Management Technology, 27*(3), 30–35. PMID:16594517

Bouchard, M. (2005). What works. ED on Track With IT. *Health Management Technology, 26*(8), 28–31. PMID:16156525

Brennan, S. (2005). *The NHS IT project: the biggest computer programme in the world ever!* Abingdon: Radcliffe.

Burton, L. C., Anderson, G. F., & Kues, I. W. (2004). Using electronic health records to help coordinate care. *The Milbank Quarterly, 82*(3), 457–481. doi:10.1111/j.0887-378X.2004.00318.x PMID:15330973

Clayton, P. D., Narus, S. P., Bowes, W. A., III, Madsen, T. S., Wilcox, A. B., & Orsmond, G., …Leckman, L. (2005). Physician use of electronic medical records: Issues and successes with direct data entry and physician productivity. In *AMIA Annual Symposium Proceedings*. Washington, DC: American Medical Informatics Association.

Coonan, K. M. (2004). Medical informatics standards applicable to emergency department information systems: Making sense of the jumble. *Academic Emergency Medicine, 11*(11), 1198–1205. doi:10.1111/j.1553-2712.2004.tb00705.x PMID:15528585

Cork, R. D., Detner, W. M., & Friedman, C. P. (1998). Academic physicians' use of, knowledge about, and attitudes toward computers: Measurement study and validation. *Journal of the American Medical Informatics Association, 5*, 164–176. doi:10.1136/jamia.1998.0050164 PMID:9524349

Da've, D. (2004). Benefits and barriers to EMR implementation. *Caring, 23*(11), 50–51. PMID:15633313

Department of Health. (2004). *Improving Emergency Care in England, Report by the Comptroller and Auditor General (HC 1075 Session 2003–2004)*. London: National Audit Office.

DeWoody, S., & Loadman, G. P. (1999). Implementing an Emergency Department Information System – How Complicated Can We Make This? *Journal of Healthcare Information Management, 13*(3), 19–30. PMID:10787597

Dinh, M., & Chu, M. (2006). Evolution of health information management and information technology in emergency medicine. *Emergency Medicine Australasia, 18*(3), 289–294. doi:10.1111/j.1742-6723.2006.00855.x PMID:16712540

Dixon-Woods, M., Agarwal, S., Jones, D., Young, B., & Sutton, A. (2005). Synthesising qualitative and quantitative evidence: A review of possible methods. *Journal of Health Services Research & Policy*, *10*(1), 45–53B. doi:10.1258/1355819052801804 PMID:15667704

Eason, K. (2005). Exploiting the potential of the NPfIT: A local design approach. *British Journal of Healthcare Computing & Information Management*, *22*, 14–15.

Estates, N. H. S. (2003). *The impact of the built environment on care within A&E departments: Key findings and recommendations*. London: The Stationery Office.

Estates, N. H. S. (2004). *A&E design evaluation. Evaluation of two proposed accident and emergency departments: Brent Emergency Care and Diagnostic centre at Central Middlesex Hospital, and an Exemplar Plan*. London: The Stationery Office.

Farley, H. L., Baumlin, K. M., Hamedani, A. G., Cheung, D. S., Edwards, M. R., Fuller, D. C., & Pines, J. M. et al. (2013). Quality and safety implications of emergency department information systems. *Annals of Emergency Medicine*, *62*(4), 399–407. doi:10.1016/j.annemergmed.2013.05.019 PMID:23796627

Fenton, S. H., Giannangelo, K., & Stanfill, M. (2006). Essential people skills for EHR implementation success. *Journal of American Health Information Management Association*, *77*, 60A–60D. PMID:16805302

Fisher, W., & Tibbs, E. W. (2003). What works. Three phases of EDIS. Installation of a comprehensive emergency department information system enables a Virginia IDN to revitalize its ED services. *Health Management Technology*, *24*, 36–40. PMID:12647615

Garvie, D. (2004). Strategic Planning Supports ED Automation. *Health Management Technology*, *25*(11), 34–36. PMID:15551708

Gordon, B. D., Flottemesch, T. J., & Asplin, B. R. (2008). Accuracy of staff-initiated emergency department tracking system timestamps in identifying actual event times. *Annals of Emergency Medicine*, *52*(5), 504–511. doi:10.1016/j.annemergmed.2007.11.036 PMID:18313799

Greenhalgh, T., Stramer, K., Bratan, T., Byrne, E., Russell, J., & Potts, H. W. (2010). Adoption and non-adoption of a shared electronic summary record in England: A mixed-method case study. *BMJ (Clinical Research Ed.)*, *340*(jun16 4), c3111. doi:10.1136/bmj.c3111 PMID:20554687

Grimson, J., & Grimson, W. (2002). Health care in the information society: Evolution or revolution? *International Journal of Medical Informatics*, *66*(1-3), 25–29. doi:10.1016/S1386-5056(02)00032-1 PMID:12453554

Handel, D. A., & Hackman, J. L. (2010). Implementing electronic health records in the emergency department. *The Journal of Emergency Medicine*, *38*(2), 257–263. doi:10.1016/j.jemermed.2008.01.020 PMID:18790591

Handel, D. A., Wears, R. L., Nathanson, L. A., & Pines, J. M. (2011). Using information technology to improve the quality and safety of emergency care. *Academic Emergency Medicine*, *18*(6), e45–e51. doi:10.1111/j.1553-2712.2011.01070.x PMID:21676049

Hendy, J., Reeves, B. C., Fulop, N., Hutchings, A., & Masseria, C. (2005). Challenges to implementing the national programme for information technology (NPfIT): A qualitative study. *BMJ (Clinical Research Ed.)*, *331*(7512), 331–336. doi:10.1136/bmj.331.7512.331 PMID:16081447

Hier, D. B., Rothschild, A., Lemaistre, A., & Keeler, J. (2005). Differing faculty and housestaff acceptance of an electronic health record. *International Journal of Medical Informatics*, *74*(7-8), 657–662. doi:10.1016/j.ijmedinf.2005.03.006 PMID:16043088

Hillestad, R., Bigelow, J., Bower, A., Girosi, F., Meili, R., Scoville, R., & Taylor, R. (2005). Can Electronic Medical Record Systems Transform Health Care? Potential Health Benefits, Savings, And Costs. *Health Affairs*, *24*(5), 1103–1117. doi:10.1377/hlthaff.24.5.1103 PMID:16162551

Hoot, N., Wright, J. C., & Aronsky, D. (2003). Factors contributing to computer system downtime in the emergency department. In *AMIA Annual Symposium Proceedings*. Washington, DC: American Medical Informatics Association.

Ingebrigtsen, T., Georgiou, A., Clay-Williams, R., Magrabi, F., Hordern, A., Prgomet, M., & Braithwaite, J. et al. (2014). The impact of clinical leadership on health information technology adoption: Systematic review. *International Journal of Medical Informatics*, *83*(6), 393–405. doi:10.1016/j.ijmedinf.2014.02.005 PMID:24656180

Inokuchi, R., Sato, H., Nakajima, S., Shinohara, K., Nakamura, K., Gunshin, M., & Yahagi, N. et al. (2013). Development of information systems and clinical decision support systems for emergency departments: A long road ahead for Japan. *Emergency Medicine Journal*, *30*(11), 914–917. doi:10.1136/emermed-2012-201869 PMID:23302505

Inokuchi, R., Sato, H., Nakamura, K., Aoki, Y., Shinohara, K., Gunshin, M., & Nakajima, S. et al. (2014). Motivations and barriers to implementing electronic health records and ED information systems in Japan. *The American Journal of Emergency Medicine*, *32*(7), 725–730. doi:10.1016/j.ajem.2014.03.035 PMID:24792932

Johnston, J. M., Leung, G. M., Wong, J. F., Ho, L. M., & Fielding, R. (2002). Physicians' attitudes towards the computerization of clinical practice in Hong Kong: A population study. *International Journal of Medical Informatics*, *65*(1), 41–49. doi:10.1016/S1386-5056(02)00005-9 PMID:11904247

Khalifa, M. (2013). Barriers to health information systems and electronic medical records implementation. A field study of Saudi Arabian hospitals. *Procedia Computer Science*, *21*, 335–342. doi:10.1016/j.procs.2013.09.044

Landman, A. B., Bernstein, S. L., Hsiao, A. L., & Desai, R. A. (2010). Emergency Department Information System Adoption in the United States. *Academic Emergency Medicine*, *17*(5), 536–544. doi:10.1111/j.1553-2712.2010.00722.x PMID:20536810

Meadors, M., Benda, N., Hettinger, A. Z., & Ratwani, R. M. (2014). Going Live Implementing an Electronic Health Record System in the Emergency Department. *Proceedings of the International Symposium of Human Factors and Ergonomics in Healthcare*, *3*, 44-49. doi:10.1177/2327857914031006

Milbank Memorial Fund. (2000). *Better Information, Better Outcomes?: The Use of Health Technology Assessment and Clinical Effectiveness Data in Health Care Purchasing Decisions in the United Kingdom and the United States*. New York: Milbank Memorial Fund.

Najaftorkaman, M., Ghapanchi, A. H., Talaei-Khoei, A., & Ray, P. (2014). A taxonomy of antecedents to user adoption of health information systems: A synthesis of thirty years of research. *Journal of the Association for Information Science and Technology*, 66(3), 576–598. doi:10.1002/asi.23181

Neal, K. (2003). ROI in the ED. *Health Management Technology*, (November): 2003. PMID:14608714

NSW Department of Health. (1998). *Emergency Department Information System: Information Management and Technology Audit*. Sydney: NSW Department of Health.

O'Connell, R. T., Cho, C., Shah, N., Brown, K., & Shiffman, R. N. (2004). Take Note(s): Differential EHR Satisfaction with Two Implementations under One Roof. *Journal of the American Medical Informatics Association*, 11(1), 43–49. doi:10.1197/jamia.M1409 PMID:14527978

Office of Government Commerce. (2012). *PRINCE2*. Retrieved from http://www.prince-officialsite.com

Righini, N. (2002). *Information Systems in the Emergency Departments. HM 816: Healthcare Information System*. Boston University School of Management.

Rogoski, R. R. (2002). IT in the ED. The nature of emergency department medicine means specific and comprehensive IT needs for clinicians. *Health Management Technology*, 23, 14–16. PMID:11842574

Rowe, B. H., Bond, K., Ospina, M. B., Blitz, S., Schull, M., Sinclair, D., & Bullard, M. (2006). Data collection on patients in emergency departments in Canada. *Canadian Journal of Emergency Medicine*, 8, 417–424. PMID:17209491

Shapiro, J. S., Baumlin, K. M., Chawla, N., Genes, N., Godbold, J., Ye, F., & Richardson, L. D. (2010). Emergency Department Information System Implementation and Process Redesign Result in Rapid and Sustained Financial Enhancement at a Large Academic Center. *Academic Emergency Medicine*, 17(5), 527–535. doi:10.1111/j.1553-2712.2010.00720.x PMID:20536809

Sheikh, A., Cornford, T., Barber, N., Avery, A., Takian, A., Lichtner, V., & Cresswell, K. et al. (2011). Implementation and adoption of nationwide electronic health records in secondary care in England: Final qualitative results from prospective national evaluation in 'early adopter' hospitals. *BMJ (Clinical Research Ed.)*, 343(1), d6054. doi:10.1136/bmj.d6054 PMID:22006942

Stuart, P. (2004). A casemix model for estimating the impact of hospital access block on the emergency department. *Emergency Medicine Australasia*, 16(3), 201–207. doi:10.1111/j.1742-6723.2004.00587.x PMID:15228462

Sujansky, W. V. (1998). The benefits and challenges of an electronic medical record: Much more than a "word-processed" patient chart. *The Western Journal of Medicine*, 169, 176–183. PMID:9771161

Svenson, J. E., Pollack, S. H., Fallat, M. E., & Drapeau, J. L. (2003). Limitations of electronic databases: A caution. *The Journal of the Kentucky State Medical Association*, 101, 109–112. PMID:12674902

Taylor, C. (2006). The Waiting Room Is Closed. *Health Management Technology*, *27*(4), 24–28. PMID:16629252

Vezyridis, P., Timmons, S., & Wharrad, H. J. (2012). Implementation of an Emergency Department Information System: A Qualitative Study of Nurses' Attitudes and Experience. *Computers, Informatics, Nursing*, *30*, 540–546. PMID:23079482

Weiner, C., Baumlin, K. M., & Shapiro, J. S. (2007). Process redesign and emergency department information system implementation improve efficiency. *Academic Emergency Medicine*, *14*(5 Supplement 1), s72. doi:10.1197/j.aem.2007.03.901

Wickramasinghe, N., Tumu, S., Bali, R. K., & Tatnall, A. (2007). Using Actor Network Theory (ANT) as an analytic tool in order to effect superior PACS implementation. *International Journal of Networking and Virtual Organisations*, *4*(3), 257–279. doi:10.1504/IJNVO.2007.015164

Wiler, J. L., Gentle, C., Halfpenny, J. M., Heins, A., Mehrotra, A., Mikhail, M. G., & Fite, D. (2010). Optimizing Emergency Department Front-End Operations. *Annals of Emergency Medicine*, *55*(2), 142–160. doi:10.1016/j.annemergmed.2009.05.021 PMID:19556030

Yoon, D., Chang, B.-C., Kang, S. W., Bae, H., & Park, R. W. (2012). Adoption of electronic health records in Korean tertiary teaching and general hospitals. *International Journal of Medical Informatics*, *81*(3), 196–203. doi:10.1016/j.ijmedinf.2011.12.002 PMID:22206619

Young, D. W. (1984). What makes doctors use computers?: Discussion paper. *Journal of the Royal Society of Medicine*, *77*, 663–667. PMID:6481741

KEY TERMS AND DEFINITIONS

4hr Wait Target: From January 2005, the English Department of Health required 98% (now 95%) of patients to be treated, admitted or discharged in four hours from the time they enter the emergency department.

Commissioning Data Sets (CDS): A basic structure for accurate data collection and analysis of clinical activity, demand forecasting and commissioning on an on-going basis (e.g. discharges, elective and emergency daily admissions, demand profiles, causes of breaches, length of stay).

Early Adoption: This strategy of IT procurement, where a system is deployed at an early stage, while it exposes an organisation to many problems and risks, it can also attract additional resources, secure more time for testing and deployment, and increase an organisation's input in the shaping of the final system to meet particular requirements. It can also foster greater enthusiasm and commitment to the success of the project.

Local Service Provider: An industry partner responsible for delivering the English NPfIT to healthcare organisations across a geographical cluster under the guidance of the NHS IT Director and a ministerial team.

National Programme for Information Technology (NPfIT): Established in 2002 in England, as one of the largest healthcare IT projects in the world, this programme aspired a common national approach in the deployment of electronic patient records, electronic prescribing, broadband networking, electronic booking for appointments, Picture Archiving and Communications Systems (PACS), GP payments and a central email and directory service across the NHS.

PRINCE (PRojects IN Controlled Environments): A de facto, flexible, standard used by governments and the private sector to establish a common language between customers, users and suppliers by addressing planning, delegation, monitoring and control of the six variables involved in any project: costs, timescales, quality, scope, risk and benefits.

Payments by Results: A public policy instrument used in the English NHS to decentralise rewards and payments in an attempt to instil concepts of self-management and accountability in hospitals. It associates carefully recorded and measured clinical activity with payments based on specific investigation and treatment coding lists.

Shop Floor: The clinical workplace where all patient assessment, treatment and management takes place.

Super Users: Enthusiastic with information systems and computer competent senior clinical staff responsible for basic troubleshooting advice and support to front users, particularly for out-of-hours. After advance training in all aspects of the system, they also act as trainers for new personnel on an on-going basis.

Winter Pressures: During winter, the cold weather and influenza as well as healthcare system's inefficiencies drive up demand for hospital admissions and trolley wait space on emergency departments, due to an increase of mortality and morbidity in the elder, very young and chronically ill population.

ENDNOTE

[1]   The Australian-based vendor of the system had a successful record of implementations in more than 145 emergency departments in Australia, Canada and the UK, making it one of the leading actors in this market.

Chapter 15

Human Interaction in the Use of Health Information Systems:
A Case of a Developing Country

Irja N. Shaanika
Namibia University of Science and Technology, Namibia

ABSTRACT

In developing countries, Health Information Systems (HISs) are increasingly used to enable and support both clinical and administrative processes for healthcare services. The use of the HISs in developing countries' healthcare centres is influenced and impacted by humans' interactions which manifests from culture and traditions. Due to the diverse nature of culture and traditions, it is near impossible to have single formula in addressing the patients' needs. As a result, the aim to improve quality of healthcare through HISs is challenged, and many stakeholders do not seem to understand the problem. The challenge continues to significantly contribute to poor service delivery, as the need for healthcare services increases. This study focused on the interaction between the healthcare professionals and the HISs, to understand how and why the challenges of using the ICT systems exist. This includes examining the implication, and how the challenges impact the recipients of healthcare services.

INTRODUCTION

In developing countries, Health Information Systems (HISs) are increasingly used to enable and support both clinical and administrative processes for healthcare services. To this extend, McDonald (2006) explored limitations to opportunities that are offered by ICTs in developing countries. This includes infrastructure availability and lack of skill among health workers, in the use of ICT tools. Due to the number of patients on the increase on daily basis and the sensitive of patients' records, healthcare services providers requires a more adequate, reliable, and accurate information. This is to support and enable healthcare workers to deliver improved services to their patients. Rodrigues (2010) argued that HISs is an ICT-based tool, to make healthcare delivery more effective and efficient.

DOI: 10.4018/978-1-4666-9446-0.ch015

Health Information Systems (HISs) is considered to be a functional computerised system, to execute healthcare related processes and activities. According to Lippeveld (2001), HIS provides specific information primarily to enable and support the processes of health organisations. In one of World Health Organization' (WHO) document of 2003, it is stated that HIS is an integrated effort to collect, process, report, and use health information and knowledge, in order to influence policy making, programme action, and research (WHO, 2003).

The use of HIS requires interaction between people, process, and technology, to support operations and management in delivering of essential information in order to improve the quality of healthcare services (Cleverley, 2009). Similar to other industries, the nature of healthcare industry has changed over time, from a relatively stable conservative industry to a dynamic one. This is attributed to the role of people, in the innovation and management of activities. The dynamism is based on the interactions with technology that people bring in from their different culture and traditions. This includes the types of technologies that are available and how they are used and managed to provide services. As stated by McDonald (2006) exploring the limitations to opportunities offered by IS in developing countries such as inadequate basic physical infrastructure availability and lack of skill among health workers for using information technology tools.

Reporting on the current states of HIS, the World Health Organisation noted that the current status of HIS varies among countries. Most developed countries have fully utilized HIS in their systems as they have the resources, expertise, and capital to implement them. While developing countries HIS are not being fully utilized yet (WHO, 2011). This could be attributed to factors such as lack of computer infrastructure, funding, technical know-how, and how culture and traditions are employed in the use and management of HISs to address health services.

This study therefore examined the impact of human interaction on HISs in a natural setting. The following questions were formulated in order to guide and collect data, to addressing the objectives of the study: (1) what are the factors which impact Human Interaction in the use of health information systems; and (2) What are the roles of Human actors in the healthcare service delivery.

The remainder of the paper is divided into five main sections. The first section presents literature review. The second section discusses the methodology used. In the third sections data analysis is presented and based on the findings the implications for the Human Interaction in the HIS are discussed.

LITERATURE REVIEW

The power of ICT is dramatically changing the ways in which the healthcare organisations operate. Istepanian (2006) explains that, networking technologies and database management systems are able to incorporate better healthcare service, faster in response, and easier to meet increasing demands for the system integration. According to Keenan et al., (2006), the implementation of information systems in hospitals has helped healthcare professionals to improve the efficiency and effectiveness of their services. Health information systems (HIS) that can record and locate important information quickly have become a standard practice in many hospital organisations. The vision of a paperless hospital is delineated as the embodiment of the future health information systems with the hope that it brings an improved promise of more reliable effectiveness and efficiency to the environment (Leppeveld, 2000).

HIS comprises of different computing applications that support the needs of healthcare organisations, clinicians, patients, and policy makers in collecting and managing all data that are related to both clinical and administrative processes (Rada, 2008). Advances in HIS are vital for our society, in that the technologies guide everyday lives, and without them life had been more difficult (Mukama, 2003). Along the same line of argument, Winter (2006) argued that the traditional recording methods of healthcare activities are limited because the captured data and information can only be kept largely in a "physical" form, and are not easily accessible, transportable, or available digitally to other expert clinicians. This makes the use of such data difficult or impossible for human interactions, in carrying out healthcare services to the needy, of different cultural and traditional affiliations.

For health information systems to provide information at the right time and when required, certain factors must be considered and understood. Sinha (2010) argued that such factors include what to collect, where to collect, whom to report to, and how the information will be used and by whom. The results of these factors are manifestations of human interactions. A poorly planned system that ignores user needs, fails to understand organisation capacities, neglects cultural constraints and ignores the local knowledge base will only result in failure for health technologies (Rodrigues & Risk, 2003). This has impact on providing services through human interaction. HIS require a process of learning and adaption from the people and systems that will use them (Steinmueller, 2001). Furthermore, technology rarely stands independently; it is rather embedded in a system of complementary technologies and capabilities and requires three key elements for success, people, process, and technology (Cleverley, 2009). The interaction between people, process and technology supports operation and management in delivering essentials information in order to improve the quality of healthcare service delivery.

Rob (2009) reported that effective use of information technologies has become a critical success factor in modern society. Yet, success is not easily achieved, hence the work in progress in many environments. John (2002) stated that many of the failures occur not in the technology, but in how technology is used in the context of the application domain and settings. This is influenced by the organisational culture and its role in IS organisational (Robey, 2007). According to Mylopoulus (2006), IS changing the social structures of the environment in which people work. In performing some aspects of work that would otherwise be performed by people, they change how tasks are allocated to individuals and groups. From the perspectives of human interactions, Lyytinen(2007) added, by his argument that each time a system is introduced or modified; responsibilities and relationships are reallocated, possibly contested and renegotiated.

The importance of social factors in information systems has long been recognised (Anshari & Almunawar, 2009). Anshari and Almunawar further argued that many systems fail or fall into disuse not because of technical failure, but in how the technology is matched to the social environment. Each time an information system is introduced within an organisational context, the corporate agenda of the target system dominates. Kahn, Aulakh and Bosworth (2006) argued that in such a case the new system is intended to improve productivity and profitability while users who are employees are expected to fit their work practices to the new system (Kahn, Aulakh, & Bosworth, 2006).

RESEARCH METHODOLOGY

The qualitative research method was adopted as the strategy for the study. The qualitative method was selected primary because it allows subjects or objects to be studied in their natural setting (Myers, 2009). Also, the qualitative method focuses on human behaviour which is considered to significantly influenced and be influenced by the setting of the environment. According to Atieno (2009), individuals and groups interpret their thoughts, feelings and actions within the qualitaive paradigm.

The case study approach was employed within the qualitaive paradigm to elicit specific answer to the problem as stated above. According to Yin (2003), a case study is an empirical inquiry that investigates a contemporary phenomenon within its real-life context. Windhoek central hospital in Namibia was used as a case. The Windhoek Central hospital in Windhoek was selected because at the time of the study it was the only public hospital in Namibia that has implemented HIS.

The semi-structured interview technique was used for the data collection. Semi structured interview implies that the researcher will have questions to guide the interview but can possibly ask any other question for clarity or to enhance data gathering process. This means that the interview questions are generally organised around a set of predetermined open-ended questions, with other questions emerging from the dialogue between interviewer and interviewees. In this way, respondents can elaborate on their responses and possibly connect them with other matters of relevance. The interviews conversations were recorded using a tape recorder and were later transcribed. A total of ten people were interviewed. The respondents included a pharmacist (1), nurses (3), network administrators (2), payroll administrator (1), administrative assistant (2) and the system administrators (1). The respondents were selected because of their lengthy years of services and their more frequent daily interaction with the HIS at the Windhoek Central hospital.

The transcribed data was analysed using a thematic analysis approach, as discussed below. The approach includes identification of patterns and themes in the data. Braun and Clarke (2006) elaborated that thematic analysis is a method for identifying, analysing, and reporting patterns (themes) within data. It is also noted by Rice and Azzy (1999) that thematic analysis process involves the identification of themes through the careful reading and re-reading of the data. According to Braun and Clarke (2006), a theme captures something important about the data in relation to the research question, and represents some level of patterned response or meaning within the data set. The thematic analysis process involved six stages as follows:

Step 1: The researcher prepared the data which was recorded data transcribed, in a summative way.

Step 2: Data classification. The data was classified in accordance to the questions, following respondents' responses as expressed in a form of single words, phrases, sentences or paragraphs.

Step 3: Develop categories and a coding scheme. In this study categories were established based on the research questions. Different colours were used in interview transcripts to identify phrases, words or statement that describes each category.

Step 4: Coded all text through sampling of data. This was done to check for consistency and revise coding rule as an interactive process. While new data continue to be analysed it was likely that new themes emerge. Step four was repeated as new themes emerged from the interviews (example: challenges).

Step 5: Draw conclusion from the coded data. "This step involves making sense of the themes or categories identified and their properties".

Step 6: report your methods of findings. Step six suggests that the researcher should report practices concerning the coding process supported by the descriptions and interpretations to provide the reader with an understanding of the phenomenon (Zhang & Wildemuth, 2009).

Table 1. Elaboration and implication of colour coding

Theme (s)	Categories	Colour Coding
ICT	Other Systems	Green
	HIS	Red
	Medical data collection	Grey
	mediation technology between offices	Purple
	Challenges on daily operations	Blue
	Service delivery	Pink

Data coding is based on the research questions in this study. Sub themes further emerged as the data analysis continues and thematic analysis steps outlined above were repeated. To determine the implication of responses, additional descriptions in different colours were pertinent.

ANALYSIS OF THE IDENTIFIED CATEGORIES

In a complementary fashion, the thematic and interpretive techniques were used in the data analysis. Thus, six categories were identified. The selection of the categories was guided by the study objectives of the study. The interpretive technique was used to analyse and better understand the categories as follows.

I. HIS and Other Systems

At the time of this study, various information systems (IS) were implemented at the hospital, in addition to the HIS. This includes the Financial Integrated System (IFMS) and the Human Resource Management Systems (HRMS).

The IFMS was used by the finance employees to carry out the hospital financial related activities. According to the payroll administrator *"the system is the same one used in all the government public services accounting activities (RS005, p5, 140-141)"*. The system is an integrated system with various financial modules. One of the respondents, an accountant stated that *"the system is working by categories, it have a payroll, SNTies and suppliers payments"* (RS0011, p9, 265-267). Additionally the system *collaborates with the IFMS system at the Ministry of Health, so whatever captured in the system, can be viewed at the Ministry of finance* (RS005, p5, 154-157).

HRMS is another information system that was used in the organisation. The system was used for supporting and enabling some activities and processes of the human resource (HR). One of the respondents shared her views as follows" *We only use the system to list employees wellness program and advertise vacancies internally but we have store room called registry where we manually keep all our employees files"*(RS001, p1,11-15).

Both the IFMS and HRMS were of importance to the hospital as they supported and enabled automation of processes and activities. The employees interacted with the systems. Also, they made use of the systems to interaction with other actors. The interactions were based on their interest as well as their technical know-how skills. As such depending on the level of expertise about the systems, employees either fully interacted with the system or were reluctant (or limited) in their use and interaction with the systems. The limited use of the systems made them white elephants in the organisation. At the hospital, skills were acquired through systems training or via previous educational background. It was the responsibility of the human resource business unit to ensure that all employees are technical know-how competent.

II. Health Information System (HIS)

The health Information system implemented at the Windhoek Central hospital is called Integrated Health Care Information Management System (IHCIMS). The system has been operating for the last two years. The system is part of The Ministry of Health and Social Services (MoHSS) initiatives to eradicate manual process and to improve healthcare service delivery. According to Suresh (personal communication, September 4, 2013) *the IHCIMS is a comprehensive web based enterprise-wide application that covers all aspects of management and day-to-day operations of a hospital.* The application modules include (i) admission - for administering patients contact details; (ii) pharmacy - for management and allocation of prescribed medications; and (iii) inpatient and outpatient – for managing patient's circulations within the hospital. The various modules are integrated and able to communicate. A pharmacist illustrated this stating that" *The doctors enter the details about the prescribed medication and when the patients collect medicine at the pharmacy, we retrieve the record using the Medical Record(MR)number in order to hand out medicines* "(RS004,p32, 115-117)

III. Medical Data Collection

The hospital did realise that they do needs reliable and accurate data in order to deliver effective and efficient services to patients. However, they employed two different systems namely (1) paper-based (2) computer-based (IHCIMS) for their activities and processes.

A. Paper-Based System

The paper-based system was the main form that was used to store and manage patients' data at the hospital. Patient data are recorded in health passport (small green and yellow booklet) that is provided by the public hospitals and clinics country wide. It is mandatory that each time a patient visit the hospital he/she is expected to have their health passport in order to receive treatment. In case a patient loses the health passport, provision for a new health passport is made. However, one of the challenges that was experienced with the use of the paper-based system was that there are no backup od patients' medical treatment, hence when a patients loses their health passport, healthcare professionals have nowhere to follow up on the patient treatments. As a result this often leads to repetition of efforts, and therefore slows down the treatment process.

B. Computer-Based System

The hospital regards this method to be the future method for data collection. With this method on the first encounter with the hospital patients are first assigned a medical record (MR) number. The record number which is automatically generated by the IHCIMS is unique henceforth it uniquely identify each patient. With this method all patients' data are recorded on the computerised system with real-time backup data available. Henceforth the system eradicates data redundancy and provides healthcare professionals with real time data required for effective service delivery. An administrative nurse shared her views stating that *"The system works with internet and each patient is allocated medical record number and then all details are being entered on the computer system and this make it easier to retrieve the in formation"(RS156,pg5,187-191).*

IV. Mediation Technology between Offices

Technologies in healthcare environment are primarily implemented to support and enable efficient and effective healthcare service delivery. Various technologies existed in the hospital environment at the time of this study. The technologies included software and hardware such as printers, scanners, servers and desktops. Technology mediation between the offices was enabled due to some of the integrated systems and systems internet connectivity. However the application of such technologies was dependent on the level of technical know-how among the employees. As such the technologies implementation, usage and maintenance depend on human interpretation and understanding. .

V. Challenges on Daily Operations

Healthcare professionals encountered challenges as they carry out their daily activities. These challenges are both technical and non-technical challenges. Both challenges hinder quality service delivery.

A. Technical Challenges

Healthcare professionals encountered technical challenges such as slow internet connectivity and system downtimes. Majority of the respondents viewed their frustration about the slow internet. As a result most of the activities were delayed due to the slow internet connectivity. Systems downtime was also a main concern among the health professionals. Most of the time the system was down due to maintenance. One of the respondents shared her dissatisfaction *"the system is not yet fully implemented"* (RS006, pg6, 195). When system is down the healthcare professionals perform their responsibilities manually. For example the doctors would write down the medicine prescription in the health passport whereby the patients will than take their passport to the pharmacist for medicines collection. In both instances there is no data recorded on the system. Also the various systems were not integrated making it difficult or impossible for employees to collaborate.

B. Non-Technical Challenges

In the organisation non-technical challenges included lack of technical know-how and lack of communication among the healthcare professionals. Most of the healthcare professionals were not able to utilise computers due to the lack of computer user skills. The use of HIS requires awareness and technical know-how. Unfortunately this was lacking among the healthcare professionals especially among the nurses. Stating her views a registers nurse said*" most of the people are not computer literate especially the nurses and then they don't have enough skills to do that"* (RS006, pg5, 193-194). As a result majority healthcare professionals preferred carrying out their activities manually. Therefore most of the computer systems were not used or rather employees found them hard to use.

Lack of sufficient training about the systems and technologies implemented at the hospital was the main factor that attributed to the lack of technical know-how. In most cases trainings are conducted but are not adequate enough for the employees to acquire the necessary skills.

There were also communication challenges within the organisation. The systems down times were most of the time not communicated on time." *When the system is being updated we are not actually informed*" stating (RS005, pg4, 144). This was attributed to the lack communication between technical people and healthcare professionals.

VI. Service Delivery

Many actors are involved in healthcare service delivery. These actors are either human or non-human. The human actors include the healthcare professionals, (such as nurses, doctors and pharmacist), administrative workers, patients and other stakeholders (Ministry of Health). The non-human actors were the ICT artefacts, medical tools and the processes used to deliver service.

Service delivery was influenced by the actors' interaction. The interaction involved human-to-human, human-to-non-human and non-human-to-non-human. The interactions were guided by rules and regulations as defined in the organisation. Based on the various interactions, it became clear that not all actors involved in the service delivery were satisfied with the processes of service delivery. For example some actors were dissatisfied with the paper based forms as most of the times files would get missing resulting in the repetition of activities that had been performed .This caused delay and response time in service delivery.

FINDINGS AND DISCUSSION

Based on the analysis of the qualitative data as presented above, there were findings from the study. This includes communicative scheme, infrastructure obsolete, system integration, systems parallel, and lack of technical know-how, data omission, and trivial use of the IHCIMS. The findings are discussed below. The discussion should be read with the Figure 1 so as to gain better understanding of how human interaction influence and impact the HIS (IHCIMS) in Windhoek Central hospital. The arrows indicates a bidirectional link among the various components.

I. Communicative Scheme

The communicative scheme in the context of this study is viewed as a form of interaction among actors. Callon (1986) defined actors as both human and non-human linked together in this network by common interest. The communicative scheme enacts the interaction between actors: human-to-human, human-to-nonhuman (such as technology), and nonhuman-to-nonhuman. The use and management of the HIS in Windhoek Central hospital is influenced by many factors as depicted in figure 1. The outcomes of the use and management of the HIS is as a result of the reproductive interaction among those factors.

Figure 1. Human Interaction with HIS

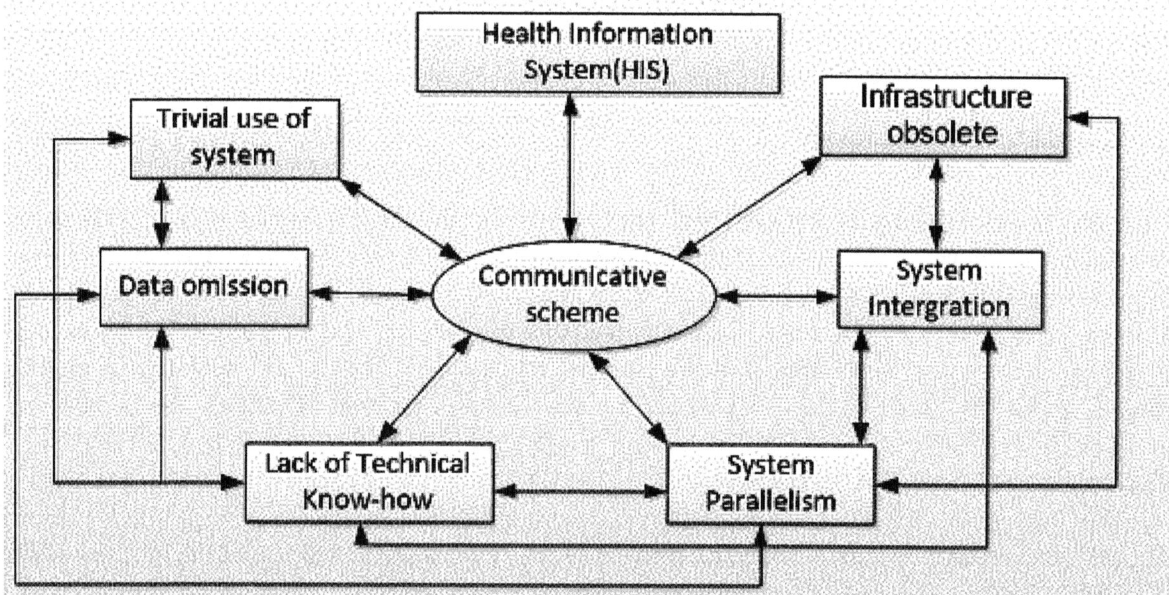

The infrastructures enabling and supporting the HIS were left, or remained obsolete primarily because of limited communication among the actors. There were lapses in the collaboration of the systems due to lack of technology-to-technology communication. Also, a more robust interaction among the actors would have eradicated parallel systems in the environment. From a more non-technical perspective, the communicative scheme facilitates, in addressing factors such as trivial use of the IHCIMS, data omission by the medical professionals, and the lack of technical know-how among the medical professionals.

II. Infrastructure Obsolete

The integrated health care information management system (IHCIMS) was web enabled, meaning the system could be accessed through the internet. This necessitated reasonable support and maintenance of the infrastructures. However, as revealed from the data, the infrastructures that were deployed to enable and support the IHCIMS were obsolete. This hampered some of the services as there was reliance on the system. For example, the -Internet connectivity was often slow, delaying services including data retrieval.

III. Systems Integration

The systems (IHCIMS, **HRMS, IFMS**) used at the Windhoek Central hospital to support the administration of employees' activities were not integrated, for their activities rather they were stand-alone systems. This leads to lack of collaboration among employees as they could not share and access real-time data. This hindered response time in providing services to co-employees as well as patients For example, during Practitioner-to-Practitioner referrals within the hospital, it becomes difficult to identify and allocate individual (as per their specialisation and availability. It gets more challenging for new practitioners who are still trying to understand the environment. Systems integration enables effective human interaction of the HIS as it minimises systems parallelism that causes implications, such as data duplications of functions. The development and implementation of integrated systems requires resources, such as personnel with technical know-how.

IV. Systems "Parallelism"

As it was revealed from data analysis, both paper-based and the IHCIMS systems were used at the Windhoek Central hospital. The use of parallel systems created data inconsistencies as some data were being recorded on the IHCIMS system and others on paper-based (manual) system. Also, the parallelism of the systems leads to implications, such as duplication of processes and activities resulting in inefficient use of resources. Integration of the systems will address the problems and challenges caused by parallelism. Otherwise, service delivery will continue be jeopardised at the Windhoek Central hospital.

V. Lack of Technical Know-How

As with other areas of expertise, technical know-how was paramount in the use of the hospital's HIS (IHCIMS). The know-how is a set of skill acquired from training and education. However, this was lacking at Windhoek Central Hospital. In the study, it was revealed that not all the system users were trained or did receive productive training to be able to use the systems to support their daily activities. Some employees were requested and expected to familiarise themselves with the functionality of the system. Thus, they lost productive time while navigating around the system. What was even more challenging was that majority of the nurses were not computer literate. As a result, they were more comfortable following the manual processes. The lack of technical know-how plays significant in human interaction with the IHCIMS, in that it contributed to data omission. Also, this contributed to trivial use of the IHCIMS in the hospital, which affected efficiency of service delivering.

VI. Data Omission

Data is an important aspect of every organisation primary because it can enable or constrain activities through its use for decision making. In lure of this, we gathered from our analysis of the data that not all patients that visit the hospital are registered on the HIS. This was because the HIS was trivially used, which was caused by lack of technical know-how. As such, some patients (or visitors) were registered manually on the paper-based forms (system). The paper-based practise contributed to patients' data incompleteness or omission. This process negatively impact service delivery due to lack of insufficient data required to make informed decisions.

VII. Trivial Use of System

At the Windhoek Central hospital, the systems, such as the HRMS were hardly used, or reluctantly used as empirically revealed. At the hospital, the HRMS was only used for internal vacancies advertisement. What was even more trivial was that the workers could not make use of the systems (HRMS) to apply for the jobs that were advertised through the system. One of the implications of this is that the system does not support online application processing. As a result, the departments mainly use manually paper forms to perform their daily activities. For example with the leave processing employees fill in their forms manually. After forms have been processed they are manually stored in cabinets in the registry. The implication is that the documentation are vulnerable to threat and disaster, such as fire and theft.

CONCLUSION

It is now hard to imagine the survival of a hospital without information and communication technologies. As known and revealed in this study, the use of HIS is critically influenced by human interaction. This means that how human interact determines the success or failure of the HIS in providing healthcare services in the Namibia. The Ministry of Health and Social Services of the Republic of Namibia thus requires a comprehensive modern Integrated Health Care Information Management System (IHCIMS) to improve the quality and effectiveness of health care for all Namibians.

The challenges of transitioning from a paper environment to an electronic environment must involve rethinking of factors, such as workflow, staff skills, availability of resources, habits and the organisational culture. Acknowledgement of this has led to a need for understanding the match between IHCIMS and existing IT infrastructure, organisational structure, and established routines. This means that the decision-making process leading to the implementation and use of ICT-based applications at the hospital has to improve generally. It should be noted that technology is an enabler and requires support from the people using it to be affective, thus the need for hospital employees to be trained and be well informed of the technology in place.

REFERENCES

Anshari, M., & Almunawar, M. N. (2009). *Health Information Systems (HIS): Concept and Technology.* Academic Press.

Atieno, O. (2009). An analysis of the strengths and limitation of qualitative and quantitative research paradigms. *Problems of Education in the 21st Century, 13,* 13-18.

Braun, V., & Clarke, V. (2006). Using thematic analysis in pyschology. *Qualitative Research in Psychology, 3*(2), 77–101. doi:10.1191/1478088706qp063oa

Callon, M. (1986). Some elements of the sociology of translation: Domestication of the scallops and the fisherman of St Brieuc Bay. In J. Law (Ed.), *A New Sociology of Knowledge, power, action and belief* (pp. 196–233). London: Routledge.

Cleverley, M. (2009). How ICT advances might help developing nations. *Communications of the ACM, 52*(9), 30–32. doi:10.1145/1562164.1562177

Goldschmidt, P. G. (2005). Implications of health information technology and medical information systems. *Communications of the ACM, 48*(10), 69–74.

Istepanian. (2006). Design and Implementation of a Mobile Diabetes Management System. *Journal of Mobile Multimedia, 1*(4), 273-284.

John, T. G. (2002). *Requirements Engineering:Social and Technical Issues*. London: Academic Press.

Kahn, J. S., Aulakh, V., & Bosworth, A. (2006). What it takes: Characteristics of the ideal personal health record. *Health Affairs*, *28*(2), 369–376. doi:10.1377/hlthaff.28.2.369 PMID:19275992

Keenan, C. R., Nguyen, H. H., & Srinivasan, M. (2006). Electronic medical records and their impact on residents and medical student education. *Academic Psychiatry*, *30*(6), 522–527. doi:10.1176/appi.ap.30.6.522 PMID:17139024

Lippeveld, T. (2001). Routine health information systems:the glue of a unified health system. *The RHINO Workshop on Issues and Innovation in Routine Health In Information in Developing Countries*.Arlington, VA: JSI Research and Training Institute.

McDonald, M. (2006). Public Health Informatics: How Information Age Technology Can Strengthen Public Health. *Annual Review of Public Health*, *4*(2), 239–252. PMID:7639873

Mukama, F. (2003). *A study of health information systems at local levels in Tanzania and Mozambique*. (MSc thesis). University of Oslo.

Myers, M. D. (2009). *Qualitative Research in Business & Management*. New Zealand: SAGE Publications Ltd.

Mylopoulus, J. (2006). Representing Knowledge About Information Systems. *ACM Transactions on Information Systems*, *3*(2), 131–140.

Rada, R. (2008). *Information Systems and Healthcare Enterprises*. Hershey, PA: IGI Publishing. doi:10.4018/978-1-59904-651-8

Rice, P., & Azzy, D. (1999). *Qualitative research methods: A health focus*. Melbourne: Oxford University Press.

Robey, D. (2007). Cultural Analysis and the Organizational Consequences of I.T. *Accounting. Management and Information Technologies*, *3*(1), 23–24.

Rodrigues, R., & Risk, A. (2003). eHealth in Latin America and the Caribbean:Development and policy issues. *Journal of Medical Internet Research*, *5*(1), 4–22. doi:10.2196/jmir.5.1.e4 PMID:12746209

Sauerborn, R., & Lippeveld, T. (2000). *What is wrong with current health information systems?* Geneva: WHO.

Sinha, R. (2010). Impact of health information technology in public health. *Sri Lanka Journal of Bio-Medical Informatics*, *1*(4), 223–236. doi:10.4038/sljbmi.v1i4.2239

Steinmueller, W. (2001). ICTs and the possibilities for leapfrogging by developing countries. *International Labour Review*, *140*(2), 193–210. doi:10.1111/j.1564-913X.2001.tb00220.x

Yin, R. (2003). *Case Study Research: Design and Methods* (3rd ed.). Sage.

KEY TERMS AND DEFINITIONS

Health Information System: A computer system used to store and process health related information.

Healthcare: The services and products offered by the hospital to the communities.

Human Interaction: The communication between the humans and computer systems as they carry out the activities and processes.

Information Systems: A computer system used to store and processes organisational information.

Chapter 16
Toward Integrating Healthcare Data and Systems:
A Study of Architectural Alternatives

Timoteus B. Ziminski
University of Connecticut, USA

Eugene Sanzi
University of Connecticut, USA

Steven A. Demurjian
University of Connecticut, USA

Thomas Agresta
University of Connecticut Health Center, USA

ABSTRACT

The adoption of health information systems and the integration of healthcare data and systems into efficient cross-institutional collaboration workflows of stakeholders (e.g., medical providers such as physicians, hospitals, clinics, labs, etc.) is a challenging problem for the healthcare domain. This chapter studies the way that well-established software engineering concepts and architectural styles can be employed to satisfy requirements of the healthcare domain and ease health information exchange (HIE) between stakeholders. Towards this goal, this chapter proposes a hybrid HIE architecture (HHIEA) that leverages the studied styles that include service-oriented architecture, grid computing, publish/ subscribe paradigm, and data warehousing to allow the health information systems of stakeholders to be integrated to facilitate collaboration among medical providers. To demonstrate the feasibility and utility of the HHIEA, a realistic regional healthcare scenario is introduced that illustrates the interactions of stakeholders across an integrated collection of health information systems.

INTRODUCTION

The healthcare domain, frequently criticized for its antiquated handling of data (e.g., by using paper-based patient registries in physician practices), has been infused with a multitude of software solutions for Health Information Exchange (HIE) that focus on the integration of patient data from multiple sources in order to improve quality of care, lower healthcare costs, and support research. Some important driving factors are programs that provide funding such as the Meaningful Use EHR Incentive Program of

DOI: 10.4018/978-1-4666-9446-0.ch016

Medicare and Medicaid (CMS, 2013) or the Strategic Health IT Advanced Research Projects (SHARP, 2013) program. For example, SHARP has already spawned highly valuable platforms such as Informatics for Integrating Biology and the Bedside (i2b2, 2004) and the Substitutable Medical Apps & Reusable Technology platform (SMART, 2011). At the same time, patient involvement has been increased by initiatives such as the Blue Button (Blue Button, 2013), which allows patients simple access to their data or the data of a cared for elderly parent or child collected from participating medical providers (e.g., physicians, nurses, clinics, hospitals, image labs, pharmacies, therapists, etc.). In addition, the fitness market has exploded with a variety of fitness devices (wearable technologies) that link to mobile applications with new initiatives by the two dominant mobile computing players, Apple and Google. Apple has proposed a new HealthKit app (Apple Health App, 2015) for a dashboard to manage health and fitness data, while Google has announced its own Google Fit fitness tracker (Google Fit, 2015). Both companies are moving strongly into the smartwatch market to track motion, heart rate, blood pressure, activity, etc. In fact, Apple just announced ResearchKit (ResearchKit, 2015), an open source framework that allows researchers/developers to create apps in support of medical research; such a transformation will strongly rely on HIE in order to gather relevant data.

Despite all of the emphasis on HIE, there have been numerous problems that have been encountered during the same time span, particularly in regards to regional or statewide networks of connected healthcare stakeholders that practice HIE. Some very promising exchanges have failed (e.g., CalRHIO (Robinson, 2010) and CareSpark (Enrado, 2011)) and the progress of the work of regional health information organizations has been described as "discouraging" and "insufficient" (President's Council of Advisors on Science and Technology, 2010). However, even though the adoption of health information systems (HIS) by medical providers is starting to approach a wider acceptance in usage, the corresponding and required integration of healthcare data and systems via HIE remains a challenging problem, technologically as well as politically. On the side of technology, factors that limit adoption of HISs and HIE have been identified

(Gomes, Ziviani, Correa, Teixeira, & Moreira, 2012): a high development cost associated with HIE; a lack of agreed upon open-standardization particularly in regard to the sharing and exchange of data; a focus on brute force technology solutions rather than a healthcare process orientation that considers the needs of patients and providers and high data availability across HISs; and, the difficulty in maintaining HIE across multiple HISs that have the potential to evolve with new capabilities. On the political side, there is concern by major medical providers (e.g., hospitals in a particular region) that sharing data may lead to losing business (patients).

The healthcare domain has significant complexity and poses unique challenges that require novel approaches as well as leveraging existing solutions to have the potential to remedy the four aforementioned factors. This chapter studies established software engineering concepts, architectural alternatives, and best practices and investigates the way that they can be utilized in support of potential HIE solutions that integrate medical data and systems. We study architectural alternatives with a four step process by exploring the varied and complex requirements of the healthcare domain for supporting HIE of HISs, and matching these requirements to solutions from the software engineering domain. The first step provides an overview of software/system architectural alternatives that can be chosen for structuring an HIE system that integrates multiple HISs. The second step describes a detailed and realistic regional healthcare scenario with multiple entities that defines the scope of stakeholders that include a sole-provider practice, a community practice, local and regional hospitals, testing laboratories (blood, scanning, etc.), pharmacies, a university academic medical center, etc.; this scenario was done in collaboration with our co-author at a medical school. Within the scenario, the collaborative links between the involved entities are identified to serve as requirements of the domain. The third step proposes a hybrid HIE architecture (HHIEA) that leverages components from all of the identified alternatives and highlights strengths for particular use cases. Finally, the fourth step maps HHIEA into the assumed scenario including the way that it satisfies identified links to demonstrate the way that the architecture could be realized in a system.

This chapter is structured in 6 sections. In the *Background* section, context information is provided on varied HISs with a focus on the benefits of HIE and on the unique challenges that an HIE system architectures has to surmount. The *Architectural Alternatives* section explores high-level alternatives for system organization from the software engineering and architecture domains (federation, replication, and centralization) and a variety of instances of those alternatives such as service-oriented architecture (Rosen, 2008), grid computing (Foster, 2002), publish/subscribe paradigm (Eugster, Felber, Guerraoui, & Kermarrec, 2003), and data warehousing (Zeh, 2003). The *Regional HIE Scenario* section details a realistic regional HIE scenario with a selection of identified stakeholders, their capacities as medical data providers and consumers, and the collaborative links that exist between them. The *Hybrid HIE Architecture (HHIEA)* section proposes an approach that leverages the studied architectural styles to address both informational and functional requirements of HIE; in the process, the architecture is aligned to the realistic regional scenario. Then, the *Future Trends* section presents future efforts and directions in HIE that are emerging that may have an impact, including app-centric plugin architectures such as the aforementioned SMART platform, abstract architecture specifications for the construction of health applications such as the Open mHealth architecture (Open mHealth, 2011), and the integration of genetic analysis and results into Electronic Medical Records and Genomics (eMERGE, 2007). Finally, the *Conclusion* section draws this chapter to a close.

BACKGROUND

This section provides background material that is required for the remainder of the chapter. To begin, health information exchange concepts are introduced and placed into context that includes their usage with other health information systems (HISs). Using this as a basis, the challenges facing health information exchanged are identified and briefly reviewed.

The Role of HIE

Medical and health data obtained at the point of care presents both a challenge and an asset. Through transformation, aggregation, and analysis, medical/health data usage can range from billing and reimbursement through insurers to clinical decision support to automatically monitor patients and issue alerts to the foundation for research to establish new knowledge and improved procedures (Shortliffe & Cimino, 2006). To support all of these possibilities, HIE has emerged as one of the major means for electronic transfer of medical data among distinct healthcare organizations and their health information systems (HISs). The goal of HIE is to make medical and health data available to healthcare stakeholders (e.g., healthcare providers, researchers in academia and industry, insurers, patients, etc.) in an efficient, cost-reducing, timely, and safe manner (Kuperman, 2011). Monetary savings can be, for example, achieved by avoiding duplicated laboratory tests and the reduction of administrative overhead. HIE also has the potential to significantly improve the quality and safety of patient care by enabling healthcare providers to react faster to a patient's needs and avoid misdiagnosis, mistreatment, and adverse effects caused by incomplete knowledge about a patient's medical and health history.

Foundationally, HIE is based on the communication of a variety of complementary HISs employed by domain stakeholders. First, electronic health records (EHRs), which are a computerized record of a patient's health-related information (e.g., physician's observations, laboratory results, treatments, etc.) which can be created, managed, and consulted by authorized clinicians and staff within one or across multiple healthcare organizations. Their purpose can be manifold (support of research, education, etc.) but usually focus on supporting continuity of care. Second, electronic medical records (EMRs), offer similar functionality as EHRs, but are usually designed to function within one larger healthcare organization such as a hospital, clinic, etc. There are various EHRs and EMRs on the software market such as the publicly available Veterans Health Information Systems and Technology Architecture (VistA, 2003) developed by the US Department of Veterans Affairs, the open source OpenEMR (OpenEMR, 2012) and OpenMRS (OpenMRS, 2004) or a vast number of commercial products (ONC, 2015). Third, Personal health records (PHRs) are electronic records of health-related information on an individual that can be drawn from multiple sources while being managed, shared, and controlled by the individual patient or their representatives. Thus, they will frequently contain a special subset of the data available in EHRs, but can be also a rich source of information such as the nutritional supplement use of a patient. However, since their control lies with the patient, PHRs do not have the best reputation among physicians in terms of the reliability of the entered data. A prominent PHR is the Microsoft HealthVault (Microsoft HealthVault, 2007) platform with many insurance companies doing their own implementations.

Other HISs of note are: Medical Laboratory Information Systems (MLIS) for supporting the laboratory workflow from the test request to the specimen labeling to the creation of the lab report; Data Repositories or Data Warehouses for structured information storage and support of research surveys in academia and industry; and, Decision support systems (DSSs) for assistance with clinical decisions through evaluation of evidence-based knowledge in the context of patient specific data. Examples of functionality are drug interaction alerts or reminders for specific guideline-based interventions during healthcare (e.g., reminders for vaccine shots during a child's physical) and the care of patients with chronic disease (e.g., reminders to check blood pressure or glucose levels). Information can be presented by a DSS in a patient-centric view of individual care or in an aggregate view in order to support population-wide health management. Practice Management Systems (PMS) are for processing financial, demographic, and non-medical information about patients as well as scheduling, claim submission to payers, and other tasks; Electronic prescribing (e-prescribing) systems for reviewing drug and formulary coverage and transmitting prescriptions electronically to a local pharmacy. Systems can be integrated into clinical information systems to also screen drug interactions and allergies; Billing systems supporting payers such as insurance companies or employer to process claims and bill patients.

Healthcare is a fundamentally collaborative discipline in which patients, particularly with chronic medical conditions, are treated by a wide range of medical providers in both outpatient (medical office or clinic) and inpatient (hospital) settings. This involvement poses a unique set of problems for data exchange including: a large number of stakeholders, workflows that routinely cross institutional boarders, and a lack of data/information standardization. Consider a case in which a patient who suffered from a heart attack presents himself with flu symptoms at a physician's office. When the physician attempts to retrieve an overview of the patient's medical history, their HIS might simultaneously obtain records from the hospital's emergency room (ER), where the patient was provided with care, the hospital clinic, where he was an inpatient during his recovery, and from his insurance company, which covered the cost of his treatments. While the record from the ER might be coding the patient's condition as *Myocardial Infarction*, the inpatient record can use the nonstandard description *Heart Attack* in combination with a decimal code, and the billing information might refer to a proprietary coding system that identifies the condition through an alphanumeric string. The significant challenge for HIE is to recognize that those three records belong to the same single individual and describe the same event (through a mapping of terms and semantics) in order to ensure that the medical history retrieved by the physician treating the patient's current flu symptoms lists the heart attack as one single incident, despite the incoherence of the source data.

This implies that in order to ensure correct and safe data transport between stakeholders, an HIE solution first has to overcome technical communication barriers between the participating systems, which can be only achieved by the establishment of nationally recognized standards for the transfer of medical data from both syntactic and semantic perspectives. In addition, an integrated HIE must not only to enable the transport of the physical data, but also to ensure that the meaning of exchanged information is maintained throughout the communication process. This second step can be achieved through a uniform utilization of medical ontology frameworks and common term databases which can translate heterogeneous names, codes, and identifiers to one common meaning (Demurjian, Saripalle, & Berhe, 2009).

Medical facilities which currently use HISs and would be involved in the above example are often not sufficiently connected to one another due to lack of HIE standards, competitive roadblocks to sharing data across enterprises, associated costs for HIE without proven cost benefits, and so on. As a result, while data is instantly available inside the physician's office system, collaboration with external providers (and their systems) is haphazard and ad-hoc. When a patient visits the majority of providers today, a hard copy paper patient chart is maintained, containing the medical records for all of the patient's visits over time. This chart grows over time as record deletion is extremely rare (unless incorrect data or lab results have been inserted); the time-oriented content (from present to past) is vital to clinicians who must not only treat the current ailment but also look back in time to have a full history of the patient and their conditions and treatments. On the path towards fully adopting HISs in all phases of a patient's treatment, the need to have a fully integrated, electronic version of this medication history (current and past) will be critical. As a result, the creation and availability of a virtual chart (VC)

(Kenny, Parsons, Gratch, & Rizzo, 2008) has been proposed to provide a consistent, complete, and historically accurate patient medical record through automatic, HIE based integration of data from various source repositories. In Figure 1, the source repositories are a patient's PHR, a physician's EHR, and a hospital's EMR; other sources would include prescription records at pharmacies, billing records of insurers, imaging/scanning and laboratory test results, etc.

In summary, the envisioned virtual chart: provides an individual patient EHR that gathers data from multiple HISs; allows for retrieval of individual EHRs facilitating communication between providers; supports extraction of anonymized patient data from for aggregation to support data mining; has data monitoring capabilities for event tracking; implements security and access control enforcement and storage of audit trails that includes privacy rules for all parts of the stored data, data de-identification, etc.; issues alerts and preventive information that is in relation to a given chart instance; and, supports system personalization for adjusting to patient and provider needs.

Figure 1. Healthcare Stakeholder Collaboration via HIE and Virtual Chart

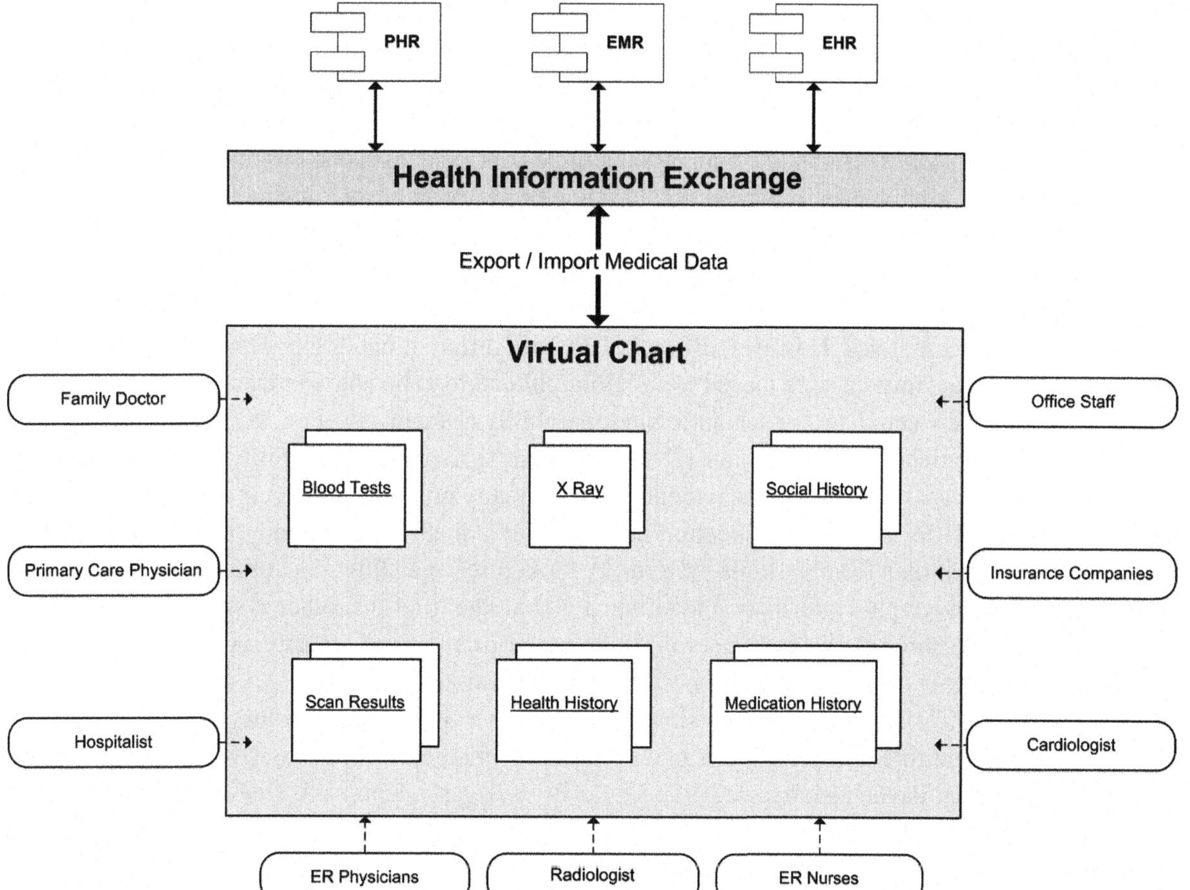

Challenges for HIE Architectures

Software designers and engineers have worked on solutions for cross-institutional communication, (legacy-) system integration, and data exchange for decades and have created a large selection of solutions, templates, and alternatives that are routinely being leveraged by software architects in various fields on a daily basis. These well accepted methods meet a significant challenge in their usage for HIE due to the extremely complex and heterogeneous nature of the healthcare domain. In a typical scenario, each group of stakeholders utilizes different types of HISs; for each of these system types there are multiple products offered by different vendors and equipped with different communication mechanisms. Software architectures for HIE must support incremental development, since systems of this scale cannot be built in one effort. Similarly, HIE must support adaption to evolving requirements, since the list of requirements are not always fully known at the start of the system construction. Furthermore, scalability in throughput and size must be at the core of a suitable architecture, since processing will be increasingly challenging with HIE growth and adaption of new technologies involved in the HIE. Finally, the chosen architectures for HIE must support heterogeneous environments, since the current HIS landscape is highly fragmented into many different types of HISs which in turn are available from different vendors. This typically hinders interoperability between systems and domain stakeholders.

Two types of interoperability are required by HIE. *Syntactic interoperability* enables interaction on a technical level (i.e., the format of the interaction) while *semantic interoperability* enables interaction on the content level (i.e., the meaning of the interaction). For example, for connecting the HISs of a physician's office, hospital, and insurance company for simple data exchange, one might establish a message format that allows the exchange of events, containing a field "event name" (syntactic interoperability). However, the same event might be recorded differently, as a cardiac arrest, a myocardial infarction, and a billing code, respectively in those HISs. The goal of semantic interoperability is then to recognize all three records as one event. To support this, a medical ontology would know that a myocardial infarction is synonymous to heart attack. However, different HISs use different ontologies and may organize their ontologies differently, thus causing a need for a HIE architecture to be able to manage different ontologies and translate between them for semantic interoperability (Demurjian et al., 2009).

Integration of patient data requires an ID Management system with the ability to identify the patient across many disparate HISs. Since patients may see many providers and their information may be stored in different HISs, the HIE architecture must provide a method to uniquely identify a patient in order to retrieve their data form multiple systems. A lookup service allows an authorized HIS to query with a patient's demographic information to obtain a global identifier that other systems can recognize. Finally, HIE architectures also require a strong support for privacy and security, since they are tasked with processing highly sensitive data that is subject to regulations such as HIPAA (HIPAA, 1996) and FERPA (FERPA, 1974). The architecture should implement a single point of entry to handle security, utilizing fine grained role and permission management for medical documents (De La Rosa Algarín, Demurjian, Berhe, & Pavlich-Mariscal, 2012; De La Rosa Algarín, Ziminski, Demurjian, Kuykendall, & Rivera Sánchez, 2013).

ARCHITECTURAL ALTERNATIVES

To set the context for the proposal of a hybrid HIE architecture, this section presents architectural styles that have the potential for usage in data integration and HIE. The first three, are collectively reviewed, namely: federation that directly utilizes in real time the data of HISs that is available for providing care; replication that off-loads data from HISs to dedicated edge servers that are then in turn federated; and, centralization that extracts data from multiple HISs into a single shared repository. Using this as a basis, a set of well-proven architectural styles and their suitability for HIE are analyzed, namely: service-oriented architecture (SOA) and grid computing, publish/subscribe architecture, data warehouse, and cloud computing.

Federation vs. Replication vs. Centralization

In the federated architectural style, shown in the right side of Figure 2, medical data remains at its HIS source(s), and is made remotely accessible on demand. In this classic approach, a global database query is submitted, broken down into constituent local queries, processed at the remote sources, with results collected and formatted for presentation to the user. There are many advantages to this style. First, since medical data remains under the governance of the HIS source(s), the central portions of such architectures can remain relatively lightweight and process ad-hoc data queries on demand. As a result, federated solutions lower the amount of sensitive data that is shared and avoid making a priori assumptions about the value of data that an exchange participant may offer. Second, the data that is provided by a federated solution should be the most up-to-date version available since the federated user is accessing the federation in real-time. Third, the nature of federated solutions promotes scalability in terms of adding new HIS sources to an exchange network. There are also some significant disadvantages. First, the availability of data depends on the availability of the providing HIS source(s) and may therefore be unpredictable., e.g., patient records stored in a physician's office EHR may be unavailable after office hours. Second, performance bottlenecks are possible, e.g., the major hospital's EMR in a region may be accessed from numerous physician offices on a daily basis; if such access impacts performance to delay patient care, the result can be catastrophic. Third, security and monitoring of activities may be challenging in federated solutions, especially controlling and restricting access to sensitive data required distributed security models.

To overcome some of the fundamental issues of the federated approach, it can be extended by replication, as shown in the middle portion of Figure 2, which introduces an additional repository for each HIS source housed on an edge server. Since each repository is periodically updated, one advantage is that there is no impact on patient care on the HIS source. A second advantage is that the data integration to the edge servers gives each participant fine-grained control about which data is shared in an exchange, therefore preserving local governance choices. Third, the replicated repositories can be optimized to-

Figure 2. The Federated, Replication, and Centralized Architectural Styles

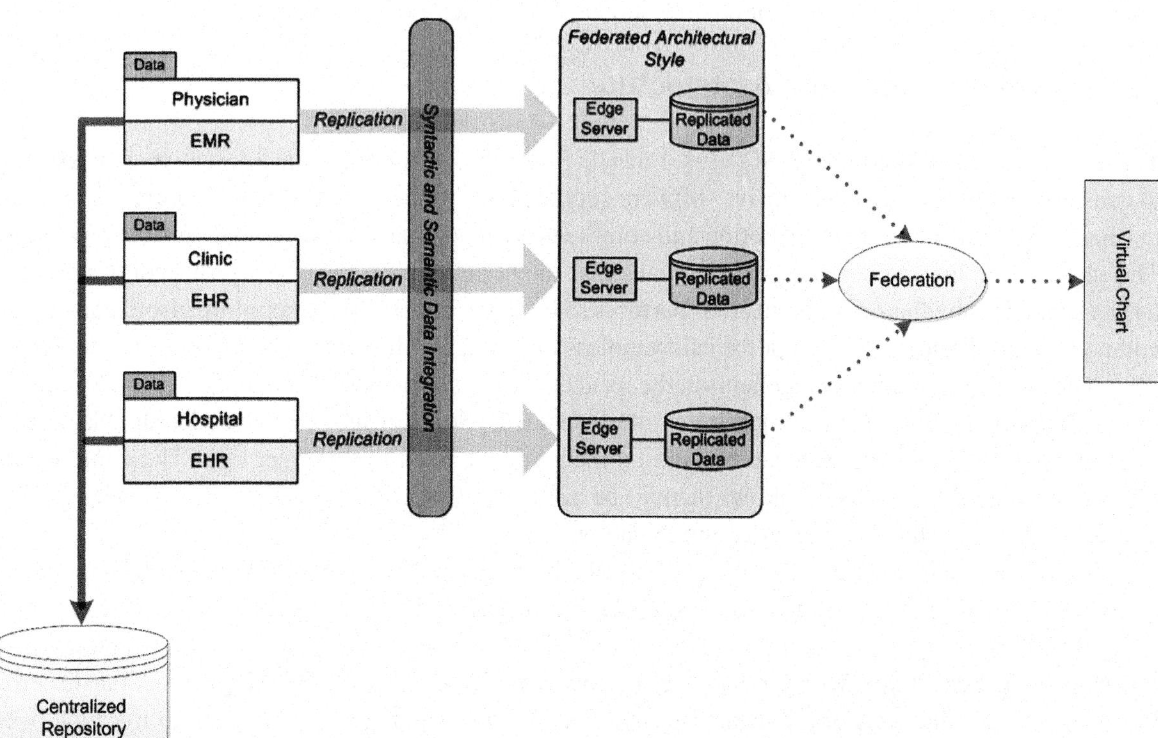

wards performance and availability, with minimal impact (typically only during offloading time) on HISs that are actively used for providing care. However, there are some disadvantages. First, the data that is offloaded from HIS source(s) may not always be up-to-date; periodic updates may be limited in order to minimize impact on the usage of the HIS source(s); for patient care, this is a problem since medical providers always require the latest patient data. Second, the information may be out of sync, e.g., the same patient that has data in two or more different HIS(s) may have an inconsistent view if the update periods differ per source. Third, security and monitoring remain just as challenging as with a federated approach.

Lastly, the centralized approach in the bottom left of Figure 2 provides a common location—a new central participant in the data exchange—to operate as a main, shared repository. Designing and implementing a centralized architecture requires the extraction and integration of existing data from the HIS source(s), either stepwise or in one major effort; this is true for both initialization and periodic updates to the repository's content. Through this integration process, a centralized approach makes it possible to attain syntactic and semantic interoperability, as discussed in the prior section. A first advantage is that one administrative governance can be utilized to control access to the shared information. Second, since the data in the central repository is available independent of HIS source(s), these source(s) are no longer impacted by external access. Third, contributors have significant control in terms of the patient that is to be shared and in what way (security). However, there are some disadvantages. First, there is a capacity factor to be considered since the data from potential hundreds of providers (e.g., hospitals, clinics, practices, labs, etc.) in a geographical region must be collected and combined; a country-wide integration would be even more difficult to achieve in practice. Second, the integration process from multiple HIS source(s) would require the need to reconcile all of the patient data to insure that the same John Smith's data has been collected from all sources without error. Third, from a system perspective, there is a probable performance bottleneck as HIS source(s) increase, the potential for fatal events if the repository goes down, and attacks or data theft that now impact a larger body of data.

Service-Oriented and Grid Architecture

The service-oriented architecture (SOA) as shown in Figure 3 is an architectural alternative which serves to construct extensible and inexpensive software support for business processes and workflows in order to supply a framework for administration and combination of software services which reflect processes. The services are loosely coupled, which means that they communicate over platform independent interfaces and assume their communication partners to be black boxes. Loose coupling also means that a component is self-sufficient except for its awareness and usage of the other components. Components offer their functions to other components in the form of services, which are similar in concept to publishing methods of an application programming interface (API). Services hide technical details (black box) and are defined functions which can be used on their own or as part of a larger task. The components connect via a mechanism which allows them to be aware of other components and their services while hiding the details of the component communication.

SOAs can be realized based on web services, which are defined by the World Wide Web Consortium (W3C) as "a software system designed to support interoperable machine-to-machine interaction over a network"

(Haas & Brown, 2004). Web services are commonly realized with HTTPS (Hypertext Transfer Protocol Secure – basic protocol for secured passing of web service data from machine to machine over the web), XML (Extensible Markup Language – a widely accepted standard for information exchange),

Figure 3. Service Communication in a Service-Oriented Architecture

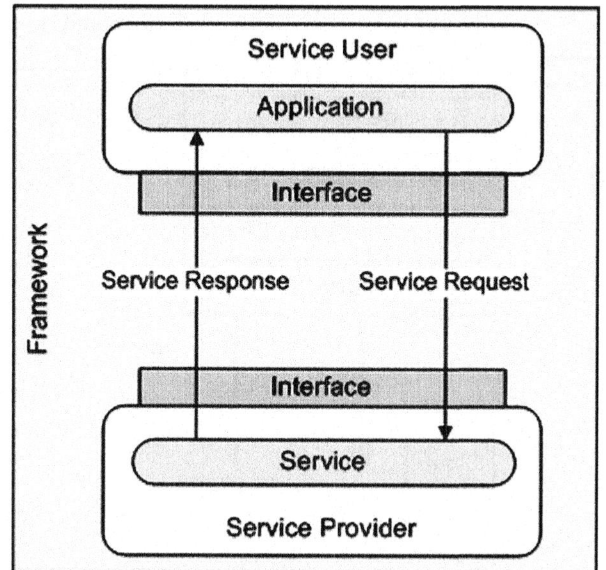

WSDL (Web Services Description Language – used to describe the functions of a web service in a machine-readable way, which allows the programmatic localization and utilization of a web service), SOAP (Simple Object Access Protocol – a lightweight communication protocol for message exchange and remote procedure calls which builds on HTTP and XML), and UDDI (Universal Description, Discovery and Integration registry – a registration directory for web service environments). Comprehensive introductions to all mentioned technologies are provided by the W3C (W3C, 2008).

SOAs manage the data of the participating components based on the federated/replicated approach. For the purpose of a healthcare SOA, this component needs to provide a set of lookup services: a *registry* for medical services, which stores references to the services that can be used through the SOA (may be based on WSDL and UDDI); a *patient identification mechanism*, which is effectively a *master patient index (MPI)* for identifying individual patients across the participating HIS sources; and, a *medical record lookup facility*, which stores of location of data, the patients index, and meta-data about the nature of the stored patient data (e.g., laboratory results, filled prescriptions, EMR, etc.) along with administrative data (e.g., creation date, last update, etc.). The meta-data will also contain information about the syntactic and semantic formats of the stored record; this allows accessing HIE participants to determine whether they can process the information automatically or not.

The lightweight central architecture means that each participating HIS source needs to implement an interface towards the SOA that is structured as depicted in Figure 4. The security component communicates with the central component of the SOA for authentication and authorization clearance. The administrative layer creates logs and audit trails for satisfying legal requirements. Transformations for semantic and syntactic interoperability are executed by the interoperability layer based on the meta-data provided with every medical record passed through the SOA. The synchronization layer is responsible for buffering or saving data for local use, signalling updates to other SOA participants, and reacting to data updates signalled from the SOA. Finally, the application interface interacts with the underlying HIS

Figure 4. Logical Components Encapsulated in the HIE Interfaces of HIS sources

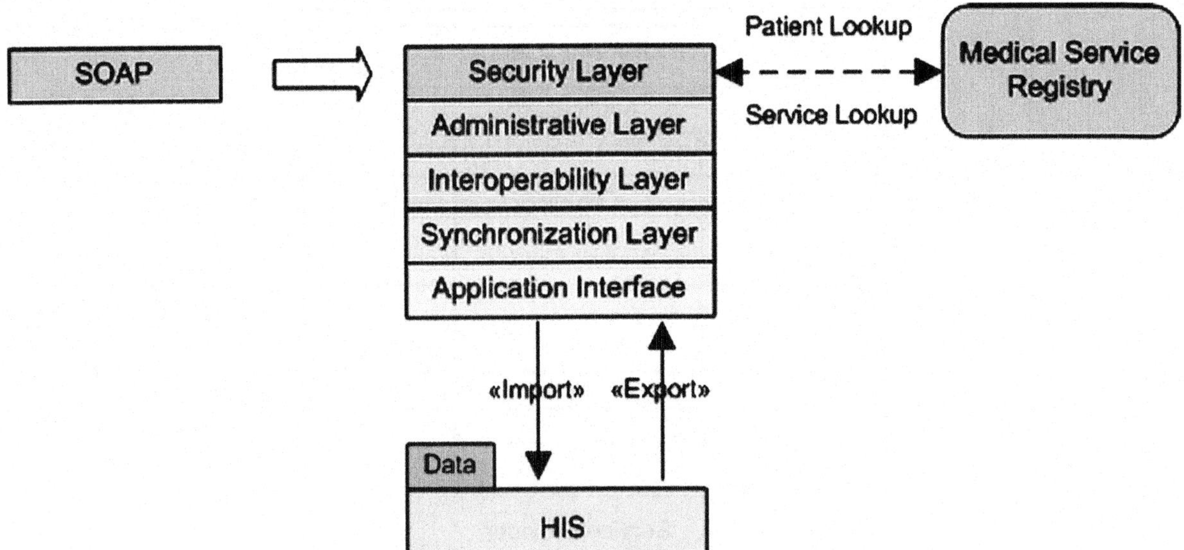

source and triggers import and export of data as well as data processing. Clearly, there is a significant set of layers that must be provided for an HIS source to successfully utilize SOA.

To deal with performance issues in SOA, for complex science and research environments with high resource demands (e.g., CPU cycles, data storage, etc.), grid computing can be utilized. Grid computing describes sharing otherwise unused resources in a cluster (grid) of independent computing nodes. This happens in a transparent way, in which the additional resources from the created virtual super computer are available, just as electricity is in a power grid, to each of the connected nodes.

(Foster, 2002) defines the grid system based on following characteristics: "A Grid is a system that coordinates resources that are not subject to centralized control, using standard, open, general-purpose protocols and interfaces to deliver nontrivial qualities of service." For the purpose of this chapter, grid computing is a realization of SOA with a selection of extremely fine-grained services. While the coarse-grained services of a SOA seem a more suitable solution for the workflow-oriented medical domain, there are emerging initiatives to utilize grid computing for healthcare improvement, medical research, and collaborative care (caBIG, 2004; World Community Grid, 2004), including: medical image processing and analysis, pharmaceutic research/development tasks, complex modelling and visualization jobs, and genomic applications. As personal genomics moves into the forward with genetic information linked to medical patient data, grid computing may be necessary to handle the potential higher volume of data.

Publish/Subscribe Architecture

Publish/subscribe is an asynchronous messaging paradigm describing the relationship of senders (publishers) and receivers (subscribers) with: *publisher* which sends out categorized messages containing relevant data and do not contain a specific target address; *subscriber* which allows a subscription to one or several feeds that cover message classes without having knowledge on publishers that process all received messages according to their needs; and, *broker* which are optional components for mediating between publishers and subscribers by encapsulating the classification of messages, the subscription process, and the message dispatch. In an HIE system that connects multiple HIS source(s), a publish/subscribe architecture could be used for: the exchange of arbitrary medical data between the stakeholders of the domain, health status and advisory notifications such as epidemic alerts, and feedback mechanisms such as drug reaction reporting.

The publisher/subscriber architecture could be applied to healthcare to provide data from multiple HIS source(s), as shown in Figure 5, by implementing the federated data storage approach without central data storage using an *enterprise service bus (ESB)* for the broker. ESB allows message-based communication and integration between components connected to the bus. This is achieved through a set of services provided by the bus, such as routing services to pass messages from a sender to one or several receivers, and transformation services which can encapsulate syntactic and semantic transformations that are needed in healthcare. Using an ESB for healthcare allows for a higher level of central governance and interoperability control, since all of the communication happens over one component, while keeping the central architecture relatively small. Several ESB products, mostly based on sets of various middleware components, are available from different vendors, in both open and closed source commercial distributions (OpenESB, 2012; WebSphere ESB, 2008; BizTalk Server, 2006; Oracle ESB, 2012; Apache ESB, 2008). Publish/subscribe for healthcare, as depicted in Figure 5, contains the following components: *Patient Identification* implements an MPI in order to identify patients across HIS source(s) by creating an index for a given patient with each source responsible for its correct usage; *Administration* and *Access Logging* contain the addresses of the registered HIS sources, their meta-data, and access rights information to log which HIE participant received which messages in the publishing process and stores records to meet legal audit requirements; *Message Feed Administration* and *Subscription Administration* that contain a list of all message feeds and their current subscribers; *Publish Service* that is the communication interface for publishers, contains syntactic and semantic transformation services for a central interoperability control, and assures that messages distributed over the ESB are readable by all related subscribers; and, *Subscription Service* that is the communication interface for subscribers, which notifies all of the subscribers of a message feed on the arrival of new related messages and maintains the messages until they are delivered to the subscribers.

In summary, the publish/subscribe architecture implements the federated approach to data storage (the broker does not persist any data after a successful dispatch), and the architecture shares the basic advantages and disadvantages as in the case of SOA. Two potential problems are the unnecessary data replication across the system and the balance which the HIS source(s) must keep between (a) signing up for too many feeds (risk of information overflow) and (b) signing up for too few (loss of relevant information). Too high a number of feeds may slow down the receiving system and have negative impact on patient care; too few feeds may mean a healthcare provider has incomplete data and cannot make a diagnosis or a researcher arrives at an invalid conclusion in a study. The central broker component of the publish/subscribe architecture can remain relatively lightweight and inexpensive, yet still incorporate a good handling of logging, access rights management, and interoperability control.

Data Warehouse

The data warehouse collects data from multiple sources to provide a uniform view on data for querying, analysis, and decision making tasks. Data warehouses (Inmon, 2005) are data collections with the following key characteristics: *subject-oriented* which describes the way that data for the warehouse is

Figure 5. Publish/Subscribe HIE

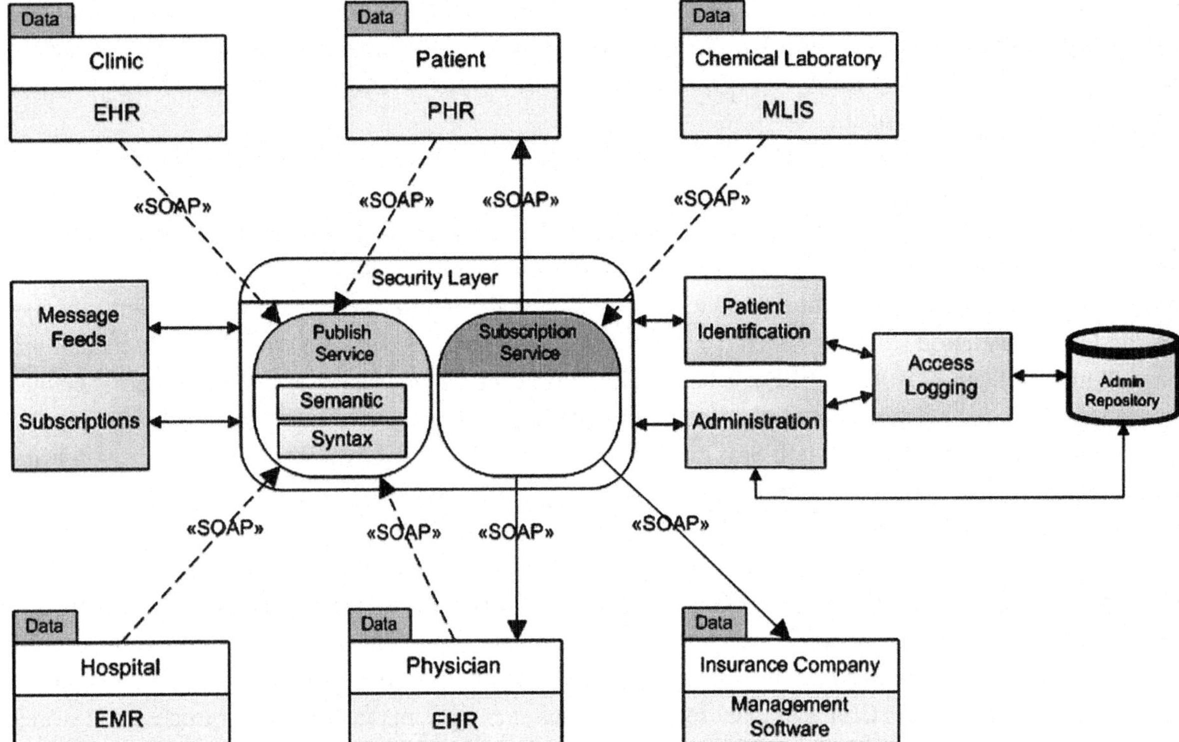

chosen, where a possible subject for the healthcare domain would be the patient or the physician; *integrated* which refers to the common schema in which the data (extracted from heterogeneous sources) is stored; *time-variant* which refers to the long-term storage of data, allowing analysis related to time; and, finally, *non-volatile* which means that once stored, data remains in the data warehouse (i.e., there are no delete or overwrite operations). For example, in healthcare, a data warehouse for emergency room patient data from hospitals throughout a country could be utilized to identify and track diseases, epidemics, etc.

Establishing a data warehouse for healthcare data includes two main tasks: extract and integrate data from multiple HIS source(s); and, make the integrated repository available to all eligible HIE participants via a query interface. Data extraction from HIS source(s) occurs periodically through scheduled pull operations (ideally in the after office hours in order to minimize impact on performance of systems used for providing care) or as push operations initiated by the sources (e.g., when low system load is detected). The extraction and integration process is complex and requires the following subtasks

(Inmon, 2005): *converting* the data into a common format (e.g., HL7 CDA (HL7, 2007) or CCR (CCR, 2012) in healthcare) with syntactical and semantic checks as well as by transformations as needed to match the utilized storage formats; *cleaning* the data of irregularities such as data entry errors, e.g., heights in meters instead of feet and inches; *integration* of the different data sets to suit the data model of the data warehouse, e.g., clearly identify the same John Smith in all sources; and, *transformation* of the data through summarizing and creating new attributes, e.g., aggregating certain medical data that may make an automated clinical decision such as finding multiple high blood pressures for the same patient over time with no appropriate medication prescribed. Note that these four steps are often a semi-automated processes requiring significant human interaction and intervention which is a negative for usage with healthcare. The healthcare data in a warehouse must separate identity with encrypted storage of patient identifiers for safe retrieval of anonymous data and identification of individuals for authorized entities, e.g., contact of suitable patient cohorts for research studies.

The data warehouse has advantages that include room for optimization, acceptable and predictable performance, and administration of security and interoperability matters under one governance structure. However, the actuality of a real-time data warehouse might be not realizable in a satisfyingly performant way for a regional or country-wide HIE. For example, in healthcare, there is a need to have high availability of data as it impacts patient care, which is not as critical for an e-commerce application. This will necessitate both frequent uploads and synchronizations which may impact HIS source(s) performance; if not, the data would be worthless to the treating medical provider. Further, a country-wide data warehouse may simply not be feasible with the large scale of systems to gather data from and the resulting volume of data. The usage of data warehouses for healthcare may be limited to non-patient care situations but might be possible to construct very large scale warehouses for offline medical and healthcare data analysis.

Cloud Computing

The formal definition of cloud computing (Mell & Grance, 2011) sums up this paradigm: "Cloud computing is a model for enabling ubiquitous, convenient, on-demand network access to a shared pool of configurable computing resources (e.g., networks, servers, storage, applications, and services) that can be rapidly provisioned and released with minimal management effort or service provider interaction". Cloud computing is an architectural concept which allows the usage of abstract resources that hide computational details and complexity from their users, much like SOA. A key feature of cloud resources is their rapid elasticity (Armbrust et al., 2009) that allows the company to grow and shrink capacities according to requirements that potentially change in real time, catering towards application fields like e-commerce with very high punctual peaks in infrastructural requirements (e.g., sales on Black Friday or Cyber Monday). Cloud computing typically provides "on-demand self-service" (Armbrust et al., 2009), which means that adjustments to the service (e.g., registration, configuration, extension) are mostly automatic and can be executed programmatically. Service will usually depend on broad network access through standard mechanisms (e.g., web service technologies) which requires a constantly available network connection with sufficient quality of service. Resource pooling and virtualization plays an important role in the background of a typical cloud computing service. However, the user deploying a service to the cloud or using it through a thing client (e.g., a smartphone) has, in most cases, no control of any physical resource instances and is protected from the complexity of that the process.

Cloud-computing solutions for enabling health information collection, exchange, and collaboration are appearing in the marketplace, e.g., Microsoft Cloud Services for Health (Microsoft Cloud Services for Health, 2015), the IBM Collaborative Care project (Andrews and Mack, 2011), Logiworks Healthcare Solutions (Logicworks, 2015), VMware vCloud (VMWare vCloud, 2015), etc. Since cloud computing platforms typically foster modular approaches, this facilitates configurable plug-in architectures with support of various extensions for healthcare tasks: decision support, note processing, voice recognition, and patient education. Furthermore, the versatility of the deployment model is capable of streamlining the realization of HIE and the integration of multiple HIS sources by installing regional clouds and enabling communication through hybrid clouds is a big plus. For example, cloud EHRs such as Practice Fusion

(Practice Fusion EHR, 2015) could be used to efficiently implement the application service provider model as described by

(Wager, Lee, & Glaser, 2009), which is important in the context of implementing EHRs in small practices that do not have the financial means to hire technical know-how for software and hardware maintenance. A third advantage is, building the virtual patient chart, as introduced earlier in this chapter, could largely benefit from a platform with some of the characteristics provided by the cloud services. There are some disadvantages. First, while HIS sources may implement federation/centralization on top of the cloud paradigm, their foundation is an abstract system under the governance of the cloud provider. This has two results: negative implications for regulatory issues since cloud providers do typically not specify where data centers are located, so that patient data may be stored outside of the patient's country and become subject to foreign laws; and, uncertainty for security particularly if sensitive data become accessible outside of an HIS source through shared hardware and faulty instance encapsulation.

A REGIONAL HIE SCENARIO

To define the canvas against which the features and components of the proposed hybrid HIE architecture to be explained in the latter portions of this chapter, this section introduces a set of HIS sources that participate in a regional HIE scenario, lists the employed HISs, and identifies selected examples for collaboration between sources. For the purpose of this discussion, a source is classified either as a data supplier or as a data consumer. Note that in order to maintain clarity, a simplified model is used, with a limited amount of sources and under the assumption that each source fits exclusively into its category. In an actual HIE scenario, suppliers naturally will consume data at the same time, and vice versa. In order to place the data suppliers and consumers into a concrete context, Figure 6 illustrates a real-life regional HIS infrastructure. The example is centered on the HISs of a physician's practice (e.g., a community practice) and explores the support for administrative tasks, clinical care, patient access, and the exchange of information in the process of providing patient care.

The core of the HIE infrastructure showcases the use of a selection of HIS sources as discussed earlier in this chapter: Administration of the practice, to manage patient demographics, appointments, billing tasks, etc. are supported by the patient management system (PMS), which interfaces with insurance companies and other payers. Clinical care is provided with the support of an EHR system in combination with a decision support system and various input devices; PMS and EMR automatically report to healthcare-related agencies. The EHR supports an e-prescribing feature as well as the electronic communication with various medical laboratories. Patients are able to access information from the practice's systems via a web-based patient portal and the PHR. The EHR system accesses information from other external providers via HIE to access a hospitals EMR or a laboratory system, and allows reviewing a patient's medical history via a virtual chart. Note that the parenthetical notation in the remainder of this section is referring to the location of each HIS source in Figure 6.

To begin, the data suppliers that are shown in Figure 6 are reviewed.

- **Community Practice (Upper Half):** A medical practice operated by several physicians (e.g., a general practitioner, a pediatrician, an internist, and a radiologist) and their staff. The HISs used in the practice are a decision support system (DSS), a practice management system, a web-based

Figure 6. Overview of a Health Information System Infrastructure

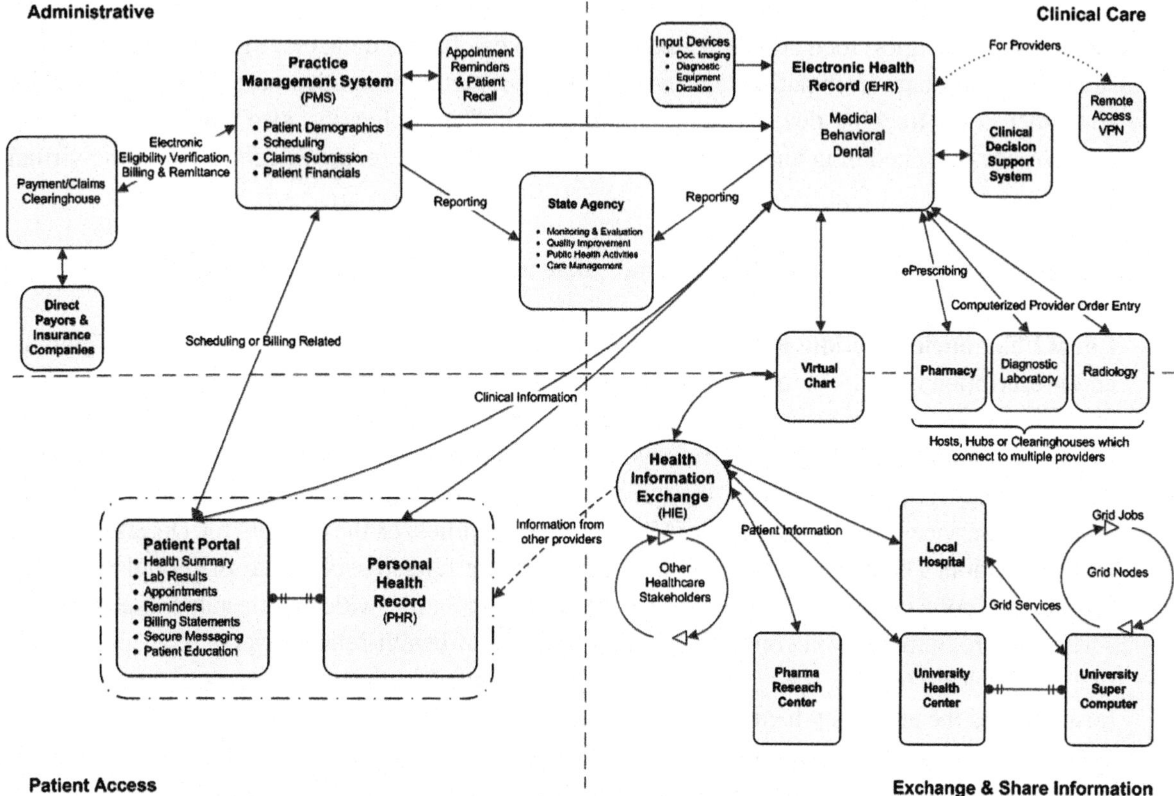

patient portal and an EHR. The practice collaborates with the virtual chart, pharmacies (e-prescriptions), and state agencies (reporting of selected diseases mandated by law).

- **Local Hospital (Lower Right):** A hospital providing healthcare to inpatients and outpatients from the local population. The hospital staff (i.e., nurses, physicians, ER personal, etc.) files patient data with an EMR and uses a DSS, where required by patient care. The hospital's radiology department participates in a large-scale breast cancer screening program and stores the resulting images in a custom database (the beginning of a data warehouse) for automatic analysis. The hospital collaborates with a university supercomputer center (automated x-ray analysis), the virtual chart, and state agencies.

- **University Health Center (Lower Right):** A research focused healthcare facility with a limited patient cohort (two hundred inpatients), maintaining an infrastructure for clinical studies, and running a human tissue and specimen bank. A medical chemistry laboratory equipped with a medical laboratory information system (MLIS) is also part of the center. The health center staff (i.e., physicians, clinical researchers, nurses, etc.) utilizes an EHR system and custom databases for the management of data related to inpatients and study participants. The EHR system supports automatic drug tolerance reporting to the pharmaceutical research center of a sponsor. The center collaborates with a university supercomputer center (for genomic research), state agencies, and a pharmaceutical research center.

- **Personal Health Record (Lower Left):** A web-based application used by patients to maintain their medical and health histories, including conditions, received treatments, current and past medications, allergies, food supplements, health markers, fitness data, etc. Significant parts of the stored data originate from patient entries (manual or recorded through smartphone apps or other consumer-grade tracking devices such as wearables). The application also supports a calendar function for the scheduling and planning of practice visits. The record is connected to the virtual chart.

To complete the discussion, the data consumers that are shown in Figure 6 are reviewed.

- **Local Pharmacies (Middle Right):** A group of pharmacies offering a variety of over-the-counter and prescription drugs. The main HIS used is a pharmacy management system (management of prescription histories, e-prescribing interface, business processes). Each pharmacy is connected to the community practice (e-prescriptions), the local hospital, and the university health center.
- **State Agency (Upper Middle):** Institution such as the Department of Mental Health and Addiction Services, the Department of Children and Families, or the Centers for Disease Control and Prevention. The agencies provide various healthcare-related services to the population such as issuing reports on health-trends, monitoring of the population-wide health status, executions of screening programs (e.g., alcohol abuse), and tracking of health-related events (e.g., in the case of a pandemic outbreak). The agency collects data generated by the community practice, the local hospital, and the university health center.
- **Insurance Company (Upper Left):** A company providing a variety of health plans for public agencies, and private and corporate customers; handles eligibility verification and billing for the local hospital and the community practice.
- **Pharmaceutical Research Center (Lower Right):** A research facility operated by a pharmaceutical company. The facility collaborates with the university health center (collection of anonymized data for research purposes) as well as with the local hospital and the community practice (recruit patients and retrieval of results from pharmaceutical studies).
- **University Supercomputer Center (Lower Right):** A virtual supercomputer operated by the university's center for transitional science. The system is based on a grid architecture, connecting grid nodes at the university and nationwide.
- **Virtual Chart (Middle Right):** An HIE application providing consistent, complete, and historically accurate patient medical records through automatic integration of data from various source repositories. The chart is linked to all HIE participants that process medical histories (such as the local hospital or the community practice).

A HYBRID HIE ARCHITECTURE (HHIEA)

The architectural alternatives studied in this chapter have many disadvantages that make their usage unsuitable for an HIE solution using only one of the alternatives. This section proposes a hybrid HIE architecture (HHIEA) at a design level, by proposing a combination of the studied architectural styles which both balances and mitigates the advantages and disadvantages. The resulting HHIEA establishes a more effective and flexible architecture that facilitates the exchange of information between multiple

HIS sources and provides a comprehensive and integrated view on healthcare data. HHIEA combines: data warehouse (Prokosch & Ganslandt, 2009; Bauer & Günzel, 2013), SOA (Rosen, 2008; Ryan & Eklund, 2008), grid computing (Dickmann et al., 2012; Foster, 2002), and the publish/subscribe paradigm (Eugster et al., 2003; Singh, Vargas, Bacon, & Moody, 2008). The proposed HHIEA, as shown in Figure 7, is presented in five logical groups in separately labeled subsections, namely: the *Data Layer* where all of the data suppliers and data consumers are logically part of this group; *ID Management* that is utilized to both identify and differentiate patients and organizations participating in the HIE; *HIE Management* that is composed of tasks related to the maintenance of medical record references; *Security* that contains components that are related to the management of audit trails, patient consents, and participant authentication; and, a *Health Service Bus* that is responsible for ensuring the precise passing messages between the HIS sources. The discussion on HHIEA is completed with a section that utilizes the realistic healthcare scenario in order to fully demonstrate the ability of HHIEA to attain and support HIE.

Data Layer

The *data layer* of the proposed HHIEA, as shown in the middle of Figure 7, is the location where information that has been extracted from each HIS source is utilized with a replicated storage style with edge servers in order to acquire information from the HIS sources. The processes for the initial loading of each HIS source (data supplier) to the replicas and subsequent incremental updates at periodic intervals are left to the administrators of the deployed HHIEA. If data of a HIS source is requested by a data consumer then it is served from the dedicated edge server within which the HIS source replicates its contents. The physical location of the replica can be at the HIS source or at a neutral location, where data from all source(s) is assembled; the location is transparent to all users. As shown in Figure 8, the *data suppliers* in the data layer are intended to provide the appropriate services that are needed in order to create both the initial replica and incrementally update from the HIS source(s). The *data consumers* in Figure 9 in the data layer provide the appropriate services for the stakeholders to access the aggregated information that spans these multiple HIS source(s) that are now replicas in the data layer. As a result, the data layer of HHIEA exploits the replication style to create and organize the replicas of the HIS source(s), leverages the publish/subscribe architecture in order to stage data in and out of the replicas, and provides data consumers with the means to make use of health information (e.g., for aggregation in a data warehouse).

This approach to the data layer insures that governing HIE participants have full control over which data is shared via HIE while simultaneously decoupling performance and security issues from the operative systems of the replicas that contain data from the HIS source(s). The combination of replication and publish/subscribe into the data layer promotes the definition of security policies, privacy regulations, and permissions at this common layer. In setting up each replica from a specific HIS source, the data owner (e.g., a hospital with an EHR) can determine what information to share, as depicted in Figure 9, where information from the EMR, patient portal, practice management system, etc., can be shared. The edge servers can enable interoperability by allowing them to enforce common standards for storage (e.g., syntactic interoperability) and to manage the stored data with common ontologies (e.g., semantic interoperability). Replication to the edge server is solved separately by each HIS source which allows for a high level of customization in order to meet special characteristics of the legacy systems. Therefore, the process of edge server deployment brings the opportunity to enforce a canonical message format and a common semantic foundation for exchanging data.

Figure 7. High Level Overview of the HHIE Architecture

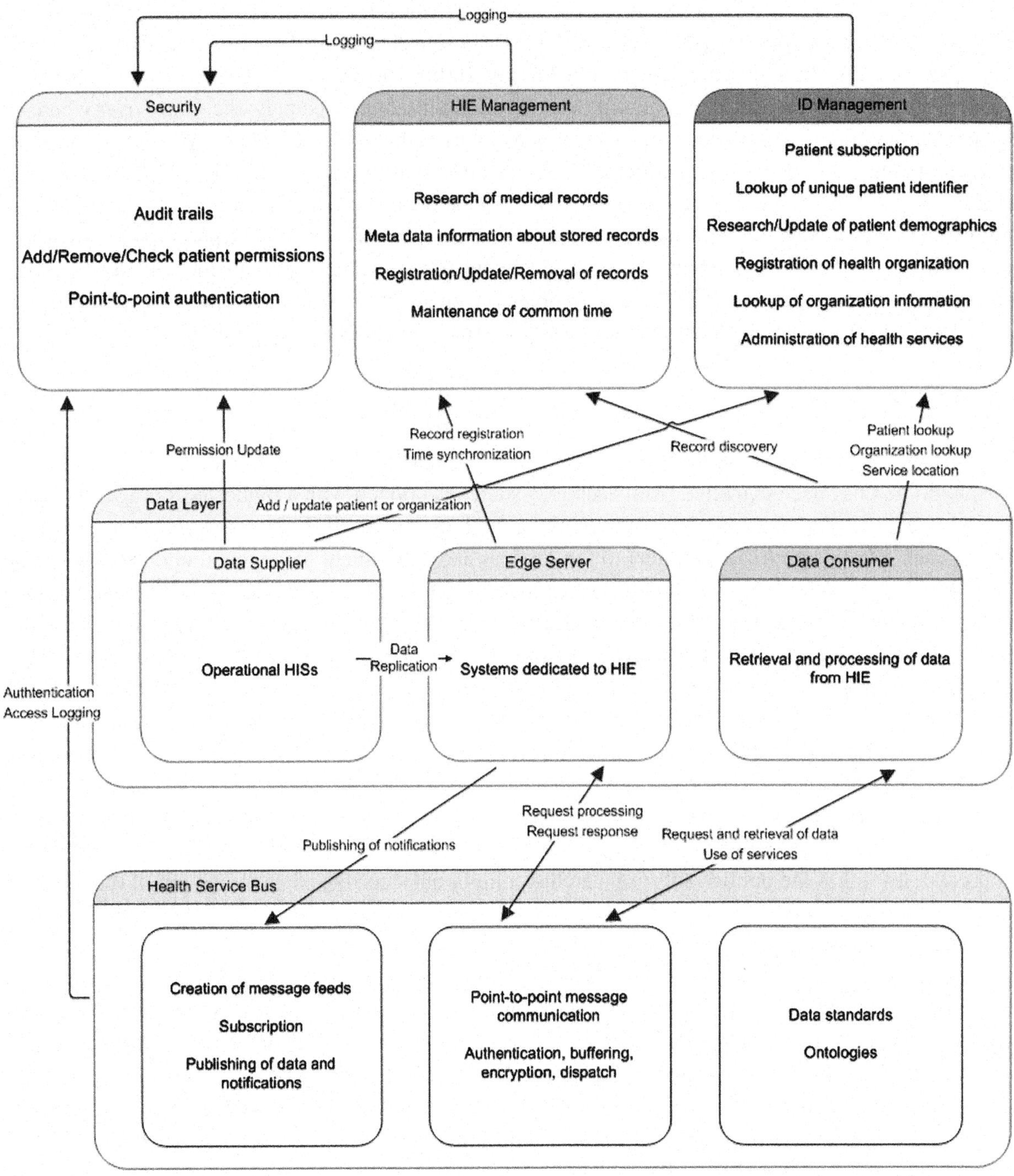

Figure 8. The Data Layer with Data Suppliers, Edge Systems, and Data Consumers

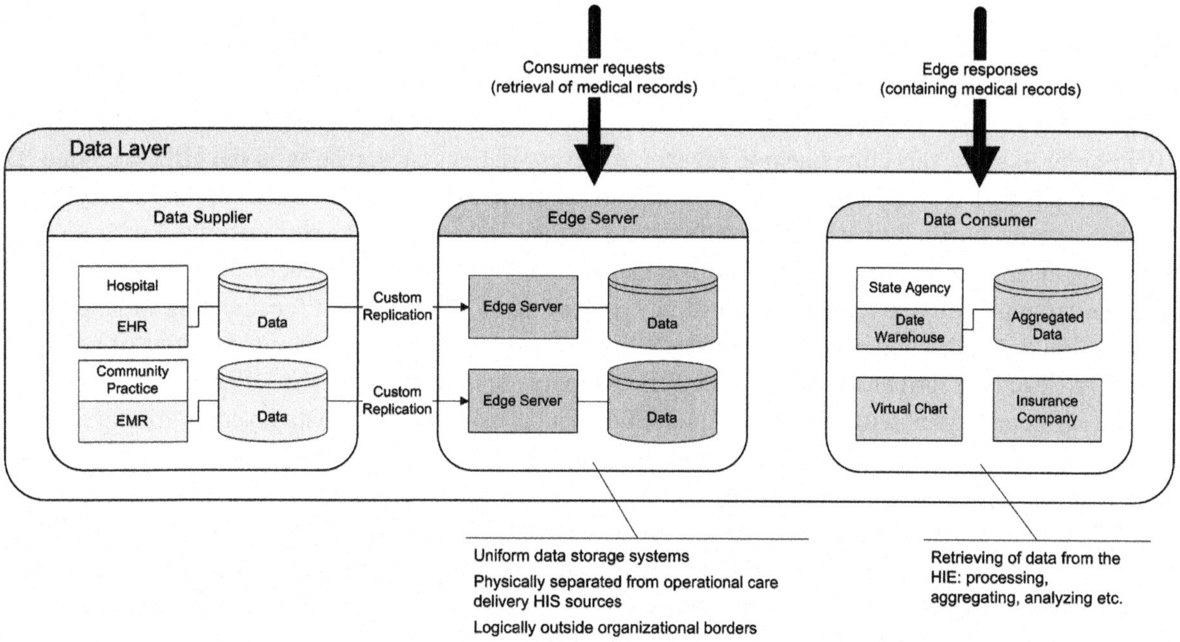

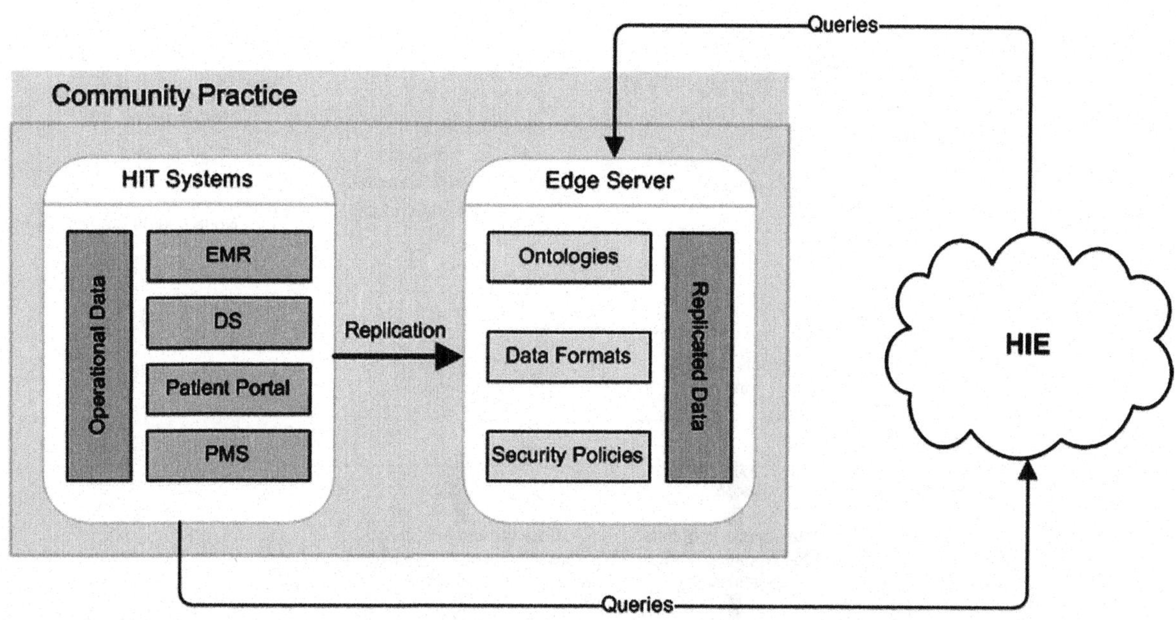

Figure 9. A Community Practice with Edge Server System and HIE Interactions

ID Management

The components in the *ID management* group, as illustrated in the upper right of Figure 7, provide the means for HHIEA to maintain cross-organizational identification of HIE participants. For the identification of patients, a *master patient index (MPI)* component must be implemented, shown in Figure 10, in order to allow this component to register, for every patient participating in the HIE, a unique ID and storing it with a set of demographic information. Furthermore, the MPI must support two types of queries: queries parameterized with a valid global patient ID, and queries parameterized with a set of demographic information (e.g., first name, last name, date of birth, and birth place). The first type returns the demographics for a given patient for identity verification purposes and for updating demographic information (e.g., changed place of residence). With the second type, the unique identifier of a patient can be retrieved for further use (or created if the patient is not registered in the HIE yet).

The MPI component will typically be queried by data consumers of the data layer in order to retrieve the MPI for a patient, which is needed to locate patient records. Data suppliers will access the component to sign up new patients (request a new MPI) and to update existing demographics. A similar component, the *HIS source registry,* is utilized for the identification of healthcare organizations (i.e., hospitals, clinics, labs, etc.) participating in the HIE. The registry maintains a globally unique ID for each HIS source, which is distributed to an organization during an adequately controlled registration process in order to avoid service violations and to ensure a secure domain. In addition to the HIS source ID, the HIS source registry stores general information about an organization (e.g., organization type, physical address, etc.) in query language form. Furthermore, each organization can offer SOA and grid services

Figure 10. The Identity Management Component

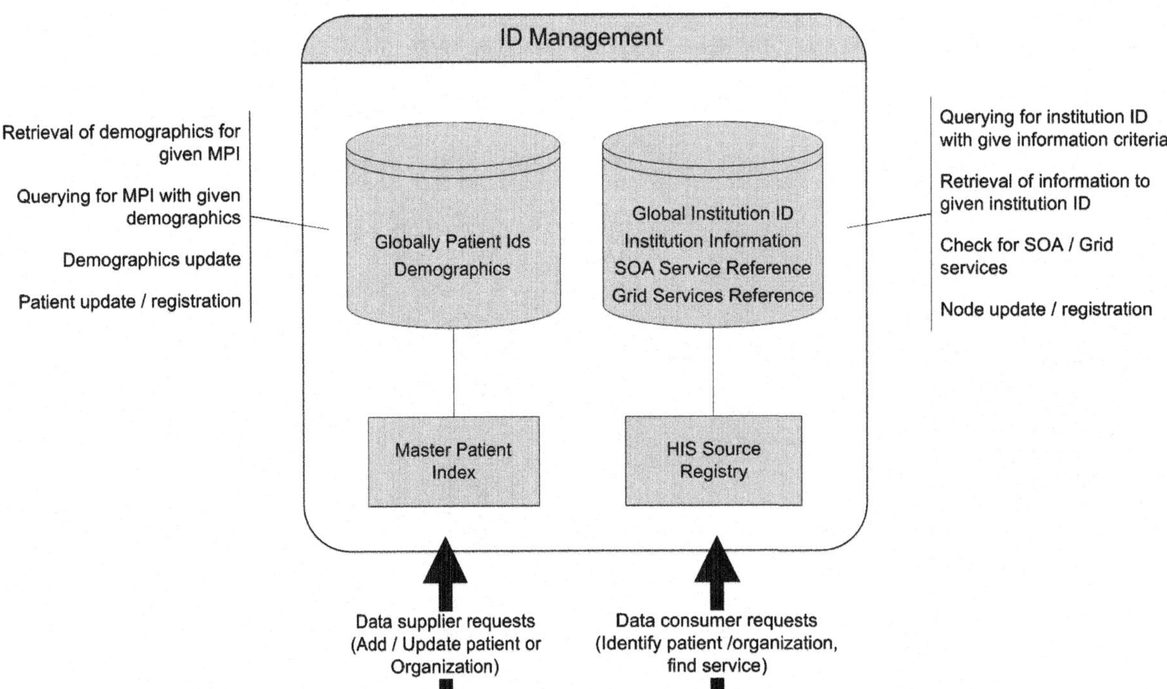

via this component; complete and machine-readable descriptions to those services are also kept in the HIS source registry. The ID Management group will, in most cases, be queried by data consumers for the lookup of services. Data suppliers will access the registry to update information about their organization.

HIE Management

The *HIE management* group of the proposed HHIEA, as shown in the upper middle of Figure 7, consists of two components: a *medical record registry* that is capable of mapping the MPI to all of the multiple replicas that may contain data for a patient; and, a *global clock* for time-stamps in order to eliminate inconsistencies in data. As shown in Figure 11, the medical record registry identifies medical records across the HIE by processing queries from data consumers; these queries must contain a valid MPI value. After receiving a query from an eligible data consumer, the registry will return a list of HIS source identifiers which reference all of the replicas that are storing records related to the MPI in question. For a baseline, a simple retrieval of all available related HIS source identifiers can be implemented that would bring in entire medical records for a patient from the HIS source replicas. A more comprehensive querying approach may be smart enough to limit the retrieval to only recently added records for the patient. With the list of identifiers, a data consumer is able to retrieve the contact information of the data suppliers storing the records and request them via an appropriate service (which will finally be served by the replica of the data supplier). In addition to the identifier, the registry stores metadata on the data formats available for the record as well as the ontologies necessary to interpret the record's content. Based on this meta-data, a requesting data consumer can determine if the processing of the record can be managed automatically or if it will require human intervention. The medical record registry will be, in most cases, accessed by data consumers during the search for records related to a patient; edge systems will also access the registry and add information each time a new record becomes available or at some periodic interval. The global clock component addresses problems arising from asynchronous/faulty timestamps in medical records. For example, if two records related to one incident are available on two different replicas and the timestamp of one of them is offset by a year due to a faulty set system time, an automatic interpretation of the records will result in the assumption that the incident occurred twice. To avoid such situations, all HIS sources and their replicas must synchronize their timestamps with the help of the global clock.

Security

In order to enable the exchange of sensitive medical data, a *security* component of the proposed HHIEA is required, as shown in the upper left of Figure 7. Security and access control in the heterogeneous and federated healthcare domain is a highly complex topic and, thus, implementation details cannot be provided in the scope of this chapter. However, to support the key requirements, a security group for the HHIEA containing the set of components illustrated in Figure 12 is proposed: an *authentication* component, an *access authorization* component, and an *audit authority* component. For secure point-to-point message communication between the participating data suppliers and data consumers, means for identity authentication of communication partners must be provided. This task is addressed by the authentication component, which is utilized as a central trusted third party.

In a healthcare setting, a medical provider (e.g., physician) would typically be authenticated to their EMR and have access to an EHR. In HHIEA, the replicas bring together multiple HIS sources, and the

Figure 11. The HIE Management Component

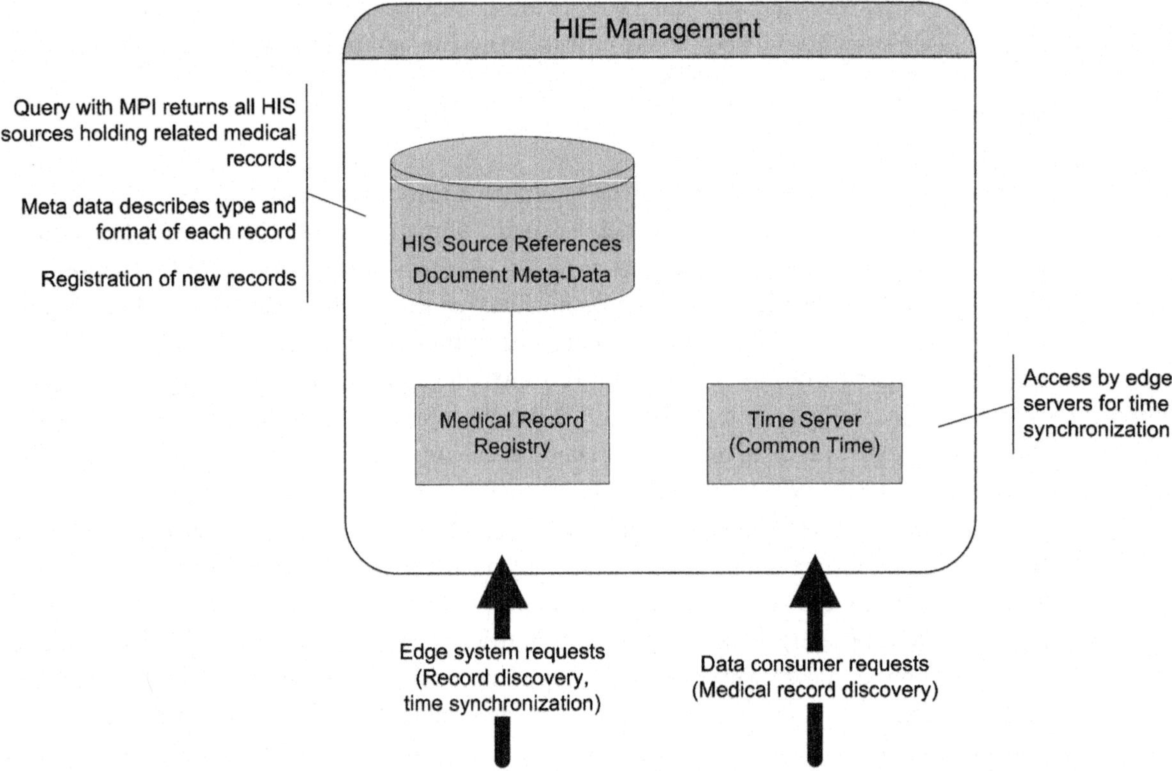

likelihood is that the physician has not been authenticated to all sources. As a result, the authentication component must be capable of reviewing a physician's authorized privileges on the HIS sources they are explicitly authorized on (EMR and EHR) and utilize this information to determine the other sources (replicas) that would also be accessible. For the authentication component, a solution based on federated business SOA approaches built around certificates and public/private key encryption could be adopted. In addition to authentication, adequate access control is a mandatory requirement for the communication between HIS sources. This would include techniques such as: role-based access control (RBAC) (Ferraiolo, Sandhu, Gavrila, Kuhn, & Chandramouli, 2001) that focuses on the responsibilities of the users for an application per role; discretionary access control (DAC) (Na & Cheon, 2000) to allow both authority and privileges to be passed from one user to another; and mandatory access control (MAC) (Bell & LaPadula, 1973) that assigns sensitivity levels to subjects (clearances) and objects (classifications) to control access to information. RBAC can set up different privileges for different categories of users such as roles for physician, nurse, therapist, etc., that differ in privileges (what can be read and/ or written). DAC can allow privileges to be passed among users such as the case where a physician delegates access to the records of their patients to the on-call physician (for nights/weekends). Lastly, MAC can classify patient data, differentiating between more generally available data (demographics, medications, tests, etc.) from very sensitive data (e.g., psychiatry records).

The access to medical records must frequently be checked against permissions given by the patient, requiring the access authorization component to store patient consents. For each request involving patient data, the authorization component has to check if the communication needs to be explicitly permitted,

Figure 12. The Security Management Component

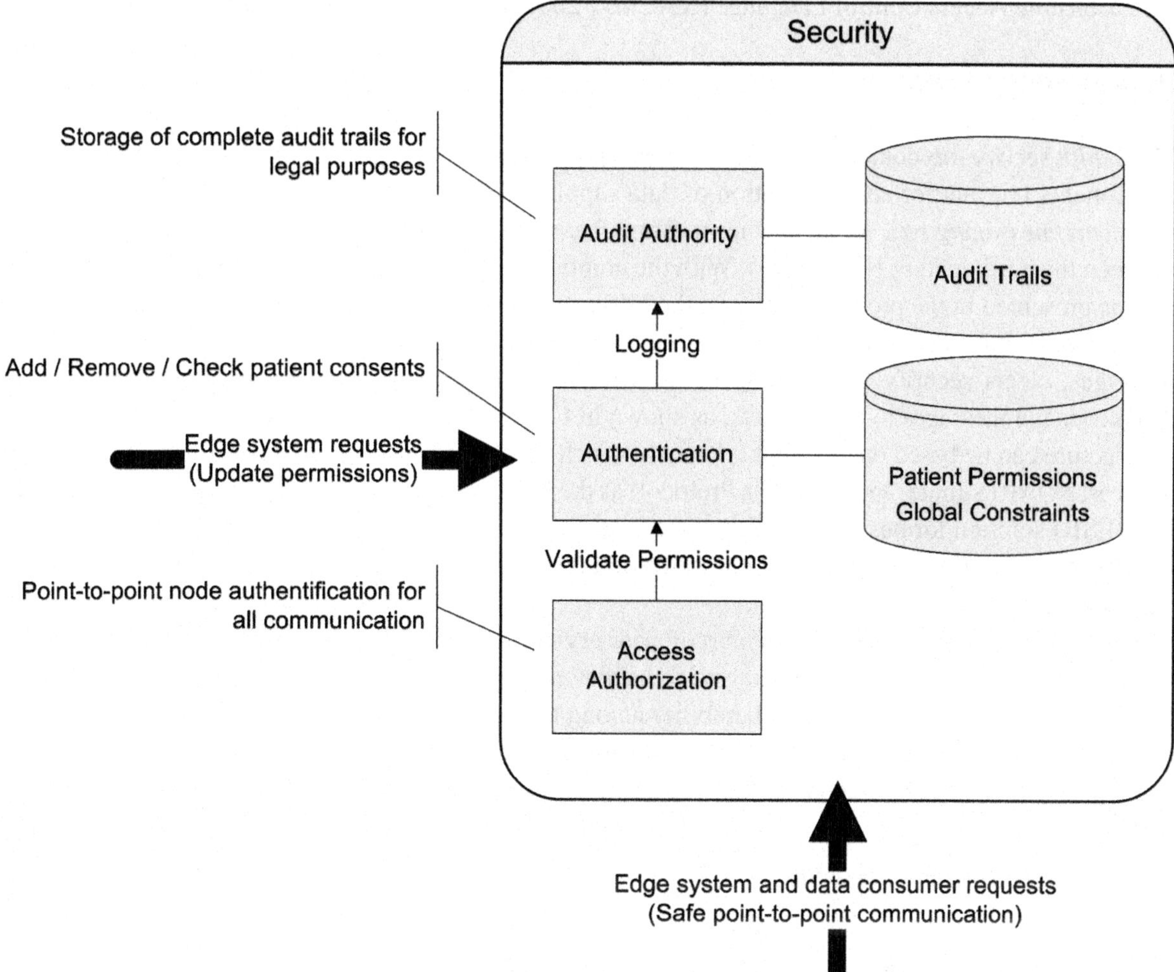

and if this is the case, it has to verify the compliance with the stored consents and global constraints. Furthermore, edge systems will access the component to update stored permissions. In this infrastructure, the security group is the point of HHIEA which is aware of all of the communication across the multiple HIS sources that form the HIE. Thus, the authentication component and the access authorization component are coupled with an audit authority, which records complete audit trails of connections between data providers and data suppliers as well as details about executed data transfers. The audit authority component provides an interface for the retrieval of those audit trails, so that they may be used to meet regulative requirements or for system maintenance and analysis. For example, while two physicians may have the same role, they may be authorized to be in charge of different patients at a hospital. As a result, most hospitals audit patient access records to insure that their employees have not been accessing patients to whom they have not been authorized (which historically has happened when a famous person is in the hospital). Note that establishing adequate security for communication in the HHIEA has significant overhead and a negative impact on the overall system performance; an estimate on complexity and the costs of this task could be attained by examining a secure multi-enterprise SOA. In addition, the Extensible Access Control Language (XACML, 2003) can be utilized to specify security policies.

Health Service Bus

The *health service bus* component of the proposed HHIEA, as shown in the bottom of Figure 7, contains components relevant for communication of data suppliers and data consumers. The key component is the *secure messaging bus*, which enables message-based, asynchronous, point-to-point communication between the participating HIS sources. With the combination of the functionalities of the other HHIEA groups presented in the previous sections, the HIS sources are able to form messages containing all of the necessary information required for the messaging bus. The service bus receives and buffers those messages, clears security and logging issues with the components of the security component, and dispatches the messages to their targets, as shown in Figure 13. The prototypical secure messaging infrastructure can be based on different approaches such as web services as interfaces for the HIS source replicas, SOAP (Simple Object Access Protocol) as the basic message format, and an Enterprise Service Bus (ESB) solution for business SOA as the connecting element (Curbera et al., 2002). The term ESB roughly describes the concept of a middleware component which allows message-based communication between entities connected to the bus.

Custom ESB extensions for the support of grid services will be required in order to minimize security overhead for messages containing anonymized and non-sensitive data. More comprehensive ESBs will require syntactic and semantic interoperability among the replicas through the support of standards and ontologies from the message bus side. This is the location to reconcile differences in healthcare nomenclature such as the need to reconcile the various medical terms for heart attack: Myocardial Infarction,

Figure 13. The Health Service Bus

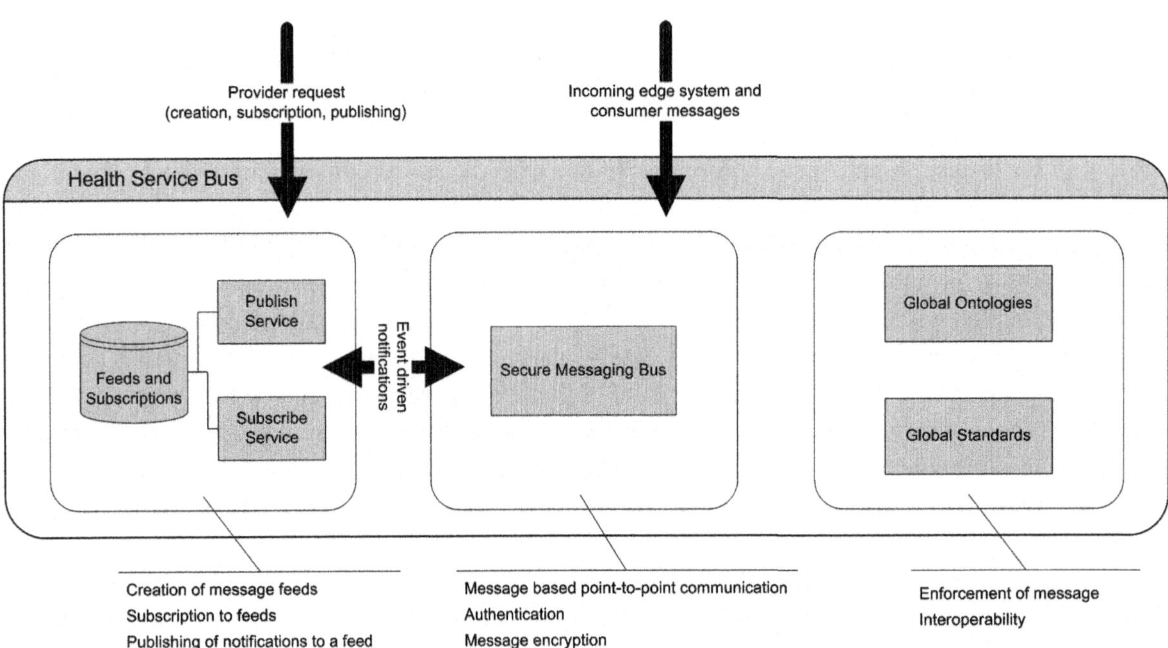

cardiac arrest, coronary infarction, etc. This means that the health service bus maintains a set of global standards and provides services for format transformations between those standards. Equally, a global ontology, alongside an ontology mapping engine, can translate between the different local ontologies utilized by the HIS sources. Finally, the health service bus can be equipped with a publisher service and a subscriber service. Both services are connected to a repository storing data related to message feeds and subscriptions, and can be used to implement the functionalities of a publish/subscribe architecture: creation of message feeds, subscription, and publishing of messages via feed (message dispatch can be realized through the secure messaging bus).

HHIEA and the Regional Scenario

This section concludes the presentation of the HHIEA by examining the identified collaborative linking of HIS sources and stakeholders, where data from each HIS source is extracted to form a replica that operates as a data supplier in the HIE, and each stakeholder is interested in accessing patient data across multiple edge servers and operates as a data consumer. The goal is to demonstrate the way that the full HHIEA architecture as shown in Figure 14 can efficiently manage an HIE scenario by providing the combined functionalities of multiple architectural styles. Figure 15 visualizes the process by complementing the previously HIS infrastructure with details from the proposed HHIEA.

HHIEA components in Figure 15 are the publish and subscribe services, which are used to realize automated reporting, and the secure messaging bus, which implements the extendable message-based communication between the various HIS sources and allows for the execution of SOA/grid services. Furthermore, each HIS source is equipped with an SOAP interface for the generation of outgoing messages and the processing of incoming messages. Data warehouses add support for data aggregation and analysis at eligible HIS sources, and may also be accessed via message bus and by services offered by the HIS source. In this infrastructure, concepts from multiple system architectures are used to resolve identified collaborative links. The following reviews the usage of the various architectures in support of the realistic scenario.

- **Service-Oriented Architecture:** By utilizing SOA, the HHIEA is designed to support service discovery, patient lookup, medical record localization, and secure point-to-point communication. In addition, a full realization of the health service bus includes comprehensive support for interoperability. In combination, these functionalities provide the means for retrieving all of the available medical records related to a certain patient and, thus, for a virtual chart. This resolves the links Community Practice – Virtual Chart, Local Hospital – Virtual Chart, and PHR – Virtual Chart. Furthermore, the SOA functionalities cover all of the links which rely on the transfer of arbitrary data, such as Community Practice – Local Pharmacy, Local Pharmacy University Health Center, Local Pharmacy – Local Hospital, Insurance Company – Community Practice, and Insurance Company – Local Hospital.
- **Publisher/Subscriber:** The proposed health service bus is equipped with a publish/subscribe service, the infrastructure for the administration of message feeds, and the means to dispatch messages containing arbitrary data. This resolves all of the links related to event-driven tasks (e.g., reporting of medical cases) such as Community Practice – State Agency, Local Hospital – State Agency, University Health Center – State Agency, Pharmaceutical Research Center – Local

Figure 14. A View of the Detailed Hybrid HIE Architecture

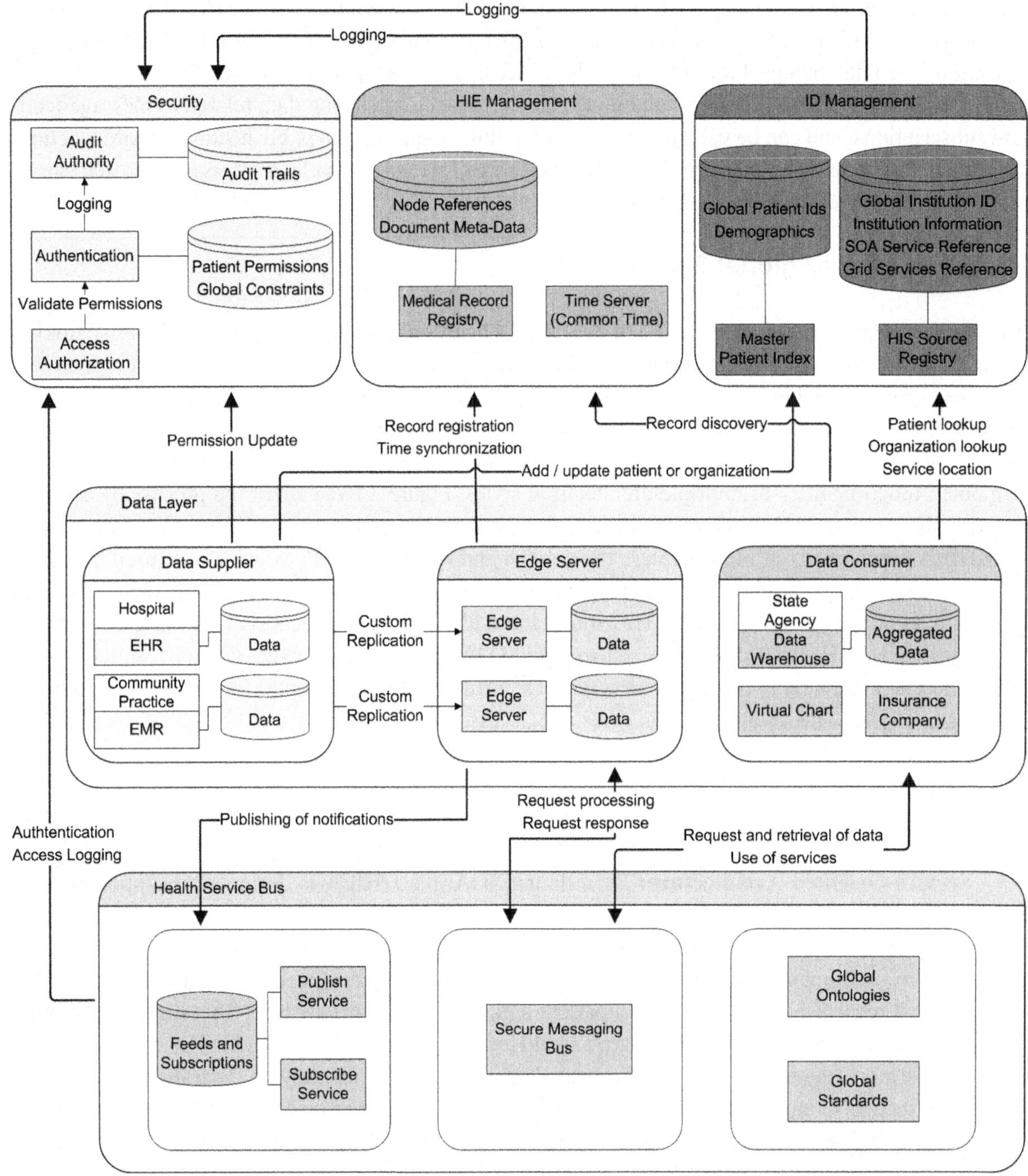

Figure 15. HHIEA Applied to HIS Infrastructure

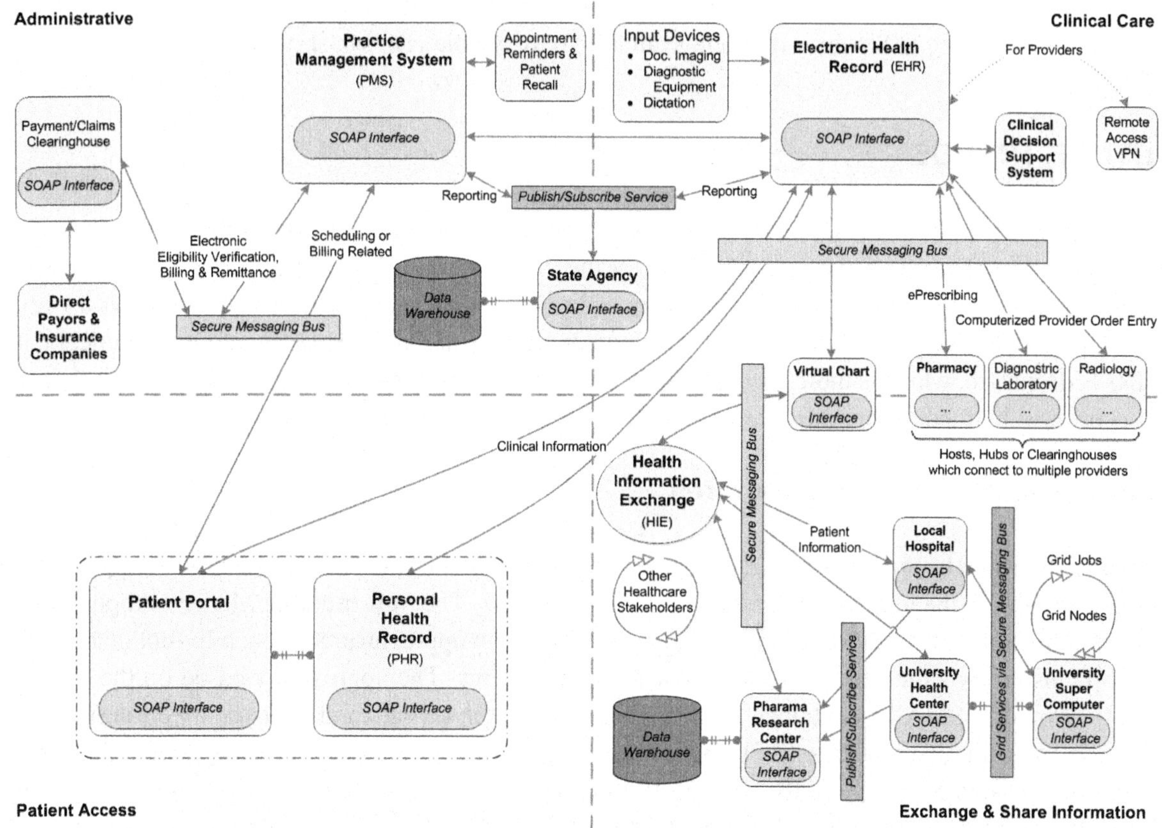

Hospital, Pharmaceutical Research Center – Community Practice, and University Health Center - Pharmaceutical Research Center.

- **Cloud Computing:** The HHIEA contains multiple components that are suitable to benefit from the cloud computing abstraction. Most importantly, the proposed edge server infrastructure can run on a cloud infrastructure with an adequate deployment model and largely benefit from its elasticity (i.e., on-the-fly relocation of resources to replicas that experience increased system load) and low up-front cost (i.e., decrease of initial implementation barriers). Further targets for the cloud model are the installed data warehouses as well as any of the dedicated HISs (e.g., EHRs, EMRs, PHRs, PMSs, etc. that are integrated).
- **Grid:** The HHIEA provides all of the means for the execution of grid applications: grid service discovery, grid service descriptions, and a secure virtual domain with point-to-point messaging. This resolves all of the links which are related to applications requiring large amounts of computational or data storage resources, such as Local Hospital - University Supercomputer Center and University Health Center – University Supercomputer Center.
- **Data Warehouse:** Since the proposed infrastructure effectively supports reporting, as well as the transfer of arbitrary medical data, data warehouses can be installed at all of the HIS sources which require the collection and analysis of large data sets, such as Stage Agency and Pharmaceutical Research Center. Note that the creation of a data warehouse can occur through incremental event-

driven reporting via publish/subscribe or through mass extraction of data from data suppliers (HIS sources) of the HIE via an adequate service. Access of the data warehouses can be either limited to the governing HIS source or made available to the whole HIE via service.

FUTURE TRENDS

This section identifies and reviews trends that will impact the evolution of HIE technologies and solution approaches. There is a two-fold emphasis for the discussion. First, the trend for modularization of healthcare applications is presented, as there are technologies that are nearing fruition towards a viable solution for HIE. Second, the need for integration genomic testing and research data with clinical care EHRs is discussed, which is more speculative in nature and represents an emerging need as genetic testing is utilized by medical providers as part of the diagnosis and treatment processes.

Modular Application Architectures

Recently there have been noteworthy efforts in developing modular frameworks for healthcare applications that are coming to the forefront as possible solutions for HIE. The Substitutable Medical Applications, Reusable Technologies (SMART, 2015) platform chooses an app-centric approach to modularization, which is inspired by the use of apps on smartphone platforms. The approach is based on the abstract specification of a SMART container that encapsulates healthcare data and exposes a well-defined application programming interface (API) that allows interaction with the data. In theory, any HIS source containing relevant data (e.g., EHRs, EMRs, PMSs, PHRs, etc.) can be turned into a SMART container by implementing the container API on top of the used HISs. The API is designed to be used by SMART apps, which perform tasks based on the containers data (e.g., detection of drug-drug interactions or the visualization of genomic test results). The apps are reusable in the sense that they only conform to the container API and are unaware of the details of the underlying HIS source and therefore can be executed by any container. They are substitutable, since the container abstraction decouples functionality from data and, thus, allows competition between different apps (e.g., there can be multiple apps for visualizing blood glucose levels). This approach lowers the complexity for software developers and fosters the creation of a quickly growing app collection (Mandl et al., 2012). From the perspective of HIE between multiple containers, the SMART architecture has to rely on functionalities implemented in its apps and will eventually require another level abstraction/synchronization (ensuring that container A and container B run compatible apps for a given task) to establish collaboration. In the SMART world, each EHR/EMR vendor could be asked to provide a SMART app to their product, where the apps would all have identical APIs in terms of the services. This would allow a developer to access multiple HISs through a similar interface thereby supporting both reuse and HIE.

Another modular approach for the healthcare domain is Open mHealth (Open mHealth 2015), which provides an architecture description based on abstract components that can be used to build healthcare applications. These components are classified as data visualization units (DVU), data processing units (DPU), and cache units (CU). By providing specifications for implementing the external behavior of the components, Open mHealth aims to define the interaction of the components. This abstraction allows for separately developing components, such as, a DVU for presenting bar charts of a fitness marker can be developed separately from the DPU aggregating the data a fitness tracking service and a PHR. As a result, these components can them be combined, such as a DVU presenting the fitness marker results as a spread sheet can replace the bar chart DVU. Here the collaboration of multiple HIS sources that are built according to the Open mHealth architecture relies on the capability of expressing HIE requirements within the specifications.

Integration of Genomics into EMRs

With the progress of genomic analysis methods and the decrease of cost for genotyping procedures, genomic data and knowledge is becoming increasingly comprehensive and available. As a result, its usage for patient diagnosis, treatment, and even medication selection, may now be based on genetic information. In support of this, the physicians must be brought into a process so that they can effectively utilized genetic information for patient care. In fact, there needs to be an HIE of genetic data with the diagnostic data found in an EHR/EMR. The major initiative of note in this area is the Electronic Medical Records and Genomics (eMERGE, 2007) Network that is striving towards the goal of providing approaches for combining and reconciling data from specialized DNA repositories with data collected in EMRs. This integration of research data and clinical data allows for advancing genetic research on the one side and significantly improving clinical care on the other side.

Genomic research investigations can benefit from this linkage by exploring a broad data set that is already available as a result of providing clinical care to patients (i.e., there are no additional costs for data collection) and contains information required for phenotype analysis (Denny, 2012). This facilitates studies that attempt to link certain genes to diseases or drug intolerances. Physicians equipped with EHRs that integrate genetic profiles have the means to provide care based on this additional dimension of knowledge. This includes options such as: better risk assessment and early prevention if the genetic profile of a patient indicates traits that research linked to diseases (Chute et al., 2013); improved diagnosis through decision support systems that make use of genetic profiles (Overby et al., 2013); and, accurate and personalized treatment based on results from pharamacogenomic research (Relling & Klein, 2011).

Integration of genomics data into EHRs and EMRs creates a new set of requirements for HIE architectures. First, data stored in the clinical care records has to be made available for data mining in the genomics context. This includes safety and privacy preserving access to the data as well as preparation of the data by establishing common formats and extraction procedures (e.g., extraction of data from free text notes) of data relevant for genomic research. Second, EHRs/ EMRs have to be redesigned to match genomics enabled workflows (e.g., preemptive ordering of tests based on a patient's health history and health markers) and to process genetic test results (frequently large and highly complex data sets); this may require sophisticated user interfaces for medical providers accompanied by education and training.

CONCLUSION

This chapter has studied the alternative approaches to data and system integration in the healthcare domain utilizing a select set of well-established software architecture styles. Towards this goal, the concept of health information exchange (HIE) has been introduced as a means to integrate data from multiple HIS sources (e.g., EHRs, EMRs, PHRs, PMSs) which required the reconciliation of a set of diverse requirements to HIE-enabled systems and a review of the challenges that HIE architectures need to overcome in order to establish interactions between these systems that facilitate the collaboration of medical providers. In support of this goal, a selection of software architectures (service-oriented architecture, grid computing, publish/subscribe paradigm, and data warehousing) was studied, presented and discussed in the context of these requirements, which allowed us to highlight strengths and weaknesses that each architecture exhibits for a given aspect of HIE. To allow a further inspection of the capabilities of the different introduced architectural styles, a regional HIE scenario was detailed around a real-life HIS infrastructure that connects multiple and diverse healthcare stakeholders and is based on significant input from our medical collaborator. From this scenario, a set of collaborative links was extracted that can be used as a benchmark for the capabilities of an HIE architecture. Utilizing the architectures and the scenario as a basis, elements from SOA, grid, publish/subscribe, data warehouse architectures, and a replication approach to data storage were subsequently utilized to propose a hybrid HIE architecture (HHIEA), which has been shown to meet the established requirements and the identified links. The usage of the studied architectural styles for the proposed HHIEA is coupled with a focus on service-oriented components which is easing the process of integrating new HIS sources over time. This chapter was concluded through a discussion of modular application architectures for healthcare that promote both abstract application development and HIE, coupled with the emerging need for integrating genetic and patient data for more effective treatment.

REFERENCES

Andrews, C., & Mack, R. (2011). IBM to Collaborate with Nuance to Apply IBM's "Watson" Analytics Technology to Healthcare. *IBM News Room*. Retrieved from http://www-03.ibm.com/press/us/en/pressrelease/33726.wss

Apache, E. S. B. (2008). *Apache Software Foundation Synapse ESB*. Retrieved from http://synapse.apache.org

Apple Health App. (2015). *Apple Health App*. Retrieved from https://www.apple.com/ios/ios8/health/

Armbrust, M., Fox, A., Griffith, R., Joseph, A. D., Katz, R. H., Konwinski, A., ... (2009). *Above the clouds: A berkeley view of cloud computing*. EECS Department, University of California, Berkeley, Tech. Rep. UCB/EECS-2009-28.

Bauer, A. & Günzel, H. (2013). *Data-Warehouse-Systeme: Architektur, Entwicklung, Anwendung*. dpunkt. verlag.

Bell, D. E., & LaPadula, L. J. (1973). *Secure computer systems: Mathematical foundations*. DTIC Document.

Booch, G., Rumbaugh, J., & Jacobson, I. (2005). *Unified Modeling Language User Guide*. Addison-Wesley Professional.

i2b2. (2004). *Informatics for Integrating Biology & the Bedside (i2b2)*. Retrieved from https://www.i2b2.org/

W3C. (2008). *World Wide Web Consortium (W3C) tutorial site*. Retrieved from http://www.w3schools.com/

BizTalk Server. (2006). *Microsoft BizTalk Server*. Retrieved from http://www.microsoft.com/biztalk/

Blue Button. (2013). *Blue Button*. Retrieved from http://www.healthit.gov/patients-families/blue-button/

caBIG. (2004). *The Cancer Biomedical Informatics Grid (caBIG)*. Retrieved from https://cabig.nci.nih.gov/

CCR. (2012). *Continuity of Care Record (CCR)*. Retrieved from http://www.aafp.org/practice-management/health-it/astm.html

Chute, C. G., Ullman-Cullere, M., Wood, G. M., Lin, S. M., He, M., & Pathak, J. (2013). Some experiences and opportunities for big data in translational research. *Genetics in Medicine, 15*(10), 802–809. doi:10.1038/gim.2013.121 PMID:24008998

CMS. (2013). *Centers of Medicare and Medicaid Electronic Health Records Incentive Programs*. Retrieved from www.cms.gov/EHRIncentivePrograms

Curbera, F., Duftler, M., Khalaf, R., Nagy, W., Mukhi, N., & Weerawarana, S. (2002). Unraveling the Web services web: An introduction to SOAP, WSDL, and UDDI. *IEEE Internet Computing, 6*(2), 86–93. doi:10.1109/4236.991449

De La Rosa Algarín, A., Demurjian, S. A., Berhe, S., & Pavlich-Mariscal, J. A. (2012). A security framework for XML schemas and documents for healthcare. *Bioinformatics and Biomedicine Workshops (BIBMW), 2012 IEEE International Conference on* (pp. 782–789). IEEE.

De La Rosa Algarín, A., Ziminski, T. B., Demurjian, S. A., Kuykendall, R., & Rivera Sánchez, Y. (2013). Defining and Enforcing XACML Role-Based Security Policies within an XML Security Framework. *Proceedings of 9th International Conference on Web Information Systems and Technologies (WEBIST 2013)* (pp. 16–25). doi:10.5220/0004366200160025

Demurjian, S. A., Saripalle, R., & Berhe, S. (2009). An Integrated Ontology Framework for Health Information Exchange. *SEKE, 09*, 575–580.

Denny, J. C. (2012). Mining electronic health records in the genomics era. *PLoS Computational Biology, 8*(12), e1002823. doi:10.1371/journal.pcbi.1002823 PMID:23300414

Dickmann, F., Falkner, J., Gunia, W., Hampe, J., Hausmann, M., Herrmann, A., & Sax, U. et al. (2012). Solutions for biomedical grid computing - case studies from the D-Grid project Services@ MediGRID. *Journal of Computational Science, 3*(5), 280–297. doi:10.1016/j.jocs.2011.06.006

eMERGE. (2007). *Electronic Medical Records and Genomics (eMERGE) Network*. Retrieved from http://emerge.mc.vanderbilt.edu/

Enrado, P. (2011). Why shuttered RHIO CareSpark's chairman is not giving up. *Government Health IT*. Retrieved from http://www.govhealthit.com/news/why-shuttered-rhio-caresparks-chairman-not-giving

Eugster, P. T., Felber, P. A., Guerraoui, R., & Kermarrec, A.-M. (2003). The many faces of publish/subscribe. *ACM Computing Surveys, 35*(2), 114–131. doi:10.1145/857076.857078

FERPA. (1974). *Family Educational Rights and Privacy Act (FERPA)*. Retrieved from http://www.ed.gov/policy/gen/guid/fpco/ferpa/

Ferraiolo, D. F., Sandhu, R., Gavrila, S., Kuhn, D. R., & Chandramouli, R. (2001). Proposed NIST standard for role-based access control. *ACM Transactions on Information and System Security, 4*(3), 224–274. doi:10.1145/501978.501980

Foster, I. (2002). What is the grid? A Three point checklist. *GRID Today, 1*(6).

Gomes, A. T. A., Ziviani, A., Correa, B. S. P. M., Teixeira, I. M., & Moreira, V. M. (2012). SPLiCE: a software product line for healthcare. *Proceedings of the 2nd ACM SIGHIT International Health Informatics Symposium* (pp. 721–726). ACM. doi:10.1145/2110363.2110447

Google Fit. (2015). *Google Fit.* Retrieved from https://developers.google.com/fit/

HL7. (2007). *HL7 Clinical Document Architecture (CDA).* Retrieved from http://www.hl7.org/implement/standards/

Haas, H., & Brown, A. (2004). *Web Services Glossary.* World Wide Web Consortium (W3C). Retrieved from http://www.w3.org/TR/ws-gloss/

HIPAA. (1996). *Health Insurance Portability and Accountability Act (HIPAA).* Retrieved from http://www.hhs.gov/ocr/privacy/

Inmon, W. H. (2005). *Building the Data Warehouse* (4th ed.). New York, NY: John Wiley & Sons, Inc.

Kenny, P., Parsons, T., Gratch, J., & Rizzo, A. (2008). Virtual humans for assisted health care. *Proceedings of the 1st international conference on Pervasive Technologies Related to Assistive Environments* (pp. 1–4). ACM. doi:10.1145/1389586.1389594

Kuperman, G. J. (2011). Health-information exchange: Why are we doing it, and what are we doing? *Journal of the American Medical Informatics Association, 18*(5), 678–682. doi:10.1136/amiajnl-2010-000021 PMID:21676940

Logicworks. (2015). *Logicworks Healthcare Solutions.* Retrieved from http://www.logicworks.net/healthcare-cloud-solutions

Mandl, K. D., Mandel, J. C., Murphy, S. N., Bernstam, E. V., Ramoni, R. L., Kreda, D. A., & Kohane, I. S. et al. (2012). The SMART Platform: Early experience enabling substitutable applications for electronic health records. *Journal of the American Medical Informatics Association, 19*(4), 597–603. doi:10.1136/amiajnl-2011-000622 PMID:22427539

Mell, P., & Grance, T. (2011). The NIST Definition of Cloud Computing (Draft) Recommendations of the National Institute of Standards and Technology. *Nist Special Publication, 145*, 1–2. Retrieved from http://csrc.nist.gov/groups/SNS/cloud-computing/cloud-def-v15.doc

Microsoft Cloud Services for Health. (2015). *Microsoft Cloud Services for Health.* Retrieved from http://www.microsoft.com/health/en-ca/initiatives/Pages/cloud-services-for-health.aspx

Microsoft HealthVault. (2007). *Microsoft HealthVault Personal Health Record.* Retrieved from https://www.healthvault.com/

Na, S., & Cheon, S. (2000). Role delegation in role-based access control. *Proceedings of the fifth ACM workshop on Role-based access control* (pp. 39–44). ACM. doi:10.1145/344287.344300

ONC. (2015). *Office of the National Coordinator for Health Information Technology Product List*. Retrieved from http://oncchpl.force.com/ehrcert

Open mHealth. (2011). *Open mHealth*. Retrieved from http://openmhealth.org/

OpenEMR. (2012). *OpenEMR electronic health record*. Retrieved from http://www.open-emr.org/

OpenESB. (2012). *Sun Microsystems OpenESB*. Retrieved from http://open-esb.dev.java.net/

OpenMRS. (2004). *OpenMRS electronic medical record system platform*. Retrieved from http://openmrs. org/

Oracle, E. S. B. (2012). *Oracle ESB*. Retrieved from http://www.oracle.com/appserver/esb.html

Overby, C. L., Kohane, I., Kannry, J. L., Williams, M. S., Starren, J., Bottinger, E., & Hripcsak, G. et al. (2013). Opportunities for genomic clinical decision support interventions. *Genetics in Medicine, 15*(10), 817–823. doi:10.1038/gim.2013.128 PMID:24051479

Practice Fusion EHR. (2015). *Practice Fusion EHR*. Retrieved from http://www.practicefusion.com/ electronic-health-record-ehr/

President's Council of Advisors on Science and Technology. (2010). *Realizing the Full Potential of Health Information Technology to Improve Healthcare for Americans: The Path Forward*. Retrieved from http:// www.whitehouse.gov/sites/default/files/microsites/ostp/pcast-health-it-report.pdf

Prokosch, H., & Ganslandt, T. (2009). Perspectives for medical informatics. Reusing the electronic medical record for clinical research. *Methods of Information in Medicine, 48*(1), 38–44. PMID:19151882

Relling, M., & Klein, T. (2011). CPIC: Clinical pharmacogenetics implementation consortium of the pharmacogenomics research network. *Clinical Pharmacology and Therapeutics, 89*(3), 464–467. doi:10.1038/clpt.2010.279 PMID:21270786

ResearchKit. (2015). *ResearchKit*. Retrieved from https://www.apple.com/researchkit/

Robinson, B. (2010). CalRHIO shuts down after missing out on HIE bid. *Government Health IT*. Retrieved from http://www.govhealthit.com/news/calrhio-shuts-down-after-missing-out-hie-bid

Rosen, M. (2008). *Applied SOA: service-oriented architecture and design strategies*. Wiley.

Ryan, A., & Eklund, P. (2008). A framework for semantic interoperability in healthcare: A service oriented architecture based on health informatics standards. *Studies in Health Technology and Informatics, 136*, 759. PMID:18487823

SHARP. (2013). *Strategic Health IT Advanced Research Projects (SHARP)*. Retrieved from http://www. healthit.gov/policy-researchers-implementers/strategic-health-it-advanced-research-projects-sharp

Shortliffe, E. H., & Cimino, J. J. (2006). *Biomedical informatics: computer applications in health care and biomedicine*. Springer Verlag. doi:10.1007/0-387-36278-9_2

Singh, J., Vargas, L., Bacon, J., & Moody, K. (2008). Policy-based information sharing in publish/subscribe middleware. *Policies for Distributed Systems and Networks, 2008. POLICY 2008. IEEE Workshop on* (pp. 137–144). IEEE.

SMART. (2011). *Substitutable Medical Apps & Reusable Technology (SMART)*. Retrieved from http://smartplatforms.org/

Vist, A. (2003). *Veterans Health Information Systems and Technology Architecture (VistA) health record and information system.* Retrieved from http://www.worldvista.org/

VMWare vCloud. (2015). *VMWare vCloud for Healthcare.* Retrieved from http://www.vmware.com/industry/healthcare/

Wager, K. A., Lee, F. W., & Glaser, J. P. (2009). *Health care information systems: a practical approach for health care management.* John Wiley and Sons.

WebSphere ESB. (2008). *IBM WebSphere Enterprise Service Bus.* Retrieved from http://www.ibm.com/software/integration/wsesb/

World Community Grid. (2004). *World Community Grid.* Retrieved from http://www.worldcommunitygrid.org/

XACML. (2003). *Introduction to XACML.* Retrieved from https://www.oasis-open.org/committees/download.php/2713/Brief_Introduction_to_XACML.html

KEY TERMS AND DEFINITIONS

Architectural Alternative: A software architecture style that is suitable for a given task (e.g., data integration) under a set of domain specific requirements.

Cloud Computing: An architectural style based on the provision of abstract computing resources, which are capable to dynamically grow and shrink depending on changing requirements.

Collaborative Link: A relationship between two domain stakeholders, in which collaboration requires the integration of systems or data.

Data Warehouse: An architectural style that collects data from multiple sources to provide a uniform view for querying, analysis, and decision making tasks.

Health Information Exchange (HIE): The electronic transfer of medical data among distinct healthcare organizations and their health information systems. HIE makes medical and health data available to healthcare stakeholders and enables collaboration.

Health Information System (HIS): A system that captures, stores, processes, or shares information about the health of individuals or supports processes and workflows of healthcare domain stakeholders.

Hybrid HIE Architecture (HHIEA): An HIE-specific system architecture incorporating multiple architectural alternatives.

Publish/Subscribe Architecture: An architectural style describing the asynchronous message passing between publishers, subscribers, and optional brokers.

Service-Oriented Architecture (SOA): An architectural style based on loosely coupled software services that collaborate through a connecting framework.

Chapter 17
On Piloting Web–Based Rabies Surveillance System for Humans and Animals:
Web–Based Rabies Surveillance System

Maulilio J. Kipanyula
Sokoine University of Agriculture, Tanzania

Anna M. Geofrey
Sokoine University of Agriculture, Tanzania

Camilius Sanga
Sokoine University of Agriculture, Tanzania

Kadeghe G. Fue
Sokoine University of Agriculture, Tanzania

ABSTRACT

Rabies is a neurodegerative viral zoonotic disease that affects all warm blooded animals. It is estimated that about 99% of human rabies cases are caused by dog bites. High prevalence of rabies has been reported in different parts of Tanzania. The disease has continued to cause public health threat to the communities due to weak passive and active surveillance systems. The data piloted in this study was based on the information gathered from Kilosa district. The geo information collected was used to develop a geospatial based system that can easily show the hotspots of rabies. The use of WEB GIS is likely to strengthen disease surveillance in Kilosa and other Districts of Tanzania. This approach offers a model for sharing both human and animal diseases surveillance information. Adoption of this approach is likely to increase awareness and timely response to rabies incidences.

INTRODUCTION

Rabies is a viral neurodegenerative zoonotic disease that affects all warm blooded animals (Fitzpatrick et al., 2012). The rabies virus belongs to the Lyssavirus genus of the family Rhabdoviridae, and order Mononegavirales (Swai et al., 2010). The disease affect not only human being and dogs, but also other domestic and wild animals such as: cattle, goats, cats, horses, pigs, hyenas, jackals, lions, wild dogs, mongoose, primates and bats (Sambo, 2012; Swai et al., 2010; Swai et al., 2011). Rabies is endemic

DOI: 10.4018/978-1-4666-9446-0.ch017

and has challenged the health systems in different developing countries; pausing a big challenge in both human and animal health systems thus calling for one health approach to manage the disease in both human and animal (Mazet et al., 2009; Rweyemamu et al., 2013). From a global public health perspective, the domestic dogs are considered to be the main target for rabies control and principal reservoir for transmission of the virus to humans and domestic livestock (Mazigo, 2011).

Poorly coordinated rabies incidences reporting system to timely identify, prevent and respond to such cases remains one of the major challenge in establishing a sustainable surveillance system in Tanzania (Mazigo, 2011, Rweyemamu et al., 2013). Certainly, human deaths due to rabies can be prevented through delivery of prompt post-exposure prophylaxis (PEP) to bite victims (Cleaveland et al, 2002). Furthermore, the transmission cycle between humans and domestic dogs can be reduced through sustained mass vaccination programs of domestic dogs, strengthening the reporting system, detection of rabid animals, mapping of endemic areas and prompt response to treatment and prevention strategies (Blanton et al., 2006; Cleaveland et al., 2001; Cleaveland et al., 2013).

The application of ICT in rabies surveillance system in Kilosa district and other parts of Tanzania is very limited (Mboera and Rumisha, 2008). However advances in ICT observed in recent years increased possibilities for community members' involvement in rabies case identification, detection, alerting, monitoring, controlling and surveillance to reduce human deaths and hence minimize its socio-economic impact (Knobel et al., 2005). Application of ICT based rabies surveillance systems is likely assist the Veterinarians to sustain mass vaccination of domestic dogs, to keep records of vaccinated domestic animals and incidences of rabies in domestic animals; to enable public health workers, to create awareness on the magnitude of risks and steps to be taken upon exposure.

Thus, the overall objective of this study was to develop an effective, efficient and cost effective real time web based surveillance system for identifying, reporting, controlling and monitoring rabies incidences in Kilosa district, Morogoro, Tanzania. Specifically the study assessed the appropriateness of the real time rabies surveillance system for instant incidence identification, reporting, control, monitoring and surveillance. Ultimately the development of web based rabies surveillance system would enhance the capacity for; identifying, collecting and reporting of incidences to a central institution, aggregating and sharing data related to national rabies control using geographic web services and social media in appropriate combinations of traditional and novel media (including Internet based Google Maps, local radio and TV); livestock based organizations and the general public (Georgiadou et al, 2011).

SITUATION ANALYSIS

Rabies is one of major public health problems in different parts of Tanzania (Mwisongo et al., 2001). In Kilosa district, rabies has remained endemic for many years despite efforts to control it in domestic dogs (Bardosh et al., 2014). The district boarders Mikumi national park thus allows interactions between humans, domestic dogs and wild animals. The presence of a human-dog-wildlife interphase in the district offers a unique environment for the persistence of the disease in the area (Sambo, 2012). In addition, lack of timely communication during vaccination campaigns has remained to be the major setback in such a way that many people especially in rural areas of Kilosa do not vaccinate their dogs on annual basis as required because such information do not reach them timely. Lack of awareness is also a problem; most people have limited knowledge on handling rabies cases and often they do not know what to do if their animals get infected (Mazigo, 2011). This is attributed to the traditional methods that are used in rabies surveillance in Kilosa District (Bardosh et al., 2014).

i. Dogs Vaccination against Rabies

Coordinated massive vaccination of domestic dogs against rabies is one of the most effect strategy for controlling the disease in communities with large dogs populations. Vaccination breaks the transmission cycle of the disease between dogs, other domestic animals and humans. Dog bites are the cause of almost all human rabies' deaths, with much smaller number of cases occurring each year from other domestic and wild animals (Hiby, 2012). Low vaccination success rate has been reported in different parts of Tanzania due to the fact that few people are aware of the vaccination campaigns thus on the day of vaccinating dogs only a small number of community members vaccinate their dogs while the majority remains un-vaccinated. This is partly caused by under reporting of the rabies incidences and lack of awareness of control measures (Mazigo, 2011).

ii. Post Exposure Prophylaxis

In humans the rabies is entirely preventable, by timely administration of Post exposure prophylaxis (PEP) to dog bite victims. Modern cell culture vaccines used in combination with rabies immunoglobulin's has been reported to be virtually 100% effective in preventing human deaths if administered promptly to rabies-exposed patients (Hampson et al, 2008). Availability of PEP in most health centers has remained a big challenge in Tanzania. For example in Kilosa district there are few health centers with PEP stocks for treating the affected dog bite victims (Mboera et al., 2001). In most cases bite victims have to travel long distances to the hospital to access PEP. This results to delayed administration of PEP and failure to adhere to treatment regimens. According to WHO guidelines, PEP is an emergency and as a general rule should not be delayed or deferred; does not have contraindications if purified rabies immunoglobulin and vaccine are used; must be applied using vaccine regimens and routes of administration that have been proven to be safe and effective. The 5 dose intramuscular regime is the most commonly used: one dose of the vaccine should be administered on days 0, 3, 7, 14 and 28 in deltoid region or, in small children, into the antero-lateral area of the thigh muscle. The 2-1-1 regimen may also be used whereby; two doses are given on day 0 in the deltoid muscle, right and left arm. In addition, one dose in the deltoid muscle on day 7 and one on day 21.

iii. Application of ICT Facilities in Diseases Surveillance Systems

For prompt detection and response to any disease outbreak, a sensitive surveillance system is indispensable. A well established communication system is the 'heart' of the surveillance system. The speed of communication which is most critical to contain or stamp out an outbreak, save lives, and prevent or minimize detrimental effect to the communities. It is challenging, however, to set up an effective communication system, and even more so in poorly established infrastructure in the developing countries like Tanzania.

Radios and Television

The media of communication to disseminate information on rabies to community members that is used in Kilosa district include the use of community radio. Kilosa community radio has played an important role in disseminating information on rabies outbreak and public health education to increase awareness of people on the disease. Despite of the use of radio and television still the disease has continued to be a public health threat. One of the reason causing difficulties to control the disease include presence of a poor link between the Veterinary and humans healthcare departments resulting to un-timely communication of the rabies incidences (Mazigo, 2011; Mboera et al., 2001; Sambo, 2012).

Mobile Phone

In recent years mobile phones usage in Tanzania has expanded so much with almost every household owning a handset. Mobile phones are very useful means of communication (Sanga et al., 2014; Pascoe et al, 2012). This technology has been used in South Africa for monitoring and surveillance of rabies outbreaks, farmers phone or send messages to the State Veterinary offices to report any rabies case and Veterinarian or Animal Health Technician gives feedback to the farmer through the mobile phone (McCrindle and Masipa, 2010). This means of communication is rarely used in Kilosa. However, it is a very useful tool such that a diversity of users have the ability to call a medical practitioner or Veterinarian to communicate rabies incidences and this reduces the cost of farmers to travel to the Veterinary office to report diseases and deaths in either livestock or human being. The challenges for this technology in Kilosa district is poverty which hinder farmers to be able to own the mobile phones and pay for the service. However, the technology has some disadvantage such as illiterate farmers cannot use; if the farmer is illiterate would find it difficult to use the technology and for poor farmers it is difficult to afford buying a mobile phone (McCrindle and Masipa, 2010). Establishment and implementation of a web based rabies surveillance system which will be more efficient and effective in commutating and disseminating rabies related information is likely to improve rabies surveillance in the country.

RABIES SURVEILLANCE SYSTEMS

The majority of animal and human exposure to rabies virus can be prevented by raising public awareness about the rabies virus and how it is transmitted and prevented (Sambo, 2012). In case there is a person or animal which has been affected by the virus then appropriate Veterinary and health care personnel should be consulted. The Veterinary and human health Departments are responsible for giving education to people through seminars, newspaper, books, articles, journals and different mass media (Mazigo, 2011). Mazigo (2011) reported increasing trend in the number of reported cases in recent years at Bugando Hospital in Tanzania that was explained as an outcome of increases awareness on the consequences of rabies which has been conducted through different stakeholders; ultimately this has raised people's level of knowledge on the disease.

According to the World Health Organization (WHO) disease surveillance is defined as the continuous, systematic collection, analysis and interpretation of health-related data needed for the planning, implementation, and evaluation of public health practice (McNabb et al., 2002; Nsubuga et al, 2002; Kimaro and Nhampossa, 2005. Recent studies have shown that the human population boom in Africa appears to correlate well with the increase in the number of domestic dogs, and by conservative estimates, however the prevalence of human rabies is considered to be under-reported due to a weak surveillance system in place (Mazigo, 2011). In Tanzania, the under-reporting is largely attributed to poor surveillance systems and people's tendency not to report human and animal cases of rabies. Furthermore, there is over-dependency on clinical diagnosis (in animals and/ or humans) that downgrade the reliability of rabies-surveillance systems. Certainly, these weaknesses have translated to poor planning of surveillance programs, resulting in shortage PEP and even when available may be accompanied with inappropriate administration, as well as delays in its administration (Mboera et al., 2001; Sambo, 2012). Although not as frequent as the inability to afford treatment, such scenarios have built a lack of trust in health facilities, as well as poor compliance with PEP regimens leading to human deaths that would otherwise be prevented.

IMPORTANCE OF RABIES SURVEILLANCE SYSTEM

Systematic collection, analysis and aggregation of quality rabies-related data is paramount to the success of all public health initiatives to fight against the disease (Cleaveland et al., 2013). This will consequently require a sound monitoring system of trends of rabies incidences and well established reporting system. The absence of correct and up-to-date data on incidences of rabies or in cases of a poor reporting system lead to futile prevention and control programs. The presence of reliable and functioning surveillance systems is necessary for the success of global health initiatives to fight against the rabies (Knobel et al., 2005). However, surveillance systems that collect useful and representative data in developing countries like Tanzania are not functioning well due to limited available resources, lack of knowledgeable staff, disorganization, and poor infrastructure for finding and reporting cases (Cleaveland et al., 2013). Furthermore, in Tanzania it has been estimated that around 23,709 humans sustained dog-bite injuries between 1990 and 1996, whereas 42,669 human dog-bite injuries were reported for the year 2000 (Mazigo, 2010; 2011; Bardosh et al., 2014). These reports suggest that there was either an increase in the number of cases or the extent of the problem was being underestimated in previous studies. However, untimely reporting and response due to poor communication networks remain to be the major obstacle for and effective and functional surveillance system (Table 1).

THE APPLICATION OF ICT IN RABIES SURVEILLANCE

In order to overcome the weaknesses of the traditional rabies surveillance system, there is a need to use the Information and Communication Technologies (ICTs) in the surveillance process. It is possible to reach a large number of people to create awareness about rabies through the use of mass communication medias such as Internet, face book, television, radios and other means of communication (Blanton et al., 2005). The ICT based rabies surveillance systems support easy awareness creation (i.e. sensitization) and a more rapid and timely reporting and response to zoonotic outbreaks (Thinyane and Foster, 2010). Furthermore, ICT facilitates communication between veterinary and human health services by making both Departments aware of rabies surveillance data. Zoonoses are certainly the most prominent example of diseases which require compulsory interaction between human and animal health Departments because of their dual affect on both livestock and humans (Zinsstag and Tanner, 2008). Introducing ICT will also be useful in determining vaccination schedules and tracking purpose.. Additionally the application of

Table 1. National Roadmap on Rabies Identification, Detection, Control, Monitoring and Surveillance System

Ministry of Livestock and Fisheries Development	• Purchase and distribute rabies vaccine • Check vaccine viability • Check vaccination coverage and certification • Ensure cold chain for storage of vaccines • Diagnosis – sample collection, submission, testing and characterization of viruses isolates • Review policy, laws regulations, guidelines, checklist and standards • Reinforce information network system from community to National level • Organize and supervise dogs population census • Law enforcement • Monitor and evaluate implementation of the rabies control strategy
Ministry of Health and Social Welfare	• Purchase and distribute human rabies vaccine • Annual supervision • Public awareness • Human rabies diagnosis • Active surveillance • Heightened awareness and training of front line workers • Policy review
Prime Minister's Office Regional Administration and Local Government	• Public awareness campaigns • Stray dog control • Support procurement of vaccines • Implement rabies vaccination campaigns • Support training of extension staff and farmers • Supervise establishment and maintenance of the Livestock Development Fund (LDF) by • Local Government Authorities • Monitor and evaluate implementation of the rabies control strategy at district level • Raise awareness on the importance of the disease to the public by LGAs • Formulate by laws, which will be used as a tool for control of the disease • Conduct regular active surveillance of the disease at village level • Involve the Standing Committee at ward level on Education, Health and Water on rabies • control • Collaborate with other stakeholders in implementing rabies control strategy
Ministry of Natural Resources and Tourism	• Improve knowledge on rabies • Capacity building at all levels • Vaccination vs rabies in interface areas (annual) • Awareness on rabies • Improve diagnostic capabilities of wildlife laboratories • Improve linkages neighbours and community • Formulation and reinforcement of Policy and Legislations • Undertaking collaborative research
Ministry of Justice and Constitutional Affairs	• Provide legal assistance in drafting by-laws and regulations regarding rabies control • Legal advice on issues related to rabies control strategy
Institutions	• Carry out operational research on rabies • Collaborate with other stakeholders in designing and implanting the rabies control strategy • Provide technical advice on rabies control • Develop and disseminate research findings • Train students in fields of rabies
Private Sector and Non Governmental Organizations	• Collaborate with other stakeholders in designing and implementing the rabies control • strategy • Support procurement of vaccines

Geographical Information System (GIS) allows mapping of rabies hotspots so that the livestock Department can easily track implement control programmes (Blanton et al., 2005). It also can present rabies data historically, which means the spread of rabies can be tracked not only based on region but also on time series (Hampson et al, 2008; Sita and Laksmita, 2012).The use of modern ICT especially GIS provide a platform for investigating the use of web GIS in supporting the report of Veterinary information during outbreaks. Such web GIS can help different stakeholders from public health and animal health as well as law enforcement agents to visualize the cases of rabies on map in real time. The idea behind Web GIS is to provide a common platform of collaboration for all entities that are significant in dealing with rabies. The importance of early awareness and response measures when dealing with rabies incidences is very important. Rabies still poses a public health threat and quick communication and collaboration between various stakeholders is an important aspect in reducing the disease burden. Example of a project which implemented Web GIS is from South Africa where it aims at improving reporting and communication mechanisms through an ICT web based system (Thinyane and Foster, 2010).

Web based application is the best option than mobile based application because early study by Steinfield and Wyche (2013) argue that even though mobile phones have potential to improve the access of agricultural information and knowledge to farmers but still there are problems which hinder its effectiveness and efficiency. According to Steinfield and Wyche (2013), these problems are:

1. Farmers lack appropriate competence in using mobile phones.
2. Many farmers speak different native language while mobile based systems are in English or Swahili and this limit comprehension of messages by end users.
3. Low levels of literacy hinder successful use of mobile based systems.
4. Some rural areas have no access to electricity to keep phones charged and also, some remote areas have not telecommunication network, thereby reducing its availability for use with mobile based system.
5. Many farmers are reluctant to use the limited airtime credit they have to access mobile based systems.
6. Some culture and norms deny women to calling or texting strangers of the opposite gender, limiting their ability to benefit from mobile based systems.

A web-based GIS application of rabies provides a new resource for the rapid mapping and displays the dissemination of data on rabies cases in order to show information about any rabies infected area. Rabies cases are shown in the points form (markers) on the map based on the coordinates of locations. Each region is being displayed in different colors according to the number of rabies cases that occurred. This application can support relevant Government authorities to make informed decisions focusing on areas which have high rabies incidences. Also it is useful in determining vaccination schedules so that the Veterinary Department can easily track and determine priority areas for controlling the disease. It also allows retrospective review of data, which means the spread of rabies can also be tracked based spatial temporal patterns (Sita and Laksmita, 2012).

The emergence of modern technologies that support geospatial information gathering is of great use now. The use of open data kit that incorporates geoinformation has brought great advancements in geo sciences. For example, geoODK application (http://geoodk.com/ accessed on 20-March-2015) can be used to collect georefenced information and update of the data can be done instantly while at the field.

Thus, the developed Web GIS improves the functionality of the existing manual systems by developing an interactive and user friendly system that aims at improving reporting and communication through web. It can also help to create awareness to the people on areas where there is an outbreak of the disease. Furthermore, it can help to provide public education on rabies in an easy way. The system can be used by people to give information on rabies incidences. The information can include animal bites, cases of animal rabies, and cases of human rabies.

PILOTING WEB BASED RABIES SURVEILLANCE SYSTEM IN KILOSA DISTRICT

This study employed a mixed research approach as well as rapid prototype technique in development web based rabies surveillance system. The study was conducted in Kilosa district which is one of the six districts of Morogoro region in Tanzania. It is bordered to the north by Manyara Region, to the northeast by the Tanga Region, to the east by Mvomero District, to the southeast by Morogoro Rural District, to the south by Kilombero District, to the southwest by the Iringa Region and to the west by the Dodoma Region. According to the 2012 national census, Kilosa district had a total population of 438,175 whereby females were 219,797 while 218,278 were males (URT, 2013). Kilosa district is divided into wards and it has 35 wards (URT, 2013). Kilosa District has climatic conditions and fertile soil that provide conducive environment for agriculture activities such as food crop production and livestock keeping. It's in this district where Mikumi National Park is allocated as described in previous sections.

REQUIREMENTS FOR DEVELOPMENT OF ICT BASED RABIES SURVEILLANCE SYSTEM

Requirements were gathered from the users first by using interviews. Interviews are a good way to collect perception data from people particularly if there are small numbers of people whose views are to be captured. Key informants in Kilosa district were interviewed focusing role of ICT in diseases surveillance and questions were probing on necessary information on the rabies in the district.

The interview was used to collect information from village executive officers from villages around Mikumi National park. Other key informants who were interviewed were: in charge for District health department, n charge for District veterinary health department, researcher from SUA Faculty of Veterinary Medicine researching on ecohealth (http://tanzaniaecohealth.com/index.html), Agricultural extension Officer from Kilosa District, Owner of rural Telecentre in Kilosa (KIRSEC) (http://www.kilosaruralservices.net/) and administrator of Kilosa Community radio. In addition semi-structured interviews were also conducted consisting of several key questions that helped to define the areas to be explored. Thus it allowed both the interviewer and interviewee to diverge in order to pursue necessary information on rabies in the district. For instance how people are aware of the disease, how is it transmitted, how is it prevented and rabies records keeping and transmission to different authorities within the district and beyond.

Also since the rapid prototype model was adopted to develop the web based rabies surveillance system thus the requirements that were missing from the prototype that was developed, both developers and the

Figure 1. Requirements for development of ICT based rabies surveillance system

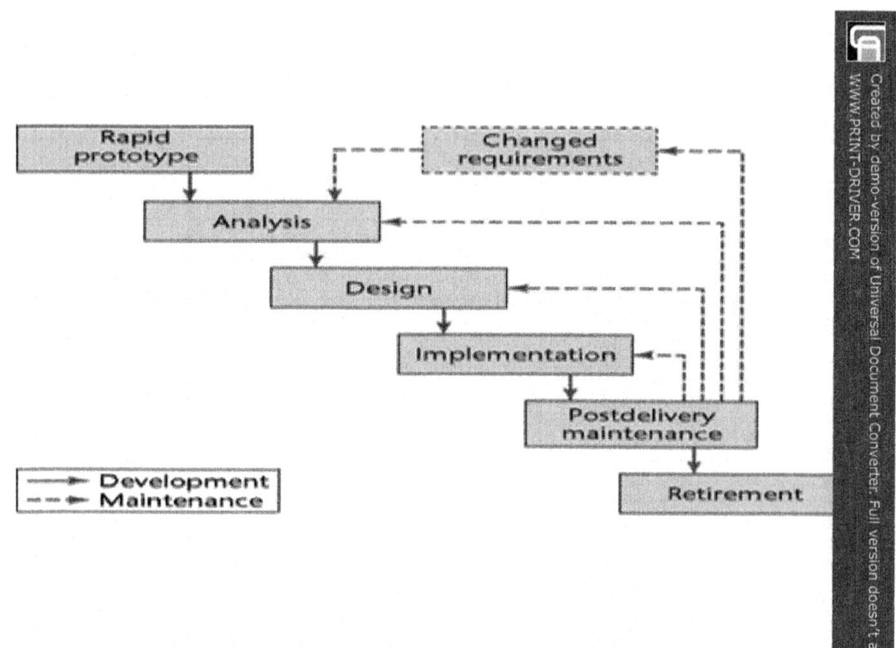

users used the prototype and determine what functionality that the prototype missed and what user and system requirements were to be added.

Interviews with key informants were used to probe the systems and user requirements which needed to be re-engineered in the prototype system during all phases of software development life cycle. The phases consist of analysis, design and implementation.

REQUIREMENT ANALYSIS

The requirements gathered from users by using interview and the prototype were analyzed to establish exactly what the system should do to solve the problem and gaps that were available within the district in respect to the disease. Thus from the analysis that was done then software requirement specification (SRS) document was prepared. Table 2 shows the data collected from secondary sources and were used to develop the system.

SYSTEM DESIGN

From the analysis above the system was designed in a way that it should answers the problems speci-fied by the SRS document. System design comprised of architectural and detailed description of the design. Architectural or high level design aims to identify the modules that should be in the system, the specifications of these modules, and the interaction between the modules in order to produce the

Table 2. Rabies Vaccination status in Kilosa District in 2012

Ward	Village	Human Population	Number of Dogs	Number of Dogs Vaccinated (% in Brackets)	Dog Bite Cases Reported	Suspected Rabid Dogs Killed
Kimamba	Kimamba "A"	7,249	177	171	12	2
	Kimamba "B"	6,271	165	0	0	0
Rudewa	Twatwatwa	2,704	905	50	9	3
Madoto	Mbwade	1,869	127	50	0	0
Tindiga	Malangali	4,247	70	0	0	0
	Tindiga	5,833	81	0	0	0
Kilangali	Kilangali	2,723	131	0	0	0
	Kiduhi	563	151	0	3	7
	Kivungu	4,179	102	0	0	0
Ulaya	Ulaya Kibaoni	3,673	189	40	0	0
	Mhenda	4,138	263	0	0	0
Mikumi	Mikumi	15,166	333	120	0	0
	Ihombwe	1,773	116	0	0	0
Kilosa town	Kilosa town	34,236	637	440	6	1
Ruhembe	Kidogobasi	4,562	227	0	0	0
Total		**99,186**	**3574**	**871**	**30**	**13**

desired results. The specifications were carefully analyzed and a module structure that has the desired functionality was produced.

Detailed design involved going deep into specific modules of the system. The system design was broken down into 3 major modules (3-tier application), namely;

1. **Front–End Design:** This comprise of the user interface which links users and the system. Users can interact with the system using the series of interactive web pages as displayed through the web browser.
2. **Application Design:** This is meant to provide communication between client and server. PHP scripting language (4 or higher) was used to fetch user queries from the browser into the database and retrieve the relevant rabies information back to the user on the web page.
3. **Back–End Design:** This comprises of the database. Database is where information about rabies is stored so that users can access them through front-end's user interface. The database was implemented using MySQL which is an open source relational database management system. It is based on the structure query language (SQL) and it is consistent, fast performance, high reliability and ease to use. ***The locations were called using postGIS technology that calls georeferenced information from the MySQL database.***

SYSTEM IMPLEMENTATION

After the design of the system then it was implemented by using the MySQL database server in the back-end while JavaScript, CSS and HTML were used in the development of user interface. In order for the user interface to connect with database, PHP scripting language was used. In the front-end of the system JavaScript and CSS were used to create an interactive user interface. Google maps API capabilities were manipulated and used to locate the interactive information using Google maps and Javascripts. AJAX technology was incorporated to improve the interactivity of the maps through the browser. Some Google API classes where used to make easy the implementation of the technology.

DESCRIPTION OF USER INTERFACE AND THE SYSTEM IN GENERAL

The web based rabies surveillance system allows users to update information that relate with rabies incidences such as reporting of areas that were affected by rabies, reporting if there was any rabid animal like dogs, etc. and viewing information on rabies. Figure 2 shows the interface of a web based rabies surveillance system.

From the interface (Figure 2), the user could view affected areas in map layer; this would let the user know which areas in Kilosa were mostly affected by rabies. These areas were identified by a green

Figure 2. The interface of the Rabies Surveillance System

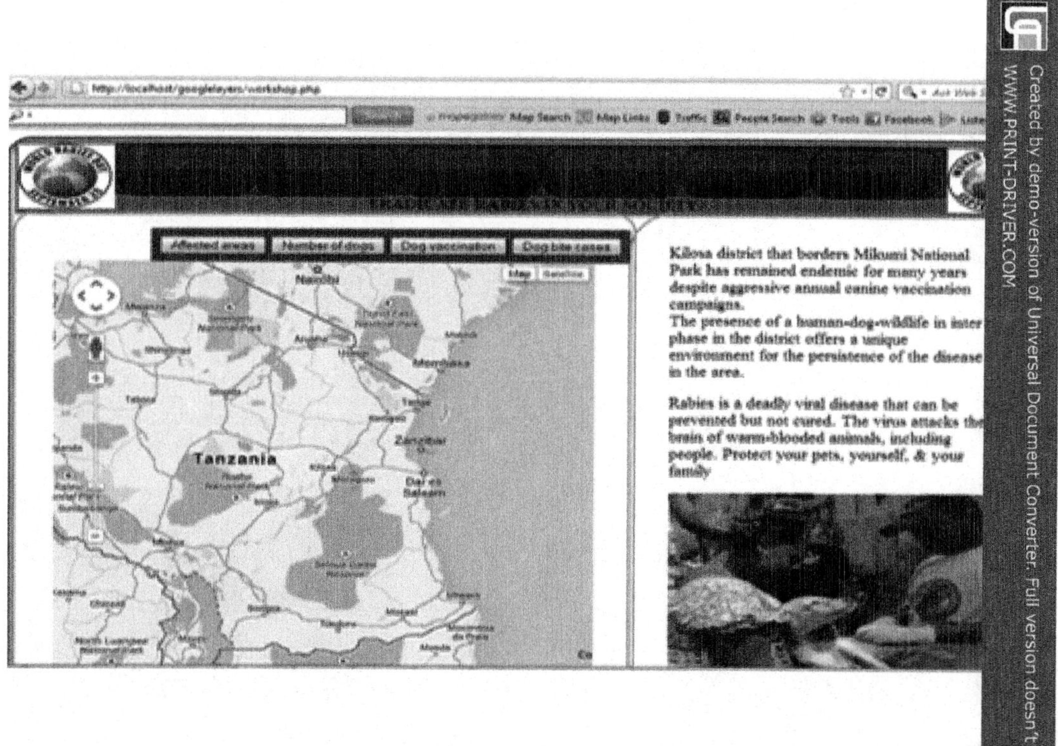

Figure 3. The highly affected areas by rabies in Kilosa

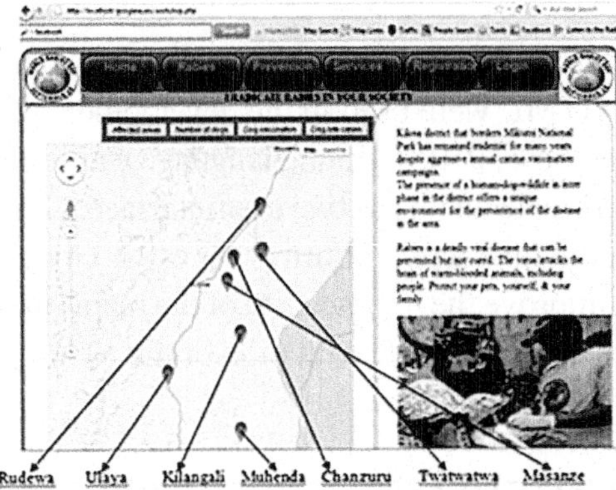

marker and by placing a cursor on it, the user could know the village name of the area. The Figure 3 below shows the snapshot for this.

From the interface (Figure 3), the user could view the number of dogs on map layer. This would let the user know how many dogs were available in a certain village. These areas were identified by a green marker and by placing a cursor on it the user could know the name of the area and by clicking the marker

Figure 4. The number of dogs within the village

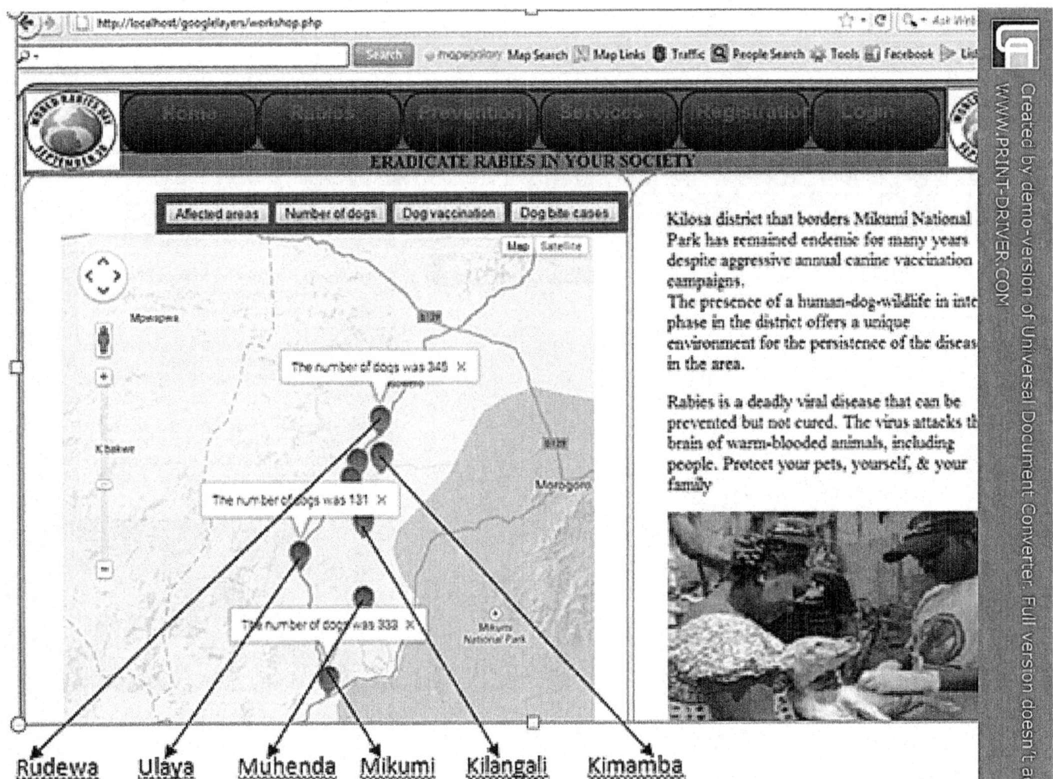

Figure 5. The villages showing the number of vaccinated dogs

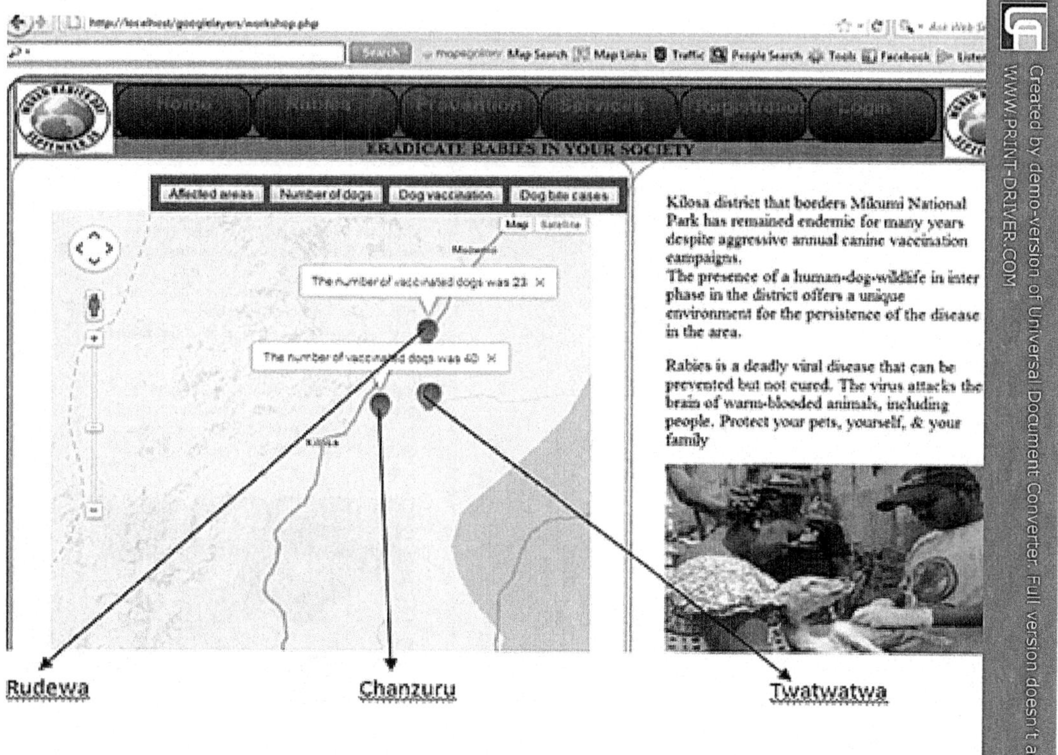

the number of dogs in the area would be displayed. The information displayed on Figure 3 relate to data collected from Kilosa presented in Table 2.

From the interface (Figure 4), the user could click the button of dog vaccination in map layer; this would let the user to know how many dogs were vaccinated in a certain village. These areas were identified by a green marker and by placing a cursor on it the user could know the name of the area and by clicking the marker the number of dogs that were vaccinated in the area would be displayed. The information displayed on Figure 4 relate to data collected from Kilosa presented in Table 2.

Also from the interface (Figure 5) the user could click the button of dog bite cases in map layer; this would let the user know how many dog bite cases were reported in a certain village. These areas were identified by a green marker and by placing a cursor on it the user could know the name of the area and by clicking the marker the number of dog bite cases reported in the area would be displayed. The information displayed on Figure 5 relate to data collected from Kilosa presented in Table 2.

Thus, from these different maps (Figure 2, Figure 3, Figure 4, Figure 5 and Figure 6) a user could make analysis on which areas were affected by rabies and determine the reasons why certain areas were highly affected. Is it due to lack of dog vaccination program or is it because of poor reporting on rabies cases such as dog bite cases?

Even though the web based surveillance system for rabies is not a new field but what has been piloted here is the applicability of web based rabies surveillance system in identification, detecting, monitoring and controlling it in Tanzania (Mwabukusi et al., 2014). The preliminary results from this pilot research carried out in Kilosa District shows promising findings which have been reported in this book chapter.

Figure 6. The number of dog bite cases reported

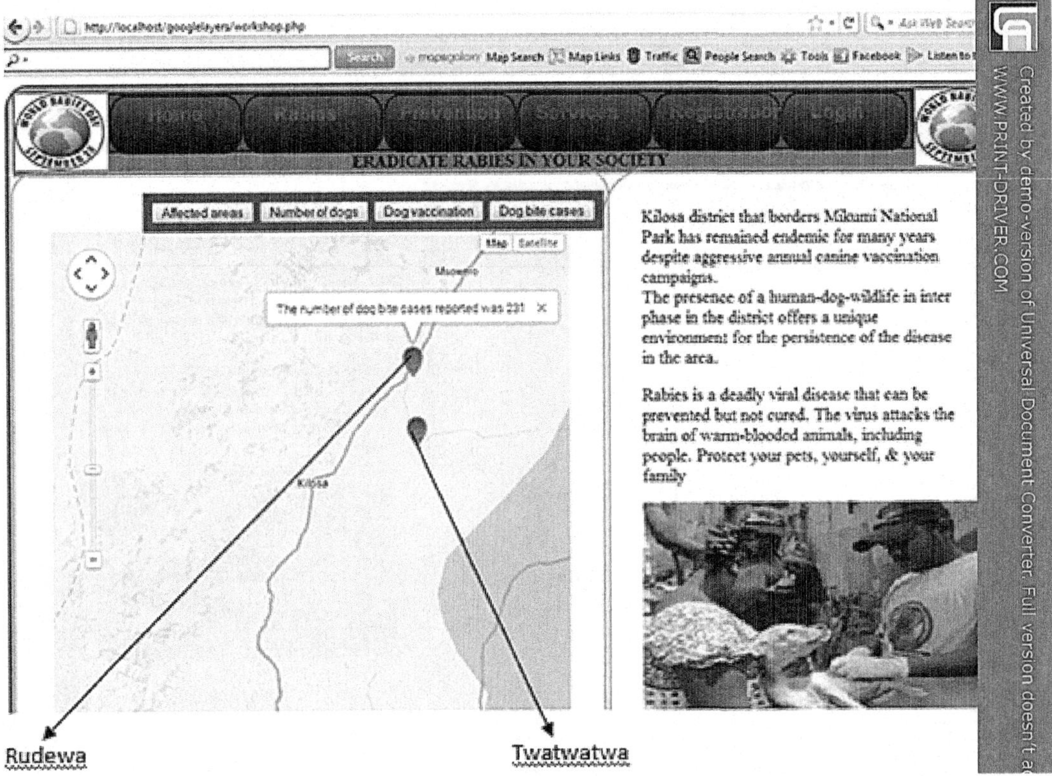

Thus, it is anticipated that new knowledge has been contributed in the areas of community informatics, health informatics and their applicability in both human and animal health (i.e. one health concept (Rock et al., 2009; Mazet et al., 2009). The developed system is different from other surveillance system for either animal health or human health which does not put human being at the centre of intervention (Brownstein et al., 2008; Rumisha et al., 2007; Mghamba et al.,2008; Mboera et al., 2001; Kimaro and Nhampossa, 2007 ; Waidyanatha and Prashant, 2010; Mwabukusi et al., 2014).

CONCLUSION

This study quantified and mapped the spatial and temporal dynamics in rabies incidences in Kilosa district, Morogoro region. Thus, the system provides rapid communication on rabies cases and it helps to increase awareness to the communities on the disease since literature shows that many people die due to rabies because of lack awareness of the disease and steps need to be followed upon encounters. The system described here allows quick communication and collaboration between Veterinary and medical Departments in Kilosa district which is very important in managing rabies at community level. Also from the web based rabies surveillance system has more unique features that includes layered maps whereby a user can navigate smoothly and make the geo-analysis of the affected areas by the disease and determine the reasons behind high infections. Also, the system administrator can use data from the database such as the village location data and the village details information to do geo-analysis of the disease impact in Kilosa. The areas with high rabies outbreak can be mapped and openly be viewed so that livestock department can easily track and set priorities for the control of the disease. The authors of this book chapter recommend that all line ministries should improve the identification, detection, alerting, monitoring, controlling and surveillance of rabies through the use of the developed web based system. The line ministries to be involved are Ministry of Livestock and Fisheries Development, Ministry of Health and Social Welfare, Ministry of Natural Resources and Tourism, Ministry of Justice and Constitutional Affairs and Prime Minister's Office - Regional Administration and Local Government as well as Private sectors and Non Governmental Organizations. Without unifying the efforts from different sectors (inter-sectoral) and disciplines (inter-disciplinary) it is difficult to address the problem of rabies (http://tanzaniaecohealth.com/index.html). Future study will focus on evaluating the adoption of the developed system in Kilosa District. The evaluation of the system will base on technology, culture related values, competence and personal values.

Another area for future research study should be on improving the performance of web based rabies surveillance system by using openlayers instead of Google layers. Google maps are too slow for real time reporting (Waidyanatha and Prashant, 2010).

REFERENCES

Bardosh, K., Sambo, M., Sikana, L., Hampson, K., & Welburn, S. C. (2014). Eliminating Rabies in Tanzania? Local Understandings and Responses to Mass Dog Vaccination in Kilombero and Ulanga Districts. *PLoS Neglected Tropical Diseases*, 8(6), 29–35. doi:10.1371/journal.pntd.0002935 PMID:24945697

Blanton, J. D., Manangan, A., Manangan, J., Hanlon, C. A., Slate, D., & Rupprecht, C. E. (2006). Development of a GIS-based, real-time Internet mapping tool for rabies surveillance. *International Journal of Health Geographics*, 5(1), 47. doi:10.1186/1476-072X-5-47 PMID:17078890

Brownstein, J. S., Freifeld, C. C., Reis, B. Y., & Mandl, K. D. (2008). Surveillance Sans Frontieres: Internet-based emerging infectious disease intelligence and the HealthMap project. *PLoS Medicine*, 5(7), e151. doi:10.1371/journal.pmed.0050151 PMID:18613747

Cerejo, L. (2010). *Design Better and Faster With Rapid Prototyping*. Germany: Smashing Media Company.

Cleaveland, S., Fevre, E. M., Kaare, M., & Coleman, P. G. (2002). Estimating human rabies mortality in the United Republic of Tanzania from dog bite injuries. *Bulletin of the World Health Organization*, 80(4), 304–310. PMID:12075367

Cleaveland, S., Lembo, T., Townsend, S., Kazwala, R., Sikana, L., Changalucha, J., & Hampson, K. (2013). *Relevance of research for development of national rabies control strategies in Africa. 11th SEARG meeting*, Dar es Salaam.

Fitzpatrick, M. C., Hampson, K., Cleaveland, S., Meyers, L. A., Townsend, J. P., & Galvani, A. P. (2012). Potential for rabies control through dog vaccination in wildlife-abundant communities of Tanzania. *PLoS Neglected Tropical Diseases, 6(8)*, e1796.

Georgiadou, Y., Bana, B., Becht, R., Hoppe, R., Ikingura, J., Kraak, M. J., & Verplanke, J. et al. (2011). Sensors, empowerment, and accountability: A Digital Earth view from East Africa. *International Journal of Digital Earth*, 4(4), 285–304. doi:10.1080/17538947.2011.585184

Hampson, K., Dobson, A., Kaare, M., Dushoff, J., Magoto, M., Sindoya, E., & Cleaveland, S. (2008). Rabies exposures, post-exposure prophylaxis and deaths in a region of endemic canine rabies. *PLoS Neglected Tropical Diseases*, 2(11), e339. doi:10.1371/journal.pntd.0000339 PMID:19030223

Hiby, E. (2012). *Vaccinate dogs to save human lives – World Rabies Day 2012. South-East Asia.* World Health Organization.

Jemberu, W. T., Molla, W., Almaw, G., & Alemu, S. (2013). Incidence of rabies in humans and domestic animals and people's awareness in North Gondar Zone, Ethiopia. *PLoS Neglected Tropical Diseases*, 7(5), e2216. doi:10.1371/journal.pntd.0002216 PMID:23675547

Kimaro, H. C., & Nhampossa, J. L. (2005). Analyzing the problem of unsustainable health information systems in less-developed economies: Case studies from Tanzania and Mozambique. *Information Technology for Development*, 11(3), 273–298. doi:10.1002/itdj.20016

Knobel, D. L., Cleaveland, S., Coleman, P. G., Fèvre, E. M., Meltzer, M. I., Miranda, M. E. G., & Meslin, F. X. (2005). Re-evaluating the burden of rabies in Africa and Asia. *Bulletin of the World Health Organization*, 83(5), 360–368. PMID:15976877

Laksmita, I. S., Sudana, A. K. O., & Buana, P. W. (2012). Design Web-based GIS Application for Rabies Spread in Bali Province. *International Journal of Informatics and Communication Technology, 1*(1), 54-62.

Lembo, T. (2012). The blueprint for rabies prevention and control: A novel operational toolkit for rabies elimination. *PLoS Neglected Tropical Diseases*, 6(2), e1388. doi:10.1371/journal.pntd.0001388 PMID:22389727

Lembo, T., Hampson, K., Kaare, M. T., Ernest, E., Knobel, D., Kazwala, R. R., & Cleaveland, S. (2010). The feasibility of canine rabies elimination in Africa: Dispelling doubts with data. *PLoS Neglected Tropical Diseases*, 4(2), e626. doi:10.1371/journal.pntd.0000626 PMID:20186330

Mazet, J. A., Clifford, D. L., Coppolillo, P. B., Deolalikar, A. B., Erickson, J. D., & Kazwala, R. R. (2009). A "one health" approach to address emerging zoonoses: The HALI project in Tanzania. *PLoS Medicine*, 6(12), e1000190. doi:10.1371/journal.pmed.1000190 PMID:20016689

Mazigo, H. D. (2011). Rabies in Tanzania: The need for a national control programme. *Tanzania Journal of Health Research, 13*(2), 88-89.

Mazigo, H. D., Okumu, F. O., Kweka, E. J., & Mnyone, L. L. (2010). Retrospective analysis of suspected rabies cases reported at Bugando Referral Hospital, Mwanza, Tanzania. *Journal of Global Infectious Diseases, 2*(3), 216.

Mboera, L. E. G., & Rumisha, S. F. (2008). The role of mass media in disease outbreak reporting in the United Republic of Tanzania. *Tanzania Journal of Health Research*, 6(2), 73–77. doi:10.4314/thrb.v6i2.14246 PMID:18846783

Mboera, L. E. G., Rumisha, S. F., & Kitua, A. Y. (2001). Strategic approach for strengthening national and regional disease surveillance system: The East African example. *Tanzania Journal of Health Research, 3*(2), 6–9. doi:10.4314/thrb.v3i2.14211

McCrindle & Masipa, A. (2010). *Rapid Spacial and Temporal Outbreak Investigations Using Cell Phone Technology*. Republic of South Africa: Farm Inn.

McNabb, S. J., Chungong, S., Ryan, M., Wuhib, T., Nsubuga, P., Alemu, W., & Rodier, G. et al. (2002). Conceptual framework of public health surveillance and action and its application in health sector reform. *BMC Public Health, 2*(1), 2. doi:10.1186/1471-2458-2-2 PMID:11846889

Mwabukusi, M., Karimuribo, E. D., Rweyemamu, M. M., & Beda, E. (2014). Mobile technologies for disease surveillance in humans and animals. *The Onderstepoort Journal of Veterinary Research, 81*(2), 5. doi:10.4102/ojvr.v81i2.737 PMID:25005126

Mwisongo, A. J., Kisoka, W. J., Mubyazi, G. M., Malebo, H., Senkoro, K. P., McHaro, J., & Kitua, A. Y. (2001). Major health problems in some selected districts of Tanzania. *Tanzania Journal of Health Research, 3*(2), 10–14. doi:10.4314/thrb.v3i2.14212

Swai, E. S., Moshy, W. E., Kaaya, J. E., & Mtui, P. F. (2010). Spatial and temporal distribution of rabies in the northern zone of Tanzania in the period of 1993-2002. *Tanzania Journal of Health Research, 12*(1), 80–85. doi:10.4314/thrb.v12i1.56335 PMID:20737833

Ncube, P. S., Thinyane, H., & Foster, G. (2010). *An Investigation into a Web Based Visualization Technique of Zoonotic Disease Outbreaks*. Rhodes University.

Sita, A. K., Nsubuga, P., Eseko, N., Tadesse, W., Ndayimirije, N., Stella, C., & McNabb, S. (2002). Structure and performance of infectious disease surveillance and response, United Republic of Tanzania, 1998. *Bulletin of the World Health Organization, 80*(3), 196–203.

Cleaveland, S., Kaare, M., Tiringa, P., & Mlengeya, T. 2001. A dog rabies vaccination campaign in rural Africa: impact on the incidence of animal rabies and human bite injuries. In *Proceedings of the Southern and Eastern African Rabies Group. World Health Organization Meeting*. WHO.

Cleaveland, S., Kaare, M., Tiringa, P., Mlengeya, T., & Barrat, J. (2003). A dog rabies vaccination campaign in rural Africa: Impact on the incidence of dog rabies and human dog-bite injuries. *Vaccine, 21*(17-18), 1965–1973. doi:10.1016/S0264-410X(02)00778-8 PMID:12706685

Georgiadou, Y., Bana, B., Becht, R., Hoppe, R., Ikingura, J., Kraak, M.-J., & Verplanke, J. et al. (2011). Sensors, empowerment, and accountability: A Digital Earth view from East Africa. *International Journal of Digital Earth, 4*(4), 285–304. doi:10.1080/17538947.2011.585184

Kimaro, H., & Nhampossa, J. (2007). The challenges of sustainability of health information systems in developing countries: Comparative case studies of Mozambique and Tanzania. *Journal of Health Informatics in Developing Countries, 1*(1).

Mboera, L. E. G., Rumisha, S. F., Magesa, S. M., & Kitua, A. Y. (2001). Utilisation of health management information system in disease surveillance in Tanzania. *Tanzania Journal of Health Research, 3*(2), 15–17. doi:10.4314/thrb.v3i2.14213

Mghamba, J. M., Mboera, L. E. G., Krekamoo, W., Senkoro, K. P., Rumisha, S. F., Shayo, E., & Mmbuji, P. (2008). Challenges of implementing an integrated disease surveillance and response strategy using the current health management information system in Tanzania. *Tanzania Journal of Health Research, 6*(2), 57–63. doi:10.4314/thrb.v6i2.14243

Pascoe, L., Lungo, J., Kaasbøll, J., & Koleleni, I. (2012, May). Collecting integrated disease surveillance and response data through mobile phones. In *Proceedings of the IST-Africa 2012 Conference and Exhibition*, (pp. 9-11). Academic Press.

Rock, M., Buntain, B. J., Hatfield, J. M., & Hallgrímsson, B. (2009). Animal–human connections,"one health," and the syndemic approach to prevention. *Social Science & Medicine, 68*(6), 991–995. doi:10.1016/j.socscimed.2008.12.047 PMID:19157669

Rumisha, S. F., Mboera, L. E., Senkoro, K. P., Gueye, D., & Mmbuji, P. K. (2007). Monitoring and evaluation of integrated disease surveillance and response in selected districts in Tanzania. *Tanzania Journal of Health Research, 9*(1), 1–11. doi:10.4314/thrb.v9i1.14285 PMID:17547094

Rweyemamu, Mmbuji, Karimuribo, Paweska, Kambarage, Neves, … Matee. (2013). The Southern African Centre for infectious disease surveillance: A one health consortium. *Emerging Health Threats Journal, 6*.

Sambo, M. B. (2012). *Epidemiological dynamics of rabies in Tanzania and its impacts on local communities* (Doctoral dissertation, University of Glasgow). Retrieved from http://theses.gla.ac.uk/3663/1/2012sambomsc.pdf

Sanga, C., Mlozi, M. R. S., Tumbo, S., Mussa, M., Muhiche, L., & Haug, R. (2014). On the Development of the Mobile based Agricultural Extension System in Tanzania: A technological perspective. *International Journal of Computing and ICT Research, 8*(1), 49–67.

Snyder, R., & Dazzo, O. (2011). *Guidelines for the Reporting Of Rabies Cases Using the Michigan Disease Surveillance System (MDSS)*. Michigan: Capitol View Building.

Steinfield, C., & Wyche, S. (2013). *Assessing the role of information and communication technologies to enhance food systems in developing countries: A FOCUS On Eastern and Southern Africa*. Retrieved from https://www.msu.edu/~steinfie/ICT4D_White_Paper_2013.pdf

Swai, E. S., Moshy, W. E., Kaaya, J. E., & Mtui, P. F. (2011). *Spatial and temporal distribution of rabies in the northern zone of Tanzania in the period of 1993-2002*. Academic Press.

URT. (2013). *2012 Population and Housing Census. Population distributed by areas. National Bureau of Statistics Ministry of Finance Dar es salaam*. Office of Chief Government Statistician President's Office, Finance, Economy and Development Planning Zanzibar.

Waidyanatha, N., & Prashant, S. (2010). User Requirements toward a Real-Time Biosurveillance Program. *Biosurveillance: Methods and Case Studies*, 239.

Zinsstag, J., & Tanner, M. (2008). *One Health: The Potential of Closer Cooperation between Human and Animal Health in Africa*. Switzerland: Swiss Tropical Institute.

KEY TERMS AND DEFINITIONS

Disease Surveillance: Is an epidemiological practice by which the spread of disease is monitored in order to establish patterns of progression (http://en.wikipedia.org/wiki/Disease_surveillance).

Information and Communications Technology (ICT): Refers to all types of technology used to handle telecommunications, broadcast media, intelligent building management systems, audiovisual processing and transmission systems, and network-based control and monitoring functions (http://en.wikipedia.org/wiki/Information_and_communications_technology).

"Stakeholder" or "User" or "Actor": Refers generically to organizations or or community or individuals who use or exploit web based rabies surveillance system. While these types of users / stakeholders may have some different interests and perhaps different concerns based on scale of data involved, generally a corporate / organization and an individual user are going to have different expectations and concerns related to web based rabies surveillance system.

Surveillance: Is the monitoring of the behavior, activities, or other changing information, usually of people for the purpose of influencing, managing, directing, or protecting them (http://en.wikipedia.org/wiki/Surveillance).

Compilation of References

ACHI. (2014). *Australasian College of Health Informatics*. Retrieved from http://www.achi.org.au

Adler-Milstein, J. R. (2011). The use of information technology in US health care delivery. *Proquest Dissertations and Theses*, 1.

Aftahi, S. R. (2013). Spirituality in a heealthcare organization: An exploratory qualitative inquiry. *Proquest Dissertations and Theses*, 52-53.

Agarwal. (2000). Individual Acceptance of Information technologies. *Educational Technology Research and Development, 40*, 90-102.

Agarwal, R., Sambamurthy, V., & Stair, R. (2000). The evolving relationship between general and specific computer efficacy: An empirical assessment. *Information Systems Research, 11*(4), 418–430. doi:10.1287/isre.11.4.418.11876

Agrawal, G. P. (2012). *Nonlinear Fiber Optics*. Retrieved from http://www.amazon.com/Nonlinear-Fiber-Optics-Edition-Photonics/dp/0123970237

AHIT blog. (2014). *U.S. Food and Drug Administration has begun collecting reports involving electronic health and IT errors, some of which have resulted in death*. Australian Health Information Technology Blog. Retrieved from http://aushealthit.blogspot.com.au/2011/08/what-is-problem-with-e-health-could-it.html

AHPRA. (n.d.). *Australian Health Practitioner Regulation Agency*. Retrieved 14 October, 2014 from https://www.ahpra.gov.au/

AIHW. (2014). Australian Institute of Human Welfare, Australian Hospital Statistics report 2013-14, Australia. AIHW.

Ajami, S., & Carter, M. W. (2013). *The advantages and disadvantages of Radio Frequency Identification (RFID) in Health-care Centers; approach in Emergency Room (ER)*. Academic Press.

Akerman, E. A. (2006). Attitudes toward computers and computerization in Canadian critical care nurses. *Proquest Dissertations and Theses*, 1.

Albarrak, A. I., Al Rashidi, E. A., & Fatani, R. K. (2014, March). Assessment of legibility and completeness of handwritten and electronic prescriptions. *Saudi Pharmaceutical Journal, 13*. doi:10.1016/j.jsps.2014.02.013

Alexander, R. C. (2009). Fostering student engagement in the history through student-created digital media: A qualitative and quantitative study of student engagement and learning outcomes in 6th-grade history instruction. *Proquest Dissertations and Theses*, 62.

Alliance for Health Policy and Systems Research. (2007). *Briefing Note 1*. Geneva: Alliance for Health Policy and Systems Research. Retrieved in January 2013, from http://www.who.int/alliance-hpsr/resources/alliancehpsr_briefingnote1.pdf

Al-Mutairi, M. S., & Mohammed, L. A. (2011). *Cases on ICT Utilization, Practice and Solutions. Tools for managing day-to-day issues*. New York: Information Science Reference. doi:10.4018/978-1-60960-015-0

Amendola, M. L. (2008). An examination of the leadership competency requirements of nurse leaders in healthcare information technology. *Proquest*, 14.

American College of Emergency Physicians. (2009). *EDIS: primer for emergency physicians, nurses, and IT professionals*. Irving, TX: ACEP SEMI.

Amershi, H. (2006). Leading information technology (IT) integration within vancouver coastal health. *Proquest Dissertations and Theses*, 2.

Anand, A., & Wamba, S. F. (2013). Business value of RFID-enabled healthcare transformation projects. *Business Process Management Journal*, *19*(1), 111–145. doi:10.1108/14637151311294895

Anderson, J. G., Jay, S. J., Schweer, H. M., & Anderson, M. M. (1986). Why doctors don't use computers: Some empirical findings. *Journal of the Royal Society of Medicine*, *79*, 142–144. PMID:3701749

Anderson, J., & Gerbing, D. (1988). Structual equation modelling in practice: A review and recommended two-step approach. *Psychological Bulletin*, *103*(3), 411–423. doi:10.1037/0033-2909.103.3.411

Anderson, O., Brodie, A., Vincent, C. A., & Hanna, G. B. (2012). A systematic proactive risk assessment of hazards in surgical wards: A quantitative study. *Annals of Surgery*, *255*(6), 1086–1092. doi:10.1097/SLA.0b013e31824f5f36 PMID:22504280

Anderson, P. (2005). Building on Success. *Health Management Technology*, *26*(5), 32–34. PMID:15932071

Andrews, C., & Mack, R. (2011). IBM to Collaborate with Nuance to Apply IBM's "Watson" Analytics Technology to Healthcare. *IBM News Room*. Retrieved from http://www-03.ibm.com/press/us/en/pressrelease/33726.wss

Anshari, M., & Almunawar, M. N. (2009). *Health Information Systems (HIS): Concept and Technology*. Academic Press.

Anthony, K., Nagel, D. M., & Goss, S. (2010). *The use of technology in mental health: Applications, ethics and practice*. Charles C Thomas Pub Limited.

Apache, E. S. B. (2008). *Apache Software Foundation Synapse ESB*. Retrieved from http://synapse.apache.org

Apple Health App. (2015). *Apple Health App*. Retrieved from https://www.apple.com/ios/ios8/health/

Armbrust, M., Fox, A., Griffith, R., Joseph, A. D., Katz, R. H., Konwinski, A., ... (2009). *Above the clouds: A berkeley view of cloud computing*. EECS Department, University of California, Berkeley, Tech. Rep. UCB/EECS-2009-28.

Arns, M., de Ridder, S., Strehl, U., Breteler, M., & Coenen, A. (2009). Efficacy of neurofeedback treatment in ADHD: the effects on inattention, impulsivity and hyperactivity: a meta-analysis. *Clinical EEG and Neuroscience*, *40*(3), 180–189. doi:10.1177/155005940904000311 PMID:19715181

Arns, M., Gunkelman, J., Breteler, M., & Spronk, D. (2008). EEG phenotypes predict treatment outcome to stimulants in children with ADHD. *Journal of Integrative Neuroscience*, *7*(03), 421–438. doi:10.1142/S0219635208001897 PMID:18988300

Aronsky, D., Jones, I., Lanaghan, K., & Slovis, C. M. (2008). Supporting Patient Care in the Emergency Department with a Computerized Whiteboard System. *Journal of the American Medical Informatics Association*, *15*(2), 184–194. doi:10.1197/jamia.M2489 PMID:18096913

Ash, J. S., Fournier, L., Stavri, P. Z., & Dykstra, R. (2003a). Principles for a Successful Computerized Physician Order Entry Implementation. In *AMIA Symposium Proceedings*. Washington, DC: American Medical Informatics Association.

Ash, J. S., Stavri, P. Z., Dykstra, R., & Fournier, L. (2003b). Implementing computerized physician order entry: The importance of special people. *International Journal of Medical Informatics*, 69(2-3), 235–250. doi:10.1016/S1386-5056(02)00107-7 PMID:12810127

Asif, Z., & Mandviwalla, M. (2005). Integrating the supply chain with RFID: A tech-nical and business analysis. *Communications of the Association for Information Systems*, 15, 393–427.

Aspden, P., Wolcott, J., Bootman, J. L., & Cronenwett, L. R. (2007). *Preventing medication errors*. National Academies Press.

Atieno, O. (2009). An analysis of the strengths and limitation of qualitative and quantitative research paradigms. *Problems of Education in the 21st Century, 13*, 13-18.

Atun, R. (2004). What are the advantages and disadvantages of restructuring a health care system to be more focused on primary care services? Geneva: WHO Regional Office for Europe's Health Evidence Network (HEN).

Australian Bureau of Statistics. (2014). *Personal internet use. 8146.0 - Household Use of Information Technology, Australia, 2012-13*. Retrieved from http://www.abs.gov.au/ausstats/abs@.nsf/Lookup/8146.0Chapter32012-13

Australian Govermment. (2012). *E-mental health strategy for Australia*. Retrieved from http://www.health.gov.au/internet/main/publishing.nsf/Content/7C7B0BFEB985D0EBCA257BF0001BB0A6/$File/emstrat.pdf

Australian Psychological Society. (n.d.). *Australian Psychological Society: Medicare and psychology*. Retrieved from http://www.psychology.org.au/medicare/

Avant. (2014). *Doctor's guide to smarter phone use*. Retrieved from http://connect.avant.org.au/i/320049

Avgar, A. C., Litwin, A. S., & Pronovost, P. J. (2012). Drivers and barriers in health IT adoption: A proposed framework. *Applied Clinical Informatics*, 3(4), 488–500. doi:10.4338/ACI-2012-07-R-0029 PMID:23646093

Aylin, P., Bottle, A., & Majeed, A. (2007). Use of administrative data or clinical databases as predictors of risk of death in hospital: Comparison of models. *BMJ: British Medical Journal*, 334(7602), 1044. doi:10.1136/bmj.39168.496366.55 PMID:17452389

Bacheldor, B. (2006). RFID Fills Security Gap at Psychiatric Ward. *RFID Journal*. Retrieved October 24, 2007 from http://www.rfidjournal.com/article/articleview/2750/1/1

Bacheldor, B. (2006, May 8). Report Sees Sharp Rise in Pharma RFID. *RFID Journal*.

Bacheldor, B. (2007a, October 29). Denver Health Adopting a Hospital-Wide RTLS System. *RFID Journal*.

Bacheldor, B. (2007b, October 9). Health Facility Uses RTLS to Provide 'Concierge' Care. *RFID Journal*.

Bacheldor, B. (2007c, April 23). Pharma RFID Adoption Still Slow. *RFID Journal*.

Bacheldor, B. (2007d, April 24). Siemens Launches RFID Pilot to Track Surgical Sponges, Procedures. *RFID Journal*.

Bacheldor, B. (2007e, April 10). Tags Track Surgical Patients at Birmingham Heartlands Hospital. *RFID Journal*.

Bacheldor, B. (2007f, December 12). Tergooi Hospital Uses RFID to Boost Efficiency. *RFID Journal*.

Bacheldor, B. (2008, February 13). BlueTag Patient-Tracking Comes to North America. *RFID Journal*.

Balas, A. E., Weingarten, S., Garb, C. T., Blumenthal, D., Boren, S., & Brown, G. D. (2000). Improving preventative care by prompting physicians. *Archives of Internal Medicine, 160*(3), 301–308. doi:10.1001/archinte.160.3.301 PMID:10668831

Bali, R. K., & Dwivedi, A. N. (2007). *Healthcare Knowledge Management.* Springer. doi:10.1007/978-0-387-49009-0

Ballon, P., & Van Heesvelde, E. (2010, August). Platform types and regulatory concerns in European ICT markets. *TPRC.*

Bardosh, K., Sambo, M., Sikana, L., Hampson, K., & Welburn, S. C. (2014). Eliminating Rabies in Tanzania? Local Understandings and Responses to Mass Dog Vaccination in Kilombero and Ulanga Districts. *PLoS Neglected Tropical Diseases, 8*(6), 29–35. doi:10.1371/journal.pntd.0002935 PMID:24945697

Barker & Badal. (2008). *Measurement of Dyshemoglobin and total Hemoglobin by pulse oximetry.* Wolters Kluwer Health | Lippincott Williams & Wilkins.

Barkley, R. A. (1997a). Behavioral inhibition, sustained attention, and executive functions: Constructing a unifying theory of ADHD. *Psychological Bulletin, 121*(1), 65–94. doi:10.1037/0033-2909.121.1.65 PMID:9000892

Barkley, R. A. (1998). *Attention deficit hyperactivity disorder: A handbook for diagnosis and treatment* (2nd ed.). New York: Guilford.

Barkley, R. A. (2006). *Attention-deficit hyperactivity disorder: A handbook for diagnosis and treatment* (3rd ed.). New York: Guilford.

Barkley, R. A. X. (1997b). *Attention-deficit Hyperactivity Disorder and the Nature of Self-control.* The Guilford Press.

Barkley, R. A., Murphy, K. R., & Fischer, M. (2008). *ADHD in adults: What the science says.* New York: Guilford.

Barrette, E. G. (2011). The impact of health information technology on demand for hospital inpatient services. *ProQuest,* 93-94.

Barry, M. J., & Edgman-Levitan, S. (2012). Shared Decision Making—The Pinnacle of Patient-Centered Care. *The New England Journal of Medicine, 366*(9), 780–781. doi:10.1056/NEJMp1109283 PMID:22375961

Bate, S. P., & Robert, G. (2002). Knowledge Management and communities of practice in the private sector: Lessons for modernizing the National Health Service in England and Wales. *Public Administration Journal, 80*(4), 643–663. doi:10.1111/1467-9299.00322

Bates, D. W., Kuperman, G. J., Wang, S., Gandhi, T., Kittler, A., Volk, L., & Middleton, B. et al. (2003). Ten commandments for effective clinical decision support: Making the practice of evidence-based medicine a reality. *Journal of the American Medical Informatics Association, 10*(6), 523–530. doi:10.1197/jamia.M1370 PMID:12925543

Bauer, A. & Günzel, H. (2013). *Data-Warehouse-Systeme: Architektur, Entwicklung, Anwendung.* dpunkt. verlag.

Baumbach, J. (2006). Nurse practitioner utilization of information technology. *Proquest Dissertations and Theses,* 7.

Baumlin, K. M., Shapiro, J. S., Weiner, C. Gottlieb, B., Chawla, N., & Richardson, L. D. (2010). Clinical Information System and Process Redesign Improves Emergency Department Efficiency. *Joint Commission Journal on Quality and Patient Safety, 36,* 179-1AP.

Baumlin, K. M., & Richardson, L. D. (2006). Emergency Department Information System (EDIS) Success: EDIS Implementation Improves Documentation and Increases Charges and Revenue. *Academic Emergency Medicine, 13*(5Supplement 1), s61. doi:10.1197/j.aem.2006.03.138

Bayo-Moriones, A., Billon, M., & Lera-Lopez, F. (2013). Perceived performance effects of ICT in manufacturing SMEs. *Industrial Management & Data Systems, 113*(1), 117–135. doi:10.1108/02635571311289700

Beck, S. J., Hanson, C. A., Puffenberger, S. S., Benninger, K. L., & Benninger, W. B. (2010). A controlled trial of working memory training for children and adolescents with ADHD. *Journal of Clinical Child and Adolescent Psychology*, *39*(6), 825–836. doi:10.1080/15374416.2010.517162 PMID:21058129

Bell, D. E., & LaPadula, L. J. (1973).*Secure computer systems: Mathematical foundations*. DTIC Document.

Ben-Arye, E., Frenkel, M., Klein, A., & Scharf, M. (2008). Attitudes toward integration of complementary and alternative medicine in primary care: Perspectives of patients, physicians and complementary practitioners. *Patient Education and Counseling*, *70*(3), 395–402. doi:10.1016/j.pec.2007.11.019 PMID:18201857

Bendavid, Y., Boeck, H., & Philippe, R. (2010). Redesigning the replenishment process of medical supplies in hospitals with RFID. *Business Process Management Journal*, *16*(6), 991–1013.

Bendavid, Y., Boeck, H., & Philippe, R. (2010). Redesigning the replenishment process of medical supplies in hospitals with RFID. *Business Process Management Journal*, *16*(6), 991–1013. doi:10.1108/14637151011093035

Bensel, P., & Gunther, O. et al.. (2008). Cost–benefit sharing in cross-company RFID applications: A case study approach. In *29th International Conference on Information Systems (ICIS)* (pp. 1–17). Paris, France.

Berghoef, H. (2006). (Good) growing pains. Michigan ED automates patient tracking, nurse documentation and charge capture to maintain excellent customer service, increase efficiencies and boost revenue. *Health Management Technology*, *27*(3), 30–35. PMID:16594517

Berg, M. (1998). Medical work and the computer-based patient record: A sociological perspective. *Methods of Information in Medicine*, *37*, 294–301. PMID:9787631

Berg, M. (2001). Implementing information systems in health care organizations: Myths and challenges. *International Journal of Medical Informatics*, *64*(2–3), 143–156. doi:10.1016/S1386-5056(01)00200-3 PMID:11734382

Berners, E. S. (Ed.). (1999). *Clinical decision supports systems*. New York: Springer-Verlag. doi:10.1007/978-1-4757-3903-9

Bhambri, V. (2011). Application of data mining in banking sector. *International Journal of Clothing Science and Technology*, *2*(2).

Bina Upaya Kesehatan Kementerian Kesehatan, R. I. (2011, November 8). *Juknis Sistem Informasi Rumah Sakit (SIRS)2011*. Retrieved from www.buk.depkes.go.id

Bina Upaya Kesehatan Kementerian Kesehatan, R. I. (2013). *Ditjen BUK Sosialisasikan SIMRS Generik Open Source*. Retrieved from http://buk.depkes.go.id/index.php?option=com_content&view=article&id=376:ditjen-buk-sosialisasikan-simrs-generik-open-source&catid=1:latest-news

Bingman, K. (2001). E-Health Solutions Series. *Cerner 2001*.

BizTalk Server. (2006). *Microsoft BizTalk Server*. Retrieved from http://www.microsoft.com/biztalk/

Blanton, J. D., Manangan, A., Manangan, J., Hanlon, C. A., Slate, D., & Rupprecht, C. E. (2006). Development of a GIS-based, real-time Internet mapping tool for rabies surveillance. *International Journal of Health Geographics*, *5*(1), 47. doi:10.1186/1476-072X-5-47 PMID:17078890

Blaya, J. A., Hamish, S. F., & Holt, B. (2010). e-Health technologies show promise in developing countries. *Health Affairs*, *29*(2), 244–251. doi:10.1377/hlthaff.2009.0894 PMID:20348068

Blue Button. (2013). *Blue Button*. Retrieved from http://www.healthit.gov/patients-families/blue-button/

Bodeker, G., & Kronenberg, F. (2002). A public health agenda for traditional, complementary, and alternative medicine. *American Journal of Public Health*, *92*(10), 1582–1591. doi:10.2105/AJPH.92.10.1582 PMID:12356597

Boerma, W.G.W., & Mulder, P. H. (2008). *Health care and general practice across Europe*. The University of Michigan.

Bogdan, R., Biklen, C., & Knopp, S. (1998). Qualitative research in education. An introduction to theory and methods. Boston: Allyn and Bacon.

Bolton, P. (1997, October). Through the looking glass. Computers & general practice. *Australian Family Physician*, *26*(10), 1167–1169. PMID:9339591

Booch, G., Rumbaugh, J., & Jacobson, I. (2005).*Unified Modeling Language User Guide*. Addison-Wesley Professional.

Booth, P., Frisch, P. H., ... (2006). Application of RFID in an integrated healthcare environment. In *Conference proceedings: Annual international conference of the IEEE Engineering in Medicine and Biology Society*. IEEE Engineering in Medicine and Biology Society. doi:10.1109/IEMBS.2006.259389

Booth, M. L., Bernard, D., Quine, S., Kang, M. S., Usherwood, T., Alperstein, G., & Bennett, D. L. (2004). Access to health care among Australian adolescents young people's perspectives and their sociodemographic distribution. *The Journal of Adolescent Health*, *34*(1), 97–103. doi:10.1016/S1054-139X(03)00304-5 PMID:14706412

Bossen, C. (2007). Test the artefact – develop the organization: The implementation of an electronic medication plan. *International Journal of Medical Informatics*, *76*(1), 13–21. doi:10.1016/j.ijmedinf.2006.01.001 PMID:16455299

Bouchard, M. (2005). What works. ED on Track With IT. *Health Management Technology*, *26*(8), 28–31. PMID:16156525

Boulard, G. (2005). RFID: Promise or Peril? It may be easier than ever to track information, but it is causing concerns over privacy and civil liberties. *State Legislatures Magazine.*, *31*(10), 22–24. PMID:16397978

Boxwala, A. A., Peleg, M., Tu, S., Ogunyemi, O., Zeng, Q. T., Wang, D., & Shortliffe, E. H. et al. (2004). GLIF3: A representation format for sharable computer-interpretable clinical practice guidelines. *Journal of Biomedical Informatics*, *37*(3), 147–161. doi:10.1016/j.jbi.2004.04.002 PMID:15196480

Braa, J., Hanseth, O., Heywood, A., Mohammed, W., & Shawn, B. (2007). Developing information systems in developing country: The flexible standards strategy. *MIS Quartely*, *31*, 1–22.

Braun, V., & Clarke, V. (2006). Using thematic analysis in pyschology. *Qualitative Research in Psychology*, *3*(2), 77–101. doi:10.1191/1478088706qp063oa

Brecht, Prough, Petrov, Petrova, Deyo, & Esenaliev. (2004). Accurate, Noninvasive measurement of total hemoglobin concentration with optoacoustic technique. In *Proceedings of the 26th Annual International Conference of the IEEE EMBS*. San Francisco, CA: IEEE.

Brennan, S. (2005). *The NHS IT project: the biggest computer programme in the world ever!* Abingdon: Radcliffe.

Brikci, N., & Green, J. (2007). *A guide to using qualitative research methodology*. Academic Press.

Brimacombe, G. G., Antunes, P., & McIntyre, J. (2001). *The future cost of health care in Canada, 2000 to 2020: balancing affordability and sustainability*. Conference Board of Canada.

Britt H, Miller GC,, Henderson J, Bayram C, Valenti L, Harrison C, Charles J, Pan Y et al. (2013). *General practice activity in Australia 2012- 13*. The Family Medicine Research Centre, General Practice Series Number 33, November 2013. Sydney University Press.

Britt, H., Miller, G. C., Charles, J., Henderson, J., Bayram, C., & Pan, Y. et al.. (2010). *General practice activity in Australia 2009-10*. Canberra: Australian Institute of Health and Welfare.

Britton, J. (2007). An investigation into the feasibility of locating portable medical devices using radio frequency identification devices and technology. *Journal of Medical Engineering & Technology, 31*(6), 450–458. doi:10.1080/03091900701292141 PMID:17994419

Brown-Davis, C. B. (2009). Managed care and minority healthcare access in Georgia: A qualitative study of the quality and accessibility of care provided to the minority elderly population of Dekalb county. *Proquest Dissertations and Theses*, 12-13.

Brownstein, J. S., Freifeld, C. C., Reis, B. Y., & Mandl, K. D. (2008). Surveillance Sans Frontieres: Internet-based emerging infectious disease intelligence and the HealthMap project. *PLoS Medicine, 5*(7), e151. doi:10.1371/journal.pmed.0050151 PMID:18613747

Burkhard, R. J., & Schooley, B. et al.. (2010). Information systems and healthcare XXXVII: When your employer provides your personal health record—Exploring employee perceptions of an employer-sponsored PHR system. *Communications of the Association for Information Systems, 27*, 323–338.

Burns, J. M., Davenport, T. A., Durkin, L. A., Luscombe, G. M., & Hickie, I. B. (2010). The internet as a setting for mental health service utilisation by young people. *The Medical Journal of Australia, 192*(11), S22. PMID:20528703

Burton, L. C., Anderson, G. F., & Kues, I. W. (2004). Using electronic health records to help coordinate care. *The Milbank Quarterly, 82*(3), 457–481. doi:10.1111/j.0887-378X.2004.00318.x PMID:15330973

Buyurgan, N., Landry, S., & Philippe, R. (2013). RFID Adoption in Healthcare and ROI Analysis. In *The Value of RFID* (pp. 81–96). Springer. doi:10.1007/978-1-4471-4345-1_7

caBIG. (2004). *The Cancer Biomedical Informatics Grid (caBIG)*. Retrieved from https://cabig.nci.nih.gov/

Callon, M. (1986). Some elements of a sociology of translation: domestication of the scallops and the fishermen of St Brieuc Bay. In *J. Law, Power, action and belief: a new sociology of knowledge?* (pp. 196–223). London: Routledge.

Callon, M. (1986). Some Elements of a Sociology of Translation: Domestication of the Scallops and the Fishermen of St Brieuc Bay. In *Power, Action and Belief: A New Sociology of Knowledge*. London: Routledge & Kegan Paul.

Callon, M. (1986). Some elements of the sociology of translation: Domestication of the scallops and the fisherman of St Brieuc Bay. In J. Law (Ed.), *A New Sociology of Knowledge, power, action and belief* (pp. 196–233). London: Routledge.

Callon, M., & Bruno, L. (1981). Unscrewing the Big Leviathan: How Actors Macro-Structure Reality and How Sociologists Help Them Do So. In K. Knorr-Cetina & A. V. Cicourel (Eds.), *Advances in Social Theory and Methodology: Toward an Integration of Micro- and Macro-Sociologies*. Boston: Routledge & Kegan Paul.

Canadian Attention Deficit Hyperactivity Disorder Resource Alliance (CADDRA). (2011). *Canadian ADHD Practice Guidelines* (3rd ed.). Toronto, Canada: CADDRA.

Cao, Q., Baker, J., Wetherbe, J., & Gu, V. (2012). *Organizational adoption of innovation: Identifying factors that influence RFID adoption in the healthcare industry*. Academic Press.

Cavoukian, A. (2008, January). *RFID and Privacy-Guidance for Health-Care Providers*. Information and Privacy Commissioner of Ontario. Retrieved from http://www.longwoods.com/articles/images/rfid-healthcare.pdf

CCR. (2012). *Continuity of Care Record (CCR)*. Retrieved from http://www.aafp.org/practice-management/health-it/astm.html

Cerejo, L. (2010). *Design Better and Faster With Rapid Prototyping.* Germany: Smashing Media Company.

Chang, J. (2007). Nursing informatics competencies required of nurses in Taiwan: A Delphi method. *Proquest Dissertations and Theses*, 1-2.

Chang, P. (2011) Modeling the Management of Electronic Health Records in Healthcare Information Systems. *2011 International Conference on Cyber-Enabled Distributed Computing and Knowledge Discovery.* doi:10.1109/CyberC.2011.98

Charles, C., Gafni, A., & Whelan, T. (1997). Shared decision-making in the medical encounter: What does it mean?(or it takes at least two to tango). *Social Science & Medicine. Social Science & Medicine, 44*(5), 681–692. doi:10.1016/S0277-9536(96)00221-3

Chaulagai, C.N, Moyo, C.M, Koot, J., & Moyo, H.B. (2005). *Design and implementation of a health management in Malawi: issues inovation and results.* Oxford University Press in association with The London School of Hygiene and Tropical Medicine.

Chen, C.C., Wu, J., Su, Y.S., & Yang, S.C. (2008). Key drivers for the continued use of RFID technology in the emergency room. *Management Research News, 31*(4), 273–288.

Cheng, C.-Y., & Chai, J.-W. (2012). Deployment of RFID in healthcare facilities—experimental design in MRI department. *Journal of Medical Systems, 36*(6), 3423–3433. doi:10.1007/s10916-011-9796-9 PMID:22072278

Chi, C. (1994). Integrating Traditional Medicine into Modern Health Care Systems: Examining the role of Chinese Medicine in Taiwan. *Pergamon, 39*(3), 307-321.

Chomsky, N. (1975). *Reflections on Language, (A good non-technical review of the extended standard theory and various philosophical issues related to generative grammar.).* New York: Pantheon.

Chowdhury, B., & Khosla, R. (2007, July). RFID based Real Time Patient Management System. Computer and Information Science, 363–368.

Christensen, H., Griffiths, K. M., & Evans, K. (2002). e-Mental health in Australia: Implications of the Internet and related technologies for policy. Canberra: Commonwealth Department of Health and Ageing Canberra.

Christensen, H., Proudfoot, J., Andrews, G., Klein, B., Kavanagh, D., O'Neil, D., . . . Graham, K. (2009). *E-mental health: a 2020 vision and strategy for Australia.* Academic Press.

Christensen, H., & Hickie, I. B. (2010). E-mental health: A new era in delivery of mental health services. *The Medical Journal of Australia, 192*(11), S2. PMID:20528702

Christensen, H., & Petrie, K. (2013). Information technology as the key to accelerating advances in mental health care. *The Australian and New Zealand Journal of Psychiatry, 47*(2), 114–116. doi:10.1177/0004867412471088 PMID:23382508

Chunharas, S. (2006). An interactive integrative approach to translating knowledge and building a "learning organisation" in health services management. *Bulletin of the World Health Organization, 84*(8), 652–657. doi:10.2471/BLT.05.026922 PMID:16917653

Churchman, C. W. (1971). *The design of inquiring systems: basic concepts of systems and organisation.* New York: Basic Books.

Chute, C. G., Ullman-Cullere, M., Wood, G. M., Lin, S. M., He, M., & Pathak, J. (2013). Some experiences and opportunities for big data in translational research. *Genetics in Medicine, 15*(10), 802–809. doi:10.1038/gim.2013.121 PMID:24008998

Cisco. (2007). *Mobility solution for healthcare: voice, text, images and information, delivered to the point of care*. Available at: http://www.cisco.com/web/strategy/docs/healthcare/07cs1084-MobForHC_062708.pdf

Clayton, P. D., Narus, S. P., Bowes, W. A., III, Madsen, T. S., Wilcox, A. B., & Orsmond, G., …Leckman, L. (2005). Physician use of electronic medical records: Issues and successes with direct data entry and physician productivity. In *AMIA Annual Symposium Proceedings*. Washington, DC: American Medical Informatics Association.

Cleaveland, S., Kaare, M., Tiringa, P., & Mlengeya, T. 2001. A dog rabies vaccination campaign in rural Africa: impact on the incidence of animal rabies and human bite injuries. In *Proceedings of the Southern and Eastern African Rabies Group. World Health Organization Meeting*. WHO.

Cleaveland, S., Fevre, E. M., Kaare, M., & Coleman, P. G. (2002). Estimating human rabies mortality in the United Republic of Tanzania from dog bite injuries. *Bulletin of the World Health Organization, 80*(4), 304–310. PMID:12075367

Cleaveland, S., Kaare, M., Tiringa, P., Mlengeya, T., & Barrat, J. (2003). A dog rabies vaccination campaign in rural Africa: Impact on the incidence of dog rabies and human dog-bite injuries. *Vaccine, 21*(17-18), 1965–1973. doi:10.1016/S0264-410X(02)00778-8 PMID:12706685

Cleaveland, S., Lembo, T., Townsend, S., Kazwala, R., Sikana, L., Changalucha, J., & Hampson, K. (2013). *Relevance of research for development of national rabies control strategies in Africa. 11th SEARG meeting*, Dar es Salaam.

Cleverley, M. (2009). How ICT advances might help developing nations. *Communications of the ACM, 52*(9), 30–32. doi:10.1145/1562164.1562177

Cline, G., & Luiz, J. (2013). Information technology systems in public sector health facilities in developing countries: the case of South Africa. *BMC Medicial informatics and decision making*, 13.

CMBA. (n.d.). *Chinese Medicine Board of Australia*. Retrieved 14 October, 2014 from http://www.chinesemedicineboard.gov.au/

CMS. (2013). *Centers of Medicare and Medicaid Electronic Health Records Incentive Programs*. Retrieved from www.cms.gov/EHRIncentivePrograms

COCIR. (2010). *The European Coordination Committee of the Radiological, Electro medical and Healthcare IT Industry: Glossary of Terms*. COCIR. Retrieved from http://www.cocir.org/uploads/documents/-883-

Codagnone, C., & Lupiañez-Villanueva, F. (2013). Benchmarking Deployment of eHealth among General Practitioners, 2013 Final report. European Commission. Doi:10.2759/24556

Collins, J. (2004a, November 16). Purdue Pharma Tags OxyContin. *RFID Journal*.

Collins, J. (2004b, November 19). Six U.K. Drug makers Pilot RFID. *RFID Journal*.

Collins, J. (2006d, June 20). Novartis Trial Shows RFID Can Boost Patient Compliance. *RFID Journal*.

Coonan, K. M. (2004). Medical informatics standards applicable to emergency department information systems: Making sense of the jumble. *Academic Emergency Medicine, 11*(11), 1198–1205. doi:10.1111/j.1553-2712.2004.tb00705.x PMID:15528585

Cork, R. D., Detner, W. M., & Friedman, C. P. (1998). Academic physicians' use of, knowledge about, and attitudes toward computers: Measurement study and validation. *Journal of the American Medical Informatics Association, 5*, 164–176. doi:10.1136/jamia.1998.0050164 PMID:9524349

Costetchi, N., Danila, C., & Stanescu, A. M. (2014). Enterprise System Architecture to Sustain Cross-Domain e-Healthcare Applications. In Enterprise Interoperability VI (pp. 271-281). Springer International Publishing. doi:10.1007/978-3-319-04948-9_23

Courtney, J. F. (2001). Decision making and knowledge management in inquiring organisations: Toward a new decision-making paradigm for DSS. *Decision Support Systems, 31*(1), 17-38.

Courtney, J. F., Haynes, J. D., & Paradice, D. B. (2005). *Inquiring organisations: moving from knowledge management to wisdom.* IGI Global. doi:10.4018/978-1-59140-309-8

Cousin, G., Schmid Mast, M., Roter, D. L., & Hall, J. A. (2012). Concordance between physician communication style and patient attitudes predicts patient satisfaction. *Patient Education and Counseling, 87*(2), 193–197. doi:10.1016/j.pec.2011.08.004 PMID:21907529

Coustasse, A., Tomblin, S., & Slack, C. (2013). A review of Radio Frequency Identification Technologies and Impacts on the Hospital Supply Chain: 2002-2012. In *Proceedings of Academic and Business Research Institute (AABRI) International Conference.* MMM Track.

Craig, H. D. (2013). Using Diffusion of Innovation theory to determine Missouri providers' perception of telemedicine. *Proquest Dissertations and Theses*, 10.

Crang, M. (1997). Analyzing qualitative material. Longman.

Cresswell, K. M., & Sheikh, A. (2008). Information technology—Based approaches toreducing repeat drug exposure in patients with known drug allergies. *Journal of Allergy and Clinical Immunology, 121*(5), 1112-1117.

Cresswell, K. M., Worth, A., & Sheikh, A. (2010). Actor-network theory and its role in understanding the implementation of information technology developments in healthcare. *BMC Medical Informatics and Decision Making, 10*(1), 67. doi:10.1186/1472-6947-10-67 PMID:21040575

Creswell, J. W. (2013). *Research design: Qualitative, quantitative, and mixed methods approaches* (4th ed.). London: Sage Publications, Incorporated.

Creswell, K., Worth, A., & Sheikh, A. (2010). Actor-Network theory and its role in understanding the implementation of information technology developments in healthcare. *BMC Medical Informatics and Decision Making*, 10–67.

Crompton, M. (2002). *Privacy, Technology and the Healthcare Sector, Federal Privacy Commissioner Report.* Paper presented at the Australian Financial Review—4th Annual Health Congress, Sydney, Australia.

Cross, M. (2006). Keeping the ER on track. *Health Data Management, 14* (9), 68–69.

Crounse, B. (2005). *RFID: Increasing patient safety, reducing healthcare costs, 2005.* Available at http://www.microsoft.com/industry/healthcare/providers/businessvalue/housecalls/rfid.mspx

Cummings, E., & Borycki, E. M. (2011). *Grounded Theory Evolution and Its Application in Health Informatics.* Paper presented at the ITCH.

Curbera, F., Duftler, M., Khalaf, R., Nagy, W., Mukhi, N., & Weerawarana, S. (2002). Unraveling the Web services web: An introduction to SOAP, WSDL, and UDDI. *IEEE Internet Computing, 6*(2), 86–93. doi:10.1109/4236.991449

Czanderna, K. H. (2013). A qualitative study on the impact of a short term global healthcare immersion experience in bachelor of science nursing students. *Proquest Dissertations and Theses*, 68-69.

Da've, D. (2004). Benefits and barriers to EMR implementation. *Caring, 23*(11), 50–51. PMID:15633313

Dahiya, S. (2008). Counterfeit medicines: The global hazard. *Latest Reviews, 6*(4), 1–4.

Daigle, M., Roychoudhury, I., Narasimhan, S., Saha, S., Saha, B., & Goebel, K. (2011). Investigating the effect of damage progression model choice on prognostics performance. In *Proceedings of the annual conference of the prognostics and health management society 2011* (pp. 323-333). Academic Press.

Daly, G. (2012). Nursing perceptions of electronic documentation. *Proquest, 3.*

Dalziel, C. A. (2007). Factors that enhance nurses' use of health information systems to support clinical decision-making. *Proquest, 1.*

Dalziel, C. A. (2008). Factors that enhance nurses use of health information systems to support clinical decision making. *Proquest dissertations and theses.*

Dalziel, C. A. (2008). *Factors that enhances nurses use of health information systems to support clinical decision making.* ProQuest Dissertations and Theses.

Das, R., & Harrop, P. (2011). *RFID Forecasts, Players and Opportunities 2011–2021.* IDTechEx.

Davis, F. (1989). Perceived usefulness, perceived ease of use, and user acceptance of information technology. *Management Information Systems Quarterly, 13*(3), 319–240. doi:10.2307/249008

Davis, S. (2004). Tagging along. RFID helps hospitals track assets and people. *Health Facilities Management, 17*(12), 20–24. PMID:15637841

De Backere, F., De Turck, F., Colpaert, K., & Decruyenaere, J. (2012). *Advanced pervasive clinical decision support for the intensive care unit.* Academic Press.

De La Rosa Algarín, A., Demurjian, S. A., Berhe, S., & Pavlich-Mariscal, J. A. (2012). A security framework for XML schemas and documents for healthcare. *Bioinformatics and Biomedicine Workshops (BIBMW), 2012 IEEE International Conference on* (pp. 782–789). IEEE.

De La Rosa Algarín, A., Ziminski, T. B., Demurjian, S. A., Kuykendall, R., & Rivera Sánchez, Y. (2013). Defining and Enforcing XACML Role-Based Security Policies within an XML Security Framework.*Proceedings of 9th International Conference on Web Information Systems and Technologies (WEBIST 2013)* (pp. 16–25). doi:10.5220/0004366200160025

Deegan, P., & Drake, R. (2006). Shared decision making and medication management in the recovery process. *Psychiatric Services (Washington, D.C.), 57*(11), 1636–1639. doi:10.1176/ps.2006.57.11.1636 PMID:17085613

Deering, P., Tatnall, A., & Burgess, S. (2010). Adoption of ICT in Rural Medical General Practices in Australia: an Actor-Network Study. *International Journal of Actor-Network Theory and Technological Innovation, 2* (1), 54-69.

DeLong, D. W., & Fahey, L. (2000). Diagnosing cultural barriers to knowledge management. *The Academy of Management Executive, 14*(4), 113–127.

Dempsey, M. (2005). Weaving through the hopes and hype surrounding RFID. *Biomedical Instrumentation and Technology Supplement,* 19–22.

Demurjian, S. A., Saripalle, R., & Berhe, S. (2009). An Integrated Ontology Framework for Health Information Exchange. *SEKE, 09,* 575–580.

Dennis, S. (2010). IS World, 2003. *Journal of International Technology.*

Denny, J. C. (2012). Mining electronic health records in the genomics era. *PLoS Computational Biology, 8*(12), e1002823. doi:10.1371/journal.pcbi.1002823 PMID:23300414

Denzin, & Lincoln. (2000). *Handbook of Qualitative Research.* London: Sage Publications.

Department of Health. (2004). *Improving Emergency Care in England, Report by the Comptroller and Auditor General (HC 1075 Session 2003–2004).* London: National Audit Office.

Department of Health. (2007). *Guidelines for Maternity Care in South Africa* [national guidelines on maternity care]. Pretoria, South Africa: Department of Health, South Africa.

Department of Health. (2008). *Confidential Enquiry into Maternal Deaths 2007* [report on enquiry into maternal deaths]. Pretoria, South Africa: Department of Health, South Africa.

Department of Health. (2012). e-Health Strategy, 2012–2016. Pretoria, South Africa: Department of Health, South Africa.

Department of Human Services Victoria. (n.d.). *Attention deficit hyperactivity disorder - adults.* Retrieved from http://www.betterhealth.vic.gov.au/bhcv2/bhcarticles.nsf/pages/Attention_deficit_hyperactivity_disorder_and_adults#

Depeoulu, A. O. (2010). College Students With ADHD: Prescriptive Concepts for Best Practices in Career Development. *Journal of Career Development.*

DeWoody, S., & Loadman, G. P. (1999). Implementing an Emergency Department Information System – How Complicated Can We Make This? *Journal of Healthcare Information Management, 13*(3), 19–30. PMID:10787597

DHS (Department of Health and Ageing). (2004). *Medicare definition of a GP.* Retrieved from http://www.health.gov.au/internet/wcms/publishing.nsf/Content/pcd-publications-gpinoz2004

DiCenso, A., Martin-Misener, R., Bryant-Lukosius, D., Bourgeault, I., Kilpatrick, K., Donald, F., & Charbonneau-Smith, R. et al. (2010, December). Advanced Practice Nursing in Canada: Overview of a decision support synthesis. *Canadian Journal of Nursing Leadership, 23*(special issue), 15–34. doi:10.12927/cjnl.2010.22267 PMID:21478685

Dickmann, F., Falkner, J., Gunia, W., Hampe, J., Hausmann, M., Herrmann, A., & Sax, U. et al. (2012). Solutions for biomedical grid computing - case studies from the D-Grid project Services@ MediGRID. *Journal of Computational Science, 3*(5), 280–297. doi:10.1016/j.jocs.2011.06.006

Dienemann, J., & Castle, B. V. (2003). The impact of healthcare informatics on the organisation. *Jona,* 557-558.

Diffusion of innovations. (1995). New York: Free Press.

Dinh, M., & Chu, M. (2006). Evolution of health information management and information technology in emergency medicine. *Emergency Medicine Australasia, 18*(3), 289–294. doi:10.1111/j.1742-6723.2006.00855.x PMID:16712540

Dixon-Woods, M., Agarwal, S., Jones, D., Young, B., & Sutton, A. (2005). Synthesising qualitative and quantitative evidence: A review of possible methods. *Journal of Health Services Research & Policy, 10*(1), 45–53B. doi:10.1258/1355819052801804 PMID:15667704

Dominguez-Péry, C., & Ageron, B. et al.. (2011). A service science framework to enhancevalue creation in service innovation projects: An RFID case study. *International Journal of Production Economics.*

Dominguez-Pery, C., Ageron, B., & Neubert, G. (2013). A service science framework to enhance value creation in service innovation projects - An RFID case study. *International Journal of Production Economics, 141*(2), 440–451. doi:10.1016/j.ijpe.2011.12.026

Doshi, & Panditrao. (n.d.). Optical Sensor System for Hemoglobin Measurement. *International Journal of Computational Engineering Research, 3.*

Dowding, D. (2013). Using computerized decision support systems. *Nursing Times, 109*(36), 23–25. PMID:24245371

Dow, S., Heddleston, K., & Klemmer, S. (2009). The Efficacy of Prototyping Under Time Constraints. In *Proceeding of ACM Conf. on Creativity and Cognition*. ACM. doi:10.1145/1640233.1640260

Duckett, S. J. (2007). *The Australian Health Care System* (3rd ed.). Australia: Oxford University Press.

Duckett, S. J., & Willcox, S. (2011). *The Australian health care system* (4th ed.). Melbourne: Oxford University Press.

Dunlevy, S. (2013). *Outrage as eHealth record sign-up squads hit Australian hospital patients in bid to boost numbers*. News.com.au. Retrieved April 30 2013 from http://www.news.com.au/national-news/outrage-as-ehealth-record-sign-up-squads-hit-australian-hospital-patients-in-bid-to-boost-numbers/story-fncynjr2-1226619874616

Dunt, D., Temple-Smith, M., & Johnson, K. A. (1991). Nursing outside hospitals: the working experience of community nurses: job characteristics. *International Journal of Nursing Studies*, 28(1), 27–37. doi:10.1016/0020-7489(91)90047-7 PMID:1856030

Eason, K. (2005). Exploiting the potential of the NPfIT: A local design approach. *British Journal of Healthcare Computing & Information Management*, 22, 14–15.

Edwards, D. (2011). Analyzing decision-Making styles and strategic planning techniques for information technology in non-profit organisations. *Proquest Dissertations and Theses*, 24.

Edwards, A., & Elwyn, G. (2009). *Shared decision-making in health care: Achieving evidence-based patient choice*. Oxford University Press.

Eisenhardt, K. M. (1989). Building theories from case study research. *Academy of Management Review*, 14(4), 532–550.

eMERGE. (2007). *Electronic Medical Records and Genomics (eMERGE) Network*. Retrieved from http://emerge.mc.vanderbilt.edu/

Enrado, P. (2011). Why shuttered RHIO CareSpark's chairman is not giving up. *Government Health IT*. Retrieved from http://www.govhealthit.com/news/why-shuttered-rhio-caresparks-chairman-not-giving

Epstein, R. M., Fiscella, K., Lesser, C. S., & Stange, K. C. (2010). Why the nation needs a policy push on patient-centered health care. *Health Affairs*, 29(8), 1489–1495. doi:10.1377/hlthaff.2009.0888 PMID:20679652

Estates, N. H. S. (2003). *The impact of the built environment on care within A&E departments: Key findings and recommendations*. London: The Stationery Office.

Estates, N. H. S. (2004). *A&E design evaluation. Evaluation of two proposed accident and emergency departments: Brent Emergency Care and Diagnostic centre at Central Middlesex Hospital, and an Exemplar Plan*. London: The Stationery Office.

Eugster, P. T., Felber, P. A., Guerraoui, R., & Kermarrec, A.-M. (2003). The many faces of publish/subscribe. *ACM Computing Surveys*, 35(2), 114–131. doi:10.1145/857076.857078

Eysenbach, G. (2001). What is e-health? *Journal of Medical Internet Research*, 3(2), e20. doi:10.2196/jmir.3.2.e20 PMID:11720962

Eysenbach, G. (2009). Infodemiology and infoveillance: Framework for an emerging set of public health informatics methods to analyze search, communication and publication behavior on the Internet. *Journal of Medical Internet Research*, 11(1), e11. doi:10.2196/jmir.1157 PMID:19329408

Farley, H. L., Baumlin, K. M., Hamedani, A. G., Cheung, D. S., Edwards, M. R., Fuller, D. C., & Pines, J. M. et al. (2013). Quality and safety implications of emergency department information systems. *Annals of Emergency Medicine*, 62(4), 399–407. doi:10.1016/j.annemergmed.2013.05.019 PMID:23796627

Farquharson, P. H. (2009). The perception of information technology investment and its impact on productivity at small private colleges. *Proquest, 6.*

Fasolino, T. (2009). *Nursing related factors influencing medication error incidence on medical surgical units.* Proquest.

Feeley, T. W., Sledge, G. W., Levit, L., & Ganz, P. A. (2013). Improving the quality of cancer care in America through health information technology. *Journal of the American Medical Informatics Association.*

Fenton, S. H., Giannangelo, K., & Stanfill, M. (2006). Essential people skills for EHR implementation success. *Journal of American Health Information Management Association, 77,* 60A–60D. PMID:16805302

Ferlie, E., Crilly, T., Jashapara, A., & Peckham, A. (2012). Knowledge mobilisation in healthcare: a critical review of health sector and generic management literature. *Social Science & Medicine, 74*(8), 1297-1304.

FERPA. (1974). *Family Educational Rights and Privacy Act (FERPA).* Retrieved from http://www.ed.gov/policy/gen/guid/fpco/ferpa/

Ferraiolo, D. F., Sandhu, R., Gavrila, S., Kuhn, D. R., & Chandramouli, R. (2001). Proposed NIST standard for role-based access control. *ACM Transactions on Information and System Security, 4*(3), 224–274. doi:10.1145/501978.501980

Fichman, R. G. (2000). The diffusion and assimilation of information technology innovations. In R. Zmud (Ed.), *Framing the domains of IT management: projec-ting the future through the past.* Cincinnati, OH: Pinnaflex Educational Resources, Incorporated.

Field, M. J., & Lohr, K. N. (1990). *Clinical practice guidelines: directions of a new paradigm.* Washington, DC: National Academy Press.

First, P. (2014). Retrieved from http://www.patientsfirst.org.nz/about

Fischer, M., Barkley, R. A., Edelbrock, C. S., & Smallish, L. (1990). The adolescent outcome of hyperactive children diagnosed by research criteria: II. Academic, attentional, and neuropsychological status. *Journal of Consulting and Clinical Psychology, 58*(5), 580–588. doi:10.1037/0022-006X.58.5.580 PMID:2254504

Fisher, J. A., & Monahan, T. (2008). Tracking the social dimensions of RFID systems in hospitals. *International Journal of Medical Informatics, 77*(3), 176–183. doi:10.1016/j.ijmedinf.2007.04.010 PMID:17544841

Fisher, W., & Tibbs, E. W. (2003). What works. Three phases of EDIS. Installation of a comprehensive emergency department information system enables a Virginia IDN to revitalize its ED services. *Health Management Technology, 24,* 36–40. PMID:12647615

Fitzpatrick, M. C., Hampson, K., Cleaveland, S., Meyers, L. A., Townsend, J. P., & Galvani, A. P. (2012). Potential for rabies control through dog vaccination in wildlife-abundant communities of Tanzania. *PLoS Neglected Tropical Diseases, 6*(8), e1796.

Flick, U. (2014). An introduction to qualitative research. *Sage (Atlanta, Ga.).*

Flight, I. H., Wilson, C. J., Zajac, I. T., Hart, E., & McGillivray, J. A. (2012). Decision support and the effectiveness of web-based delivery and information tailoring for bowel cancer screening: an exploratory study. *JMIR Research Protocols, 1*(2), e12.

Fortinsky, R. H., Iannuzzi-Sucich, M., Baker, D. I., Gottschalk, M., King, M. B., Brown, C. J., & Tinetti, M. E. (2004). Fall-Risk Assessment and Management in Clinical Practice: Views from Healthcare Providers. *Journal of the American Geriatrics Society, 52*(9), 1522–1526. doi:10.1111/j.1532-5415.2004.52416.x PMID:15341555

Fosso Wamba, S., & Ngai, E. W. T. (2011). Unveiling the potential of RFID-enabled intelligent patient management: Results of a Delphi study. In *44th Hawaii international conference on systems science*. Koloa, HI: IEEE.

Fosso Wamba, S. (2011). Positioning RFID technology into the innovation theorylandscape: A multidimensional perspective integrating case study approach. In *Proceedings of the 15th Pacific Asia Conference on Information systems (PACIS)*. Brisbane, Australia: PACIS.

Fosso Wamba, S., Anand, A., & Carter, L. (2013). A literature review of RFID-enabled healthcare applications and issues. *International Journal of Information Management*, *33*(5), 875–891. doi:10.1016/j.ijinfomgt.2013.07.005

Fosso Wamba, S., & Chatfield, A. T. (2009). A contingency model for creating value from RFID supply chain network projects in logistics and manufacturing environments. *European Journal of Information Systems*, *18*(6), 615–636. doi:10.1057/ejis.2009.44

Fosso Wamba, S., Lefebvre, L. A., Bendavid, Y., & Lefebvre, E. (2008). Exploring the impact of RFID technology and the EPC network on mobile B2B eCommerce: A case study in the retail industry. *International Journal of Production Economics*, *112*(2), 614–629. doi:10.1016/j.ijpe.2007.05.010

Foster, I. (2002). What is the grid? A Three point checklist. *GRID Today, 1*(6).

Friedlos, D. (2010, December). Australia's Bendigo Health Improves Efficiency Through RFID. *RFID Journal.*

Fuhrer, P., & Guinard, D. (2006). Building a smart hospital using RFID technologies. In *European conference on eHealth* (pp. 131–142). Fribourg, Switzerland: Academic Press.

Gabbitas, O., & Jeffs, C. (2007). *Assessing productivity in the delivery of health systems in Australia: some experimental estimates*. Paper presented to the ABS-PC Productivity Perspectives 2007 Conference. Retrieved from http://www.pc.gov.au/research/conference-papers/health-service-productivity

Gagne, R., Bridges, L., & Wagne, W. (1998). *Principles of Instructional Design*. Orlando, FL: Holt, Rinehart and Winston, Inc.

Gambon, J. (2006, August 28). RFID Frees Up Patient Beds. *RFID Journal.*

Gambrill, E., & Shlonsky, A. (2000). Risk assessment in context. *Children and Youth Services Review, 22*(11), 813–837. doi:10.1016/S0190-7409(00)00123-7

Gandevia, B. (1971). A History of General Practice in Australia. *Canadian Family Physician Medecin de Famille Canadien*, (October), 51–59. PMID:20468689

Garfinkel, S., & Rosenberg, B. (2006). *RFID: Applications, security, and privacy*. Pearson Education India.

Garvie, D. (2004). Strategic Planning Supports ED Automation. *Health Management Technology, 25*(11), 34–36. PMID:15551708

Gearon, C. (2005). Technology. Behind the hype. *Hospitals & Health Networks, 79*(6), 22, 24.

Georgiadou, Y., Bana, B., Becht, R., Hoppe, R., Ikingura, J., Kraak, M. J., & Verplanke, J. et al. (2011). Sensors, empowerment, and accountability: A Digital Earth view from East Africa. *International Journal of Digital Earth, 4*(4), 285–304. doi:10.1080/17538947.2011.585184

Gevensleben, H., Holl, B., Albrecht, B., Vogel, C., Schlamp, D., Kratz, O., & Heinrich, H. et al. (2009). Is neurofeedback an efficacious treatment for ADHD? A randomised controlled clinical trial. *Journal of Child Psychology and Psychiatry, and Allied Disciplines, 50*(7), 780–789. doi:10.1111/j.1469-7610.2008.02033.x PMID:19207632

Giddens, A. (1984). *The Constitution of society: Outline of the theory of Structuration.* Berkeley, CA: University of California Press.

Giddens, A. (1986). *Situation of society: Outline of the theory of structuration.* Uninversity of Carlifornia Press.

Glaser, B., & Strauss, A. (1967). *The discovery of grounded theory: strategies for qualitative research.* New York: Aldine.

Gleitman, L., & Papafragou, A. (2012). New perspectives on language and thought. In K. Holyoak & R. Morrison (Eds.), *Cambridge Handbook of Thinking and Reasoning* (2nd ed.). New York: Oxford University Press. doi:10.1093/oxfordhb/9780199734689.013.0028

Goldschmidt, P. G. (2005). Implications of health information technology and medical information systems. *Communications of the ACM, 48*(10), 69–74.

Gomes, A. T. A., Ziviani, A., Correa, B. S. P. M., Teixeira, I. M., & Moreira, V. M. (2012). SPLiCE: a software product line for healthcare. *Proceedings of the 2nd ACM SIGHIT International Health Informatics Symposium* (pp. 721–726). ACM. doi:10.1145/2110363.2110447

Goodwin, C. S. (2013). Healthcare organizational metaphors and implications for leadership. *Proquest Dissertations and Theses*, 1.

Google Fit. (2015). *Google Fit.* Retrieved from https://developers.google.com/fit/

Goossens, E., Apers, S., Gewillig, M., Budts, W., & Moons, P. (2013). *Evaluating quality of life after correction of a cardiac defect.* Academic Press.

Gordon, B. D., Flottemesch, T. J., & Asplin, B. R. (2008). Accuracy of staff-initiated emergency department tracking system timestamps in identifying actual event times. *Annals of Emergency Medicine, 52*(5), 504–511. doi:10.1016/j.annemergmed.2007.11.036 PMID:18313799

Gosain, A., & Kumar, A. (2009). *Analysis of health care data using different data mining techniques.* Paper presented at the Intelligent Agent & Multi-Agent Systems, 2009. IAMA 2009. International Conference on. doi:10.1109/IAMA.2009.5228051

Goss, J. (2008). *Projection of Australian health care expenditure by disease, 2003–2033, Cat. No. HWE 43.* Canberra: Australian Institute of Health and Welfare.

GP NSW. (2011). *A Guide to understanding and working with General Practice in New South Wales.* Retrieved 14 October, 2014 from http://www.gpnsw.com.au/__data/assets/pdf_file/0015/3444/AND145_GPNSW_Guide_WEB.pdf

Gp2Gp. (2014). Retrieved from http://systems.hscic.gov.uk/gp2gp/implementation/gp2gpfactsheet.pdf–

Gran, B. A., Fredriksen, R., & Thunem, A. P.-J. (2004). *An approach for model-based risk assessment. In Computer Safety, Reliability, and Security* (pp. 311–324). Springer. doi:10.1007/978-3-540-30138-7_26

Greenhalgh, T., Stramer, K., Bratan, T., Byrne, E., Russell, J., & Potts, H. W. (2010). Adoption and non-adoption of a shared electronic summary record in England: A mixed-method case study. *BMJ (Clinical Research Ed.), 340*(jun16 4), c3111. doi:10.1136/bmj.c3111 PMID:20554687

Greenland, P. (2012). Should the resting electrocardiogram be ordered as a routine risk assessment test in healthy asymptomatic adults? *Journal of the American Medical Association, 307*(14), 1530–1531. doi:10.1001/jama.2012.441 PMID:22496268

Grenwald-Mayes, G. (2001). Relationship between current quality of life and family of origin dynamics for college students with attention-deficit/hyperactivity disorder. *Journal of Attention Disorders, 5*(4), 211–222. doi:10.1177/108705470100500403 PMID:11967477

Grgurović, M. (2010). Technology-enhanced blended language learning in an ESL class: A description of a model and an application of the diffusion of innovations theory. *Proquest Dissertations and Theses*, 21-25.

Grimshaw, J. M., Thomas, R. E., MacLennan, G., Fraser, C., Ramsay, C. R., Vale, L., & Donaldson, C. et al. (2004). Effectiveness and effeciency of guideline dissemination and implementation strategies[technical report, health systems research agency]. *Health Technology Assessment, 8*(6). doi:10.3310/hta8060 PMID:14960256

Grimson, J., & Grimson, W. (2002). Health care in the information society: Evolution or revolution? *International Journal of Medical Informatics, 66*(1-3), 25–29. doi:10.1016/S1386-5056(02)00032-1 PMID:12453554

Grint, K., & Woolgar, S. (1997). *The machine at work- technology, work and organisation.* Cambridge: Polity Press.

Gropper, R. J., & Tannock, R. (2009). A pilot study of working memory and academic achievement in college students with ADHD. *Journal of Attention Disorders, 12*(6), 574–581. doi:10.1177/1087054708320390 PMID:19380519

Grossman, C. S. (2014). Succession planning and knowledge transfer in higher education. *Proquest Dissertations and Theses*, 70.

GS1-Australia (2010). *Healthcare industry.* Author.

GS1-Australia. (2010). *Healthcare Industry Report.* Author.

Haas, H., & Brown, A. (2004). *Web Services Glossary.* World Wide Web Consortium (W3C). Retrieved from http://www.w3.org/TR/ws-gloss/

Haga, Y., Ikejiri, K., Takeuchi, H., Ikenaga, M., & Wada, Y. (2012). Value of general surgical risk models for predicting postoperative liver failure and mortality following liver surgery. *Journal of Surgical Oncology, 106*(7), 898–904. doi:10.1002/jso.23160 PMID:22605669

Hagland, M. (2005). Nine tech trends: Bar coding and RFID. *Healthcare Informatics.*

Halamka, J., Juels, J., Stubblefield, A., & Westhues, J. (2006). *The security implications of RFID for Healthcare and Pharmaceuticals 2008-2018.* IDTechEx. Retrieved from http://www.idtechex.com/research/reports/rfid_for_healthcare_and_ pharmaceuticals_2008_2018_000146.asp

Hall, B. H., & Khan, B. (2003). Adoption of new technology. In D. C. Jones (Ed.), *The New Economy Handbook.* San Diego, CA: Elsevier/ Academic Press.

Hall, D. J., & Croasdell, D. (2005). *Inquiring organisations: an organisational form perspective.* IGI Global. doi:10.4018/978-1-59140-309-8.ch001

Hall, E. (2005). The 'geneticisation' of heart disease: A network analysis of the production of new genetic knowledge. *Social Science & Medicine, 60*(12), 2673–2683. doi:10.1016/j.socscimed.2004.11.024 PMID:15820579

Hampson, K., Dobson, A., Kaare, M., Dushoff, J., Magoto, M., Sindoya, E., & Cleaveland, S. (2008). Rabies exposures, post-exposure prophylaxis and deaths in a region of endemic canine rabies. *PLoS Neglected Tropical Diseases, 2*(11), e339. doi:10.1371/journal.pntd.0000339 PMID:19030223

Hamunyela, S., & Iyamu, T. (2013). Readness Assessment model for the deployment of health information systems in the Namibian MoH. International Federation for Information Processing, *12*th *Internation Conference on Social Implications of Computer in Developing countries.*

Handayani, P. W., Hidayanto, A. N., Sandhyaduhita, P. I., Pinem, A. A., Fajrina, H. R., & Trisnanty, I. A. K. (2014). Critical Success Factors in Implementing Hospital Information System in Indonesia: Case Study Public Hospitals. In *Proceedings of the International Conference for Diversity, Technology and Innovation for Operational Competitiveness* (TIIM). Academic Press.

Handel, D. A., & Hackman, J. L. (2010). Implementing electronic health records in the emergency department. *The Journal of Emergency Medicine*, *38*(2), 257–263. doi:10.1016/j.jemermed.2008.01.020 PMID:18790591

Handel, D. A., Wears, R. L., Nathanson, L. A., & Pines, J. M. (2011). Using information technology to improve the quality and safety of emergency care. *Academic Emergency Medicine*, *18*(6), e45–e51. doi:10.1111/j.1553-2712.2011.01070.x PMID:21676049

Hanson, G., & Price, B. (1992). Academic Program Review. In M. A. Wjitley, J. D. Porter, & R. H. Fenske (Eds.), *The Primer for Institutional Research*. Tallahassee, FL: Association for Institutional Research.

Haoses-Gorases, L. (2005). *Utilisation of health information system (HIS) in Namibia: focus on challenges and opportunities faced by health care delivery system*. Academic Press.

Harder, & Boshkov. (n.d.). *The optimal Hematocrit.* Department of Pulmonary and Critical Care Medicine, Oregon Health and Sciences University.

Harrop, P., Das R., et al. (2009). *RFID for Healthcare and Pharmaceuticals 2009–2019*. IDTechEx.

Harshberger, C. A., Harper, A. J., Carro, G. W., Spath, W. E., Hui, W. C., Lawton, J. M., & Brockstein, B. E. (2011). Outcomes of computerized physician order entry in an electronic health record after implementation in an outpatient oncology setting. *Journal of Oncology Practice*, *7*(4), 233–237. doi:10.1200/JOP.2011.000261 PMID:22043187

Hasanali, F. (2002*). Critical success factors of Knowledge Management*. Available online: http://polaris.umuc.edu/mts/TMAN/TMAN_636/articles/csfs.pdf

Haug, P. J., Gardner, R. M., Evans, R. S., Rocha, B. H., & Rocha, R. A. (2007). Clinical decision support at Intermountain Healthcare. *Clinical Decision Support Systems*, 159-189.

Haux, R. (2006). Health information systems- past, present, future. *International Journal of Medical Informatics*, *75*(3-4), 268–281. doi:10.1016/j.ijmedinf.2005.08.002 PMID:16169771

Health and Hospitals Reform Commission. (2009). *A healthier future for all Australians: Final Report*. Canberra: Commonwealth of Australia. doi:10.4018/978-1-60960-197-3.ch004

Health Metrics Network. (2008). Retrieved from http://www.who.int/healthmetrics/library/countries/HMN_KEN_Assess_Final_2008_06_en.pdf

Heiligenstein, E., Greta Guenther Msn, M. S., Levy, A., Savino, F. P., & Fulwiler, J. P. (1999). Psychological and academic functioning in college students with attention deficit hyperactivity disorder. *Journal of American College Health*, *47*(4), 181–185. doi:10.1080/07448489909595644 PMID:9919849

Heiligenstein, E., & Keeling, R. P. (1995). Presentation of unrecognized attention deficit hyperactivity disorder in college students. *Journal of American College Health*, *43*(5), 226–228. doi:10.1080/07448481.1995.9940481 PMID:7499637

Hendy, J., Reeves, B. C., Fulop, N., Hutchings, A., & Masseria, C. (2005). Challenges to implementing the national programme for information technology (NPfIT): A qualitative study. *BMJ (Clinical Research Ed.)*, *331*(7512), 331–336. doi:10.1136/bmj.331.7512.331 PMID:16081447

Hersh, W. (2009). A stimulus to define informatics and health information technology. *BMC Medical Informatics and Decision Making, 9*(1), 24. doi:10.1186/1472-6947-9-24 PMID:19445665

Hersh, W. R. (1995, December). The electronic medical record: Promises and problems. *Journal of the American Society for Information Science, 46*(10), 772–776. doi:10.1002/(SICI)1097-4571(199512)46:10<772::AID-ASI9>3.0.CO;2-0

Hesketh, T., & Zhu, W. X. (1997). Traditional Chinese Medicine: One country, two systems. *British Medical Journal, 315*(7100), 115–117. doi:10.1136/bmj.315.7100.115 PMID:9240055

Hevner, A. R., March, S.T., Park, J., & Ram, S. (2004). Design Science in Information Systems Research. *MIS Quarterly, 28*(1), 75 - 105.

Hiby, E. (2012). *Vaccinate dogs to save human lives – World Rabies Day 2012. South-East Asia.* World Health Organization.

Hier, D. B., Rothschild, A., Lemaistre, A., & Keeler, J. (2005). Differing faculty and housestaff acceptance of an electronic health record. *International Journal of Medical Informatics, 74*(7-8), 657–662. doi:10.1016/j.ijmedinf.2005.03.006 PMID:16043088

Hillestad, R., Bigelow, J., Bower, A., Girosi, F., Meili, R., Scoville, R., & Taylor, R. (2005). Can Electronic Medical Record Systems Transform Health Care? Potential Health Benefits, Savings, And Costs. *Health Affairs, 24*(5), 1103–1117. doi:10.1377/hlthaff.24.5.1103 PMID:16162551

HIPAA. (1996). *Health Insurance Portability and Accountability Act (HIPAA).* Retrieved from http://www.hhs.gov/ocr/privacy/

HISA. (2014). *Health Informatics Society of Australia.* Retrieved from http://www.hisa.org.au

HL7. (2007). *HL7 Clinical Document Architecture (CDA).* Retrieved from http://www.hl7.org/implement/standards/

Ho, G. (2012, April 27). *Can technology help overcome Australia's healthcare challenges?* Australian Broadcasting Corporation (ABC) - Technology and Games.

Hobbs, S. D. (2007). Clinical nurses' perception of nursing informatics competencies. *Proquest Dissertations and Theses, 1.*

Hoffman, J. I., & Kaplan, S. (2002). The incidence of congenital heart disease. *Journal of the American College of Cardiology, 39*(12), 1890–1900. doi:10.1016/S0735-1097(02)01886-7 PMID:12084585

Hofler, L. D. (2007). A case study of the relationship between the North Carolina center for nursing and nursing workforce issues in the state of North Carolina through the lens of planned change. *Proquest Dissertations and Theses, 33.*

Hojabri, R., & Manafi, M. (2012). Impact of using telemedicine on knowledge management in healthcare organisations: A case study. *African Journal of Business Management, 6*(4), 1604-1613.

Hoot, N., Wright, J. C., & Aronsky, D. (2003). Factors contributing to computer system downtime in the emergency department. In *AMIA Annual Symposium Proceedings.* Washington, DC: American Medical Informatics Association.

Horner, V. (2013). *Development and piloting of an e-health decision support system for improving compliance of primary health care staff to the maternity care guidelines and protocols.* (PhD thesis). University of Limpopo, Medunsa Medical Campus, Garankua, South Africa.

Horner, V., Rautenbach, P., Mbananga, N., Mashamba, T., & Kwinda, H. (2013). An e-health decision support system for improving compliance of health workers to the maternity care protocols in South Africa. *Appl.Clin.Inf., 4*(1), 25–36. doi:10.4338/ACI-2012-10-RA-0044 PMID:23650485

Horner, V., Rautenbach, P., Mbananga, N., Mashamba, T., Olurunju, S., Kwinda, H., & Ramahlo, T. (2014). Audit of antenatal care at a community health centre in Tshwane North sub-district, Gauteng Province. *South African Family Practice Journal, 56*(2), 153–158. doi:10.1080/20786204.2014.10855354

Horwitz, R. I., Abell, J. E., Christian, J. B., & Wivel, A. E. (2014). Right answers, wrong questions in clinical research. *Science Translational Medicine, 6*(221), 221fs225-221fs225.

Hoskins, R. (2006). *InfoLogix Announces HealthTrax RFID Asset Tracking Software for Hospital Mobile Assets Management.* Retrieved 12 February 2006 from http://www.bbwexchange.com/pubs/2006/02/11/page1395-98309.asp

Hsu, E. (Ed.). (2001). *Innovation in Chinese medicine* (Vol. 3). Cambridge University Press.

Hsu, W.-K., Tseng, C.-P., Chiang, W.-L., & Chen, C.-W. (2012). Risk and uncertainty analysis in the planning stages of a risk decision-making process. *Natural Hazards, 61*(3), 1355–1365. doi:10.1007/s11069-011-0032-1

Huang, M. J. & Chen, M. Y. (2007). Integrated Design of the Intelligent Web-based Chinese Medical Diagnostic System (CMDS) - Systematic Development for Digestive Health. *Expert Systems with Applications, 32*(2), 658-673.

i2b2. (2004). *Informatics for Integrating Biology & the Bedside (i2b2).* Retrieved from https://www.i2b2.org/

Iacono, J., Brown, A., & Holtham, C. (2009). Research methods: A case example of participant observation. *Electronic Journal of Business Research Methods*, 40.

Iakovidis, D. K., Tsevas, S., Savelonas, M. A., & Papamichalis, G. (2012). Image analysis framework for infection monitoring. *Biomedical Engineering. IEEE Transactions on, 59*(4), 1135–1144.

IDTechEx (2006). *Rapid adoption of RFID in healthcare.* Author.

IEEE. (2000). *IEEE Recommended Practice for Architectural Description of Software Intensive Systems.* IEEE Std 1471- 2000.

Ingebrigtsen, T., Georgiou, A., Clay-Williams, R., Magrabi, F., Hordern, A., Pigonet, M., & Braithwaite, J. et al. (2014). The impact of clinical leadership on health information technology adoption: Systematic review. *International Journal of Medical Informatics, 83*(6), 393–405. doi:10.1016/j.ijmedinf.2014.02.005 PMID:24656180

Inmon, W. H. (2005). *Building the Data Warehouse* (4th ed.). New York, NY: John Wiley & Sons, Inc.

Inokuchi, R., Sato, H., Nakajima, S., Shinohara, K., Nakamura, K., Gunshin, M., & Yahagi, N. et al. (2013). Development of information systems and clinical decision support systems for emergency departments: A long road ahead for Japan. *Emergency Medicine Journal, 30*(11), 914–917. doi:10.1136/emermed-2012-201869 PMID:23302505

Inokuchi, R., Sato, H., Nakamura, K., Aoki, Y., Shinohara, K., Gunshin, M., & Nakajima, S. et al. (2014). Motivations and barriers to implementing electronic health records and ED information systems in Japan. *The American Journal of Emergency Medicine, 32*(7), 725–730. doi:10.1016/j.ajem.2014.03.035 PMID:24792932

Ioan, T., Turcu, C., Turcu, C., & Cerlinc, M. (2010). RFID-based Information System for Patients and Medical Staff Identification and Tracking. In C. Turcu (Ed.), *Sustainable Radio Frequency Identification Solutions.* InTech. Retrieved from http://www.intechopen.com/books/sustainable-radio-frequency-identification-solutions/rfid-based-information-system-for-patients-and-medical-staff-identification-and-tracking

ISO9241-11. (1998). *Ergonomic requirements for office work with visual display terminals (VDT) – Part II: Guidance on usability.* International Organisation for Standardisation.

Istepanian. (2006). Design and Implementation of a Mobile Diabetes Management System. *Journal of Mobile Multimedia, 1*(4), 273-284.

Istepanian, R. J., Jovanov, E., & Zhang, Y. T. (2004). Guest Editorial Introduction to the Specialon M-Health: Beyond Seamless Mobility and Global Wireless Health-Care Connectivity. *IEEE Transactions on Information Technology in Biomedicine, 8*(4), 405–414. doi:10.1109/TITB.2004.840019 PMID:15615031

ITU. (2012). *International Telecommunication Union, CH-1211*. Retrieved from http://www.itu.int/en/ITU-D/Statistics/Documents/publications/mis2012/MIS2012_without_Annex_4.pdf

Iyamu, T., & Adelakun, O. 2008. The impact of non-technical factors on Information Technology Strategy and E-business. In *Proceedings of the 12th Pacific Asia Conference on Information Systems (PACIS)*. Academic Press.

Iyamu, T., & Tatnall, A. (2009). *An actor-network analysis of a case of development and implementation of IT strategy*. Paper presented at the Information systems conference. Retrieved doi:10.4018/jantti.2009062303

Iyamu, T. (2010). Theoretical Analysis of the Implementation of Enterprise Architecture. *International Journal of Actor-Network Theory and Technological Innovation, 2*(3), 27–38.

Iyamu, T. (2011). Institutionalisation of the enterprise architecture: The actor-network perspective. *International Journal of Actor-Network Theory and Technological Innovation, 3*(1), 27–38. doi:10.4018/jantti.2011010103

Iyamu, T., & Roode, D. (2010). The use of Structuration and Actor Network Theory for analysis: A case study of a financial institution in South Africa. *International Journal of Actor-Network Theory and Technological Innovation, 2*(1), 1–26. doi:10.4018/jantti.2010071601

Iyamu, T., & Tatnall, A. (2011). *The impact of netwrork of actors on the infomation technology. In Actor network theory and technology innovation: advancements and new concepts journal*. Hershey, PA: Information Science Reference.

Jackson, A. C. (2014). The effect of suspension as a deterrent to student misconduct. *Proquest Dissertations and Theses*, 110.

Jackson, A. S. (2013). Impact of electronic health records on nurses' information seeking and discriminating skills for critical thinking. *ProQuest*, 4-5.

Jacobs, E., Punt, C., & Bothloko, C. (2009). *A profile of the North West Province: demographics, poverty, income, inequality and unemployment* [technical report; Internet]. PROVIDE Project. North West Provincial Government, South Africa. Retrieved in 2012, from: http://ideas.repec.org/p/ags/provbp/58055.html

Jemberu, W. T., Molla, W., Almaw, G., & Alemu, S. (2013). Incidence of rabies in humans and domestic animals and people's awareness in North Gondar Zone, Ethiopia. *PLoS Neglected Tropical Diseases, 7*(5), e2216. doi:10.1371/journal.pntd.0002216 PMID:23675547

Jensen, C. T., Cline, O., & Owen, M. (2011, March). *Combining Business Process Management and Enterprise Architecture for Better Business Outcomes*. IBM Redbook.

Jensen, T. A. (2013). Nurses' perceptions of nursing care documentation in the electronic health record. *Proquest Dissertations and Theses*, 1.

Joe. (2010). Securing Mobile Devices! *Security Professionals 2011 Preconference Seminar*.

Johnson, B., & Christensen, L. (2008). *Qualitative Research Educational research: Quantitative, qualitative, and mixed approaches* (3rd ed.). London: Sage.

Johnston, J. M., Leung, G. M., Wong, J. F., Ho, L. M., & Fielding, R. (2002). Physicians' attitudes towards the computerization of clinical practice in Hong Kong: A population study. *International Journal of Medical Informatics, 65*(1), 41–49. doi:10.1016/S1386-5056(02)00005-9 PMID:11904247

John, T. G. (2002). *Requirements Engineering:Social and Technical Issues*. London: Academic Press.

Jones, S. M. (2012). The development of trust in the nurse-patient relationship with hospitalized Mexican American patients. *Proquest Dissertations and Theses*, 179.

Jones-Zeigler, C. M. (2011). Computerization in practice: The lived experience of experienced nurses. *Proquest*, 1-2.

Jorm, A. F., Wright, A., & Morgan, A. J. (2007). Where to seek help for a mental disorder? *The Medical Journal of Australia*, *187*(10), 556–560. PMID:18021042

Jowett, M., & Danielyan, E. (2010). Is there a role for user charges? Thoughts on health system reform in Armenia. *Bulletin of the World Health Organization*, *88*(6), 472–473. doi:10.2471/BLT.09.074765 PMID:20539867

Kabupaten Bogor, P. P. I. D. (2013). *Profil RSUD Cibinong*. Retrieved from Pejabat Pengelola Informasi dan Dokumentasi (PPID) Kabupaten Bogor: http://ppid.bogorkab.go.id/?site=27

Kahn, J. S., Aulakh, V., & Bosworth, A. (2006). What it takes: Characteristics of the ideal personal health record. *Health Affairs*, *28*(2), 369–376. doi:10.1377/hlthaff.28.2.369 PMID:19275992

Kaltenthaler, E., Brazier, J., De Nigris, E., Tumur, I., Ferriter, M., Beverley, C., & Sutcliffe, P. A. et al. (2006). Computerised cognitive behaviour therapy for depression and anxiety update: A systematic review and economic evaluation. *Health Technology Assessment*, *10*(33), 1–186. doi:10.3310/hta10330 PMID:16959169

Kaplan, R. S., & Porter, M. E. (2011). How to solve the cost crisis in health care. *Harvard Business Review*, *89*(9), 46–64. PMID:21939127

Kaptchuk, T. J. (2000). *Chinese Medicine - The Web That Has No Weaver*. An Imprint of Elbury Press, Random House, Rider.

Karahanna, E., Straub, D., & Chervany, N. (1999). *Information technology adoption across time: A cross-sectional comparison of pre-adoption and post-adoption beliefs*. MIS Quarterly.

Kaur, Kumar, Sardana, Bhatnagar, & Mehla. (n.d.). *Non Invasive Blood Glucose Measurement Using Optical Method: Feasibility Study And Design Issues*. Central Scientific Instruments Organization, Chandigarh (A Lab. of Council of Scientific and Industrial Research, New Delhi).

Keenan, C. R., Nguyen, H. H., & Srinivasan, M. (2006). Electronic medical records and their impact on residents and medical student education. *Academic Psychiatry*, *30*(6), 522–527. doi:10.1176/appi.ap.30.6.522 PMID:17139024

Kelley, T. F. (2012). Information use with paper and electronic nursing documentation by nurses caring for pediatric patients. *Proquest Dissertations and Theses*, 15.

Kementrian Kesehatan, R. I. (2011, November 10). *Pertemuan Koordinasi Teknis IT Dalam Rangka E-Health*. Retrieved from http://buk.depkes.go.id/index.php?option=com_content&view=article&id=224:pertemuan-koordinasi-teknis-it-dalam-rangka-e-health

Kenny, P., Parsons, T., Gratch, J., & Rizzo, A. (2008). Virtual humans for assisted health care.*Proceedings of the 1st international conference on Pervasive Technologies Related to Assistive Environments* (pp. 1–4). ACM. doi:10.1145/1389586.1389594

Khalifa, M. (2013). Barriers to health information systems and electronic medical records implementation. A field study of Saudi Arabian hospitals. *Procedia Computer Science*, *21*, 335–342. doi:10.1016/j.procs.2013.09.044

Khawaja, N. G., & Dempsey, J. (2008). A comparison of international and domestic tertiary students in Australia. *Australian Journal of Guidance & Counselling*, *18*(1), 30–46. doi:10.1375/ajgc.18.1.30

Khorasani, E., Darab, M. G., Yarmohammadian, M., & Afshari, S. (2012). Knowledge based health system in the age of Knowledge Management.*Proceedings of the 3rd International Conference on Information Management and Evaluation*. Ankara, Turkey: Academic Press.

Kimaro, H. C., & Nhampossa, J. L. (2005). Analyzing the problem of unsustainable health information systems in less-developed economies: Case studies from Tanzania and Mozambique. *Information Technology for Development, 11*(3), 273–298. doi:10.1002/itdj.20016

Kimaro, H., & Nhampossa, J. (2007). The challenges of sustainability of health information systems in developing countries: Comparative case studies of Mozambique and Tanzania. *Journal of Health Informatics in Developing Countries, 1*(1).

King, G., O'Donnell, C., Boddy, D., Smith, F., Heaney, D., & Mair, F. (2012). Boundaries and e-health implementation in health and social care. *BMC Medical Informatics and Decision Making, 12*(100).

Klingberg, T., Fernell, E., Olesen, P. J., Johnson, M., Gustafsson, P., Dahlström, K., & Westerberg, H. et al. (2005). Computerized training of working memory in children with ADHD-A randomized, controlled trial. *Journal of the American Academy of Child and Adolescent Psychiatry, 44*(2), 177–186. doi:10.1097/00004583-200502000-00010 PMID:15689731

Knobel, D. L., Cleaveland, S., Coleman, P. G., Fèvre, E. M., Meltzer, M. I., Miranda, M. E. G., & Meslin, F. X. (2005). Re-evaluating the burden of rabies in Africa and Asia. *Bulletin of the World Health Organization, 83*(5), 360–368. PMID:15976877

Kuhn, K., Wurst, S., Bott, O., & Giuse, D. (2006). Expanding the scope of health information systems. *IMIA Yearbook of Medical Informatics*, 43-52.

Kulkarni, V. A. (2006). *Implementation of electronic health records: Modeling and evaluating healthcare information systems for quality improvements in the U.S. healthcare industry*. Academic Press.

Kuperman, G. J. (2011). Health-information exchange: Why are we doing it, and what are we doing? *Journal of the American Medical Informatics Association, 18*(5), 678–682. doi:10.1136/amiajnl-2010-000021 PMID:21676940

Kvale, S. (1996). *Interviews: An introduction to qualitative research interviewing*. London, UK: Sage.

Kvale, S. (2007). *Doing interviews*. Thousand Oaks, CA: Sage.

Lahey, K. (2003). *The cost of dropping out: The economic impact of early school leaving*. Australia: Business Council of Australia.

Lai, P. (2012). Shared decision making. *Surgical Practice, 16*(4), 127–127. doi:10.1111/j.1744-1633.2012.00623.x

Laksmita, I. S., Sudana, A. K. O., & Buana, P. W. (2012). Design Web-based GIS Application for Rabies Spread in Bali Province. *International Journal of Informatics and Communication Technology, 1*(1), 54-62.

Lam, C. F. D., Leung, K. S., Heng, P. A., Lim, C. E. D., & Wong, F. W. S. (2012). Chinese Acupuncture Expert System (CAES) - A useful tool to practice and Learn Medical Acupuncture. *Journal of Medical Systems, 36*(3), 1883-1890.

Landman, A. B., Bernstein, S. L., Hsiao, A. L., & Desai, R. A. (2010). Emergency Department Information System Adoption in the United States. *Academic Emergency Medicine, 17*(5), 536–544. doi:10.1111/j.1553-2712.2010.00722.x PMID:20536810

Landolt, M. A., Buechel, E. V., & Latal, B. (2011). Predictors of parental quality of life after child open heart surgery: A 6-month prospective study. *The Journal of Pediatrics, 158*(1), 37–43. doi:10.1016/j.jpeds.2010.06.037 PMID:20688338

Lange, M., & Mendling, J. (2011). An Experts' Perspective on Enterprise Architecture Goals, Framework Adoption and Benefit Assessment.*15th IEEE International Enterprise Distributed Object Computing Conference Workshops (EDOCW)*. Helsinki: IEEE.

Lansbergen, M., van Dongen-Boomsma, M., Buitelaar, J., & Slaats-Willemse, D. (2011). ADHD and EEG-neurofeedback: A double-blind randomized placebo-controlled feasibility study. *Journal of Neural Transmission, 118*(2), 275–284. doi:10.1007/s00702-010-0524-2 PMID:21165661

Lapan, S. D., Quartaroli, M. T., & Riemer, F. J. (2011). *Qualitative research: An introduction to methods and designs* (Vol. 37). Wiley.com.

Larrazabal, L. A., Jenkins, K. J., Gauvreau, K., Vida, V. L., Benavidez, O. J., Gaitán, G. A., . . . Castañeda, A. R. (2007). Improvement in Congenital Heart Surgery in a Developing Country: The Guatemalan Experience. *Circulation is published by the American Heart Association, 116*, 1872-1877.

Latour, B. (1986). Article. In J. Law (Ed.), The power of association, Power, Action and Belief – a new Sociology of Knowledge, Sociological Review Monograph 32 (pp. 264–280). London: Routledge and Kegan Paul.

Law, J. (1992). *Notes on the theory of the Actor Network: ordering, strategy and heterogeneity*. Available at: http://comp. lancs.ac.uk/sociology/soc054jl.html

Law, J., & Callon, M. (1988). Engineering and Sociology in a Military Aircraft project: A network analysis of Technological Change. *Social Problems, 35*(3), 284–297. doi:10.2307/800623

Lee, K. C., Lee, S., & Kang, I. W. (2005). KMPI: Measuring knowledge management performance. *Information & Management Journal, 42*(3), 469–482. doi:10.1016/j.im.2004.02.003

Lee, Y. C., & Lee, S. K. (2007). Capabilities, processes and performance of knowledge management: A structural approach. Research Articles. *Human Factors Ergonomics and Manufacturing Journal, 17*(1), 21–41. doi:10.1002/hfm.20065

Lefebvre, F., Castro, L., & Lefebvre, L. A. (2011). Assessing the prevailing implementation issues of RFID in healthcare: A five-phase implementation model. *Int. J. Electron. Comput. Comm. Tech, 5*(2), 110–117.

Lefebvre, E., & Romero, A. et al.. (2011). Technological strategies to deal with counter-feit medicines: The European and North-American perspectives. *International Journal of Education and Information Technologies, 5*(3), 275–284.

Légaré, F., Stacey, D., Pouliot, S., Gauvin, F. P., Desroches, S., Kryworuchko, J., & Gagnon, M. P. et al. (2011). Inter-professionalism and shared decision-making in primary care: A stepwise approach towards a new model. *Journal of Interprofessional Care, 25*(1), 18–25. doi:10.3109/13561820.2010.490502 PMID:20795835

Lembo, T. (2012). The blueprint for rabies prevention and control: A novel operational toolkit for rabies elimination. *PLoS Neglected Tropical Diseases, 6*(2), e1388. doi:10.1371/journal.pntd.0001388 PMID:22389727

Lembo, T., Hampson, K., Kaare, M. T., Ernest, E., Knobel, D., Kazwala, R. R., & Cleaveland, S. (2010). The feasibility of canine rabies elimination in Africa: Dispelling doubts with data. *PLoS Neglected Tropical Diseases, 4*(2), e626. doi:10.1371/journal.pntd.0000626 PMID:20186330

LeRouge, C., Mantzana, V., & Wilson, E. V. (2007). Healthcare information systems research, revelations and visions. *European Journal of Information Systems, 16*(6), 669–671. doi:10.1057/palgrave.ejis.3000712

Lewis, M. O., Sankaranarayanan, B., ... (2009). RFID-enabled process capabilities and its impacts on healthcare process performance: A multi-level analysis. In ECIS 2009 proceedings. Verona, Italy: ECIS.

Liao, S. H. (2003). Knowledge management technologies and applications - literature review from 1995 to 2002. *Expert Systems with Applications, 25*(2), 155-164.

Liao, Y. Q. (2011). *Traditional Chinese Medicine*. Cambridge University Press.

Lichter, H., Schneider-Hufschmidt, M., & Zullighoven, H. (1994). Prototyping in Industrial Software Projects: Bridging the Gap between Theory and Practice. *IEEE Transactions on Software Engineering, 20*(11), 11,825–842. doi:10.1109/32.368126

Lin, C. H., Yang, A. W. H., Pittayachawan, S., & Wickramasinghe, N. (2013). Using IS/IT to support the delivery of Chinese medicine: The design of a Chinese medicine clinic system. In *Proceedings of Australasian Conference on Information Systems*. Academic Press.

Lin, C. H., Yang, A. W. H., Pittayachawan, S., Vogel, D., & Wickramasinghe, N. (2014a). Investigating the possibility for IS/IT to support the delivery of Chinese medicine. In *Proceedings of The First AIS-Journals Joint Author Workshop in ECIS*. Tel Aviv, Israel: ECIS.

Lin, C. H., Yang, A. W. H., Pittayachawan, S., Vogel, D., & Wickramasinghe, N. (2014b). Inquiring Knowledge Management Systems - A Chinese Medicine Perspective. In *Proceedings of the 2015 48th Hawaii International Conference on System Sciences (HICSS 2015)*. IEEE.

Lin, C. H., Yang, A. W. H., Pittayachawan, S., & Wickramasinghe, N. (2014c). *Using IS/IT to support the delivery of Chinese medicine: a Chinese medicine clinic management system. International Journal of Biomedical Engineering and Technology*.

Link, H. (2014). Retrieved from https://www.healthlink.net/en_AU/about-us/company-profile/-

Linton, N. (2010). *Connecting: the use of information and communication technologies by older adults in a retirement community*. Academic Press.

Liong, A. S. (2008). Descriptions of nurses experiences with electronic health records (EHR): A phenomenological study. *Proquest Dissertations and Theses*, 1-2.

Liong, A. S. (2008, March). *Descriptions of nurses experiences with electronic health records (EHR): A phenomenological study*. Academic Press.

Lippeveld, T. (2001). Routine health information systems:the glue of a unified health system.*The RHINO Workshop on Issues and Innovation in Routine Health In Information in Developing Countries*.Arlington, VA: JSI Research and Training Institute.

Liu, Z. W., & Liu, L. (2009). *Essentials of Chinese Medicine*. Springer.

Lobach, D. F., & Hammond, W. E. (1997). Computerized decision support based on a clinical practice guideline improves compliance with care standards. *The American Journal of Medicine, 102*(1), 89–98. doi:10.1016/S0002-9343(96)00382-8 PMID:9209205

Logicworks. (2015). *Logicworks Healthcare Solutions*. Retrieved from http://www.logicworks.net/healthcare-cloud-solutions

Long, S. H., Galea, M. P., Eldridge, B. J., & Harris, S. R. (2012). Performance of 2-year-old children after early surgery for congenital heart disease on the Bayley Scales of Infant and Toddler Development. *Early Human Development, 88*(8), 603–607. doi:10.1016/j.earlhumdev.2012.01.007 PMID:22336496

Lorenzi, N., & Riley, R. (2004). *Managing technological change: organizational aspects*. New York: Springer. doi:10.1007/978-1-4757-4116-2

Lu, A. P., Jia, H. W., Xiao, C., & Lu, Q. P. (2004). Theory of Traditional Chinese Medicine and Therapeutic Method of Diseases. *World Journal of Gastroenterology, 10*(13), 1854-1856.

Lukman, S., He, Y., & Hui, S. C. (2007). *Computational methods for Traditional Chinese Medicine: A survey.* Elsevier.

Lu, X., Duan, H., Li, H., Zhao, C., & An, J. (2005). The Architecture of Enterprise Hospital Information.*Proceeding of the 2005 IEEE Engineering in Medicine and Biology 27th Annual Conference,* (pp. 6957-6960). IEEE.

MacGregor, R. C., Hyland, P. N., Harvie, C., & Lee, B. C. (2006). An Examination of the Driving Forces Behind ICT Adoption in Australian Rural and Regional Medical Practices. In Proceedings of IIT06 Conference. Dubai, UAE: IEEE.

Macinko, J., Starfield, B., & Shi, L. (2003). The contribution of Primary Care Systems to health outcomes within Organisation for Economic Cooperation & Development (OECD) countries, 1970 – 1998. *Health Services Research, 38*(3), 831 – 865. DOI: 10.1111/1475-6773.00149

Maerten, E. (2009). Study of the first woman president hired by a board of regents in Oklahoma president Emerita of Southwestern Oklahoma state university Dr. Joe Anna Hibler. *ProQuest Dissertations and Theses,* 65-66.

Magazine, P. (2012, May 3). Prototyping Definition. *PC Magazine.*

Maier, R. (2007). *Knowledge management systems: Information and communication technologies for knowledge management.* Springer.

Maier, R., & Hädrich, T. (2011). *Knowledge Management Systems.* IGI.

Makoul, G., & Clayman, M. L. (2006). An integrative model of shared decision making in medical encounters. *Patient Education and Counseling, 60*(3), 301–312. doi:10.1016/j.pec.2005.06.010 PMID:16051459

Mallet, R. K. (2014). The influence of organizational subculture on information technology project success in the healthcare sector: A qualitative, multi-case study. *Proquest Dissertations and Theses,* 57.

Malviya, A., Martin, K., Harper, I., Muller, S. D., Emmerson, K. P., Partington, P. F., & Reed, M. R. (2011). Enhanced recovery program for hip and knee replacement reduces death rate: A study of 4,500 consecutive primary hip and knee replacements. *Acta Orthopaedica, 82*(5), 577–581. doi:10.3109/17453674.2011.618911 PMID:21895500

Mandl, K. D., Mandel, J. C., Murphy, S. N., Bernstam, E. V., Ramoni, R. L., Kreda, D. A., & Kohane, I. S. et al. (2012). The SMART Platform: Early experience enabling substitutable applications for electronic health records. *Journal of the American Medical Informatics Association, 19*(4), 597–603. doi:10.1136/amiajnl-2011-000622 PMID:22427539

Mann, C. (2013). Experience of adjunct novice clinical nursing faculty: An interpretive case study. *Proquest Dissertations and Theses,* 88-89.

Mannuzza, S., Klein, R. G., Bessler, A., Malloy, P., & LaPadula, M. (1998). Adult psychiatric status of hyperactive boys grown up. *The American Journal of Psychiatry, 155*(4), 493–498. doi:10.1176/ajp.155.4.493 PMID:9545994

Marconi, J. (2002, May). E-Health: Navigating the Internet for Health Information Healthcare. Advocacy White Paper. *Healthcare Information and Management Systems Society.*

Marcus, A. (1989, February 4). Computers and general practice. *Lancet, 1*(8632), 278. doi:10.1016/S0140-6736(89)91288-9 PMID:2563438

Marino, B. S., Lipkin, P. H., Newburger, J. W., Peacock, G., Gerdes, M., Gaynor, J. W., & Johnson, W. H. et al. (2012). Neurodevelopmental Outcomes in Children With Congenital Heart Disease: Evaluation and Management A Scientific Statement From the American Heart Association. *Circulation, 126*(9), 1143–1172. doi:10.1161/CIR.0b013e318265ee8a PMID:22851541

MarketResearch.com. (2011). *RFID readers and tags? A global market overview*. Author.

Marschollek, M., Gövercin, M., Rust, S., Gietzelt, M., Schulze, M., Wolf, K.-H., & Steinhagen-Thiessen, E. (2012). Mining geriatric assessment data for in-patient fall prediction models and high-risk subgroups. *BMC Medical Informatics and Decision Making, 12*(1), 19. doi:10.1186/1472-6947-12-19 PMID:22417403

Martin, C.M., & Sturmberg, J.P. (2005). General practice — chaos, complexity and innovation. *MJA, 183*(2), 106-109.

Maselli, J. (2003, May 27). Xtag Unveils Infant Security System. *RFID Journal.*

Mason, R. O., & Mitroff, I. I. (1973). A program for research on management information systems. *Management Science, 19*(5), 475-487.

Massyn, N., Day, C., & Dombo, M et al. (Eds.). (2004). *District health barometer*. Durban, South Africa: Health Systems Trust.

Mayes, S. D., Calhoun, S. L., & Crowell, E. W. (2000). Learning Disabilities and ADHD Overlapping Spectrum Disorders. *Journal of Learning Disabilities, 33*(5), 417–424. doi:10.1177/002221940003300502 PMID:15495544

Mazet, J. A., Clifford, D. L., Coppolillo, P. B., Deolalikar, A. B., Erickson, J. D., & Kazwala, R. R. (2009). A "one health" approach to address emerging zoonoses: The HALI project in Tanzania. *PLoS Medicine, 6*(12), e1000190. doi:10.1371/journal.pmed.1000190 PMID:20016689

Mazigo, H. D. (2011). Rabies in Tanzania: The need for a national control programme. *Tanzania Journal of Health Research, 13*(2), 88-89.

Mazigo, H. D., Okumu, F. O., Kweka, E. J., & Mnyone, L. L. (2010). Retrospective analysis of suspected rabies cases reported at Bugando Referral Hospital, Mwanza, Tanzania. *Journal of Global Infectious Diseases, 2*(3), 216.

Mboera, L. E. G., & Rumisha, S. F. (2008). The role of mass media in disease outbreak reporting in the United Republic of Tanzania. *Tanzania Journal of Health Research, 6*(2), 73–77. doi:10.4314/thrb.v6i2.14246 PMID:18846783

Mboera, L. E. G., Rumisha, S. F., & Kitua, A. Y. (2001). Strategic approach for strengthening national and regional disease surveillance system: The East African example. *Tanzania Journal of Health Research, 3*(2), 6–9. doi:10.4314/thrb.v3i2.14211

Mboera, L. E. G., Rumisha, S. F., Magesa, S. M., & Kitua, A. Y. (2001). Utilisation of health management information system in disease surveillance in Tanzania. *Tanzania Journal of Health Research, 3*(2), 15–17. doi:10.4314/thrb.v3i2.14213

McCrindle & Masipa, A. (2010). *Rapid Spacial and Temporal Outbreak Investigations Using Cell Phone Technology*. Republic of South Africa: Farm Inn.

McDonald, M. (2006). Public Health Informatics: How Information Age Technology Can Strengthen Public Health. *Annual Review of Public Health, 4*(2), 239–252. PMID:7639873

McInnes, D. (2006). General practitioners' use of computers for prescribing and electronic health records: Results from a national survey. *The Medical Journal of Australia, 185*(2), 88–91. PMID:16842064

McMaster, T., Vidgen, R. T., & Wastell, D. G. (1997). *Towards an understanding of technology in transition - Two conflicting theories*. Paper presented at Information Systems research in Scandinavia, IRIS20 Conference, Hanko, Norway.

McNabb, S. J., Chungong, S., Ryan, M., Wuhib, T., Nsubuga, P., Alemu, W., & Rodier, G. et al. (2002). Conceptual framework of public health surveillance and action and its application in health sector reform. *BMC Public Health, 2*(1), 2. doi:10.1186/1471-2458-2-2 PMID:11846889

McSweeney, A. (2000). *Enterprise Architecture and TOGAF*. The Open Group Architecture Framework.

Meadors, M., Benda, N., Hettinger, A. Z., & Ratwani, R. M. (2014). Going Live Implementing an Electronic Health Record System in the Emergency Department.*Proceedings of the International Symposium of Human Factors and Ergonomics in Healthcare, 3,*44-49. doi:10.1177/2327857914031006

Means, C. (2008). *Mobile technology gets boost with vendor collaboration.* Retrieved from http://healthcareitnews.eu/content/view/765/45

Meaux, J. B., Green, A., & Broussard, L. (2009). ADHD in the college student: A block in the road. *Journal of Psychiatric and Mental Health Nursing, 16*(3), 248–256. doi:10.1111/j.1365-2850.2008.01349.x PMID:19291153

Meho, L. I. (2006). E-mail interviewing in qualitative research: A methodological discussion. *Journal of the American Society for Information Science and Technology, 57*(10), 1284–1295. doi:10.1002/asi.20416

Mehrjerdi, Y. Z. (2010). RFID-enabled healthcare systems: Risk-benefit analysis. *International Journal of Pharmaceutical and Healthcare Marketing, 4*(3), 282–300. doi:10.1108/17506121011076192

Melesse, M. (2010). Gender, equity and access to health care: The Case of Ghana's Health Financing Reform. *ProQuest,* 11.

Mell, P., & Grance, T. (2011). The NIST Definition of Cloud Computing (Draft) Recommendations of the National Institute of Standards and Technology. *Nist Special Publication, 145,* 1–2. Retrieved from http://csrc.nist.gov/groups/SNS/cloud-computing/cloud-def-v15.doc

Menachemi, N., & Brooks, R. G. (2006). EHR and other IT adoption among physicians: Results of a large-scale state wide analysis. *Journal of Healthcare Information Management, 20*(3), 79–87. PMID:16903665

Mghamba, J. M., Mboera, L. E. G., Krekamoo, W., Senkoro, K. P., Rumisha, S. F., Shayo, E., & Mmbuji, P. (2008). Challenges of implementing an integrated disease surveillance and response strategy using the current health management information system in Tanzania. *Tanzania Journal of Health Research, 6*(2), 57–63. doi:10.4314/thrb.v6i2.14243

Michael, M. G., Fusco, S. J., & Michael, K. (2008). A research note on ethics in the emerging age of überveillance. *Computer Communications, 31*(6), 1192–1199. doi:10.1016/j.comcom.2008.01.023

Microsoft Cloud Services for Health. (2015). *Microsoft Cloud Services for Health.* Retrieved from http://www.microsoft.com/health/en-ca/initiatives/Pages/cloud-services-for-health.aspx

Microsoft Health Vault. (2007). *Microsoft Health Vault Personal Health Record.* Retrieved from https://www.healthvault.com/

Middleton, B. (2009). *Re-engineering U. S. health care with healthcare information technology- promises and peril.* Academic Press.

Milbank Memorial Fund. (2000). *Better Information, Better Outcomes?: The Use of Health Technology Assessment and Clinical Effectiveness Data in Health Care Purchasing Decisions in the United Kingdom and the United States.* New York: Milbank Memorial Fund.

Millennium Project. (2006). *Goals.* United Nations. Retrieved in Jan 2013 December, from: http://www.milleniumproject.org/goals

Miller, B. A. (2008). Exploring the use of information technology for enhancing interagency coordination. *Proguest,* 10.

Miller, G. C., Britt, H. C., & Valenti, L. (2006). Adverse drug events in general practice patients in Australia. *The Medical Journal of Australia, 184,* 321–324. PMID:16584364

Minor, M. O. (2009). What is the efficacy of using an integrated model in measuring sense of community (SOC) in accelerated degree completion programs? *Proquest Dissertations and Theses*, 8.

Mithas, S., & Ramasubbu, N. et al.. (2011). How information management capability influences firm performance. *Management Information Systems Quarterly*, *35*(1), 237–256.

Moghimi, H., Schaffer, J., & Wickramasinghe, N. (2014). *Exploring The Possibilities For Intelligent Risk Detection In Healthcare Contexts* Paper presented at the ECIS Workshop, Tel Aviv.

Moghimi, H., Seif Zadeh, H., Cheung, M., & Wickramasinghe, N. (2011). *An intelligent risk detection framework using business intelligence tools to improve decision efficiency in healthcare contexts.* Paper presented at the Seventeenth Americas Conference on Information Systems (AMCIS).

Moghimi, H., & Wickramasinghe, N. (2012).*Improving e-performance management in healthcare using intelligent IT solutions. In Critical Issues for the Development of Sustainable E-health Solutions* (pp. 3–15). Springer. doi:10.1007/978-1-4614-1536-7_1

Moghimi, H., Zadeh, H., Schaffer, J., & Wickramasinghe, N. (2012). Incorporating intelligent risk detection to enable superior decision support: The example of orthopaedic surgeries. *Health Technology*, *2*(1), 33–41. doi:10.1007/s12553-011-0014-z

MoHSS. (2012). *Integrated healthcare delivery the challenge and implementations.* Available at: http://www.healthnet.org.na/documents.html

Monier, J. P. (2011). Community development in rural America: The power to exchange capital resources in Norton county, Kansas. *Proquest Dissertations and Theses*, 11.

Moody, D. L., & Shanks, G. G. (1999). Using knowledge management and the internet to support evidence based practice: a medical case study. In *Proceedings of the 10th Australasian Conference on Information Systems* (pp. 660-676). Academic Press.

Morr, C. E., & Subercaze, J. (2010). *Handbook of Research on Developments in E-Health and Telemedicine: Technological and Social Perspectives.* IGI Global.

Motorola. (2013). *RFID solutions for healthcare reducing costs and improving operational efficiency.* Retrieved from http://www.motorolasolutions.com/web/Business/Solutions/Industry%20Solutions/RFID%20Solutions/RFID_in_Healthcare/_documents/_staticfiles/Application_Brief_RFID_in_Healthcare.pdf

Moumtzoglou, A. (2011). E-Health: A Bridge to People-Centered Health Care. *E-health Systems Quality and Reliability: Models and Standards, 47.*

Muhammad, I., Moghimi, F. H., Taylor, N. J., Redley, B., Nguyen, L., Stein, M., & Wickramasinghe, N. et al. (2013). Using ANT to uncover the full potential of an intelligent operational planning and support tool (IOPST) for acute healthcare contexts. *International Journal of Actor-Network Theory and Technological Innovation*, *5*(2), 29–49. doi:10.4018/jantti.2013040103

Muhammed, I., Teoh, S., & Wickramasinghe, N. (2012). Why Using Actor Network Theory (ANT) Can Help to Understand the Personally Controlled Electronic Health Record (PCEHR) in Australia. *International Journal of Actor-Network Theory and Technological Innovation*, *4*(2), 44–60. doi:10.4018/jantti.2012040105

Muhmmed, I., Zwicker, M., & Wickramasinghe, N. (2013). How Using ANT Can Assist to Understand Key Issues for Successful e-Health Solutions. *International Journal of Actor-Network Theory and Technological Innovation*, *5*(3), 1–17.

Mukama, F. (2003). *A study of health information systems at local levels in Tanzania and Mozambique.* (MSc thesis). University of Oslo.

Murphy, D. (2006). Is RFID right for your organization? Understand your process before implementing a solution. *Materials Management in Health Care, 15*(6), 28–33. PMID:16859241

Murphy, K. R., Barkley, R. A., & Bush, T. (2002). Young adults with attention deficit hyperactivity disorder: Subtype differences in comorbidity, educational, and clinical history. *The Journal of Nervous and Mental Disease, 190*(3), 147–157. doi:10.1097/00005053-200203000-00003 PMID:11923649

Murray, T. S. (1991, August). Computer assisted learning for general practice. *The British Journal of General Practice, 41*(349), 344–345. PMID:1777283

Mwabukusi, M., Karimuribo, E. D., Rweyemamu, M. M., & Beda, E. (2014). Mobile technologies for disease surveillance in humans and animals. *The Onderstepoort Journal of Veterinary Research, 81*(2), 5. doi:10.4102/ojvr.v81i2.737 PMID:25005126

Mwisongo, A. J., Kisoka, W. J., Mubyazi, G. M., Malebo, H., Senkoro, K. P., McHaro, J., & Kitua, A. Y. (2001). Major health problems in some selected districts of Tanzania. *Tanzania Journal of Health Research, 3*(2), 10–14. doi:10.4314/thrb.v3i2.14212

Myers. (2002). Qualitative research and the generalizability question: Standing firm with Proteus. *The Qualitative Report, 4*(3/4). Retrieved from http://www.nova.edu/ssss/QR/QR4-3/myers.html

Myers, M. D. (2009). *Qualitative Research in Business & Management.* New Zealand: SAGE Publications Ltd.

Mylopoulus, J. (2006). Representing Knowledge About Information Systems. *ACM Transactions on Information Systems, 3*(2), 131–140.

Najaftorkaman, M., Ghapanchi, A. H., Talaei-Khoei, A., & Ray, P. (2014). A taxonomy of antecedents to user adoption of health information systems: A synthesis of thirty years of research. *Journal of the Association for Information Science and Technology, 66*(3), 576–598. doi:10.1002/asi.23181

Najera, P., Lopez, J., & Roman, R. (2011). Real-time location and inpatient care systems based on passive RFID. *Journal of Network and Computer Applications, 34*(3), 980–989. doi:10.1016/j.jnca.2010.04.011

Namibia, M. (2007). *Community-based healtcare policy.* Windhoek: MoHSS.

Narang, J. K. (2011). Quality of Healthcare Services in Rural India: The User Perspective. *VIKALPA*, 51-60.

Na, S., & Cheon, S. (2000). Role delegation in role-based access control. *Proceedings of the fifth ACM workshop on Role-based access control* (pp. 39–44). ACM. doi:10.1145/344287.344300

National Association of Boards of Pharmacy. (2009). *National Association of Boards of Pharmacy (NABP), About the issue.* Available at http://www.dangerouspill.com/about_the_issue.html

National Institutes of Health. (2011, November 8). *Benefits of Enterprise Architecture.* Retrieved from https://enterprisearchitecture.nih.gov/Pages/BenefitsEnterpriseArchitecture.aspx

National-Academy-of-Sciences (2007). *Preventing medication errors: Quality chasm series.* Author.

Ncube, P. S., Thinyane, H., & Foster, G. (2010). *An Investigation into a Web Based Visualization Technique of Zoonotic Disease Outbreaks.* Rhodes University.

Neal, K. (2003). ROI in the ED. *Health Management Technology,* (November): 2003. PMID:14608714

NEHTA. (2014). *National E-Health Transition Authority of Australia*. Retrieved from http://www.nehta.gov.au

Newell, S. (2011). Special section on healthcare information systems. *The Journal of Strategic Information Systems*, *20*(2), 158–160. doi:10.1016/j.jsis.2011.05.002

Ngafeeson, M. N. (2013). Understanding user resistance to information technology: Toward a comprehensive model in health information technology. *Proquest Dissertations and Theses*, 113.

Ngai, E. W. T., Moon, K. K. L., Riggins, F. J., & Yi, C. Y. (2008). RFID research: An academic literature review (1995–2005) and future research directions. *International Journal of Production Economics*, *112*(2), 510–520. doi:10.1016/j.ijpe.2007.05.004

Ngai, E. W. T., Poon, J. K. L., Suk, F. F. C., & Ng, C. C. (2009). Design of an RFID-based Healthcare Management System using an Information System Design Theory. *Information Systems Frontiers*, *11*(4), 405–417. doi:10.1007/s10796-009-9154-3

Ngai, E. W. T., Xiu, L., & Chau, D. C. K. (2009b). Application of data mining techniques in customer relationship management: A literature review and classification. *Expert Systems with Applications*, *36*(2, Part 2), 2592–2602. doi:10.1016/j.eswa.2008.02.021

Niemi, E. (2006). Enterprise Architecture Benefits: Perceptions from Literature and Practice.*Proceedings of the 7th IBIMA Conference Internet & Information Systems in the Digital Age*. IBIMA.

Noble, E. (2012). The role mentoring plays in a white female novice teacher's perceptions of her enculturation into a culturally diverse campus. *ProQuest Dissertations and Theses*, 11-12.

Nonaka, I., Reinmoeller, P., & Senoo, D. (1998). Management Focus The 'ART' of Knowledge: Systems to Capitalize on Market Knowledge. *European Management Journal, 16*(6), 673-684.

North, N. (2008). *Immigrant doctors practising non-Western medicine: a study of self-employed immigrant Chinese and Indian doctors practising non-biomedical traditions of medicine, New Settlers Programme*. Massey University.

Noseworthy, J. (2012). A solitary journey: Interpretive description of women's experiences of perinatal loss in labour. *Proquest Dissertations and Theses*, 40.

Novak, J., & Judah, A. (2011). *Towards a health productivity reform agenda for Australia*. South Melbourne: Australian Centre for Health Research.

Noyes, J., Masakowski, Y., & Cook, M. (2012). *Decision making in complex environments*. Ashgate Publishing, Ltd.

NPC. (2012). *Namibia 2011 population and housing census*. Available at: www.npc.gov.na

NSW Department of Health. (1998). *Emergency Department Information System: Information Management and Technology Audit*. Sydney: NSW Department of Health.

Nyrhinen, M. (2006). *IT Infrastructure: Structure, properties and processes*. Helsinki School of Economics, Finland. Working paper, W-403. HSE Print.

O'Brien, M. S., Crickard, E. L., Rapp, C., Holmes, C., & McDonald, T. (2011). Critical issues for psychiatric medication shared decision making with youth and families. *Families in Society*, *93*(3), 310–316. doi:10.1606/1044-3894.4135

O'connor, A., Bennett, C., Stacey, D., Barry, M., Col, N., Eden, K., . . . Khangura, S. (2009). Decision aids for people facing health treatment or screening decisions (Review). *The Cochrane Collaboration published in the Cochrane Library, 3*.

O'Connor, M. C. (2005, February 17). Surveys Reveal Dubious Consumers. *RFID Journal*.

O'Connor, M. C. (2007, February 6). RFID Tidies Up Distribution of Hospital Scrubs. *RFID Journal.*

O'Dell, C., & Grayson, C. J. (1998). If only we knew what we know: Identification and transfer of internal best practices. *California Management Review, 40*(3), 154–174. doi:10.2307/41165948

O'Brien, J. (2011). *Revenue up despite drop-off in international students.* Retrieved from http://www-public.jcu.edu.au/news/current/JCU_101879

O'Brien, E., Coats, A., Owens, P., Petrie, J., Padfield, P. L., Littler, W. A., & Mee, F. (2000). Use and interpretation of ambulatory blood pressure monitoring: Recommendations of the British Hypertension Society. *BMJ: British Medical Journal, 320*(7242), 1128–1134. doi:10.1136/bmj.320.7242.1128 PMID:10775227

O'Connell, R. T., Cho, C., Shah, N., Brown, K., & Shiffman, R. N. (2004). Take Note(s): Differential EHR Satisfaction with Two Implementations under One Roof. *Journal of the American Medical Informatics Association, 11*(1), 43–49. doi:10.1197/jamia.M1409 PMID:14527978

Office of Government Commerce. (2012). *PRINCE2.* Retrieved from http://www.prince-officialsite.com

Omary, Z., Lupiana, D., Mtenzi, F. & Wu, B. (2009). *Challenges to E-Healthcare Adoption in Developing Countries: A Case Study of Tanzania.* Academic Press.

ONC. (2015). *Office of the National Coordinator for Health Information Technology Product List.* Retrieved from http://oncchpl.force.com/ehrcert

Onion, D. K., & Berrington, R. M. (1999, March-April). Comparioson of UK General Practice and US Family Practice. *ABFP, 12*(2), 164–172.

Open mHealth. (2011). *Open mHealth.* Retrieved from http://openmhealth.org/

OpenEMR. (2012). *OpenEMR electronic health record.* Retrieved from http://www.open-emr.org/

OpenESB. (2012). *Sun Microsystems OpenESB.* Retrieved from http://open-esb.dev.java.net/

OpenMRS. (2004). *OpenMRS electronic medical record system platform.* Retrieved from http://openmrs.org/

Oracle, E. S. B. (2012). *Oracle ESB.* Retrieved from http://www.oracle.com/appserver/esb.html

Overby, C. L., Kohane, I., Kannry, J. L., Williams, M. S., Starren, J., Bottinger, E., & Hripcsak, G. et al. (2013). Opportunities for genomic clinical decision support interventions. *Genetics in Medicine, 15*(10), 817–823. doi:10.1038/gim.2013.128 PMID:24051479

Ozaki. (n.d.). *Near-Infrared Spectroscopy—Its Versatility in Analytical Chemistry.* Department of Chemistry, School of Science and Technology, Kwansei Gakuin University.

Oztekin, A., Foad, M. P., Delen, D., & Swim, L. K. (2010). An RFID network design methodology for asset tracking in healthcare. *Decision Support Systems, 49*(1), 100–109. doi:10.1016/j.dss.2010.01.007

Oztekin, A., Mahdavi, F., Erande, K., Kong, Z. J., Swim, L. K., & Bukkapatnam, S. T. S. (2010a). Criticality index analysis based optimal RFID reader placement models for asset tracking. *International Journal of Production Research, 48*(9), 2679–2698. doi:10.1080/00207540903565006

Pack, J. (2011). Multiple intelligences and experiential learning styles: A mixed method study of registered nurses' attitudes toward computers and web-based learning. *Proquest,* 1.

Pagano, M. W. (2013). Toward improved security and privacy in modern healthcare. *Proquest Dissertations and Theses,* 10.

Page, L. (2007). Testing gives way to implementation. Hospitals tune in to RFID. *Materials Management in Health Care, 16*(5), 18–20. PMID:17552344

Pancorbo-Hidalgo, P. L., Garcia-Fernandez, F. P., Lopez-Medina, I. M., & Alvarez-Nieto, C. (2006). Risk assessment scales for pressure ulcer prevention: A systematic review. *Journal of Advanced Nursing, 54*(1), 94–110. doi:10.1111/j.1365-2648.2006.03794.x PMID:16553695

Parrish, J. L. Jr, & Courtney, J. F. (2012). Inquiring Systems: Theoretical Foundations for Current and Future Information Systems, Information Systems Theory. *Springer New York, 2012*, 387–396.

Parsons, S., Harding, G., Breen, A., Foster, N., Pincus, T., Vogel, S., & Underwood, M. (2012). Will shared decision making between patients with chronic musculoskeletal pain and physiotherapists, osteopaths and chiropractors improve patient care? *Family Practice, 29*(2), 203–212. doi:10.1093/fampra/cmr083 PMID:21982810

Pascoe, L., Lungo, J., Kaasbøll, J., & Koleleni, I. (2012, May). Collecting integrated disease surveillance and response data through mobile phones. In *Proceedings of the IST-Africa 2012 Conference and Exhibition*, (pp. 9-11). Academic Press.

Patel, V. L., Allen, V. G., Arocha, J. F., Jose, B. A., & Shortliffe, E. H. (1998). Representing clinical guidelines in GLIF: Individual and collaborative expertise. *Journal of the American Medical Informatics Association, 5*(5), 467–483. doi:10.1136/jamia.1998.0050467 PMID:9760394

Pattinson, R. C. (2004). Maternal health. [report by health systems research agency] In *South African Health Review 2003/2004* (pp. 89–99). Durban, South Africa: Health Systems Trust, South Africa.

Pattinson, R. C. (2007). *Basic Antenatal Care (BANC) Handbook* [training manual for nurses]. Pretoria, South Africa: University of Pretoria, South Africa.

Payton, F. C., & Pare, G. et al.. (2011). Health care IT: Process, people, patients and inter-disciplinary considerations. *Journal of the Association for Information Systems, 12*(2/3), i–xiii.

Payton, F. C., Pare, G., Le Rouge, C. M., & Reddy, M. (2011). Health care IT: Process, people, patients and interdisciplinary considerations. *Journal of the Association for Information Systems, 12*(2), 3.

Payton, F. C., Pare, G., LeRouge, C., & Reddy, M. (2011). Health care IT: Process, people, patients and interdisciplinary considerations. *Journal of the Association for Information Systems, 12*(2), i–xiii.

PCAST. (2010). *Report to the President realizing the full potential of the health information technology to improve healthcare for Americans: The path forward. President's Council of Advisors on Science and Technology (PCAST)*. Executive Office of the President.

Perron, M. D. (2014). Residential substance abuse treatment experiences of baby boomers: A qualitative study. *Proquest Dissertations and Theses*, 6-39.

Perron, M. D. (2014). Residential substance abuse treatment experiences of baby boomers: A qualitative study. *Proquest Dissertations and Theses*, 6-51.

Peterson, L. A. (2006). Information technology use in nursing and nursing education as reported by beginning nurses. *Proquest Dissertations and Theses*, 2.

Peterson, L. A. (2006). Information technology use in nursing and nursing education as reported by beginning nurses. *Proquest*, 2.

Petroudi, D., & Giannakakis, N. (2011). New Technologies in Hospital Information System. In Clinical Technologies: Concepts, Methodologies, Tools and Applications, (pp. 2029-2034). IGI Global. doi:10.4018/978-1-60960-561-2.ch801

PHCRIS. (2006-07). *PHCRIS Fast Fact - IM/IT use in Australian general practices, 2003-04 to 2006-07; Annual Survey of Divisions (ASD) Report series, 2003-04 to 2006-07.* Retrieved from http://www.phcris.org.au/fastfacts/fact.php?id=5029

Pilot, D., & Beck, C. (2014). *Study Guide for Essentials of Nursing Research: Appraising Evidence for Nursing Practice* (8th ed.). Philadelphia: Lippincott Williams & Wilkins.

PIP. (2014). *Practice Incentive Programme.* Retrieved from http://www.medicareaustralia.gov.au/provider/incentives/pip/-

Pisk, R. M. (2010). *Physician satisfaction and workflow intergration factors associated with electronic medical record implementation in a pediatric hospital.* Proquest.

Pleshek, J. (2011). *RFID will see double-digit growth in the healthcare market.* Retrieved 21 December, 2011, from http://wtnnews.com/articles/8824/

Plianbangchang, S. (2011). *Regional Consultation on Strengthening Role of Family/Community Physicians in Primary Health Care.* Jakarta, Indonesia: Academic Press.

Porter, M. E. (1985). *Competitive advantage: creating and sustaining competitive performance.* New York: The Free Press.

Practice Fusion EHR. (2015). *Practice Fusion EHR.* Retrieved from http://www.practicefusion.com/electronic-health-record-ehr/

President's Council of Advisors on Science and Technology. (2010). *Realizing the Full Potential of Health Information Technology to Improve Healthcare for Americans: The Path Forward.* Retrieved from http://www.whitehouse.gov/sites/default/files/microsites/ostp/pcast-health-it-report.pdf

Prevatt, F., Lampropoulos, G. K., Bowles, V., & Garrett, L. (2011). The use of between session assignments in ADHD coaching with college students. *Journal of Attention Disorders, 15*(1), 18–27. doi:10.1177/1087054709356181 PMID:20019381

Privacy Act of Australia. (1988). Retrieved from http://www.privacy.gov.au/law/act

Privacy.Gov. (2013). *State and Territory Laws.* Office of the Australian Privacy Commissioner, Australia. Retrieved from http://www.privacy.gov.au/law/states

Productivity Commission (2006). *Potential benefits of the National Reform Agenda, Report to the Council of Australian Governments.* Canberra: Commonwealth of Australia.

Productivity Commission. (2005). *Impacts of advances in medical technology in Australia.* Productivity Commission Research Report. Retrieved from http://www.pc.gov.au/study/medicaltechnology/finalreport/medicaltechnology.pdf

Prokosch, H., & Ganslandt, T. (2009). Perspectives for medical informatics. Reusing the electronic medical record for clinical research. *Methods of Information in Medicine, 48*(1), 38–44. PMID:19151882

Puffenberger, S. S. (2011). *The Efficacy of Working Memory Training for Children and Adolescents with Attention-Deficit/Hyperactivity Disorder-Combined type compared to Children and Adolescents with Attention-Deficit/Hyperactivity Disorder-Primarily Inattentive type.* Ohio State University.

Pulakkazhy, S., & Balan, R. (2013). Data mining in banking and its applications-a review. *Journal of Computer Science, 9*(10), 1252–1259. doi:10.3844/jcssp.2013.1252.1259

Pusat Data dan Informasi Kementerian Kesehatan RI. (2012). *Roadmap Sistem Informasi Kesehatan tahun 2011-2014.* Jakarta: Kemenkes RI.

Quinn, G. P., & Keough, M. J. (2002). *Experimental Design and Data Analysis for Biologists.* Cambridge University Press. Retrieved from http://books.google.com.au/books?hl=en&lr=&id=VtU3-y7LaLYC&oi=fnd&pg=PP17&dq=GP+and+IT&ots=czom2Bqkiy&sig=iVsd0AsJx11cM5WmUIwSU8nh21I#v=onepage&q=GP%20and%20IT&f=false

Quinn, J. A., Reardon, D. A., Friedman, A. H., Rich, J. N., Sampson, J. H., & Provenzale, J. M. et al.. (2003). Phase II trial of temozolomide in patients with progressive low-grade glioma. *Journal of Clinical Oncology, 21*(4), 646–651. doi:10.1200/JCO.2003.01.009 PMID:12586801

Quinn, P. O. (2001). *ADD and the college student: A guide for high school and college students with attention deficit disorde.* Washington, DC: Magination Press.

RACGP. (2014). Retrieved from http://www.racgp.org.au/becomingagp/what-is-a-gp/what-is-general-practice/

Rada, R. (2008). *Information Systems and Healthcare Enterprises.* Hershey, PA: IGI Publishing. doi:10.4018/978-1-59904-651-8

Ramli, D. (2014). Telstra inks eHealth deal with Medgate. *The Australian Financial Review.* Retrieved from http://www.afr.com/p/technology/telstra_inks_ehealth_deal_with_medgate_dfUoP2yhYylu0uxVskoPDI

Ramsay, J. R. (2012). "Without a Net" CBT Without Medications for an Adult With ADHD. *Clinical Case Studies, 11*(1), 48–65. doi:10.1177/1534650112440741

Rawabdeh, A. A. A. (2007). An E-health Trend Plan for the Jordanian Health Care System. *International Journal of Health Care Quality Assurance, 20*(6), 516–531. doi:10.1108/09526860710819459 PMID:18030969

Relling, M., & Klein, T. (2011). CPIC: Clinical pharmacogenetics implementation consortium of the pharmacogenomics research network. *Clinical Pharmacology and Therapeutics, 89*(3), 464–467. doi:10.1038/clpt.2010.279 PMID:21270786

ResearchKit. (2015). *ResearchKit.* Retrieved from https://www.apple.com/researchkit/

Reyes, P. M., Li, S., et al. (2011). Accessing antecedents and outcomes of RFID implementation in health care. *International Journal of Production Economics.*

Reynolds, J., Griffiths, K., & Christensen, H. (2011). Anxiety and depression-online resources and management tools. *Australian Family Physician, 40*(6), 382. PMID:21655483

Rice, P., & Azzy, D. (1999). *Qualitative research methods: A health focus.* Melbourne: Oxford University Press.

Riggins, F. J., & Mukhopadhyay, T. (1994). Interdependent benefits from interorganizational systems: Opportunities for business partner reengineering. *Journal of Management Information Systems, 11*(2), 37–57.

Righini, N. (2002). *Information Systems in the Emergency Departments. HM 816: Healthcare Information System.* Boston University School of Management.

Rizzo, V. M., & Kintner, E. (2013). The utility of the behavioral risk factor surveillance system (BRFSS) in testing quality of life theory: An evaluation using structural equation modeling. *Quality of Life Research: An International Journal of Quality of Life Aspects of Treatment, Care and Rehabilitation, 22*(5), 987–995. doi:10.1007/s11136-012-0228-1 PMID:22797867

Roark, D. C., & Miguel, K. (2006). Bar coding's replacement? *Nursing Management, 37*(2), 29–31. doi:10.1097/00006247-200602000-00009 PMID:16452888

Roberts, S. A. (2007). The impact of Information Technology on small, medium, and large hospitals: quality, safety and financial metrics. *Proquest Dissertations and Theses,* 14.

Roberts, S. A. (2007). The impact of Information Technology on small, medium, and large hospitals: quality, safety and financial metrics. *Proquest*, 14.

Robey, D. (2007). Cultural Analysis and the Organizational Consequences of I.T. *Accounting. Management and Information Technologies*, *3*(1), 23–24.

Robinson, B. (2010). CalRHIO shuts down after missing out on HIE bid. *Government Health IT*. Retrieved from http://www.govhealthit.com/news/calrhio-shuts-down-after-missing-out-hie-bid

Robinson, Eaton, Haaland, Koepp, Thomas, Stallard, & Robinson. (n.d.). *Noninvasive Glucose Monitoring in Diabetic Patients: A Preliminary Evaluation.* Academic Press.

Rock, M., Buntain, B. J., Hatfield, J. M., & Hallgrímsson, B. (2009). Animal–human connections,"one health," and the syndemic approach to prevention. *Social Science & Medicine*, *68*(6), 991–995. doi:10.1016/j.socscimed.2008.12.047 PMID:19157669

Rodrigues, R., & Risk, A. (2003). eHealth in Latin America and the Caribbean:Development and policy issues. *Journal of Medical Internet Research*, *5*(1), 4–22. doi:10.2196/jmir.5.1.e4 PMID:12746209

Rogoski, R. R. (2002). IT in the ED. The nature of emergency department medicine means specific and comprehensive IT needs for clinicians. *Health Management Technology*, *23*, 14–16. PMID:11842574

Rood, M. A. (1994). Enterprise Architecture: Definition, Content, and Utility.*Proceedings of the IEEE Third Workshop on Enabling Technologies: Infrastructure for Collaborative Enterprises*, (pp. 106-111). IEEE.

Rose, J. (1998). Evaluating the contribution of Structuration Theory to the Information Systems discipline, In *Proceedings of the 6th European Conference on Information Systems (ECIS)*, Aix-en-Provence, France.

Rosen, M. (2008). *Applied SOA: service-oriented architecture and design strategies.* Wiley.

Rouse, M. (2005). *ICT (information and communications technology - or technologies).* Retrieved from http://searchcio-midmarket.techtarget.com/definition/ICT

Rowe, B. H., Bond, K., Ospina, M. B., Blitz, S., Schull, M., Sinclair, D., & Bullard, M. (2006). Data collection on patients in emergency departments in Canada. *Canadian Journal of Emergency Medicine*, *8*, 417–424. PMID:17209491

Royce, M. (2008). A step beyond inclusion: A case study of what one principle did to improve achievement for students with disabilities. *Proquest Dissertations and Theses*, 63-69.

Rumisha, S. F., Mboera, L. E., Senkoro, K. P., Gueye, D., & Mmbuji, P. K. (2007). Monitoring and evaluation of integrated disease surveillance and response in selected districts in Tanzania. *Tanzania Journal of Health Research*, *9*(1), 1–11. doi:10.4314/thrb.v9i1.14285 PMID:17547094

Rweyemamu, Mmbuji, Karimuribo, Paweska, Kambarage, Neves, … Matee. (2013). The Southern African Centre for infectious disease surveillance: A one health consortium. *Emerging Health Threats Journal, 6.*

Ryan, A., & Eklund, P. (2008). A framework for semantic interoperability in healthcare: A service oriented architecture based on health informatics standards. *Studies in Health Technology and Informatics*, *136*, 759. PMID:18487823

Ryan, M. P. (1989, May). A system for general practice computing in Scotland. *Health Bulletin*, *47*(3), 110–119. PMID:2807896

Ryan, P. B., Madigan, D., Stang, P. E., Marc Overhage, J., Racoosin, J. A., & Hartzema, A. G. (2012). Empirical assessment of methods for risk identification in healthcare data: Results from the experiments of the Observational Medical Outcomes Partnership. *Statistics in Medicine*, *31*(30), 4401–4415. PMID:23015364

Rygh, E. M., & Hjortdahl, P. H. (2007). Continuous and integrated health care services in rural areas. A literature study. The International Electronic Journal of Rural and Remote Health Research, Education Practice and Policy, 7(766), 1-10.

Safran, C., Bloomrosen, M., Hammond, W. E., Labkoff, S., Markel-Fox, S., Tang, P. C., & Detmer, D. E. (2007). Toward a national framework for the secondary use of health data: An American Medical Informatics Association White Paper. *Journal of the American Medical Informatics Association*, 14(1), 1–9. doi:10.1197/jamia.M2273 PMID:17077452

Safren, S. A., Otto, M. W., Sprich, S., Winett, C. L., Wilens, T. E., & Biederman, J. (2005). Cognitive-behavioral therapy for ADHD in medication-treated adults with continued symptoms. *Behaviour Research and Therapy*, 43(7), 831–842. doi:10.1016/j.brat.2004.07.001 PMID:15896281

Sajid, M., & Ahsan, K. (2014). Enterprise Architecture for Healthcare Organizations. *World Applied Sciences Journal*, 30(10), 1330–1333.

Sambo, M. B. (2012). *Epidemiological dynamics of rabies in Tanzania and its impacts on local communities* (Doctoral dissertation, University of Glasgow). Retrieved from http://theses.gla.ac.uk/3663/1/2012sambomsc.pdf

Sander Granlien, M., & Hertzum, M. (2012). Confirmatory factor analysis of service quality dimensions within mobile telephony industry in Ghana. *The Electronic Journal Information Systems Evaluation*, 15(2), pp197–pp227.

Sanga, C., Mlozi, M. R. S., Tumbo, S., Mussa, M., Muhiche, L., & Haug, R. (2014). On the Development of the Mobile based Agricultural Extension System in Tanzania: A technological perspective. *International Journal of Computing and ICT Research*, 8(1), 49–67.

Satterly, D. (1989). *Assessment in schools*. Oxford, UK: Basil Blackwell Ltd.

Sauerborn, R., & Lippeveld, T. (2000). *What is wrong with current health information systems?* Geneva: WHO.

Schauer, C., Everett, A., del Vecchio, P., & Anderson, L. (2007). Promoting the value and practice of shared decision-making in mental health care. *Psychiatric Rehabilitation Journal*, 31(1), 54–61. doi:10.2975/31.1.2007.54.61 PMID:17694716

Scholl, I., Loon, M. K., Sepucha, K., Elwyn, G., Légaré, F., Härter, M., & Dirmaier, J. (2011). Measurement of shared decision making–a review of instruments. *Zeitschrift für Evidenz. Fortbildung und Qualität im Gesundheitswesen*, 105(4), 313–324. doi:10.1016/j.zefq.2011.04.012

Shapiro, J. S., Baumlin, K. M., Chawla, N., Genes, N., Godbold, J., Ye, F., & Richardson, L. D. (2010). Emergency Department Information System Implementation and Process Redesign Result in Rapid and Sustained Financial Enhancement at a Large Academic Center. *Academic Emergency Medicine*, 17(5), 527–535. doi:10.1111/j.1553-2712.2010.00720.x PMID:20536809

SHARP. (2013). *Strategic Health IT Advanced Research Projects (SHARP)*. Retrieved from http://www.healthit.gov/policy-researchers-implementers/strategic-health-it-advanced-research-projects-sharp

Shaughnessy, J., Zechmeister, E., & Jeanne, Z. (2011). *Research methods in psychology* (9th ed.). McGraw Hill.

Sheikh, A., Cornford, T., Barber, N., Avery, A., Takian, A., Lichtner, V., & Cresswell, K. et al. (2011). Implementation and adoption of nationwide electronic health records in secondary care in England: Final qualitative results from prospective national evaluation in 'early adopter' hospitals. *BMJ (Clinical Research Ed.)*, 343(1), d6054. doi:10.1136/bmj.d6054 PMID:22006942

Sherer, S. (2010). Information systems and healthcare: An institutional theory per-spective on physician adoption of electronic health records. *Communications of the Association for Information Systems*, 27(7), 127–140.

Sheridan, S. L., Harris, R. P., & Woolf, S. H. (2004). Shared decision making about screening and chemoprevention. *American Journal of Preventive Medicine, 26*(1), 56–66. doi:10.1016/j.amepre.2003.09.011 PMID:14700714

Shinde. (n.d.). Non Invasive Blood Glucose Measurement using NIR technique based on occlusion spectroscopy. *International Journal of Engineering Science and Technology.*

Shortliffe, E. H., & Cimino, J. J. (2006). *Biomedical informatics: computer applications in health care and biomedicine.* Springer Verlag. doi:10.1007/0-387-36278-9_2

Simon, C. (2009). From Generalism to Specialty—A Short History of General Practice. InnovAiT.

Singh, J., Vargas, L., Bacon, J., & Moody, K. (2008). Policy-based information sharing in publish/subscribe middleware. *Policies for Distributed Systems and Networks, 2008. POLICY 2008. IEEE Workshop on* (pp. 137–144). IEEE.

Singleton, V., & Michael, M. (1993). Actor-Networks and Ambivalence: General practitioners in the UK Cervical Screening Programme. *Social Studies of Science, 23*(2), 227–264. doi:10.1177/030631293023002001

Sinha, R. K. (2010). Impact of Health Information Technology in Public Health. *Sri Lanka Journal of Bio-Medical Informatics, 1*(4), 223–236. doi:10.4038/sljbmi.v1i4.2239

Sini, E., Locatelli, P., & Restifo, N. (2008). Making the clinical process safe and efficient using RFID in healthcare. *European Journal of ePractice, 2.* Available at http://www.epractice.eu/en/document/287903

Sita, A. K., Nsubuga, P., Eseko, N., Tadesse, W., Ndayimirije, N., Stella, C., & McNabb, S. (2002).Structure and performance of infectious disease surveillance and response, United Republic of Tanzania, 1998. *Bulletin of the World Health Organization, 80*(3), 196–203.

Slettemeås, D. (2009). RFID—the "Next Step" in Consumer–Product Relations or Orwellian Nightmare? *Challenges for Research and Policy, 32*(3), 219–244. doi:10.1007/s10603-009-9103-z

SMART. (2011). *Substitutable Medical Apps & Reusable Technology (SMART).* Retrieved from http://smartplatforms.org/

Snyder, R., & Dazzo, O. (2011). *Guidelines for the Reporting Of Rabies Cases Using the Michigan Disease Surveillance System (MDSS).* Michigan: Capitol View Building.

Sondheimer, N., Katsh, E., Clarke, L., Osterweil, L., & Rainey, D. (2009). *Dispute prevention and dispute resolution in networked.* Academic Press.

Southard, P. B., Chandra, C., & Kumar, S. (2012). RFID in healthcare: A Six Sigma DMAIC and simulation case study. *International Journal of Health Care Quality Assurance, 25*(4), 291–321. doi:10.1108/09526861211221491 PMID:22755482

Sox, H. C., Higgins, M. C., & Owens, D. K. (2013). *Medical decision making.* John Wiley & Sons. doi:10.1002/9781118341544

Soy, S. (1997). *The case study as a research method: Uses and users of Information–LIS 391D.* Unpublished.

Spoelstra, S. (2006). Asking the question: What is organization? *Proquest Dissertations and Theses, 18.*

Staal, I. I., Hermanns, J., Schrijvers, A. J., & van Stel, H. F. (2013). Risk assessment of parents' concerns at 18 months in preventive child health care predicted child abuse and neglect. *Child Abuse & Neglect, 37*(7), 475–484. doi:10.1016/j.chiabu.2012.12.002 PMID:23352082

Stake, R. E. (1995). *The art of case study research.* Academic Press.

Starfield, B., Shi, L., & Macinko, J. (2005, September). Contribution of Primary Care to Health Systems and Health. *The Milbank Quarterly, 83*(3), 457–502. doi:10.1111/j.1468-0009.2005.00409.x PMID:16202000

State of Illinois. (2009). *Department of Central Management Services Bureau of Communication and Computer Services Effective October 01, 2009Version 1*. Author.

Steinfield, C., & Wyche, S. (2013). *Assessing the role of information and communication technologies to enhance food systems in developing countries: A FOCUS On Eastern and Southern Africa*. Retrieved from https://www.msu.edu/~steinfie/ICT4D_White_Paper_2013.pdf

Steinmueller, W. (2001). ICTs and the possibilities for leapfrogging by developing countries. *International Labour Review, 140*(2), 193–210. doi:10.1111/j.1564-913X.2001.tb00220.x

Stuart, P. (2004). A casemix model for estimating the impact of hospital access block on the emergency department. *Emergency Medicine Australasia, 16*(3), 201–207. doi:10.1111/j.1742-6723.2004.00587.x PMID:15228462

Sujansky, W. V. (1998). The benefits and challenges of an electronic medical record: Much more than a "word-processed" patient chart. *The Western Journal of Medicine, 169*, 176–183. PMID:9771161

Sullivan, L. (2006). *Medline Markets RFID System for Surgical Sponges*. RFID Journal.

Svenson, J. E., Pollack, S. H., Fallat, M. E., & Drapeau, J. L. (2003). Limitations of electronic databases: A caution. *The Journal of the Kentucky State Medical Association, 101*, 109–112. PMID:12674902

Swai, E. S., Moshy, W. E., Kaaya, J. E., & Mtui, P. F. (2011). *Spatial and temporal distribution of rabies in the northern zone of Tanzania in the period of 1993-2002*. Academic Press.

Swai, E. S., Moshy, W. E., Kaaya, J. E., & Mtui, P. F. (2010). Spatial and temporal distribution of rabies in the northern zone of Tanzania in the period of 1993-2002. *Tanzania Journal of Health Research, 12*(1), 80–85. doi:10.4314/thrb.v12i1.56335 PMID:20737833

Swan, D. (2014). *Telstra targets healthcare with new deals*. Business Spectator. Retrieved from http://www.businessspectator.com.au/news/2014/10/22/technology/telstra-targets-healthcare-new-deals

Swartz, N. (2005). FDA Okays Implanted Chip for Health Care. Information Management Journal. *Lenexa, 39*(1), 16.

Swartz, S. L., Prevatt, F., & Proctor, B. E. (2005). A coaching intervention for college students with Attention Deficit/Hyperactivity Disorder. *Psychology in the Schools, 42*(6), 647–656. doi:10.1002/pits.20101

Swedberg, C. (2005, September 12). Pittsburgh Hospital Pilots Hybrid System. *RFID Journal.*

Swedberg, C. (2007, February 16). MedicAlert Aims to RFID-Enable Medical Records. *RFID Journal.*

Swedberg, C. (2008a, January 3). Medical Center Set to Grow With RFID. *RFID Journal.*

Swedberg, C. (2008b, March 18). Surgeon Designs System to Monitor Orthopedic Implants and Promote Healing. *RFID Journal.*

Swisher, J. R., Jacobson, S. H., Jun, J. B., & Balci, O. (2001). Modeling and analyzing a physician clinic environment using discrete-event (visual) simulation. *Computers & Operations Research, 28*(2), 105-125.

Symonds, J., & Parry, D. et al.. (2007). An RFID-based system for assisted living:Challenges and solutions. *The Journal on Information Technology in Healthcare, 5*(6), 387–398. PMID:17901606

Tabbutt, S., Ghanayem, N., Ravishankar, C., Sleeper, L. A., Cooper, D. S., Frank, D. U., & Goldberg, C. S. et al. (2012). Risk factors for hospital morbidity and mortality after the Norwood procedure: A report from the Pediatric Heart Network Single Ventricle Reconstruction trial. *The Journal of Thoracic and Cardiovascular Surgery, 144*(4), 882–895. doi:10.1016/j.jtcvs.2012.05.019 PMID:22704284

Tatnall, A. (2011). Innovation Translation, Innovation Diffusion, and the Technology Acceptance Model: Comparing three different approaches to Theorising Technological Innovation. In *Actor–Network Theory and Technology Innovation: Advancements and New Concepts*. IGI Global.

Tatnall, A., & Burgess, S. (2002). Using Actor-Network to research the implementation of a B-B Portal for Regional SME in Melbourne.*15th Bled Electronic Commerce Conference.*

Taylor, C. (2006). The Waiting Room Is Closed. *Health Management Technology, 27*(4), 24–28. PMID:16629252

Telstra. (2014a). *Our partners in health.* Retrieved from http://www.telstra.com.au/personal/telstra-health/about/our-partners/-

Telstra. (2014b). *Readycare and Healthengine will transform how Australians connect with healthcare.* Retrieved from http://www.telstra.com.au/personal/telstra-health/products/telehealth/clinical-consultation/

The Royal Australian College of Physicians. (2009). *Australian Guidelines on Attention Deficit Hyperactivity Disorder (ADHD) (draft).* Canberra, NH: MRC.

Thomas, R. K. (2006). The History of Health Communication. In Health Communication. Springer US. Doi:10.1007/0-387-26116-8_4

Thompson, C. D. (2014). Benefits and risks of electronic medical record (EMR): An interpretive analysis of Healthcare consumers' perceptions of an evolving health information systems technology. *Proquest Dissertations and Theses, 43.*

Thuemmler, C., Buchanan, W., & Kumar, V. (2007). Setting safety standards by designing a low budget and compatible patient identification system based on passive RFID technology. *International Journal of Healthcare Technology and Management, 8*(5), 571–583. doi:10.1504/IJHTM.2007.013524

Tian, R. (2013). Effect of work complexity and individual differences on nursing IT utilization. *Proquest Dissertations and Theses, 19.*

Ting, S. L., Kwok, S. K., Tsang, A. H., & Lee, W. B. (2011). Critical elements and lessons learnt from the implementation of an RFID-enabled healthcare management system in a medical organization. *Journal of Medical Systems, 35*(4), 657–669. doi:10.1007/s10916-009-9403-5 PMID:20703523

TOGAF 9.1. (2013). Retrieved from http://pubs.opengroup.org/architecture/togaf9-doc/arch/index.html

Toland, B. (2011, August 7). Electronic records no panacea for health care industry. *Pittsburgh Post-Gazette.* Retrieved from http://old.post-gazette.com/pg/11219/1165767-114-0.stm?cmpid=nationworld.xml

Tonge, S. I. (2014). Exploring juvenile delinquency and the justice system: Social workers' perspective. *Proquest Dissertations and Theses, 55-57.*

Trucco, P., & Cavallin, M. (2006). A quantitative approach to clinical risk assessment: The CREA method. *Safety Science, 44*(6), 491–513. doi:10.1016/j.ssci.2006.01.003

Tucker, M. T. (2009). Application of the Diffusion of Innovations theory and the health believe model to describe the EMR use among Alabama family medicine physicians: A rural and urban analysis. *Proquest Dissertations and Theses, 29-34.*

Tuckman, A. (2009). *More attention, less deficit success strategies for adults with ADHD.* Plantation, FL: Specialty Press.

Tu, Y. J., Zhou, W., & Piramuthu, S. (2009). Identifying RFID-embedded objects in pervasive healthcare applications. *Decision Support Systems, 46*(2), 586–593. doi:10.1016/j.dss.2008.10.001

Twetman, S., Fontana, M., & Featherstone, J. D. (2013). Risk assessment–can we achieve consensus? *Community Dentistry and Oral Epidemiology, 41*(1), e64–e70. doi:10.1111/cdoe.12026 PMID:24916679

Uden, L., & Francis, J. (2011). *Service Innovation using Actor-Network theory. In Actor-network theory and technology innovation: advancements and new concepts journal, Advancements and new concepts journal.* Hershey, PA: Information Science Reference.

United-States-Department-of-Labor. (2010). Healthcare: Career guide to industries U.S.D. o. labor. VeriChip cloning. *Journal of the American Medical Informatics Association, 13*(6), 601–607.

Unnithan C, Tatnall A (2014). Actor-Network Theory (ANT) based visualisation of Socio-Technical Facets of RFID Technology Translation: An Australian Hospital Scenario. *International Journal of Actor-Network Theory and Technology Innovation, 2*(2).

URT. (2013). *2012 Population and Housing Census. Population distributed by areas. National Bureau of Statistics Ministry of Finance Dar es salaam.* Office of Chief Government Statistician President's Office, Finance, Economy and Development Planning Zanzibar.

Van Beveren, J. 2003. Does health care for knowledge management? *Journal of Knowledge Management, 7* (1), 90-95.

van der Weijden, T., van Veenendaal, H., Drenthen, T., Versluijs, M., Stalmeier, P., Loon, M. K., & Timmermans, D. (2011). Shared decision making in the Netherlands, is the time ripe for nationwide, structural implementation? *Zeitschrift für Evidenz. Fortbildung und Qualität im Gesundheitswesen, 105*(4), 283–288. doi:10.1016/j.zefq.2011.04.005

Vezyridis, P., Timmons, S., & Wharrad, H. J. (2012). Implementation of an Emergency Department Information System: A Qualitative Study of Nurses' Attitudes and Experience. *Computers, Informatics, Nursing, 30*, 540–546. PMID:23079482

Vichianin, Y. (2007). *How to healthcare information and communication technology (HICT) interventions affect access to public sector healthcare delivery in a developing country? A case study of professionals' perception in saraburi province.* Thailand: ProQuest.

Vilamovska, A. M., Hatziandreu, E., Schindler, R., Oranje, C., Vries, H., & Krapels, J. (2008). *Study on the requirements and options for RFID application in healthcare, July 2008.* Retrieved from http://ec.europa.eu/information_society/activities/health/docs/studies/200807-rfid-ehealth.pdf

Vist, A. (2003). *Veterans Health Information Systems and Technology Architecture (VistA) health record and information system.* Retrieved from http://www.worldvista.org/

VMWare vCloud. (2015). *VMWare vCloud for Healthcare.* Retrieved from http://www.vmware.com/industry/healthcare/

W3C. (2008). *World Wide Web Consortium (W3C) tutorial site.* Retrieved from http://www.w3schools.com/

Waegemann, C. (2010). mHealth: The next generation of telemedicine?. *Telemedicine Journal and e-Health, 16*(1), 23–25. doi:10.1089/tmj.2010.9990 PMID:20070168

Wager, K. A., Lee, F. W., & Glaser, J. P. (2009). *Health care information systems: a practical approach for health care management.* John Wiley and Sons.

Waidyanatha, N., & Prashant, S. (2010). User Requirements toward a Real-Time Biosurveillance Program. *Biosurveillance: Methods and Case Studies*, 239.

Wallace, B. A., & Winsler, A., & NeSmith, P. (1999). Factors Associated with Success for College Students with ADHD: Are Standard Accommodations Helping? Wang, J.-R., & Hsieh, S. (2013). Neurofeedback training improves attention and working memory performance. *Clinical Neurophysiology.*

Walley, T., & Mantgani, A. (1997, October11). The UK General Practice Research Database. *Lancet, 350*(9084), 1097–1099. doi:10.1016/S0140-6736(97)04248-7 PMID:10213569

Wamba, S. F. (2012). RFID-enabled healthcare applications, issues and benefits: An archival analysis (1997–2011). *Journal of Medical Systems, 36*(6), 3393–3398. doi:10.1007/s10916-011-9807-x PMID:22109670

Wang, Z. G., Chen, P., & Xie, P. P. (1999). *History and development of traditional Chinese medicine.* Science Press.

Warshawsky, S. (1993, December). General practitioner records on computer. *Family Practice, 10*(4), 474. doi:10.1093/fampra/10.4.474 PMID:8031369

Webb, P., & Bain, C. (2011). *Essential epidemiology.* Cambridge: Cambridge University Press.

Weber, R. O. (2007). Knowledge Management in Call Centres. *Electronic Journal of Knowledge Management, 5*(3), 333–346.

WebSphere ESB. (2008). *IBM WebSphere Enterprise Service Bus.* Retrieved from http://www.ibm.com/software/integration/wsesb/

Weiner, C., Baumlin, K. M., & Shapiro, J. S. (2007). Process redesign and emergency department information system implementation improve efficiency. *Academic Emergency Medicine, 14*(5 Supplement 1), s72. doi:10.1197/j.aem.2007.03.901

Welman, J., & Kruger, S. (2001). Research Methodology: for the Business and administrative sciences (2nd Ed.). Oxford University Press.

Wender, P. H., Wolf, L. E., & Wasserstein, J. (2001). Adults with ADHD. *Annals of the New York Academy of Sciences, 931*(1), 1–16. doi:10.1111/j.1749-6632.2001.tb05770.x PMID:11462736

Weng, S.-J. (2008). A framework for efficient resource allocation in healthcare. *Proquest Dissertations and Theses*, 1.

Wessel, R. (2006a, February 27). German Clinic Uses RFID to Track Blood. *RFID Journal.*

Wessel, R. (2006b, June 9). German Hospital Expects RFID to Eradicate Drug Errors. *RFID Journal.*

Wessel, R. (2006c, September 26). RFID-enabled Locks Secure Bags of Blood. *RFID Journal.*

Wessel, R. (2007, June 1). Jena University Hospital Prescribes RFID to Reduce Medication Errors. *RFID Journal.*

Westerberg, H., Jacobaeus, H., Hirvikoski, T., Clevberger, P., Östensson, M.-L., Bartfai, A., & Klingberg, T. (2007). Computerized working memory training after stroke-A pilot study. *Brain Injury: [BI], 21*(1), 21–29. doi:10.1080/02699050601148726 PMID:17364516

Whetton, S. (2005). *Health Informatics.* Australia: Oxford University Press.

Whitney, S. N., McGuire, A. L., & McCullough, L. B. (2003). A typology of shared decision making, informed consent, and simple consent. *Annals of Internal Medicine, 140*(1), 54–59. doi:10.7326/0003-4819-140-1-200401060-00012 PMID:14706973

Whittaker, R., Merry, S., Stasiak, K., McDowell, H., Doherty, I., Shepherd, M., & Rodgers, A. et al. (2012). MEMO—A mobile phone depression prevention intervention for adolescents: Development process and postprogram findings on acceptability from a randomized controlled trial. *Journal of Medical Internet Research, 14*(1), e13. doi:10.2196/jmir.1857 PMID:22278284

WHO. (2013). *WHO Traditional Medicine Strategy 2014 – 2023.* World Health Organisation. Retrieved 14 October, 2014 from: http://www.who.int/medicines/publications/traditional/trm_strategy14_23/en/

WHO. (2014). *Brochure.* Retrieved from http://www.who.int/hrh/documents/strategy_brochure9-20-14.pdf

Wickramasinghe, N., Chalasani, S., & Koritala, S. (2012). *The role of healthcare system of systems and collaborative technologies in providing superior healthcare delivery to native american patients.* Paper presented at the System Science (HICSS), 2012 45th Hawaii International Conference. doi:10.1109/HICSS.2012.582

Wickramasinghe, N. (2005). The phenomenon of duality: A key to facilitate the transition from knowledge management to wisdom for inquiring organisations. In *Inquiring organisations: moving from knowledge management to wisdom* (pp. 272–315). IGI Global. doi:10.4018/978-1-59140-309-8.ch013

Wickramasinghe, N. (2013). Implicit and Explicit Knowledge Assets in Healthcare. In *Pervasive Health Knowledge Management* (pp. 15–26). Springer New York. doi:10.1007/978-1-4614-4514-2_3

Wickramasinghe, N. S., Fadlalla, A. M. A., Geisler, E., & Schaffer, J. L. (2005). A framework for assessing e-health preparedness. *International Journal of Electronic Healthcare, 1*(3), 316–334. doi:10.1504/IJEH.2005.006478 PMID:18048213

Wickramasinghe, N., Bali, R., & Tatnall, A. (2012). A Manifesto for e-health Success- The Key Role for ANT. *International Journal of Actor-Network Theory and Technological Innovation, 4*(3), 24–35. doi:10.4018/jantti.2012070103

Wickramasinghe, N., Geisler, E., & Schaffer, J. (2005). *Assessing e-health. E-Health Systems Diffusion and Use: The Innovation, the User and the USE IT model.* Hershey, PA: Idea Group.

Wickramasinghe, N., Gupta, J. N. D., & Sharma, S. K. (2005). *Creating Knowledge-Based Healthcare Organizations.* Idea Group Inc. doi:10.4018/978-1-59140-459-0

Wickramasinghe, N., & Misra, S. K. (2004). A wireless trust model for healthcare. *International Journal of Electronic Healthcare, 1*(1), 60–77. doi:10.1504/IJEH.2004.004658 PMID:18048204

Wickramasinghe, N., Tumu, S., Bali, R. K., & Tatnall, A. (2007). Using Actor Network Theory (ANT) as an analytic tool in order to effect superior PACS implementation. *International Journal of Networking and Virtual Organisations, 4*(3), 257–279. doi:10.1504/IJNVO.2007.015164

Wiener, J. M., & Tilly, J. (2002). Population ageing in the United States of America: Implications for public programmes. *International Journal of Epidemiology, 31*(4), 776–781. doi:10.1093/ije/31.4.776 PMID:12177018

Wikipedia. (2014). *General Practitioner.* Retrieved from http://en.wikipedia.org/wiki/General_practitioner

Wilens, T. E., Adler, L. A., Adams, J., Sgambati, S., Rotrosen, J., Sawtelle, R., & Fusillo, S. et al. (2008). Misuse and diversion of stimulants prescribed for ADHD: A systematic review of the literature. *Journal of the American Academy of Child and Adolescent Psychiatry, 47*(1), 21–31. doi:10.1097/chi.0b013e31815a56f1 PMID:18174822

Wilens, T. E., McDermott, S. P., Biederman, J., Abrantes, A., Hahesy, A., & Spencer, T. J. (1999). Cognitive therapy in the treatment of adults with ADHD: A systematic chart review of 26 cases. *Journal of Cognitive Psychotherapy, 13*(3), 215–226.

Wiler, J. L., Gentle, C., Halfpenny, J. M., Heins, A., Mehrotra, A., Mikhail, M. G., & Fite, D. (2010). Optimizing Emergency Department Front-End Operations. *Annals of Emergency Medicine, 55*(2), 142–160. doi:10.1016/j.annemergmed.2009.05.021 PMID:19556030

Wilkerson, J. L., & McDonald Jr, C. L. (2007). RFID in Healthcare. *The Journal of Organizational Leadership & Business*, 1–8.

Winter, R., & Fischer, R. (2007). Essential Layers, Artifacts, and Dependencies of Enterprise Architecture. *Journal of Enterprise Architecture*, 1-12.

Winter, A., Haux, R., Ammenwerth, E., Brigl, B., Hellrung, N., & Jahn, F. (2011). *Health Information System Architectures and Strategies*. London: Springer-Verlag London Limited. doi:10.1007/978-1-84996-441-8

Winzenreid, J. E. (2009). Exploring cultural norms and behaviors that define an ethical environment in charitable non-profit organizations. *Proquest Dissertations and Theses*, 21.

Wolf, L. E. (2001). College students with ADHD and other hidden disabilities. *Annals of the New York Academy of Sciences*, *931*(1), 385–395. doi:10.1111/j.1749-6632.2001.tb05792.x PMID:11462755

WONCA. (2014). *WONCA in brief*. Retrieved from http://www.globalfamilydoctor.com/AboutWonca/brief.aspx

World Community Grid. (2004). *World Community Grid*. Retrieved from http://www.worldcommunitygrid.org/

World Economic Forum. (2013). *Global Information Technology Report 2013*. Retrieved from http://www.weforum.org/reports/global-information-technology-report-2013

World Health Organisation. (2012). *Health systems*. Geneva: WHO.

World Health Organization. (2001). *Medical Records Manual A Guide for Developing Countries*. World Health Organization.

World Health Organization. (2011, November 8). *Key Components of a Well-Functioning Health System*. Retrieved from http://www.who.int/healthsystems/EN_HSSkeycomponents.pdf

World Medical Association. (2001). World Medical Association Declaration of Helsinki: Ethical principles for medical research involving human subject. *Bulletin of the World Health Organization*, 79(4), 373–374. PMID:11357217

Wu, S., & Hall, F. (2012). A Panel Analysis of the Strategic Association between Information and Communication Technology and Public Health Delivery. Journal of Medical Research, 14(5).

Wu, S., Chaudhry, B., Wang, J., Maglione, M., Mojica, W., Roth, E., et al. (2006). *Systematic review: impact of health information technology on quality, efficiency, and costs of medical care*. Academic Press.

Wurster, C. J., Lichtenstein, B. B., & Hogeboom, T. (2008). Strategic, political, and cultural aspects of IT implementation: improving the efficacy of an IT system in a large hospital. *Journal of Healthcare Management, 54*(3), 191–206, discussion 206–7.

Wurster, C., & Lichtenstein, B. P. et al.. (2009). Strategic, political, and cultural aspectsof IT implementation: Improving the efficacy of an IT system in a large hospital. *Journal of Healthcare Management, 54*(3), 191. PMID:19554799

XACML. (2003). *Introduction to XACML*. Retrieved from https://www.oasis-open.org/committees/download.php/2713/Brief_Introduction_to_XACML.html

Xiao, N. (2012). Essay on the impact of health information technology on healthcare providers and patients. *ProQuest*, 1-2.

Xue, C. C., & O'Brien, K. A. (2003). A Comprehensive Guide to Chinese Medicine Chapter 2: Modalities of Chinese Medicine. World Scientific Publishing.

Xue, C.L, Zhang, A. L., Lin, V., Costa, C. D., & Story, D. F. (2007). Complementary and Alternative Medicine Use in Australia: A National Population-Based Survey. *The Journal of Alternative and Complementary Medicine, 13*(6), 643-650.

Xue, Y., Liang, H., Boulton, W. R., & Snyder, C. A. (2005). ERP implementation failures in China: case studies with implications for ERP vendors. *International Journal of Production Economics, 97*(3), 279-295.

Xue, C. C., Zhang, A. L., Lin, V., Myers, R., Polus, B., & Story, D. F. (2008). Acupuncture, chiropractic and osteopathy use in Australia: A national population survey. *BMC Public Health*, 8(1), 105. doi:10.1186/1471-2458-8-105 PMID:18377663

Yang, A. W., Allan, G., Li, C. G., & Xue, C. C. (2009). Effective Application of Knowledge Management in Evidence-based Chinese Medicine: A Case Study. *eCam, 6*(3), 393-398.

Yang, B., & Halvorsen, P. (2010). *Use of RFID to enhance the patient experience, increase safety and eliminate treatment errors, RFID in Oncology Clinics*. White Paper. Alliance Oncology.

Yao, W., Chu, C.-H., & Li, Z. (2010). The use of RFID in healthcare: Benefits and barriers. In *RFID-Technology and Applications (RFID-TA), 2010 IEEE International Conference on* (pp. 128–134). IEEE.

Yao, W., Chu, C.-H., & Li, Z. (2012). The Adoption and Implementation of RFID technologies in Healthcare: A literature review. *Journal of Medical Systems, 36*(6), 3507–3525. doi:10.1007/s10916-011-9789-8 PMID:22009254

Yen Y, Lo N, Wu T (2012). *Two RFID based solutions for secure inpatient medication*. Academic Press.

Yen-Han, L. (2013). Healthcare reform in mainland China: The relationship of healthcare reform and economic development in Chinese rural and urban areas. *ProQuest Dissertations and Theses, 1*.

Yin, R. K. (1999). Enhancing the quality of case studies in Health Services Research. *Health Services Research, 34*(5), 1209.

Yin. (2009). *Case Study Research: Design and Methods*. SAGE.

Yin, R. K. (2002). *Case Study Research: Design and Methods*. SAGE Publications.

Yin, R. K. (2009). *Case Study Research, Design and Methods* (3rd ed.). Newbury Park, CA: Sage Publications.

Yin, R. K. (2009). *Case study research: Design and methods* (Vol. 5). Sage.

Yoon, D., Chang, B.-C., Kang, S. W., Bae, H., & Park, R. W. (2012). Adoption of electronic health records in Korean tertiary teaching and general hospitals. *International Journal of Medical Informatics, 81*(3), 196–203. doi:10.1016/j.ijmedinf.2011.12.002 PMID:22206619

Young, D. W. (1984). What makes doctors use computers?: Discussion paper. *Journal of the Royal Society of Medicine, 77*, 663–667. PMID:6481741

Yu, Y. C. Y., Hou, T. W. T., & Chiang, T. C. T. (2012). Low cost RFID real lightweight binding proof protocol for medication errors and patient safety. *Journal of Medical Systems, 36*(2), 823–828. doi:10.1007/s10916-010-9546-4 PMID:20703651

Zhao, Y. K., Tsursui, T. Endo, A. Minato, K., & Takahashi, T. (1994). Design and development of an expert system to assist diagnosis and treatment of chronic hepatitis using traditional Chinese medicine. *Informatics for Health and Social Care, 19*(1), 37-45.

Zheng, Z. (2014). *Acupuncture in Australia: regulation, education, practice, and research*. Integrative Medicine Research.

Zhu, B., & Wang, H. C. (2011). *Basic Theories of Traditional Chinese Medicine*. Jessica Kingsley Publishers.

Zielstorff, R. D. (1998). Online practice guidelines: Issues, obstacles, and future prospects. *Journal of the American Medical Informatics Association, 5*(3), 227–236. doi:10.1136/jamia.1998.0050227 PMID:9609492

Zinsstag, J., & Tanner, M. (2008). *One Health: The Potential of Closer Cooperation between Human and Animal Health in Africa*. Switzerland: Swiss Tropical Institute.

Zwar, N., & Davis, G. P. (2012). General Practice. In Understanding the Australian Health Care System (2nd ed.). Elsevier Health Sciences.

About the Contributors

Tiko Iyamu holds a PhD in Information Systems. He is currently a Professor of Information Technology at Cape Peninsula University of Technology, Cape Town, South Africa. He was a Professor of Informatics Tshwane University of Technology. Thereafter, he was a Professor of Informatics, Chair of Health Informatics at the Namibia University of Science and Technology, Windhoek, Namibia. He also serves as a Professor Extraordinaire at the Department of Computer Science, University of the Western Cape, South Africa. In 2013 and 2014, he was a visiting professor at Flensburg University of Applied Sciences, Germany. Prior to his fulltime appointment in academic in 2009, Professor Iyamu held several positions in both Public and Private Institutions in South Africa. He was System Analyst and Technologist at both Nedcor Investment Bank and Metropolitan Life, respectively. He became the Chief Architect at the City of Cape Town in 1999. Thereafter, he joined Old Mutual as IT Architect, from 2001 to 2008. Iyamu's last corporate experience was at a MWeb, as Head of IT Architecture & Governance. Iyamu is the author of books, such as *Enterprise Architecture: From Concept to Practice* (First and Second editions) and *Application of Underpinning Theories in Information Systems*. He has published widely, over seventy-four research articles in book chapters, journals and conference proceedings. Professor Iyamu is an *Associate Editor* of the International Journal of Actor-Network Theory and Technological Innovation (IJANTTI), USA.

Arthur Tatnall is an Associate Professor in Information Systems at Victoria University, Melbourne, Australia. Before taking up his university position he was a secondary school teacher, computer education consultant and educational computer systems analyst at the Victorian State Computer Education Centre. In his PhD he used actor-network theory to investigate adoption of Visual Basic in the curriculum of an Australian university. Arthur's research interests include technological innovation, history of technology, computers in education, IT in educational management, information systems curriculum, project management and electronic business. Much of his research is based on the use of actor-network theory. Arthur is a Fellow of the Australian Computer Society and is active in the International Federation for Information Processing (IFIP) as Chair of IFIP WG9.7 – History of Computing, Chair of IFIP WG3.4 – ICT in Professional and Vocational Education and a member of IFIP WG3.7 – Information Technology in Educational Management. He has published widely in journals, books and book chapters.

* * *

Thomas Agresta is Full Professor and Director of Medical Informatics in the Department of Family Medicine at the University of Connecticut Health Center, Director of Clinical Informatics for the

Biomedical Informatics Division of the Center for Quantitative Medicine and is the Section Leader for Informatics at the Connecticut Institute for Primary Care Innovation. He is a family physician with more than 25 years experience caring for patients at Asylum Hill Family Medicine Center in Hartford, CT. He is Board Certified in Clinical Informatics and is nationally known for his innovative approach to teaching students, residents and physicians to use technology at point of care to provide patient-entered, evidence-based care.

Ajit N. Babu is Clinical Professor of Internal Medicine at Saint Louis University and a staff physician at the St. Louis VA Medical Center. He is also the Director of the Center for Advancement of Global Health, an NGO based in Kochi, India which focuses on the judicious use of technology for promoting resource optimization and better outcomes in public health.

Bader Binhadyan is a PhD candidate at RMIT University, Australia. He holds a master degree in Business Information Systems from Monash University, majoring in Enterprise Resource Planning (ERP), and a bachelor degree in Information Technology from La Trobe, Australia as well as two diplomas in IT, University of California, San Diego and Imam Saud University in Riyadh. He Worked at Saudi Arabian Monetary Agency (SAMA) for just over 8 years as asst. computer programmer. Because Bader has worked and studied in Australia, the Middle East and North America, It helps him to get insight into different cultures and crafted his ability to adapt new environments and introduce new ideas. He has interests in psychology,human behaviour, and technology which have had the most influence on his research.

Indra Budi received the Doctoral degree in Computer Science in 2008 from University of Indonesia. Currently, he is an academic staff at the University of Indonesia. His research interest includes information extraction, Natural Language processing, e-government and it-governance.

Alfred Coleman has a PhD in Information Systems. The topic of his PhD was "E-health readiness assessment for e-health framework in developing countries". He is a member of IEEE, ACM and SAICSIT (South African Institute of Computer Scientists and Information Technology). Alfred is presently an associate professor at the School of Computing, University of South Africa. In the school his responsibilities are the following: tuition of software development, chair of the school's advisory board, and head of its health informatics group. He has published extensively in accredited journals and participated in many conferences.

Steven A. Demurjian is a Full Professor in Computer Science & Engineering at the University of Connecticut, and co-Director of Research Informatics for the Biomedical Informatics Division of the Center for Quantitative Medicine, with research interests of: cross-domain systems, software architectures for health information exchange, secure-software engineering, security for biomedical applications, and security-web architectures. Dr. Demurjian has over 150 archival publications, in the following categories: 1 book, 2 edited collections, 58 journal articles and book chapters, and 98 refereed conference/workshop articles.

Haya Rizqi Fajrina obtained her bachelor degree in Information Systems from Universitas Indonesia. Currently, she is pursuing her master study at the Faculty of Computer Science Universitas Indonesia.

Her research interests are related to knowledge management, supply chain management and customer relationship management.

Kadeghe G. Fue received his Master of Science from the University of Florida, USA in the summer of 2014. He studied precision agriculture, information systems and automation. He was sponsored by iAGRI under USAID feed the future program. He received Borlaug LEAP fellowship award in the fall 2013. After then, He received the Pan African Conference on Science, Computing and Telecommunications (PACT) 2014 best student paper award in Arusha, Tanzania for the paper entitled "A Solar-powered, Wi-Fi Re-programmable Precision Irrigation Controller" on 17th July, 2014. Before joining the University of Florida, he received Bachelor of Science in computer engineering and information technology and attained honors degree from the University of Dar es Salaam, Tanzania in October, 2011. Then, he joined Sokoine University of Agriculture in 2011 as the member of academic staff. He teaches several courses in Computer programming languages and algorithms, Networking, Microcomputer systems, instrumentation, electronics, geoinformatics and database management systems.

Suama Hamunyela holds a Masters in Information Technology. Currently, he is a Lecturer of Informatics, at the Namibia University of Science and Technology, Windhoek, Namibia. Prior to his fulltime appointment in academic in 2010, Suama led an IT department in a Public Institution in Namibia. She was an IT technician and Systems Administrator at the ministry of Gender Equality and Child Welfare Services. Suama's research interests and focus areas include Health Informatics, Enterprise Architecture, Information Technology Strategy, Actor Network Theory and Structuration Theory. She published book chapters, journals articles and conference proceedings.

Catherine Han-Lin has worked in the IS/IT profession for more than 20 years with many well-known international companies at various positions including: System Analyst, BI/BA, ICT Manager, Research Assistant, and IS/IT Lecturer. Her research interest include: Information Systems, Information Management, Health Informatics, IS/IT in Complementary and Alternative Medicine especially Chinese Medicine.

Putu Wuri Handayani is a lecture in Faculty of Computer Science Universitas Indonesia. She obtained her master degree in electronic business from University of Applied Science Fulda, Germany. She is currently pursuing her doctoral study at the Faculty of Computer Science Universitas Indonesia. Her research interest are related to information system/information technology such as e-commerce, enterprise resource planning, supply chain manaegement, customer relationship management and healthcare information system.

Achmad Nizar Hidayanto is the Head of Information Systems/Information Technology Stream, the Faculty of Computer Science, Universitas Indonesia. He received his PhD in Computer Science from Universitas Indonesia. His research interests are information systems/information technology, e-learning, information systems security, change management, distributed systems and information retrieval.

Vincent Horner has a Master's Degree in Computer Science from the University of Pretoria, South Africa. His Master's degree was on a topic in the interdisciplinary field of health informatics. Vincent has recently completed a PhD in the health discipline of Community Health, which he obtained from the University of Limpopo, Medunsa Medical Campus. The topic of his PhD has expanded on the themes of health informatics and public health studies in South Africa. Professionally: Vincent is currently working for the University of South Africa, School of Computing, as a lecturer. His duties include tuition, supervision of postgraduate students, and research. Prior to joining UNISA Vincent worked as a scientists and research fellow at the South African Medical Research Council (MRC) for nine years. He has also worked in the private sector for large as well as start-up organisations.

Kasiyah M. Junus is a Lecturer in Faculty of Computer Science Universitas Indonesia. Currently, she is pursuing her doctoral study at the Faculty of Computer Science Universitas Indonesia. Her research interest is related to information system/information technology such as e-learning.

Ronald Karon is a staff member at the Namibia University of Science and Technology (NU). He is currently tasked to be the coordinator for computer courses for non-Computer Science students in the institution. He has extensive lecturing experience at both undergraduate and post-graduate levels. He holds a Bachelor's degree in Systems Administration and Networks and an Honours degree in Business Computing from the NU. He is currently enrolled for a Masters program in Informatics at the same institution.

Maulilio Kipanyula is a Veterinarian with specialization in tropical livestock diseases, with keen interests in integrating ICT in advisory systems for surveillance and management of livestock diseases. He has researched extensively on One Health approach with application of ICT in surveillance of zoonotic diseases such as rabies. He is a co-project leader in a Project titled: Characterization of Tanzania Zebu Cattle for Tolerance to Ticks and East Coast Fever. Also, he is a Deputy coordinator in a Project titled: Capacity Building for Training and Research in Aquatic and Environmental Health in Eastern and Southern Africa (TRAHESA), funded by NORAD through NORHED programme. Furthermore, he participated in year 2008 in a Training of Trainers; A consultancy to evaluate a manual on Improved and Safe Poultry Production based on the training manual by FAO.

Amir Manzoor holds a bachelor's degree in engineering from NED University, Karachi, an MBA from Lahore University of Management Sciences (LUMS), and an MBA from Bangor University, United Kingdom. He has many years of diverse professional and teaching experience working at many renowned national and internal organizations and higher education institutions.

Sharol Sibongile Mkhomazi received her Master's degree in Business Information Systems from Tshwane University of Technology, Pretoria, South Africa in 2009 and her Doctoral Degree in Computer Science and Data Processing in 2013 from the same institution. She is currently an HOD in the Department of Office Management and Technology, Faculty of Management Sciences at Tshwane University of Technology. Her main research activities involve Telecommunication Infrastructure management, Knowledge Management and Research methodology. She has published articles in book chapters and international conferences.

Hoda Moghimi is a strategic and tactical professional with over 10 years experience in lecturing, research, consulting, solution transformation and project management including the delivery of large business analytics, Big Data and information management projects. Dr. Moghimi also has over 30 peer-reviewed scholarly publications and she is the author of several book chapters in Health Informatics contexts.

Phathutshedzo Nemutanzhela is a PhD student. She holds a Masters Degree from Tshwane University of Technology, South Africa. Her principle research interest is Competitive Intelligence and Information Systems, Diffusion of Innovation theory and also developed an interest on mobile health (mHealth) and e-health.

Sandeep Patil completed Bachelor of engineering in Biomedical Engineering(BIET) and Masters in Embedded System, Manipal University. Currently Working as a Project manager and also playing vital role in industry-academic relationship development at Applied Cognition Systems and pursuing my part time PhD in Manipal University in the field of Image Processing. I also work as guest faculty at school of information sciences, Manipal University. I am also a external member to the board of studies to school of information sciences, Manipal University.

Ave Adriana Pinem obtained her master degree in Computer Science from Universitas Indonesia. Her research interests are related to enterprise resource planning, knowledge management, supply chain management and customer relationship management.

P. S. Ramkumar is functioning currently the Founding director of Applied Cognition Systems, an R&D company developing innovative technology solutions for Governance, Health and Education. He is also currently an AICTE Distinguished Visiting Professor for Vishweshariah Technological University and Adjunct professor at Manipal University and Advisor to Providence Education Group at Thailand. He also serves as an empaneled expert of the Cyber-Security division in ITU wing of United Nations. Dr. P.S. Ramkumar has over 30 years of experience in various roles as a scientist, teacher, entrepreneur, business and corporate manager. Dr.Ram grew from a Lab-assistant to a Scientist heading Signal Processing Labs at the Raman Research Institute, and from a Diploma to M.Tech and Ph.D degrees along with his job. With several publications and 8 patent filings, he has been a research guide for over 100 PG students. Dr. Ram has held several important positions in the Industry as the Director of Innovation and Research Program at Intel Corp., as founding director of VxTel-India, as CTO at SRIT, as General Manager at Nuntius Systems Inc., etc. Dr Ramkumar was a special invitee to Health IT standards advisory committee of central ministry of IT. He has been an advisory to boards of several companies and an active member of IETE, IEEE, IAMI, TSI. In recognition of his contributions, he was awarded Young Scientist Membership by Indian Academy of Sciences and received several excellence awards from Intel and industry in general.

Puspa Indahati Sandhyaduhita is a lecturer at the Faculty of Computer Science, Universitas Indonesia. She received her master degree from TU Delft, the Netherlands. Her research interests include information systems, requirements engineering, business process modeling, enterprise architecture, enterprise resource planning, and supply chain management.

Camilius Sanga is an Associate Professor of Informatics in the Department of Informatics at Sokoine University of Agriculture (SUA), Tanzania. He is a head of Department of Informatics in the Faculty of Science, SUA. He has PhD in Computer Science from University of the Western Cape, South Africa.

Also, he holds MSc. Computer Science and BSc. in Computer Science from Osmania University and University of Dar es Salaam respectively. His research interest is in the area of Information and Communication Technology for Development (ICT4D). He has published papers in a number of International journals. He has also published articles in local and International conferences in the field of ICT4D. Furthermore, he has co-authored two books as well as a number of book chapters. Some of the research projects which Sanga has been involved are: (i) Development of Monitoring and Evaluation system for Projects under Enhancing Pro-poor Innovations in Natural Resources and Agricultural Value-chains (EPINAV) at SUA, (ii) Promoting participation of female students in Science, Technology, Engineering and Mathematics using e-learning and (iii) Farmer Voice Radio (FVR) Project - Building a radio - based, impact driven small farmer extension service system. Currently, he is an assistant project leader for the research titled "The role of mobile phones towards improving coverage of agricultural extension services: a case study of maize value chain". Lastly, he is involved in the project titled "Assessing the impacts of climate variability and change on agricultural systems in Eastern Africa while enhancing the region's capacity to undertake integrated assessment of vulnerabilities to future changes in climate" (2012-2014) (http://www.agmip.org/).

Eugene Sanzi is a Ph.D. student at the Computer Science & Engineering department at the University of Connecticut. His research interests include the usage of credentials to define user profiles that can be utilized to provide authentication to a system that a user has never been authorized to utilize for time-critical situations.

Jonathan L. Schaffer is the managing director in the Information Technology Division and of the Distance Health team at Cleveland Clinic where he manages the eClevelandClinic effort to connect the participants in the care process. Cleveland Clinic's MyConsult program, an online second medical opinion program, is used by consumers and corporations worldwide to provide access to care while removing the geographic barriers. He also leads the DrConnect series of portals which securely connect referring physicians and facilities to their patient's care at Cleveland Clinic. Dr Schaffer is also an active board certified joint replacement surgeon and the Program Director for the Advanced Operative Technology Group in the Orthopaedic and Rheumatologic Research Center. Jonathan is a graduate of Haverford College, Case Western Reserve University's School of Medicine, University of Pennsylvania's Orthopaedic Surgery Residency program, the Adult Reconstructive Orthopaedic Surgery Fellowship program at Brigham and Women's Hospital and holds an MBA from the Kellogg School of Management at Northwestern University in Evanston, Illinois.

Irja N. Shaanika is a student at the university of Science and Technology, currently enrolled for the Master of Informatics.Her research areas include health informatics and enterprise architecture.

Chandana Unnithan is a higher education professional (academic) in Australian Universities. Her academic portfolio intersects teaching and research in Information Communication Technologies (ICTs), Informatics/Analytics, Business Management and Public Health. She has also spent a few years in the ICT sector, handling international projects with multinational corporations such as IBM. A passionate researcher with over 70 peer reviewed publications, her current focus is on leveraging social media for citizen engagement and public health, the development of health informatics discipline. She is an invited speaker, panelist and member of many international program committees for conferences in the information systems and management discipline.

Paraskevas Vezyridis is a Research Fellow at the University of Nottingham, UK. His research focuses on the socio-technical examination of the implementation and use of clinical information systems. His research interests also include new technologies in education and practice of health professionals, the operation of the emergency department, ethics and culture in healthcare.

Nilmini Wickramasinghe has an internationally recognized research record in the area of healthcare and technology management. Her expertise is in the strategic application and management of technology for effecting superior healthcare solutions. As of 13th Dec 2009 she was appointed the professor of information management and library science in the school of Business IT and Logistics at RMIT University. Prior Prof. Wickramasinghe currently has over 200 peer-reviewed scholarly publications and is the author of several books and an Encyclopedia in Healthcare and Technology. In addition, she is the Editor-in-Chief of two scholarly international peer-reviewed scholarly journals published by InderScience.

Angela Wei Hong Yang has been teaching, researching and practicing Chinese medicine for nearly 20 years. Her research specialty is to investigate the quality, safety and effectiveness of Chinese medicine, particularly Chinese herbal medicine, for the ageing population and those with chronic diseases (e.g. diseases of immune system and endocrine system). Her research expertise includes the development of systematic reviews and clinical trials as well as instruments for quality assessment of Chinese medicine studies. She is also specialising in using the interdisciplinary approach (e.g. information systems) to promote, manage and analyse Chinese medicine knowledge.

Timoteus B. Ziminski is a Ph.D. student at the Computer Science & Engineering department at the University of Connecticut. His research interests include software architectures with a focus on data and system integration, emphasizing on solutions that are suitable for application in the biomedical and healthcare domains. Next to pursuing research, he holds the degree Diplom-Informatiker from the Technical University of Dortmund and is a full time software developer in industry.

Index

S

T

U

W

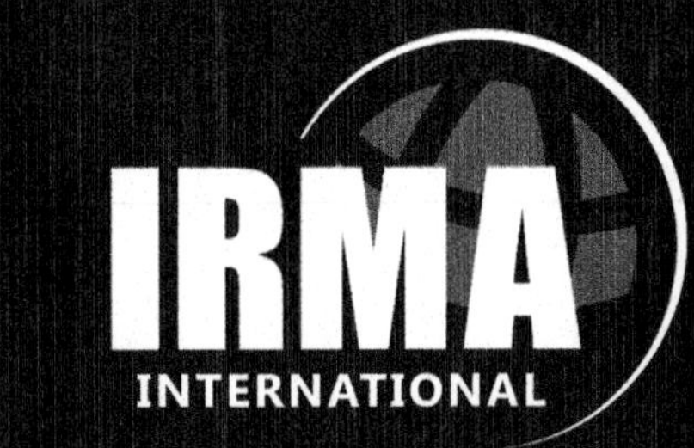

Become an IRMA Member

Members of the **Information Resources Management Association (IRMA)** understand the importance of community within their field of study. The Information Resources Management Association is an ideal venue through which professionals, students, and academicians can convene and share the latest industry innovations and scholarly research that is changing the field of information science and technology. Become a member today and enjoy the benefits of membership as well as the opportunity to collaborate and network with fellow experts in the field.

IRMA Membership Benefits:

- **One FREE Journal Subscription**
- **30% Off Additional Journal Subscriptions**
- **20% Off Book Purchases**
- Updates on the latest events and research on Information Resources Management through the IRMA-L listserv.
- Updates on new open access and downloadable content added to Research IRM.
- A copy of the Information Technology Management Newsletter twice a year.
- A certificate of membership.

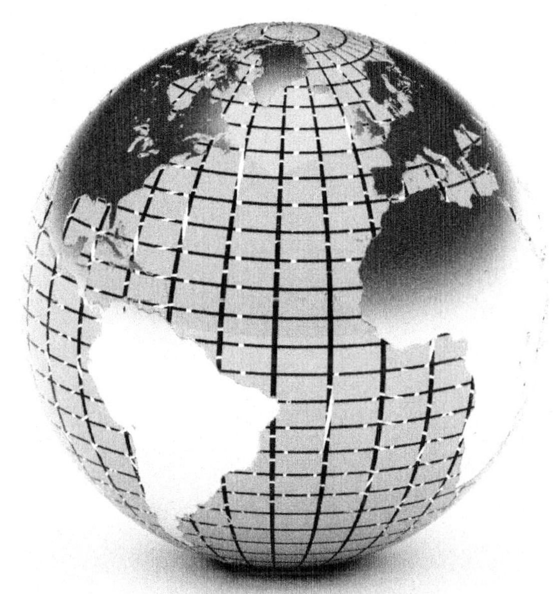

IRMA Membership $195

Scan code to visit irma-international.org and begin by selecting your free journal subscription.

Membership is good for one full year.

CPSIA information can be obtained at www.ICGtesting.com
Printed in the USA
LVOW05*2301080915

453380LV00015B/122/P